Children's Health Issues in Historical Perspective

ℭℛ

Children's Health Issues in Historical Perspective

☙

CHERYL KRASNICK WARSH AND
VERONICA STRONG-BOAG, EDITORS

Wilfrid Laurier University Press
WLU

We acknowledge the financial support of the Government of Canada through the Book Publishing Industry Development Program for our publishing activities. We acknowledge the financial support of Associated Medical Services, Inc. (AMS) which was established in 1936 by Dr. Jason Hannah as a pioneer prepaid not-for-profit health care organization in Ontario. With the advent of Medicare AMS became a charitable organization supporting innovations in academic medicine and health services, specifically the history of medicine and health care, as well as innovations in health professional education and bioethics.

Library and Archives Canada Cataloguing in Publication

Children's health issues in historical perspective / Cheryl Krasnick Warsh and Veronica Strong-Boag, editors.

Includes bibliographical references and index.
ISBN 0-88920-474-8

1. Child health services—History. 2. Children—Health and hygiene—History.
I. Warsh, Cheryl Lynn Krasnick, 1957– II. Strong-Boag, Veronica Jane, 1947–

RJ101.C44 2005   362.198'92'0009   C2005-905034-9

Cover: pictures from *Child Health Alphabet* by Mrs. Frederick Peterson (New York: Macmillan, 1922). Back cover: top, nurse with young patient (MCH Archives); bottom, Inuit woman with child, Aklavik, 1926 (Canada, Department of Interior). Cover design by P.J. Woodland. Text design by Catharine Bonas-Taylor.

Divider pages: p. 21, from *Our Health Habits* by Whitcomb and Beveridge (Chicago: Rand McNally, 1926); p. 129, from *Health Education in an American City* by Louise Franklin Bache (Garden City, NJ: Doubleday, Doran, 1934); p.207, from Fleming/ NWT Archives; p. 325, from the Carpenter Collection; p. 409, courtesy of Annmarie Adams.

Printed in Canada

To Our Children* With Love

> Sarah Rachel Warsh
> Christopher Nicholas Bridges Ross
> Dominic Angus Bridges Ross
> Gabriel Andrew Bridges Ross
> Nat Warner
> Dory Warner
> Esperanza Francesca Nikolaevna Birn
>   Mendels Krementsova
> Hadrien Baillargeon
> Andréanne Marleau
> Audrey Marleau
> Caroline Marleau
> Sébastien Marleau
> Marilou Nadeau
> Alexander Bruno Ly
> Theodore Ownby
> Lachlan Bradley Macdermid
> Kathryn Moore-Ostry
> Beth Rachel Markel
> Samantha Louise Markel
> Sophie Lapierre Bragg
> William Ian Bragg
> Ella Agnew Sorscher
> Nathan Swift Sorscher
> Lincoln Finch Sorscher
> Andrew James Angus Rutherdale
> Alex Schneider
> Ben Schneider
> Charlie Adams-Gossage
> Katie Adams-Gossage
> Taylor Poirier

*This list includes children, grandchildren, nieces, nephews, and even an infant *in utero* whom we hold dear!

Miss Lucy

Miss Lucy had a baby,
She named him Tiny Tim.
She put him in the bathtub
To see if he could swim.
He drank up all the water,
He ate up all the soap,
He tried to eat the bathtub
But it wouldn't go down his throat.

Miss Lucy called the doctor,
Miss Lucy called the nurse,
Miss Lucy called the lady
With the alligator purse.

"Mumps," said the doctor,
"Measles," said the nurse,
"Nothing," said the lady
With the alligator purse.

Miss Lucy punched the doctor,
Miss Lucy knocked the nurse,
Miss Lucy paid the Lady
With the alligator purse.

> — Traditional child's song game
> still popular in playgrounds

Contents

☙

INSTITUTIONS

Acknowledgements

CR

W e would like to thank the editors and reviewers who have assisted us in the production of this book, including Carroll Klein and Heather Blain-Yanke of Wilfrid Laurier University Press. We also thank Heather MacDougall, Paul Potter, Jacques Bérnier, Othmar Keel, Guy Grenier, Helen Brown, Darcey Kaluza, and Michael Warsh. The financial support of the Canadian Society for the History of Medicine, Associated Medical Services Inc., and Malaspina University-College is gratefully acknowledged.

The following articles, originally published in the *Canadian Bulletin of Medical History/ Bulletin canadien d'histoire de la médicine* (volume 19, number 1, 2002), were revised for inclusion in this collection: Veronica Strong-Boag, "The Spotlight on Children"; Anne-Emanuelle Birn, "'No More Surprising Than a Broken Pitcher': Maternal and Child Health in the Early Years of the Pan American Sanitary Bureau"; Denyse Baillargeon, "Entre la «Revanche» et la «Veillée» des berceaux : Les médecins québécois francophones, la mortalité infantile, et la question nationale, 1910–1940"; Laurence Monnais, "La médicalisation de la mere et de son enfant: L'exemple du Vietnam sous domination française, 1860–1939"; Margaret Tennant, "Complicating Childhood: Gender, Ethnicity, and 'Disadvantage' within the New Zealand Children's Health Camps Movement"; Mona Gleason, "Race, Class, and Health: School Medical Inspection and 'Healthy' Children in British Columbia, 1890–1930"; Cynthia Comacchio, "'Living Symptoms': Adolescent Health Care in English Canada, 1920–1970"; Annmarie Adams and David Theodore, "The Architecture of Children's Hospitals in Toronto and Montreal, 1875–2010"; Sharon L. Richardson, "Frontier Health Services for Children: Alberta's Provincial Travelling Clinic, 1924–1942."

Introduction

The Spotlight on Children

∞

Cheryl Krasnick Warsh and
Veronica Strong-Boag

Children's health regularly concerns parents and family. It also receives intermittent attention from communities and nations. At the 1990 World Summit for Children, seventy-one countries signed the World Declaration on Survival, Protection and Development of Children and adopted a Plan of Action. That plan promised to improve "living conditions for children and their chances for survival by increasing access to health services for women and children," "reducing the spread of preventable diseases," "creating more opportunities for education," "providing better sanitation and greater food supply; and protecting children in danger."[1] During the 1990s some progress occurred with respect to polio, neonatal tetanus, diarrhea, and Vitamin A and iodine deficiency. Overall, however, as the UN Report *We the Children: Meeting the Promises of the World Summit for Children* (2002) observed, "Over 600 million children continue to live in dire poverty, over 10 million die each year from preventable diseases, 149 million are malnourished, 113 million are not in school (two thirds of whom are girls), and 250 million work as children labourers. Over half a million children have died from AIDS, 2.7 million live with the virus, and over 12 million have been orphaned by it."[2]

Governments have an immense role in determining children's opportunities for good health. For example, while Sweden, Canada, and the United States have similar "market" poverty rates before government intervention, only 2.6 per cent of Sweden's children live in relative poverty, compared to 15.5 per cent in Canada, and 22.4 per cent in the United States. Only Mexico fares worse than the United States among twenty-three of the world's richest nations.[3] The United States also continues to display questionable commitment to child health by its refusal to sign international conventions on everything from the banning of landmines (that injure many thousands of children) to child slavery and the elimination of discrimination against women.[4]

1

In May 2002 (postponed from September 2001) the UN General Assembly hosted an unprecedented Special Session on Children. Government leaders, heads of state, NGOs, children's advocates, and young people met to update the 1990 agenda. Their goals were to ensure the best possible start in life, a quality basic education for all children, and opportunities for all children, especially adolescents, to participate meaningfully in their communities. In preparation for this session, Canada, like other nations, presented UNICEF with a review of its progress in achieving 1990 goals.[5] As the co-chair on the 1990 conference, as well as an early ratifier (1991) of the *Convention on the Rights of the Child* (1989), Canada prepared a self-evaluation that was largely self-congratulatory. The national review deftly evaded noting ongoing cuts in federal and provincial programs in health, welfare, and education that substantially threatened gains in children's well-being won after the Second World War. Notably absent was mention of the federal government's failure to keep its long-standing promise to eliminate child poverty. Neo-conservative provincial administrations, notably in Alberta, Ontario, and British Columbia, like similar governments in the United States and Australia, only worsened matters. They could take instruction from majority world nations such as Kenya and Colombia who, in the face of terrible disadvantage, still strive to maintain "community-based" programs for their children.[6]

In Canada, on November 24, 1999 (the tenth anniversary of the 1989 unanimous House of Commons resolution to end child poverty within a decade), Campaign 2000, a coalition of national, provincial, and community partners, issued a report card. The number of young Canadians in poverty had increased from about one in seven to one in five. For some communities the news was still worse. In 2001 40.0 per cent of Aboriginal children, 33.6 per cent of visible minority kids, and 27.7 per cent of those with disabilities lived in poverty. In March 2003 more than 306,000 children relied on food banks. *The Progress of Canada's Children*, published yearly by the Canadian Council on Social Development, continues to document the extent of such failure, as do advocacy groups in other nations.[7]

Today, the overall record of English-speaking countries on levels of child poverty is notably worse than other OECD nations. Although no jurisdiction entirely escapes the costs, especially high levels of teen pregnancy in the United States consign many girls and their offspring to a lifetime of low income and ill-health.[8] And Aboriginal youngsters everywhere generally fare worse than their counterparts. The 2002 report *Australia's Children: Their Health and Well-Being* typically concludes that Aboriginal and Torres Strait Islander children were worse off. So too were those living in rural and remote areas, an experience again readily matched in different sites the world over.[9]

Many children can name the problems they face. One 1992 study, part of a sixteen-nation investigation coordinated by the World Health Organization, consulted 4500 eleven-, thirteen-, and fifteen-year-old Canadians. Respondents revealed a wide variety of "health-risk factors" (smoking, alcohol, and drugs), "exercise/leisure-time activity," "nutrition and dental care," "ailments and medication," and "relationships with others."[10] In a 2001 survey, more than 1,200 Canadian young people identified "poverty, abuse, safety and a clean environment as the most important issues in their lives today." While many kids mentioned good experiences in matters from recreation to teachers, 50.6 per cent "responded that they wished adults would listen, understand and believe them." A fourteen-year-old girl from Burnaby, BC, put it this way: "We have a voice but sometimes don't know how to get it out to everyone. Please help us speak out."[11] Children elsewhere are similarly asking for a hearing. Unfortunately, the observation of one American AIDS orphan is commonplace: "'Not many people pay attention to me.'"[12]

Studying Children

This collection doesn't go as far as such respondents would wish. Young voices and opinions remain for the most part missing. As editors, we very much wished for their inclusion and we deeply regret their ultimate omission.[13] However, in children's history, a field of historical inquiry still significantly undeveloped and often regarded as lacking legitimacy comparable to more familiar scholarly preoccupations, our contributors have worked hard to stake out new ground. Their interrogation of issues as diverse as gender, race, class, professional monopolies, discourses of normalization, and institutional space lay valuable foundations for anyone seeking to explore the history of children and health.

In their common ignorance of the past, Canadians and others in the Western world readily succumb to notions of the "natural" child, one who supposedly develops in response to almost universal biological and psychological imperatives. From this only too popular perspective, rooted in longstanding ethnocentrism and the functionalist theories of the 1950s social sciences, children and childhood are essentially timeless in their nature and demands. Health and welfare initiatives that assume that children develop normally and best only within a nuclear, heterosexual, and breadwinner family flourish, in spite of all evidence to the contrary. A vision of middle-class children of European origin, that ignores even the diversity of that group, is largely taken for granted as the appropriate measure of normality. This narrow perspective hobbles even well-meaning efforts to succour children all around the globe.[14]

All efforts to reconstruct the past, whether from "knee-high" or adult perspectives, need to address the reality that *children* and their *health* are not homogeneous categories. Youngsters, like adults, live lives of multiple identities in which they may variously, even simultaneously, experience both power and oppression. Historians, like health care providers and policy-makers, need to appreciate much better the implications of these various identities, whether of age, (dis)ability, class, race, religion, or sexuality. We need to ask what it means to be considered normal in society. Who and what set the criteria? What does it mean for individuals and communities in general, when winners and losers can be identified from their earliest years, or even, increasingly with the new reproductive technologies, before birth itself?[15] As we begin to consider such questions, we will come closer to understanding how the health of various groups of children has been variously constructed both now and in times before our own.

Children and Health in the Past

When biological families fail, extended kin or neighbours have sometimes been there to help, but it is dangerously easy to romanticize those prospects in the past. In fact, there has never been a golden age for all families. Kin might offer sympathy and support, but violence, incest, and neglect are also there to be documented.[16] Support for children in biological, fictive, and adoptive families has been highly contingent on good health, physical proximity, intimate relations, resources of capital and labour, and the relative power of women and men.

Communities have also differed tremendously in how they regard immature members. North American Native nations have, for example, been as diverse in child–adult relations as they have been in their traditions and practices in social hierarchy and gender. Evidence of early child-rearing practices gentler than those of Europeans certainly exists.[17] Whether kindness determined the dominant experience of children on the margins—such as those of low status generally, or enslaved populations on Canada's Pacific Coast, for example—is, however, yet unknown. Native legends, for example, sometimes suggest that children might not always be equally or sensitively treated, and their well-being suffered accordingly.[18] Whatever the state of pre-Contact societies, the lives of indigenous youngsters, like those of adults, deteriorated with the arrival of European empires around the world. More and different diseases left unprecedented numbers dead, orphaned, or injured. Resource depletion and loss brought more hunger and disability. Direct assaults on Aboriginal culture and traditions undermined long-standing obligations and exchanges that might have comforted the vulnerable.

While their own nations were decreasingly able to nurture them, Aboriginal children had good reason to expect worse from white visitors or settlers who had little to offer the poor or the marginal of any race.[19]

As the operations of Poor Laws in the British colonies of Nova Scotia and New Brunswick demonstrated, disease and premature death regularly compromised even the nurture of European children in new settlements. Life was little better for the transplanted poor than it had been in European homelands. In the Canadian Maritime colonies, "the sick, the mentally ill, the mentally retarded, infants and children, tramps and vagrants," like many of the elderly, typically passed their days in almshouses or found themselves auctioned off to the lowest bidder.[20]

In its expectation that frontier families and private charity could cope with distress, the British colony of Upper Canada rejected the Elizabethan Poor Law whose terrible institutions were so well commemorated by Charles Dickens. In fact, jails, asylums, and hospitals became the crowded refuges of the poor of all ages. Private charity and religious institutions provided equally cold comfort in colonial Quebec. Canada's long, harsh winters, with their special threat to health, employment, and fortune in general, made destitution and distress all the more painful.[21] Infant and child mortality was correspondingly high. With the union of the British North American colonies in 1867 and subsequent industrialization and urbanization, the spread of European settlement, and increased immigration, older makeshift responses appeared even less adequate. The situation in other colonies of European settlement was much the same.

In the late nineteenth century, Canada, like most countries, was youthful: children under the age of fifteen made up some 40 per cent of a population that numbered about four million. These youngsters were vulnerable to disease and discipline in ways that are difficult to imagine today. Again vulnerability was not shared equally. Gender, ethnicity, race, class, and ability determined options. Many thousands of girls and boys, native-born and immigrant, experienced want and abuse on the uncertain road to adulthood. If the offspring of the Victorian era lived increasingly with a "cult of childhood" that emphasized and celebrated their difference from adults, the same inheritance made critical distinctions among the young themselves. Some, those closest in character and potential to society's powerful, received the fullest benefits of shifting sensibilities. White, able-bodied, attractive youngsters were permitted the longest and the greatest degree of "dependence, protection, segregation and delayed responsibilities."[22]

Informed as they were by shifting sensibilities regarding children and childhood, nineteenth- and early twentieth-century Canadian and other child-savers were equally associated with elite efforts to direct and discipline multi-class and increasingly multi-ethnic states in which subordinated communities were regularly restive. Opportunities for different groups of youngsters were central to many conflicts. Native parents objected to residential schools. Feminists targeted the abuse of girls. Workers demanded better education for their kids. North Americans of African descent both formed their own schools and fought segregation. Yet for all the fundamental questions that all asked about justice and fairness, such diverse critics were rarely allies.[23] They often battled alone, unable or unwilling to look beyond their own ranks. The offspring of the most vulnerable of citizens continued to suffer as the powerful in settled and long-settled societies readily channeled often genuine humanitarian impulses into nineteenth-and twentieth-century programs that ultimately did little to threaten existing social relations.

The problems of many natal families produced two major responses. On the one hand, children have been apprehended, sometimes at the request of families, and sometimes mandated by external authority, to be placed into institutions and other people's families. On the other hand, parents, most commonly mothers, and children have been supported, with various degrees of monitoring, by private charities and public services, at home.[24] In both cases, the state, real and imagined, of children's physical and moral health was central to the social calculation that determined state and private investment.

The historic problems created by institutionalizing vulnerable children and young people have been devastatingly summed up in the Law Commission of Canada's *Restoring Dignity: Responding to Child Abuse in Canadian Institutions* (2000). This report describes how authorities, ranging from parents and legal guardians to courts and child welfare agencies, have consigned the vulnerable to a wide variety of "total institutions."[25] The commission chronicled the painful histories of "special needs schools; child welfare facilities; youth detention facilities; and residential schools for Aboriginal children,"[26] and at least some of the children's hospitals described in this volume might have been added to this list. Their inmates, often casualties of poverty and prejudice, are not anybody's children. Almost without exception, they have been drawn from historically disadvantaged populations. Reports from institutions like the Mount Cashel orphanage—run by the Christian Brothers in St. John's, NL—sound remarkably like those of both the Alberni Indian school and BC's Boys' Industrial School on Canada's West Coast.

Early recognition of the health and other problems associated with institutional care, not to mention their expense, provoked continuing interest in alternatives. The children's aid societies set up first in the 1890s in Ontario, and comparable state and private initiatives in many jurisdictions, reflected growing enthusiasm for fostering and adoption.

But these too early revealed shortcomings. Good homes, like good sum-mer camps as one article here confirms, have always been difficult to guarantee. Over the years children have only too frequently shifted from one site of mistreatment to another. The now infamous 1960s scoop of Native children from poverty-stricken homes to placements in non-Abo-riginal families in Canada, like the Indian Adoption Project of the Child Welfare League of America (1958–67) in the United States, illustrated only too well how policies meant to side-step institutions could be every bit as arbitrary and damaging.[27]

From the nineteenth century on, Canada, like the developed world in general, has experimented with universal public services to head off child welfare problems. A massive expansion, first of primary and then of secondary schools, which became increasingly both free and compul-sory, brought unprecedented opportunities. Public health improvements often concentrated on infants and young children. The expansion of social security throughout much of the Western world in the twentieth century, especially after the Second World War, promised better prospects and working-class, immigrant, and Native parents actively used gains to improve the lives of their offspring.[28] It seems fair to argue, as does Neil Sutherland in *Children in English-Canadian Society*, that youngsters' physical well-being, with the critical exception often of First Nations children, has generally improved. Today's greatly enhanced life expectancy reminds us that death and disability no longer so commonly stalk cradles and classrooms.

Yet for all the undeniable and hard-won progress, universal entitle-ment to schooling, fundamental medical care, and social assistance have been regularly compromised. Special treatment, regulated access, and individual prejudice have been matter-of-course. Working-class and Native girls have routinely been directed to training, whether in com-mercial or domestic subjects, that helps limit their options as adults.[29] Poor kids who come hungry or poorly clothed to classes have frequently found little to keep them in attendance. Impoverished students have been unlikely to stay long enough or do well enough to bring hope into their lives.

In the past and today, explanations and solutions for poverty, dis-ease, and mistreatment have matter-of-factly criticized the parenting qualifications of single mothers, of the First Nations, of non-Anglo-Celtic communities, of ethnic and racial minorities, and of the working class in general. Failure to measure up to dominant normative stan-dards has been ascribed to individual and community shortcomings rather than the logic of the economic and social system. While girls and boys might be admitted to be the unfortunate casualties of parental incompetence and misfortune, the vast majority of help has been intended to assist the needy at an economic level well below that secured by the lowest-waged adult male worker. The iron rule of "lesser eligibility" ensured that children, no more than adults, were to escape the stern lessons of the survival of the fittest. Furthermore, childhood has been made more difficult by inadequate wages, unsafe working conditions, prejudice of every sort, and lack of economic opportunity facing too many parents. When contributions to paid labour increasingly became the central basis for claims of full citizenship in the twentieth century, as manifested in eligibility for social security ranging from old age pensions to maternity benefits, the suffering of a wide range of families was ignored.[30]

Ultimately, less privileged youngsters[31] have had to compare their very different experiences with what they might read about Anne of Green Gables, Pollyanna, and Mary Lennox (the popular girl heroines respectively of the 1908 bestseller by Lucy Maud Montgomery, its 1913 American rival by Eleanor Porter, and *The Secret Garden*, 1911, by Frances Hodgson Burnett) or saw later of most of their equally untypical mass-marketed successors. In the 1930s the provincial government in Ontario, Canada, and medical authorities concocted a fairy tale around the Dionne quintuplets to distract North Americans during the Great Depression. The tourist destination "Quintland," like the dolls and films depicting the five identical girls, ignored exploitation.[32] The lifestyle marketed to teenagers by modern consumer culture is often similarly divorced from reality.[33]

Bringing the Past to the
Aid of the Present

It is clear in the pages that follow that for all the bleak stories, new ideas about children pervade modern sensibilities. The singling out of the young for protection has become a benchmark of civilized society. Child labour, sexual slavery, and poverty, all inspire research and efforts at eradication. Today it is fair to conclude, "Not since the 19th-century social and legislative actions that removed children from the sweatshops of Europe and North America has such reform zeal been demonstrated on behalf of children."[34]

Scholars and activists have turned to international collaborations to expose problems and suggest solutions. For some time, Florence's Instituto degli Innocenti and UNICEF's International Child Development Centre have sponsored an influential series, Historical Perspectives on Childhood. These include publications on breastfeeding, infant mortality in Europe, and child labour, all issues of central concern to those interested in the health of the world's youngsters.[35] As Giuseppe Arpioni, president of the Instituto, and James R. Himes, director of the centre, reminded readers in 1996,

> a greater understanding of the history of childhood, especially problems of children and families suffering from various forms of deprivations, might help shed light on the quest for improved policies and programs for dealing with contemporary child-related social issues. Avoiding the mistakes of the past is also an important though often frustrated aspiration of policy makers and reflective practitioners seeking to learn lessons from history.[36]

New Research, New Perspectives

The essays that follow describe the malleability of children in the rhetoric of child educators, public health officials, and political leaders. Children were like clay, to be moulded into permanent creations of harmony and beauty. Yet clay also could be pummelled, ripped apart, and abandoned, and no less a fate was experienced by countless, equally brutalized children. Furthermore, the agents of creation and brutality were often one and the same. Acts or omissions that were perpetrated for children's "own good" demonstrated the essential powerlessness of youngsters. This was particularly apparent when the institutions of power, such as the state, the church, and the medical professions, confronted children.

Historians, anthropologists, sociologists, and political scientists are among the contributors to the growing field of the history of children's health, and to the recognition that childhood issues, far from being marginal to society, run through all veins of the commonweal. In "Politics," the first section of this collection, the rhetoric and practices of child rearing as adjuncts of nation building are examined. In chapter 1, Naomi Rogers discusses the American government's interest in child health during the interwar period as a consequence of the national scandal of the poor health of wartime recruits. While the government paid lip service to the internationalist focus of the Red Cross and other shared wartime experiences of child health advocates, the liberal, individualistic ideology of pre-Depression America was an uncomfortable fit with the collectivities of public health measures. That good child health was an essential component of an emergent powerhouse on the international scene was a view shared by child advocates on both the Left and Right.

Many of these views, as well as the pundits themselves, influenced child health measures in other parts of the world, as Anne-Emmanuelle Birn, in chapter 2, demonstrates in her study of the Pan-American Sanitary Boards directed, yet not completely overrun by American imperialism. Latin American health officials were more influenced by the

French model of socialized medicine and puericulture (which included prenatal and postnatal clinics, milk depots, and other measures to reduce infant mortality), although part of the raison d'être for these measures, at least in the old country, was to protect the nation's economic and military future. Latin America also declined to follow the American interwar model of negative eugenics, or targeted population control, to promote child health; it preferred, at least in theory, the French/Catholic/ southern Europe model of ameliorating health problems encountered by mothers and their infants.

In Quebec, as Denyse Baillargeon recounts in chapter 3, the exceptionally high infant mortality rate was an embarrassing blight that nationalists—both clergy and lay—were forced to confront. To accept, as the Americans did, the full public health agenda of instilling sanitary propaganda in the young, or, as the Latin Americans did, promote state-enforced sanitary measures, would be to admit that the public health initiatives embraced by the anglophone population in Quebec and Ontario were superior to traditional francophone values—a concession that nationalists in the early twentieth century were loath to give. They were forced to make the insubstantial arguments that while lackadaisical enforcement of pasteurization regulations might be a leading killer of babies, it reflected the independent spirit of the French Canadian, and that while infant mortality in French Quebec far exceeded the rest of Canada and immigrants and anglophones within its own borders, at least the birth rate equally exceeded the national average.

Nutrition

The theme of infants as human capital is continued in the second section, "Nutrition," commencing with Lisa Featherstone's examination, in chapter 4, of the medicalization of infant care in Australia at the turn of the twentieth century. The role of the pediatrician was to protect the capital against the purportedly ignorant, selfish, and recalcitrant actions of mothers, whose role was reduced to the biological act of breastfeeding, an act that nevertheless required the careful supervision of physicians to be performed correctly. The special challenges of impoverished women who were required to be in the paid labour force, and the widespread lack of clean, inexpensive, and safe alternatives to breast milk were overlooked in the prescriptive literature.

In the United States, Charles R. King, in *Children's Health in America: A History*, and Rima D. Apple, in *Mothers and Medicine: A Social History of Infant Feeding, 1890–1950*, have considered the growth of a variety of professional and commercial experts in the area of infant feeding. That prescriptive literature could be contradictory and confusing is noted as well in chapter 5, with Judith Sealander's survey of American nutritional advice for children in the twentieth century. The "American science" of nutrition (although with origins in Germany) generated a new profession and a revolutionary way of seeing foods as the sum of their parts (i.e., fats, carbohydrates, minerals, vitamins, and proteins). The pediatricians, nutritionists, government bureaucrats, and food industry lobbyists, each with a personal agendas, argued about the purity of milk, the proper composition of formulae, and the ideal diet for children. A common theme throughout the century, however, was that malnutrition among the poor was often blamed on the spendthrift or ignorant habits of parents, especially mothers.

In Canada, government initiatives regarding infant feeding were the bailiwick of Dr. Helen MacMurchy of the Canadian Child Welfare Division, a public health office she helped to create. Her endeavours and influence upon generations of mothers have been examined by Katherine Arnup in *Education for Motherhood: Advice for Mothers in Twentieth-Century Canada*, and Cynthia R. Comacchio in *"Nations Are Built of Babies": Saving Ontario's Mothers and Children, 1900–1940*. In chapter 6, Aleck Ostry investigates the influence of the economic agenda of government and industry officials in determining advice to mothers on breastfeeding, and on consumption of cows' milk. At the same time as the Canadian Child Welfare Division's *Canadian Mothers Book* was encouraging breast milk consumption to the age of nine months, the dairy industry and public health officials were trumpeting the protective qualities of the vitamin and mineral content of cows' milk. The "new knowledge" preceded the availability of a national uncontaminated milk supply, thereby contributing to a continued, excessively high infant mortality rate.

Racial and Ethnic Dimensions

When poverty takes on an ethnic dimension, as investigated in the third section, "Racial and Ethnic Dimensions," the difficulties associated with culture clashes are added to the mix. There have been several important studies on American immigrant and child health, including Evelynn Maxine Hammonds's *Childhood's Deadly Scourge: The Campaign to Control Diphtheria in New York City, 1880–1930*, as well as several selections in Alexandra M. Stern and Howard Markel's edited collection, *Formative Years: Children's Health in America, 1880–2000*. In chapter 7, Howard Markel's study of the health of immigrant children to the United States at the turn of the twentieth century reveals the extreme hardships and tragedies associated with the most densely populated, filthy, and disease-ridden immigrant ghettoes. Acculturation, including public health education, was seen as the key in combating high infant and child mortality and abandonment, and this acculturation was facilitated not simply by native-born social reformers but organized immigrant groups themselves. Nevertheless, many of the reformers shared their compatriots' disdain and mistrust of the immigrants they served.

Colonialism was a complex experience when it related to maternal and child health, as narrated by Laurence Monnais in chapter 8, in her study of Vietnam under French rule. As noted in the earlier study on Latin American public health initiatives, members of the francophonie incorporated the French model of combating infant mortality, through the Roussel law of the late nineteenth century. In Vietnam, the imperatives of Catholicism (through religious orders), empire (through philanthropies), scientific medicine (through government health officials), and local customs and religion (through midwives and other lay healers) all played roles in the care of mothers and infants. As Jennifer Beinart has noted in her study of photographic images of African children in the early twentieth century, however, colonized children tended to be rendered invisible through the lens of the colonizers.[37]

Changing social concerns played out upon the bodies of children with the establishment of fresh air schools and camps in the early twentieth century. In England, as Linda Bryder points out, the avowed goal of the open-air school movement was to fight tuberculosis among debilitated urban children, yet in practice, the inculcation of traditional liberal ideals of self-help and self-discipline were equally as important.[38] In New Zealand's health camps in the twentieth century, as demonstrated by Margaret Tennant in chapter 9, class, gender, and racial preoccupations influenced their mandates. The camps first targeted poor housebound girls whose lack of fresh air and physical exercise weakened their capacities to be breeders of healthy white stock. Later generations of reformers focused first upon insufficiently masculine boys, and then overly masculinized/delinquent boys, and finally upon an urbanized, insufficiently assimilated Maori population.

The public health experiences in the province of British Columbia, newly settled with deep racial divisions, exemplified the ethnic and class divisions of public health, as discussed by Mona Gleason in chapter 10. Medical inspections in early twentieth-century BC public schools characterized the impoverished descendant children of Asians, Aboriginals, and Europeans as filthy carriers of contagion improperly supervised by ignorant and neglectful parents. The children and parents, for their part, regarded the public health inspectors and nurses as authoritarian and uncaring.

In chapter 11, Myra Rutherdale similarly describes the contestation for the bodies of parturient mothers and children between missionaries and the peoples of the Far North. The missionaries, since their first contact in the 1860s, criticized and attempted to alter traditional patterns of childbirth, sleeping habits, hygiene, and clothing. Yet missionaries, who arrived after the mid-twentieth century, particularly female nurses, displayed some sensitivity towards local folkways.

Experts

Experts ranging from public health nurses to pediatricians, and factory inspectors to psychoanalysts placed their professional imprimaturs upon the determination of the physical, psychological, and behavioural health of children.[39] One international phenomenon of the early twentieth century was the Better Baby Contests to find the "perfect" child, as Annette Vance Dorey recounts, through the use of detailed (and arbitrary) standardized measurements at state fairs.[40] These partly public health/partly carnivalesque competitions often ran counter to attempts by the new field of pediatrics, exemplified by its founder, New York's Abraham Jacobi, to establish itself as a serious medical specialty.[41] Yet the experts failed many children. The fact that cultural, medical, and socioeconomic forces played out upon the bodies of children was epitomized by medical reactions to evidence of child sexual abuse. As recounted in chapter 12 by Hughes Evans, American physicians commonly were confronted with evidence of abuse, such as gonorrheal vaginitis, but wrote hundreds of articles denying the possibility that the venereal infection could be caused by child abuse. When attempts to differentiate between adult and pediatric gonorrhea failed in the laboratory, physicians resorted to downplaying the results or passing the blame onto the victims, often abetted by mothers who could not bear the loss of the family breadwinner. Thus patriarchal, professional imperatives overwhelmed the individual rights of children over their bodies.

Propping up existing power structures also was at the heart of the mental hygiene and child guidance movements in North America. Indeed, as Theresa Richardson and Margo Horn relate in their respective studies, both movements owed their existence to the corporate agendas of vast philanthropies such as the Rockefeller and Harkness Foundations.[42] Maintaining power structures also is the focus of chapter 13, as Cynthia Comacchio investigates the mixed success of the new sub-specialty of pediatrics and child psychology in casting their professional nets over adolescence. Since adolescents tend to be physiologically the healthiest age cohort, the problems identified were based upon behavioural "symptoms" such as rebelliousness, sexual expression, and idleness. The health of adolescents, like that of infants, was constructed in terms of a national resource to be nurtured and guided for the civic good.

In chapter 14, Janet Golden examines the practice of one leading pediatrician, Philadelphian Howard Childs Carpenter, who compiled an extensive collection of slides and pictures to promote child-saving and disease prevention programs to the general public. Progressive reformers often used the powerful immediacy of photographs to take middle-class audiences into impoverished ghettoes, thereby encouraging remedial action. Child health photography, however, was more ambivalent in assigning blame for disease and hardship; bad parenting was targeted along with socio-economic causes.

Institutions

Institutions ranging from the concrete—such as children's hospitals and reformatories—to the itinerant—travelling health and screening clinics— were created to fight childhood illnesses, but all were affected by political and financial exigencies. In chapter 15, Marie-Josée Fleury and Guy Grenier demonstrate that, despite the defensive rhetoric used by Quebec nationalists to justify exceptionally high infant mortality rates at the turn of the twentieth century, provincial politicians, public health officials, and pediatricians combated contagious childhood diseases through the establishment of two modern hospitals in Montreal: Hôpital Saint-Paul and Alexandra Hospital. Built as parallel institutions to serve the French and English populations respectively, both institutions embraced innovations in diagnostics and bacteriology, and both serviced a clientele that crossed religious and language lines.

Similarly, as Annemarie Adams and David Theodore illustrate in chapter 16, it would be the premier French children's hospital in Montreal—Hôpital Ste-Justine—rather than the English Children's Memorial Hospital that would be the leading innovator in incorporating twentieth-century scientific design in hospital construction. The healing power of architecture has been a tenet of charitable institutions since at least the establishment of the first asylum, the York Retreat. This remains a guiding principle, particularly in the creation of children's hospitals. From the ornate Victorian castles to the postmodern cartoonesque complexes, children's hospitals were conceived as part medical centres and part welfare refuges—reflecting the dual nature of child health (protective and curative) in general.

Political and financial considerations determined the fate of mega-initiatives, such as the American federal government's Early and Periodic Screening, Diagnosis and Treatment Program of Medicaid as analyzed by Anne-Marie Foltz.[43] But smaller projects, such as the travelling clinic discussed by Sharon Richardson in chapter 17, similarly were affected. Richardson recounts the adventures of intrepid physicians, dentists, and nurses who fought mud and flies to offer seasonal medical care to the children of isolated communities in northern Alberta over a period of almost twenty years. At minimal expense to (albeit to the public acclaim of) the provincial government, the travelling clinics replaced a system of public health clinics drastically cut in a depressed economy.

What do all these stories tell us? First, they regularly present children's vulnerability. Second, they confirm adults' assertion of fundamental rights over young bodies and minds. Third, they demonstrate the diversity of children and their varying susceptibility to the control of the powerful. Finally, however, the story is not entirely dreary: infant mortality has fallen and life expectancy risen in most communities, and abuse is no longer readily taken for granted as the necessary fate of any group of youngsters. In closing, we hope that the contradictory history described in the following pages may assist today's policy-makers, professionals, and citizens as they think more critically about how to improve the health and well-being of *all* children.

Notes

1 See the UNICEF website: http://www.unicef.org/wsc/plan.htm.
2 Michael Udy and Ruth Annis, "A World Fit for Children: Unfinished Business from the United Nations Special Session on Children," First Call BC: Child & Youth Advocacy Coalition, http://www.firstcallbc.org/publications/publications_home.htm. For the UN report, see http://www.unicef.org/specialsession/about/sg-report.htm
3 See UNICEF, *A League Table of Child Poverty in Rich Nations*, p. 4, http://www.unicef-icdc.org/research.
4 On the U.S. refusal to sign international conventions and treaties, see Christopher Hitchens, "Rogue Nation U.S.A.," *Mother Jones* 26, 3 (May–June 2001): 32–37.
5 See Canada, *National Report—Canada: Ten-Year Review of the World Summit for Children* (Ottawa: Public Health Agency of Canada, c2001), http://www.phac-aspc.gc.ca/dca-dea/publications/wsc_e.html.
6 Jessica Ball, Alan Pence, and Allison Benner, "Quality Child Care and Community Development: What Is the Connection?" in *Too Small To See, Too Big To Ignore: Child Health and Well-being in British Columbia*, ed. Michael V. Hayes and Leslie T. Foster, Canadian Western Geographical Series 35 (Victoria: Western Geographical Press, 2002), 92–95.
7 See http://www.campaign2000.ca.
8 In April 2001, experienced child advocates such as UNICEF, World Vision, and Save the Children initiated the Say Yes for Children Campaign in order to lobby the UN's member governments and attempt to hold them accountable for progress in children's rights, including health care. See John Micklewright, "Child Poverty in English-speaking Countries" (Innocenti Working Paper 94, June 2003). See also Bruce Bradbury, Stephen P. Jenkins, and John Micklewright, *The Dynamics of Child Poverty in Industrialised Countries* (Cambridge and New York: Cambridge University Press, 2001); V. Susan Dahinten and J. Douglas Willms, "The Effects of Adolescent Child-bearing on Children's Outcomes," in *Vulnerable Children: Findings from Canada's National Longitudinal Survey of Children and*

Youth, ed. J. Douglas Willms (Edmonton: University of Alberta Press, 2002), 243–58; and Thomas L. Whitman, John G. Borkowski, Deborah A. Keogh, and Ken Weed, *Interwoven Lives: Adolescent Mothers and Their Children* (Mahwah, NJ: Lawrence Erlbaum Associates, 2001). See also Veronica Strong-Boag and Gillian Creese, "Canada," in *The Greenwood Encyclopedia of Women's Issues Worldwide: North America and the Caribbean*, ed. Cheryl T. Kalny (Westport and London: Greenwood Press, 2003), 62.

 9 Fodwa Al-Yaman and Meredith Bryant, *Australia's Children: Their Health and Well-being* (Canberra: Australian Institute of Health and Welfare, 2002). See also Cynthia Duncan, *Worlds Apart: Why Poverty Persists in Rural America* (New Haven: Yale University Press, 1999). Youngsters without health insurance in the so-called developed world, as is the case with many American farm workers, are also especially vulnerable. See Hilary Sargeant, *Fingers to the Bone: United Failure To Protect Child Farm Workers* (New York: Human Rights Watch, 2000).

10 Alan J. C. King and Beverly Coles, *The Health of Canada's Youth: Views and Behaviours of 11-, 13- and 15-Year-Olds from 11 Countries* (Ottawa: National Health and Welfare, 1992), 6. Sixteen countries participated in the 1990 survey of school children: Austria, Belgium, Canada, Finland, Iceland, Norway, Poland, Scotland, Spain, Sweden, Wales, France, Hungry, Latvia, the Netherlands, and Switzerland.

11 Darren Yourk, "Poverty, abuse the main concerns of children," *Globe and Mail*, August 14, 2001. This article considered the report released that day by Save the Children Canada.

12 Quoted in Shelley Geballe and Janice Gruendel, "The Crisis within the Crisis: The Growing Epidemic of AIDS Orphans," in *Invisible Children in the Society and Its Schools*, ed. Sue Books (Mahwah, NJ, and London: Lawrence Erlbaum Associates, 1998), 47.

13 On the difficulty of getting children's perspectives and voices, see Neil Sutherland, "When You Listen to the Winds of Childhood, How Much Can You Believe?" *Curriculum Inquiry* 22, 3 (1992): 235–56.

14 See Catherine Panter-Brick, "Nobody's Children? A Reconsideration of Child Abandonment," in *Abandoned Children*, ed. Catherine Panter-Brick and Malcolm T. Smith (Cambridge, UK: Cambridge University Press, 2000), 1–26, for its important assessment of some of the tragic results of Western ethnocentrism.

15 The literature on the implications of NRTs is expanding rapidly. See, inter alia, Tom Shakespeare, "Manifesto for Genetic Justice," *Social Alternatives* 18, 1 (January 1999): 29–32; Alan Petersen, "The New Genetics and the Politics of Public Health," *Critical Public Health* 8, 1 (March 1998): 59–71; Erica V. Haimes, "When Transgressions Become Transparent: Limiting Family Forms in Assisted Conception." *Journal of Law and Medicine* 9, 4 (2000): 438–48; and Mariana Valverde and Lorna Weir, "Regulating New Reproductive and Genetic Technologies: A Feminist View of Recent Canadian Government Initiatives," *Feminist Studies* 23, 2 (Summer 1997): 419–23.

16 See Joan Sangster, "Masking and Unmasking the Sexual Abuse of Children: Perceptions of Violence against Children in 'The Badlands' of Ontario, 1916–1930," *Journal of Family History* 25, 4 (October 2000): 504–26, and Marie-Aimé Cliche, "Un Secret bien gardé: l'inceste dans la société, traditionnelle québeçoise, 1858–1938," *Revue d'histoire d'Amérique française* 50, 2 (1996): 201–26.

17 See, for example, Sylvia Van Kirk, *Many Tender Ties: Women in Fur Trade Society in Western Canada, 1670–1830* (Winnipeg: Watson & Dwyer, 1980).

18 See, for example, the treatment of a nephew in "The Gifts of the Little People," in J. Burgeron, *Iroquois Stories* (Trumansurg, NY: Crossing Press, 1985).

19 See Tina Moffat and Ann Herring, "The Historical Roots of High Rates of Infant Death in Aboriginal Communities in Canada in the Early Twentieth Century: The Case of Fisher River, Manitoba," *Social Science & Medicine* 48 (1999): 1821–32; Megan Sproule-Jones, "Crusading for the Forgotten: Dr. Peter Bryce, Public Health, and Prairie Native Residential Schools," *Canadian Bulletin of Medical History / Bulletin canadien de l'histoire de la médecine* 13, 2 (1996): 199–224.

20 Dennis Guest, *The Emergence of Social Security in Canada* (Vancouver: University of British Columbia Press, 1980), 10.

21 See Judy Fingard, "'The Winter's Tale': The Seasonal Contours of Pre-Industrial Poverty in British North America, 1815–1860," Canadian Historical Association, *Historical Papers* (1974): 65–94.

22 Patricia Rooke and R. L. Schnell, *Discarding the Asylum: From Child Rescue to the Welfare State in English Canada (1800–1950)* (Lanham, MD: University Press of America, 1983), 8.

23 See Veronica Strong-Boag, "Claiming a Place in the Nation: Citizenship Education and the Challenge of Feminists, Natives, and Workers in Post-Confederation Canada," ed. Alan Sears, special issue, *Canadian and International Education* (December 1996): 128–45.

24 See Karen Murray, "Upsetting the Public–Private Divide: The Third Sector and the Governance of Single Mothers in 20th-Century Canada" (PhD thesis, University of British Columbia, 2001) for an important reminder of the similarities between governance of the poor by the third, private, or philanthropic sector and that by governments.

25 Law Commission of Canada, *Restoring Dignity: Responding to Child Abuse in Canadian Institutions* (Ottawa: Law Commission of Canada, 2000). Total institutions are those "that seek to re-socialize people by instilling them with new roles, skills or values...[where] every aspect of his or her life is determined and controlled" (p. 2).

26 Law Commission of Canada, *Restoring Dignity*, 27.

27 See S. Fournier and E. Crey, Jr., *Stolen from Our Embrace: The Abduction of First Nations Children and the Restoration of Aboriginal Communities* (Vancouver: Douglas & McIntyre, 1997). See also Marilyn Irvin Holt, *Indian Orphanages* (Lawrence: University Press of Kansas, 2001); James T. Carroll, *Catholic Indian Boarding Schools* (New York: Garland, 2000); and Andrew Armitage, *Comparing the Policy of Aboriginal Assimilation Australia, Canada and New Zealand* (Vancouver: UBC Press, 1995).

28 See Margaret Little, *No Car, No Radio, No Liquor Permit: The Moral Regulation of Single Mothers in Ontario, 1920–1997* (Toronto: University of Toronto Press, 1998); and Dominique Marshall, *Aux origines sociales de l'État-providence* (Montreal: Les Presses de l'Université de Montréal, 1998).

29 See Jane Gaskell, *Gender Matters from School to Work* (Philadelphia: Open University Press, 1982); J. R. Miller, *Shingwauk's Vision: A History of Native Residential Schools* (Toronto: University of Toronto Press, 1996); and Jo-Anne Fiske, "Carrier Women and the Politics of Mothering," in *Rethinking Canada: The Promise of Women's History*, ed. Veronica Strong-Boag, Mona Gleason, and Adele Perry (Toronto: Oxford University Press, 2002), 235–48.

30 The tragic failure of provincial children's services in British Columbia to avert the 1992 death of five-year-old Matthew Vaudreuil at the hands of a impoverished mother, herself the victim of abuse, illustrated how Canadians, like too many others, remain ill-equipped to assist youngsters in direst distress. See Thomas Gove, *Gove Inquiry into Child Protection: Final Report.* Vol. 1, *Matthew's Story.* Vol. 2,

Matthew's Legacy (Victoria: Queen's Printer, 1995). See also Andrew Armitage, "Lost Vision: Children and the Ministry for Children and Families," *BC Studies* 118 (Summer 1998): 93–108, the commentaries by Richard Sullivan and Kelly A. MacDonald, the reply by Armitage, pp. 109–14, 114–19, and 120–22; and C. Morton, "Learning from the Past: Improving Child-Serving Systems," in *Too Small To See*, Hayes and Foster, 161–92.

31 See Maureen Baker and David Tippin, "Fighting 'Child Poverty': The Discourse of Restructuring in Canada and Australia," *Australia-Canadian Studies*, 17, 2 (1998): 121–31. See also N. Scheper-Hugers and C. Sargent, "Introduction: The Cultural Politics of Childhood," in *Small Wars: The Cultural Politics of Childhood*, eds. N. Scheper-Hughes and C. Sargent (Berkeley: University of California Press, 1998), 20, 28.

32 See Veronica Strong-Boag, "Intruders in the Nursery: Childcare Professionals Reshape the Years from One to Five, 1920–1940," in *Childhood and Family in Canadian History*, ed. Joy Parr (Toronto: McClelland & Stewart, 1982).

33 See Dawn Currie, *Girl Talk: Adolescent Magazines and Their Readers* (Toronto: University of Toronto Press, 1999) for a relatively optimistic view of the capacity of young women to "read" pop culture critically, and the more pessimistic observations of the journalist Myrna Kostash, *No Kidding: Inside the World of Teenage Girls* (Toronto: McClelland & Stewart, 1987). The gritty, award-winning, Canadian-produced but globally marketed television series of the 1980s–2000s, *Degrassi High*, provided rare portrayal of real-life situations ranging from drug and alcohol abuse to teen pregnancy and AIDS.

34 Maggie Black, *Children First: The Story of Unicef, Past and Present* (Oxford: Oxford University Press and UNICEF, 1996), 5.

35 Carlo A. Corsini and Sara Matthews Grieco, *Historical Perspectives on Breastfeeding* (Florence: Istituto degli Innocenti, 1991) and Pier Paolo Viazzo and Carlo A. Corsini, *The Decline of Infant Mortality in Europe* (1993), and Hugh Cunningham and Pier Paolo Viazzo, eds., *Child Labour in Historical Perspective, 1800–1985: Case Studies from Europe, Japan and Colombia* (Florence: UNICEF and the Instituto degli Innocenti, 1996).

36 Giuseppe Arpioni and James R. Himes, foreword to *Child Labour in Historical Perspective*, Cunningham and Viazzo, eds., 7.

37 Jennifer Beinart, "Darkly through a Lens: Changing Perceptions of the African Child in Sickness and Health, 1900–1945," in *In the Name of the Child: Health and Welfare, 1880–1940*, ed. Roger Cooter (London: Routledge, 1992): 220–43.

38 Linda Bryder, "Wonderlands of Buttercup, Clover and Daisies: Tuberculosis and the Open-Air School Movement in Britain, 1907–39," in *In the Name of the Child*, ed. Cooter, 72–95.

39 Sources on Canadian experts include Robert McIntosh, *Boys in the Pits: Child Labour in Coal Mines* (Montreal: McGill-Queen's University Press, 2000) [factory inspectors]; Neil Sutherland, *Children in English-Canadian Society: Framing the 20th-Century Consensus* (Waterloo: Wilfrid Laurier University Press, 2000); Norah Lewis, "Physical Perfection for Spiritual Welfare: Health Care for the Urban Child, 1900–1939," in *Studies in Childhood History: A Canadian Perspective*, ed. Patricia T. Rooke and R. L. Schnell (Calgary: Detselig, 1982), 135–66 [educators and public health officials]; Strong-Boag, "Intruders in the Nursery," 160–78; and Larry Prochner, "The Development of the Day Treatment Centre for Emotionally Disturbed Children at the West End Creche, Toronto," *Canadian Bulletin of Medical History* 14, 2 (1997), 215–40 [pediatric and mental health professionals]. American contributions include Anthony M. Platt, *The Child Savers: The*

Invention of Delinquency (Chicago: University of Chicago Press, 1977) [juvenile courts]; Howard Markel, "For the Welfare of Children: The Origins of the Relationship between U.S. Public Health Workers and Pediatricians," and Jeffrey P. Brosco, "Weight Charts and Well Child Care: When the Pediatrician Became the Expert in Child Health," in *Formative Years: Children's Health in America, 1880–2000*, ed. Alexandra M. Stern and Howard Markel (Ann Arbor: University of Michigan Press, 2002), 47–65 and 66–88 respectively [pediatricians]; and in Britain, Cathy Urwin and Elaine Sharland, "From Bodies to Minds in Childcare Literature: Advice to Parents in Inter-War Britain," in *In the Name of the Child*, ed. Cooter, 174–99 [childcare and child guidance experts].

40 Annette K. Vance Dorey, *Better Baby Contests: The Scientific Quest for Perfect Childhood Health in the Early 20th Century* (Jefferson, NC: McFarland, 1999).

41 Russel Viner, "Abraham Jacobi and the Origins of Scientific Pediatrics in America," in *Formative Years*, eds. Stern and Markel, 23–46.

42 Theresa R. Richardson, *The Century of the Child: The Mental Hygiene Movement and Social Policy in the United States and Canada* (Albany: State University of New York Press, 1989); Margo Horn, *Before It's Too Late: The Child Guidance Movement in the United States, 1922–1945* (Philadelphia: Temple University Press, 1989); Lewis, "Physical Perfection" [educators and public health officials]; Strong-Boag, "Intruders in the Nursery"; and Prochner, "West End Creche" [pediatric and mental health professionals]. American contributions include Platt, *The Child Savers* [juvenile courts]; Markel, "For the Welfare of Children"; and Brosco, "Weight Charts" [pediatricians]; and in Britain, Urwin and Sharland, "From Bodies to Minds" [childcare and child guidance experts].

43 Anne-Marie Foltz, *An Ounce of Prevention: Child Health Politics under Medicaid* (Cambridge, MA: MIT Press, 1982).

Politics

ର

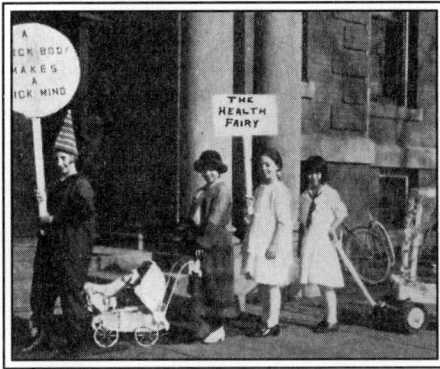

Vegetables on Parade
American Medicine and the Child Health Movement in the Jazz Age

ભ

Naomi Rogers

Amerian Progressives' dream of an efficient, humane, and harmonious nation was shattered by the First World War and its aftermath. During the war patriotic outbursts reinforced by crude propaganda from Woodrow Wilson's administration often turned into violent attacks on pacifist, socialist, and immigrant dissenters. Racism, nativism, and class conflict intensified after the war with strikes, the Red Scare, and the Ku Klux Klan. Even the smug sense that families in the United States were protected from the ravages of famine in Europe was jolted by the news that almost a third of American military recruits during the war had been rejected for physical defects that could have been prevented in childhood. This evidence became a mantra for politicians and reformers, but its lessons were ambiguous. Clearly many young men had come of age without adequate medical care, nutrition, or sanitation. But in the conservative 1920s these "revelations of the Selective Service Act," as one writer termed them, were interpreted not as demonstrating a need to reorganize the nation's fee-for-service medical system or to address the insidious links between poverty and disease, but as indicating the general public's lack of "a conscious, active organized interest in health and physical fitness."[1] American schools had been teaching physiology, hygiene, and domestic science for decades, yet "those young men who were found to be physically unfit for military duty were the same boys who were in our schools only a few years ago," nurse-educator Sally Lucas Jean observed at a social work conference in 1920. "We taught them how many bones were in their bodies, but did we teach them how to live?"[2]

During the interwar years policy makers and health reformers tried to address this question and transform public outrage over the rejected recruits into a force for change.[3] But in the immediate postwar political climate, health activism had to be designed cautiously, especially by reformers whose reputations were already tarnished by their association with socialism, pacifism, and internationalism. The health reform work proposed in the interwar period therefore was consciously designed with only a limited role for government: the maintenance of the nation's sanitary infrastructure. Officials were to make sure there were pipes for sewage disposal, filtration systems for clean drinking water, and sanitation workers to remove garbage.[4] Reformers used as their model the experience of American soldiers in army camps, who were exposed to a regimented hygienic infrastructure "where indifference, disobedience, or insubordination were not tolerated," and disease (other than the devastating influenza pandemic at the end of the war) was prevented through systematic exercise, compulsory rest, and obligatory cleanliness. Each soldier, South Carolina's state health director James Hayne reflected in 1919, learnt "how dependent was each individual upon the proper conduct of every other individual if a camp or a community was to be kept free from disease. Their sanitary conscience was awakened."[5] The new goal of the interwar health movement, thus, was not coercion but the inculcation of hygienic self-discipline and what came to be termed a "sanitary consciousness." Public health work now involved convincing members of the public to fill their homes with the technology of personal hygiene (washbasins, toilets, toothbrushes, soap, and tissues) and then making sure that these products were used. It was the job for a new kind of expert: a professional health educator.

Schoolchildren were considered the most promising recipients for such messages, and they became the new target of interwar health work. The hungry European orphan was contrasted with the happy, well-nourished American child, whose confident outlook promised to banish the shadows of war. "Children are the material with which we must build the world of to-morrow," physician Sara Josephine Baker argued in her 1925 text *Child Hygiene*, a work that both summarized and gave direction to a new field. "The preventive part of public-health work, to be effective, must begin at the time of life when habits of health are early established. The child is plastic material."[6] Boosted by the science of behavioural psychology, reformers' faith in the possibility of teaching children healthy habits that would last into adulthood counterbalanced a growing pessimism about their immutable parents. For example, after discovering that every man and woman he met had ignored the 40,000 anti-tuberculosis circulars his department had mailed out, an exasperated health official concluded that "anything official coming to the public ear does not enter the brain. We have decided, therefore, to give up the old people and get after the next generation."[7]

Three main premises animated this movement: individuals, no matter how limited their resources, could monitor their own bodies to maintain good health and inspire others to do the same; preventive health care based on good habits of eating, sleeping, and keeping clean could obviate much interventionist medical care; and the new "sanitary consciousness" could be achieved through an activist pedagogy based on learning through participation. Health precepts were kept simple—sunshine, fresh air, cleanliness, sleep, and proper nutrition—so that they could easily be summed up in songs, stories, and plays. To avoid what they considered the pitfalls of the pre-war Progressive era, child health activists left most medical technologies safely in the doctor's private office and refrained from criticizing the structure of the American health care system.[8] Messages that were designed to be apolitical and consensual, and to ignore divisions of class and race, also helped protect child health groups from entanglements with suspicious private practitioners, conservative local politicians, and intransigent school boards.

The movement to popularize science at a child's level, valuing the popular and straightforward over the obscure and intricate, has been little explored by historians who have instead focused on reformist efforts to educate and regulate adults, especially mothers, soldiers, and midwives.[9] Science popularizers have been easily dismissed as propagandistic hucksters, exploiting the gap between "real" science and its popular forms.[10] But just as the work of advertising agents has gained a critical place in recent cultural history, so we must take seriously the work of these health propagandists. Interwar child health organizers did try to "sell" health to children, but it was a campaign motivated by complex and sometimes altruistic motives.

Of the complicated networks of proponents and ideologies that comprised the interwar child health movement, I will trace here only a few strands. Ambitious in intent and wide-ranging in scope, the interwar child health movement brought its messages to classrooms, school boards, city halls, teachers colleges, medical and nursing schools, health departments, and homes. Aided by federal agencies like the Children's Bureau, by philanthropies that funded health demonstration projects, and by enthusiastic soap manufacturers and food producers, organizers created and distributed pamphlets, posters, play scripts, songs, textbooks, and guides to community celebrations. Here I focus on the *tools* of the Child Health Organization (later the American Child Health Organization), founded in 1918 and active until 1935: the plays, the parades, the storybooks and the songs.[11] These sources demonstrate the broader movement's distinctive goals: a commitment to activism but an avoidance of political controversy; an individualistic approach to health issues combined with an assumption of civic responsibility; a comfortable integration of voluntary reform and government resources; the adoption of the forms and methods of popular culture; and a modernist professionalism in organization structure and health propaganda. Peak-

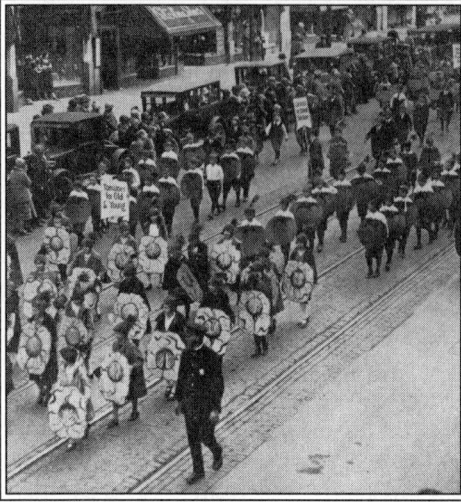

Vegetables on parade in Syracuse during Health Week in the 1920s; Louise Franklin Bache, *Health Education in an American City: An Account of a Five-Year Program in Syracuse, New York* (Garden City: Doubleday, Doran, 1934)

ing in the late 1920s, the movement declined by the mid-1930s as its methods became no longer innovative but conventional. And during the depths of the Great Depression the reluctance of its proponents to question the extent that any individual, no matter how poor, could improve his or her health turned the movement's faith in apolitical voluntarism into naive politics.

Although the health activism that developed after the First World War involved many of the same men and women who had worked in voluntary agencies and government bureaus during the 1900s and 1910s, the movement was self-consciously post-Progressive. More pragmatic and less idealistic, its methods drew on the culture of the jazz era—its popular songs, its sophisticated advertising campaigns, its whimsical graphics—and left behind stark, politically charged images of forlorn child mill workers. Interwar organizers also embraced many of the values of the Jazz Age, especially a modernist aesthetic and an unreflective consumerist optimism that an individual's life could be transformed with the purchase of commercial products. Their posters' clarity and their colourful, orderly parades contrasted with the cluttered lists of bones and muscles in hygiene lessons and the dusty Victorian parlours of an older generation.[12] Thus, to show the success of the five-year health demonstration in Syracuse, New York, Milbank Memorial Fund organizer Louise Bache used a photograph of a children's parade, with children dressed as tomatoes and other fruits and vegetables.[13] Vegetables on parade came to epitomize the methods of this movement, encapsulating as they did a kind of "stripped down" science of catchy precepts that complemented the pristine bathrooms in the family home.

From Military Marches to
Children's Crusades

Propaganda came of age during the Great War, and children were a crucial means of selling war to the public. Heart-rending pictures of the
homeless and malnourished European orphans were placed beside the
precious and vulnerable American child, symbol of New World democracy. Offering a sentimental, sometimes comical parallel to military
marches, child-centred civic celebrations allowed the youngest Americans
to transform school and civic associations into part of the war machine.
By the end of the war, child propagandists were employed to sell everything from patriotism and soap to breakfast cereal and health reform.

As Woodrow Wilson's food administrator during the war, millionaire
engineer Herbert Hoover used children as small agents of patriotism,
whose simple empathy led them to want to help the children of Europe
and American soldiers abroad. A crucial part of his successful voluntary
domestic rationing system (known as "Hooverizing"), children were able
to transform food conservation into a patriotic act. In a magazine story
published in 1917, for example, a father tries to coax his daughter out
of the idea of a Hoover-style Thanksgiving dinner by saying, "You have
been Hooverizing so long that I grow positively sentimental over the
memory of broiled sirloin." "Aren't you all ashamed," Estelle assails her
family in reply, "to be talking about things to eat, after the pictures you
have seen of those starving French and Belgian children? You know we
should all save every ounce of sugar, fats, meat and wheat that we can
spare to those children and to our own soldiers who are fighting for
them."[14]

After the war, Hoover directed the private American Relief Association's European Children's Fund, supported initially by $100 million that
Congress had provided for postwar restoration. Hoover then raised
around $30 million privately, with clever techniques such as "invisible
guest" dinners, where patrons paid to dine at tables serving "relief
rations" next to an empty high chair symbolizing the hungry European
child.[15] During the 1920s, as secretary of commerce in both Warren
Harding's and Calvin Coolidge's Republican administrations and then
as president himself, Hoover continued to promote child health as a
civic responsibility that could ensure a strong and healthy nation,
although his political preference was for voluntary action rather than government bureaucracy.

For critics of the war, child welfare work provided a safe haven for
inculcating internationalism with a dose of patriotic pride. The American branch of the Junior Red Cross was organized in 1917 under the
direction of Henry Noble MacCracken, the pacifist president of Vassar

College. Boys and girls sewed clothing for hospitalized American veterans, made red currant jelly for patients in French hospitals, and sent "Friendship Boxes" to children in Europe.[16] After the war, with the new motto "Happy Childhood the World Over," American Junior Red Cross members raised money for victims of the influenza pandemic, school lunch programs in Flanders, Greek child health centres, and schools for Beirut war orphans. "Now that the war against the Germans is won," a Junior Red Cross manual explained, "it is time to take up with renewed vigor the fight against germs and apply to them the motto of Verdun: 'they shall not pass.'"[17] The assumption that the Junior Red Cross programs were humane and politically neutral was, however, challenged on occasion by its recipients. In former Czechoslovakia, a country that was, readers of *Ladies Home Journal* were assured in the early 1920s, "just emerging from a period of starvation and misery which we in this country can barely imagine," an American health educator had begun to explain the ideals of child health work to a group of Prague schoolteachers, when "one excited man teacher, rushing down the room, shook a fragment of black bread in her face. 'This is what we want from America,' he shouted. 'Bread, not foolish ideas!'" The Red Cross organizers calmed him down, and the lecture continued.[18]

During the war, suffragists and other feminists also used parades and pageants featuring children to raise civic consciousness and to expand the politics of the sentimental. In April 1918 the Children's Bureau and the new Woman's Committee, established as part of the National Council of Defense, organized "Children's Year" in order to stimulate the "civil population…to protect the children of this nation as a patriotic duty." Financed by a special defence fund from Woodrow Wilson's administration, and building on the successful national Baby Week of 1916, Children's Year was intended to inspire the public to demand child health divisions in their health departments and state laws to restrict child labour. In a typical "patriotic pageant" some children were dressed in festive red, white, and blue, while others representing the "suffering children" were "draped in grey" with "a sorrowful appearance." The campaign concluded in May 1919 with a White House Conference on Children attended by child welfare activists from Britain, France, Belgium, Japan, and Serbia.[19] Children's Year was a critical part of the feminist appropriation of American patriotic fervour, an example of war-related welfare activism sheltered in sentimental child-centred celebrations. Suffragists judged its success by two postwar legislative milestones: the passage of the Eighteenth Amendment giving adult women the right to vote in federal elections, and then the new Maternity and Infancy Protection (Sheppard-Towner) Act of 1921. This legislation, providing matching federal grants to states for maternal and infant health programs, infused the Children's Bureau with money and political clout, and enabled it by the mid-1920s to become "a world leader in the child welfare movement."[20] Although mothers, midwives, health officials. and physicians remained the bureau's major targets, director Grace Abbott provided child health organizers with publicity and limited funding throughout the interwar period.[21]

The Child Health Organization (CHO), which would become the era's most influential child health group, was founded on the established themes of protecting the vulnerable American child and therefore guarding against the threat that war might pose to national resources and future civic strength. Before the war, Luther Emmett Holt—one of a small group of elite New York physicians specializing in pediatrics, and a researcher in the science of artificial infant-feeding—was best known as the author of two best sellers: a child care book for mothers and a pediatrics textbook for medical students. During the war, Holt's interests shifted from infant feeding to child nutrition more broadly. In 1917, a survey of 170,000 New York public school children by the New York Association for Improvement of Conditions of the Poor (AICP) revealed that one child in five was seriously malnourished. Holt and six other pediatricians responded by forming a Committee of War-Time Problems in Childhood. Working with the AICP, they set up a "Food Scout Demonstration" in a single public school and then convinced local officials to establish a school hot-lunch program across the city. The committee's success interested Franklin Lane, Woodrow Wilson's secretary of the interior, who suggested it expand into a national organization and promised that his department would print and distribute its literature.[22] In March 1918 this group became the Child Health Organization, with Holt as president and Sally Lucas Jean, the committee's secretary, as director. Jean had nursed in army hospitals during the Spanish-American war, tried and disliked private duty nursing, and made public health education her career with such creative projects as a children's Toothbrush League at the Baltimore Summer Playgrounds.[23]

Holt's position as CHO's president led to an invitation to be one of nineteen American delegates—including Herman Biggs, William Welch, and Lillian Wald—to a meeting in Cannes in April 1919 of some fifty international health experts from North America, Britain, France, Italy, and Japan, a group described as "a veritable 'who's who' of medicine, public health and philanthropy."[24] Onboard ship to Cannes, Holt proudly handed around CHO pamphlets that were "admired very much." In Cannes he was elected general secretary, and his own report on child health had the largest audience and was, Biggs and Welch told him later, "the best report thus far presented."[25] The conference delegates voted to establish a new League of Red Cross Societies (to counterbal-

ance the already highly politicized League of Nations) and an affiliated
international Bureau of Hygiene and Public Health. The new League's
Bureau would help war-torn nations set up stable health infrastructures,
thereby alleviating "social deprivation" and acting as a force for world
peace.[26] The most active part of the new global health organization was
its child welfare program, based on the CHO methods Holt had
described, and intended to help the world's most vulnerable and least
politically controversial subjects.[27] In 1921 Yale public health activist
Charles-Edward Amory Winslow spent eight months in Geneva as director of the League's Health Bureau, and, like Holt, brought back with him
a vision of health reform as the "moral extension of the victory just won
in the world war."[28] By the end of that year, however, the League's headquarters had shifted from Geneva to Paris, and was left "at the periphery of the intergovernmental health regime."[29] Its influence lingered,
however, in American child health work, like the children's book Winslow
and children's author Grace Hallock wrote in 1922, which featured child
citizens of the Land of Health using fly swatters, toothbrushes, bars of
soap, and other weapons to defend their country from the invading
"airplanes of the enemy" (flies and mosquitoes) that carry "germs of
sickness."[30]

The lessons of the Great War, thus, were rewritten into child health
work. The war at home had demonstrated the ways that publicizing the
disabilities and ill health of youth, especially of future soldiers, could
inspire the general public with outrage, an outrage that could be transformed into reformist health politics. Wartime propaganda had also
shown how effective patriotism paraded in the streets was as a selling technique. The child-centred work of the Junior Red Cross and the Children's
Year suggested that, shorn of the taint of socialism and Bolshevism,
domestic health activism with a dose of sentimentalism could turn vulnerable American children into the means for expanding government
and private resources. In short, parades of school-age girls and boys
could teach the public lessons of personal and civic health, and sweeten
the message through the adorable, apolitical messengers.

Health Modernism in a Jazz Age

Child health organizers in the interwar period prided themselves not just
on integrating the latest scientific and educational theories, but being
able to package them in contemporary garb. Indeed, the most striking
element of this movement was its proponents' willingness—in fact eager-
ness—to embrace popular culture. Unlike Progressive reformers' typically skeptical attitude to mass culture, interwar activists sought out the
Jazz Age, and used the expanding film, advertising, and radio industries

as both models and tools.[31] Virginia's director of child hygiene rewrote the blues song "Lazy Bones":

> Lazy bones
> Didn't clean his teeth
> Wouldn't brush 'em up and underneath
> Now he's got a mean ole pain
> Dentist chair for him again![32]

In *What Price Flies?* a prize-winning play written by high school girls in Atlanta, there were health lyrics to "Yes Sir, That's My Baby," and "If You Knew Susie" with the verse

> All we did was give the kiddies typhoid,
> And enjoy the garbage in the store.
> Now it's clean
> It's clear to be seen
> Flies can't live here any more.[33]

Even popular wartime songs appeared, like this extract from *The Brownie's Health Book*:

> What's the use of lollypops?
> They've just a foolish style,
> So, eat up the vegetables and fruit and bread,
> And smile, smile, smile.[34]

In 1915 Charles de Forest of the National Association for the Study and Prevention of Tuberculosis, later the National Tuberculosis Association (NTA) had developed a distinctive campaign to encourage children to sell the NTA's Christmas Seal stamps. The NTA's Modern Health Crusade, a combination of Christian symbolism, medieval militarism, and consumerist sentimentalism, was the most influential domestic child-centred health work.[35] Parading through streets to inspire local communities to undertake anti-tuberculosis work, "little crusaders" dressed in white capes and hats with a double-barrelled cross became, in Nancy Tomes's words, "a sort of human figure trademark."[36] By 1917 the crusade combined anti-tuberculosis fundraising with the completion of simple health tasks. Child Crusaders followed a set of health rules recorded on a chore card, and were rewarded by a progression of titles from page to knight. Promoted by special posters, plays, stories, and weight tables designed and distributed by the NTA, the crusade turned children into health advocates, making their own lives safe through proper habits of sleeping, eating, and hygiene. Not only were crusaders to change their own behaviour, but they were also supposed to function as child health police, as Georgina Feldberg has pointed out, surveying their own neighbourhoods and identifying any "unhygienic" homes. Endorsed by the

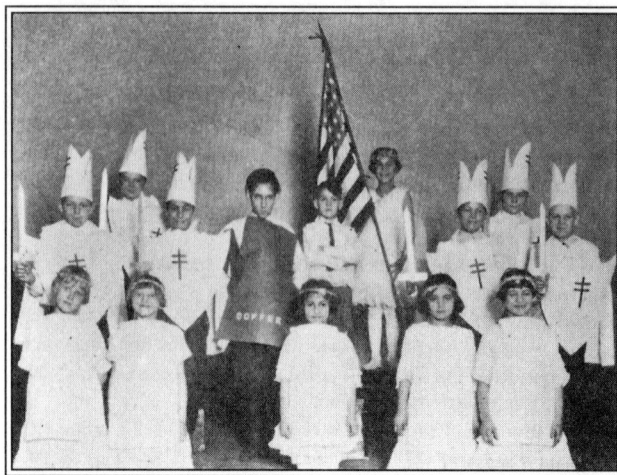

"A Band of [Modern Health] Crusaders" surrounding the evil Coffee character; Charlotte Townsend Whitcomb and John H. Beveridge, *Our Health Habits: A Complete Course in Child Hygiene for the Grades* (Chicago: Rand McNally, 1926)

National Education Association, the crusade was adopted by many schools, and in Washington, DC, it was even made compulsory for all third to eighth grade classes in the public schools.[37] This mixture of disease prevention, health consumerism, and child-oriented entertainment became the model for the postwar child health movement.

CHO transformed the NTA's Modern Health Crusade into a Rules of Health game, dropping the NTA's crusading knights and emphasis on the prevention of a particular disease. Under its own slogan "Health in Education—Education in Health," CHO focused on the child in school, and institutionalized the approval of teachers and peers to promote "training in health habits rather than teaching of health facts."[38] As teachers, according to Sally Lucas Jean, began "begging for more stories, more plays," CHO responded not only with additional materials but with special characters to make the Rules of Health concrete and entertaining for both students and teachers. The clown Cho-Cho was trained to "teach health, sugar coated with all the nonsense and fun of the sawdust ring." The Health Fairy, a public health nurse, told "delightful stories," and a cartoonist drew "a white loaf of bread into a sourfaced boy,…a brown loaf into a round-faced smiling boy," and "vegetables weeping great tears because children do not eat them." All three travelled to elementary and secondary schools, as well as exhibitions, fairs, and "any place where children were gathered together."[39] A less traditional figure was CHO's pseudo-professor Happy (played by Clifford Goldsmith), who entertained child and adult audiences with snappy

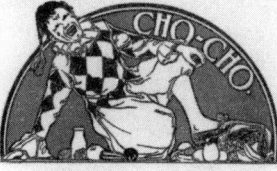

CHO-CHO

A clown who, in a 45-minute performance that rings with mirth, makes children enthusiastic about following his Rules of the Game of Health. One child wrote to him, "Most people just talk and talk, but you make it so plain and so interesting." When CHO-CHO leaves, it seems desirable to clean one's teeth, to bathe, to drink milk, and to eat vegetables, because it is the way of health and the way of happiness. It becomes a game with CHO-CHO.

If you want CHO-CHO to perform for you, he will come for $25 a day for one performance; $35 a day for two performances; living and traveling expenses. But if you want two performances they must not be more than two hours apart.

How to order a performance by Cho-Cho who "makes children enthusiastic about following his Rules of the Game of Health," in CHO pamphlet *Open the Door for Child Health* [c. 1922] (Harvey Cushing/John Jay Whitney Medical Library, Yale University School of Medicine)

health maxims. Happy, the Health Fairy, and the cartoonist worked well within the boundaries of CHO's program, but when the clown who played Cho-Cho began to regard himself "as a real authority on diet, hygiene, and even the morals of childhood," and deviated from his "carefully learned lines," the organization had to find a new Cho-Cho.[40]

During the first four years of its organization life, CHO's work contrasted sharply with the American Child Hygiene Association, which, unlike CHO, was directed primarily by physicians and focused on improving the health of mothers and infants. First called the American Association for the Study and Prevention of Infant Mortality (AASPIM), the group had been established in 1909 during a conference on infant mortality organized by the American Academy of Medicine. Organizers of AASPIM were a significant force behind the creation of the U.S. Children's Bureau in 1912, and by 1914 the group led a national network of around 140 similarly oriented voluntary health agencies promoting the decline of maternal and infant mortality.[41] In 1918 the name was altered by the association's new president and one of its founders, Sara Josephine Baker, a 1898 graduate of Elizabeth Blackwell's New York Women's Medical College.

Baker had built her career in pediatric preventive care and health reform, and in 1908 had convinced New York City's Department of Health to establish a Bureau of Child Hygiene under her direction. During the war Baker linked infant health activism to work at the front, with her slogan, "It's six times safer to be a soldier in the trenches in France than to be born a baby in the United States," and her bureau in New York City was a frequent stop for North American and European public health visitors.[42] When Baker became president of the AASPIM, she gave a strong speech about the "lessons from the draft." Uncomfortable with the group's awkward long name and aware of the renewed public interest in the health of school-age children, she renamed it the American Child Hygiene Association.[43]

In 1923 CHO merged with the Child Hygiene Association to form the American Child Health Association (ACHA), and chose Herbert Hoover as its president and political patron, Holt as one of its vice-presidents, and Jean as director of health education.[44] The ACHA's official announcement claimed the new group had a "humble willingness to learn...how best we may apply the facts and principles of science to make them function in the actual lives of children."[45] Some reformers worried, however, that in the merger science would be swallowed up by health enthusiasm. CHO's health program had been "purely a matter of health habits, without, at the same time, laying a sufficiently broad foundation of scientific information on which those habits might be based," one physician complained to Winslow, cautioning that, in the new association, CHO's "excellent propaganda work" must be subordinated to "the scientific ideals and attitude of the American Child Hygiene Association."[46] The ACHA board of directors maintained a careful balance between health professionals and educators, including Arnold Gesell, Lee Frankel, Josephine Baker, Grace Abbott, William Welch, Homer Folks, Philip Van Ingen, and Winslow himself.[47] But the concern that the ACHA was more propaganda than science never disappeared. Johns Hopkins bacteriologist William Welch, who years earlier had worked with Emmett Holt in the laboratories of Bellevue Hospital, used to remark to his students, "What fun Holt is having with that new toy of his!"[48]

CHO's Rules of Health game as well as its posters, health alphabets, plays, and guides for teachers became part of the ACHA's national program. Working with the Commonwealth Fund and Milbank Memorial Fund, the ACHA helped to coordinate a number of regional health demonstrations, and with the backing of the U.S. Bureau of Education and the Children's Bureau, the organization rapidly became a national resource providing teaching aids to urban, small town, and rural communities.[49] The ACHA also promoted its distinctive style of health pedagogy by providing teaching guides and special scholarships to teachers colleges. The numbers of health teaching courses and health education specialists rose significantly during the interwar years.[50]

Child health education in the American school curriculum had been used as an activist tool since the 1880s and 1890s, when the Women's Christian Temperance Union successfully pressured state legislators to require school courses on physiology and hygiene that dramatized the dangers of alcohol, tobacco, animal vivisection, and sexual experimen-

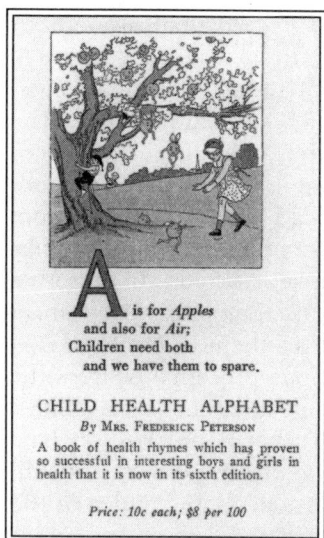

"A is for Apples"; notice for sixth edition of *Child Health Alphabet* (1918) by Mrs Frederick Peterson in CHO pamphlet *Open the Door for Child Health* [c. 1922] (Harvey Cushing/John Jay Whitney Medical Library, Yale University School of Medicine)

tation.[51] These textbooks included lists of rules and facts to be learnt by rote (although historians know little about how the subjects were actually taught), and the lessons were clearly animated by a middle-class Victorian suspicion of both the dangers and pleasures of urban living. In the 1920s these books provided a wonderful foil for child health reformers, who dismissed them as old-fashioned and antithetical to modern knowledge of child development and psychology.[52] In one health play, a boy explains to the Health Fairy why he "hooked" school: "My teacher's awful nice, but I got so tired hearing about how many bones were mixed up inside of me when we had our physiology lesson this morning that I didn't go back after dinner [lunch]."[53] The new health teacher was expected, in the words of an ACHA health survey, to become "the Apostle of Health," to "sell" the principles of health in a catchy, imaginative way that would spill over from the excited child to his or her family and neighbours.[54] "ARE YOU a Health Enthusiast?" an ACHA scholarship application form for graduate teacher training typically asked "DO YOU BELIEVE...that the formation of Health habits is more important than the mere acquisition of facts in physiology and hygiene? That in order to teach Health effectively we must capture the interest and imagination of the child, and help him to express his new enthusiasm originally and creatively?"[55] This style was epitomized in distinctive teaching aids like "Happy's Calendar" and "Happy's Vanity Case," which, a California ACHA organizer boasted, "have been responsible for more classroom teaching of Health than all the hygiene [books] and physiologies that have ever been written."[56]

The child health movement developed its pedagogical methods from child psychology experts. "The child must be instructed in *how* to do the right thing in health, rather than *why* to do it," leading psychologist Lewis Terman explained in his own school health guide. "The right thing in health will be done by children only when they are so educated that they do not have to think about it."[57] In turn, child guidance experts seeking to popularize their field used techniques from CHO and ACHA. In *The Story of Mother Wise*, a pamphlet produced by the Massachusetts Society for Mental Hygiene in 1926, Mr. and Mrs. Want-To-Do-Right, the parents of a toddler with temper tantrums, meet Smilio the health sprite. This fairy introduces them to Mother Wise, whose simple advice (based on child guidance precepts) enables the parents to establish good mental health habits and tame their child.[58] Pamphlets like this were directed at parents, but popularized behaviourist psychology linking the mind and body was also directed at children. Mental illness could result from improper maintenance of the body, one school health text warned, for untreated defective adenoids could cause the "slowing of mental process" and lead to "truancy, incorrigibility and actually immoral actions."[59]

The Commercial Side of Child Health

Selling health worked even better, child health organizers discovered, with the resources of the business world. Department stores, dairies, and other food producers and retailers found myriad opportunities to do well by doing good. The burgeoning radio and film industries also quickly recognized the commercial appeal of child health–oriented products and the utility of the movement's methods. Denver's two radio stations invited experts to talk about children's teeth, eyes, mental health, tuberculosis, and posture during the city's 1927 Health Week.[60]

Health films had been produced by voluntary health agencies like the NTA since the 1910s, but in the 1920s they became a thriving business, combining professional promotion, public entertainment, and civic education.[61] Schools, welfare agencies, and health departments could now rent the American Dental Association's *Tommy Tucker's Tooth* and *Clara Cleans Her Teeth*, and the American Medical Association's *The Magic Fluid* (on diphtheria antitoxin), and *The Trial of Jimmy the Germ*.[62] The National Dairy Council produced the films *Healthland* (a trip through the Land of Health) and *The Romance of the White Bottle* (featuring milk fairies), and worked with the ACHA's Professor Happy Goldsmith to design a "Healthland Exhibit" for a Health Exposition sponsored by the council.[63] The Metropolitan Life Insurance Company, a pioneer in health education, eagerly sent its subscribers CHO and ACHA publica-

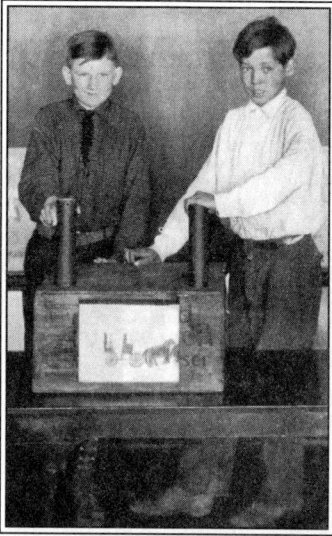

Fifth-grade boys with their health movie project, Fargo, North Dakota; Maud A. Brown, *Teaching Health in Fargo* (New York: Commonwealth Fund, 1929)

tions as well its own *The Metropolitan Mother Goose*, organized a children's Health and Happiness League, and distributed its films, *One Scar or Many* on smallpox and *New Ways for Old* on diphtheria.[64] Not only watching movies but also creating them became a central part of the new health teaching. To demonstrate the success of a child health demonstration funded by the Commonwealth Fund in Fargo, North Dakota, Maud Brown showed a photograph of two boys posing proudly beside their own "health movie" and mock projector.[65]

These efforts adopted the methods of the child health movement and relied on its endorsement. Health activists defended this cooperation by claiming that commercial companies shared their understanding of child health goals. Advertisers were being "influenced by the propaganda of the health organizations," a CHO organizer argued, so "we can safely welcome their advance."[66] But how far should reformers cooperate with companies whose motives were first to sell a product and only secondarily to promote healthful habits? At one point members of CHO's executive board wanted to refuse a contribution from milk companies offered "in payment of work done by our association in advertising milk." CHO's president Emmett Holt disagreed. While such dealers were of course "actuated by motives of self-interest only," Holt told his board, he did not view such contributions as "tainted money," because CHO was "only incidentally helping their business." Holt urged the board not to jeopardize the "good will and cooperation" of these companies "by taking a position which would seem to impugn their motives."[67] The ACHA's executive was even more confident that "wide-

awake commercial enterprises whose products contribute to Child
Health" should send those products "into homes where thousands and
boys and girls will be cleaner and better-fed."[68] The blurring of distinctions between the work of commercial advertisers and child health promoters was made concrete by the baskets that the children of Owyhee
County, Idaho, presented during a school parade "loaded with good
health advertisements cut from magazines."[69]

Image was thus a critical element in the child health movement.
Organizations cultivated a sophisticated professional look, reflected in
their crisp artistic letterheads and whimsical illustrations. The ACHA
urged health officials to spruce up their weekly department bulletins with
modern graphic designs and clever slogans.[70] Teachers were even expected
to look as if they lived by the health rules they taught. Sally Lucas Jean
announced proudly that "one large teaching institution" did not give references to its graduates unless they demonstrated "a fair standard of personal health...[for] a clear complexion is recognized as well as knowledge of the circulatory system."[71] Sometimes, though, embracing the new
made for an awkward fit with older public health traditions. This was
especially true in the case of the still controversial female professional. In
1922 the Children's Bureau sent physician Ethel Watters to tour child
health projects in the Midwest. Writing back to a colleague in Washington, Watters praised one nurse in Kansas who, although "not wholly sound
in the modern public health teaching," had "white hair and her dignity
and manner lend prestige to the [exhibit] car." While this traditional
image seemed likely to Watters to prove an asset to child health work, the
flapper look did not. Another nurse who was, Watters believed, "older than
I am" wore "her hair bobbed and her skirts up to her knees. She knows
prof.[essional] health work but her appearance detracts."[72]

Although American child health organizers clearly sought to capture
the bodies and minds of participant and viewer through magical, dramatic, comical, and sentimental means, it is important to recognize that
they did not see themselves as pandering to the public. In the 1910s, for
example, officials at the Children's Bureau had resisted using the popular baby contest. They had tried at first to co-opt baby shows by adding
health standards to those of physical beauty, and then by discouraging
prizes for the "best" baby.[73] But their efforts to create "health conferences" as a non-competitive alternative failed, and baby contests
remained wildly popular. Further, public interest in Fitter Family and
other eugenic competitions stood as a competitor to interwar child
health work, for they implicitly undermined the message that defects were
not immutable and that physical and mental health could be improved.[74]

By the 1920s, most child health activists had few qualms about competitions or prizes. The whole premise of the CHO's Rules of Health

game, after all, was children working for publicly recognized rewards. Teachers were expected to ensure conformity by the threat of social ostracism and academic failure. At the end of every lunch at a summer health school in Los Angeles, for example, the dietitian called roll. Instead of saying "present," each child, seated in teams at three long tables, was asked to respond "clean plate," as the teams competed for a clean plate trophy. "If food is left uneaten," reported one observer, "there is a dead silence."[75] Peer pressure was also used to spur children to bypass reluctant parents who neglected their children's health defects and therefore threatened their success in school. In one story a girl with painful adenoids ignored her parents' fears that her family doctor would hurt her, walked into his office, and asked him to take them out. Subsequently "she began to grow well and fat and strong so fast that she soon 'caught up' in her classes."[76]

There were still child health advocates who feared that these methods created froth rather than substance. At one CHO meeting Sally Lucas Jean faced such concerted opposition to her proposals that she had to phone Emmett Holt to come and explain to the rest of the committee that "the clowns, prestidigitators and nursery rhymes" were "only the brass band" compared to CHO's "real objectives"—extracting money from "recalcitrant politicians" for school lunches and health education, and convincing teaching colleges to introduce the new health pedagogy.[77] After CHO's merger with the Child Hygiene Association, Jean stayed on only a few months as ACHA's director of health education. She and the eight members of her division resigned to protest Herbert Hoover's open distaste for her style of health propaganda—he had called projects like *Professor Happy's Official Rule Book* "claptrap"—and his cost-cutting measures directed at her staff.[78]

Jean was replaced by Kansas physician Samuel Crumbine, the former secretary of his state's board of health, whose flamboyant campaigns Swat the Fly and Bat the Rat had gained him national attention. Crumbine's new prominence in the child health movement, however, tended to reinforce critics' fear that science would be trumped by health propaganda. One searing critic was Sinclair Lewis. In his 1925 novel *Arrowsmith* Lewis ridiculed officials like Crumbine with his character Almus Pickerbaugh, a city health commissioner who spends his time not fighting tuberculosis-ridden tenements, diseased cows, or filthy drinking water, but bullying the public with what Lewis called "holy frenzy and bogus statistics." Pickerbaugh's Swat the Fly week was boosted by posters that read "Hang onto the old fly-swatter/ if you don't want disease sneaking into the Home/ Then to kill the fly you gotter!" and his campaign to give prizes to the children who caught the most flies.[79]

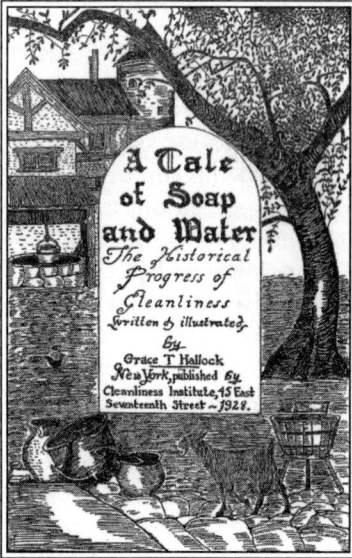

Title page of *A Tale of Soap and Water* (1928) published by the Cleanliness Institute; Grace T. Hallock, *A Tale of Soap and Water: The Historical Progress of Cleanliness* (New York: Cleanliness Institute, 1928)

Jean was widely respected as a child health organizer, and by the mid-1920s she was working as a freelance health consultant, organizing health programs for the National Dairy Council, the Metropolitan Life Insurance Company, Quaker Oats, and the Cleanliness Institute.[80] Her swift transition from voluntary health work to the corporate world demonstrates how easy it was for commercial companies to integrate the messages and methods of the child health movement. The Cleanliness Institute, for example, founded in 1927 by the Association of American Soap and Glycerine Producers, produced children's books, posters, and teachers' guides, claiming that "the object should be not merely to make children clean, but to make them love to be clean."[81] The Institute relied not only on Sally Lucas Jean as a consultant but also hired former CHO Professor Happy Goldsmith who was touted as the "author" of *Learn the Art of Magic*, a fourteen-page pamphlet showing how hygiene could be fun.[82] The link between happiness and soap was best expressed in an American history of cleanliness that the Institute published in 1931. The story begins with American pioneers in log cabins making their own soap, and ends in a modern New York City apartment with a "beautiful and artistic bathroom," the floor and the wall "made of gleaming tiles in cool blue-green like the sea," the faucets "a sculptured fish," and the shower curtains and bath mat green with flecks of "bright red-gold."[83] Here, beauty, consumerism, happiness, success, and health are encapsulated for child readers in the modern bathroom.

Building on the NTA's Modern Health Crusade, CHO and the ACHA combined disease prevention with health promotion. Children could develop a sanitary conscience, organizers argued, through simple and repeatable health habits. The school teacher became health propagandist, teaching her students to become propagandists themselves. Outside the school, the example of welfare capitalism in the 1920s suggested to these consensus-seeking reformers that employers could be made to recognize their responsibilities to the health needs of their community. Child health organizers also believed that the advertising industry could be used as a model and resource, that its messages were controllable, and that the transformation of children into health consumers was an unalloyed good. Their faith in integrating the consumerist culture of the Jazz Age into schools and health departments was a distinctive characteristic of the interwar movement, where soap brought happiness, slogans became inspiration, and radio shows and movies provided a new, more effective health text.

What Kind of Medicine? The Problem of the Doctor's Office

Although the ACHA and other child health groups sought to develop good relations with health professionals, they recognized that their work could also antagonize them. Already suspicious of the growing numbers of municipal venereal disease and tuberculosis clinics, many general practitioners disliked the new maternal and infant health programs that states were setting up with Sheppard-Towner Act funding, and the public health nurses, infant care pamphlets, and letters of advice sent out by the Children's Bureau.[84] A Colorado nurse wryly reported to the Children's Bureau that "a doctor in a rural community expressing his opinion of public health work states that after the Community Health Conference had been in his town teaching the children to drink milk, eat vegetables, and take their naps each day, it took him just <u>MONTHS</u> to get those mothers and children back again into their old routine."[85]

To defuse controversy, the ACHA was careful to have its booklets approved by medical and nursing groups, and avoided including material on alcohol, tobacco, or sex.[86] The directors of health education at Syracuse's public and parochial schools, "serving as self-appointed critics," reviewed health stories to be broadcast on the local radio.[87] But on the whole, the movement's organizers made a sharp division between learning health habits and the doctor's office, between individual disease prevention and medical treatment. "Demonstration workers scrupulously kept their hands off the relations between practitioners and their patients," Commonwealth Fund organizers noted in 1930, for they had promised local doctors and dentists to "protect and preserve the professional interests of the private practitioner."[88] Child health popularizers also kept their distance from hospitals; indeed, complicated medical technologies were rarely mentioned. Instead, small operations like tonsillectomies and teeth extraction were presented as simple techniques that could fix "defects." During Child Health Days in Tennessee, Virginia, Indiana, Missouri, Ohio, and Kentucky so-called Blue Ribbon children who had not only completed their health chores but also had all their defects fixed rode on special floats and received special certificates and prizes.[89]

Although many doctors and dentists remained skeptical of the propaganda excesses of child health work, the major professional organizations had nevertheless begun to adopt the movement's methods. In plays like *The Bad Baby Molar*, as well as posters, slides, and films, the American Dental Association (ADA) explained the importance of combining preventive dental care with regular visits to the dentist.[90] In 1921 the American Medical Association (AMA) and the National Education Association formalized their shared interest in school health by forming a Joint Committee on Health Problems in Education headed by Columbia University health educator Thomas Wood.[91] In an adroit mixture of medical politics and health propaganda, AMA posters, pamphlets, and films warned of the dangers of superstition, alternative medicine, and too much free medical care. In 1923 the AMA founded its own popular health magazine, *Hygeia*, to try to gain control of the spiralling health popularization movement. Edited by Morris Fishbein, the AMA's leading professional promoter and powerful general secretary, *Hygeia* published many articles about CHO and ACHA and found that costumed children on parade made great illustrations.

Although the methods were similar, the *content* of the plays, posters, parades, and children's books demonstrated significant differences between the child health movement and AMA and ADA propaganda.[92] In most child health storybooks, for example, doctors and dentists played largely tangential roles. In *All Through the Day the Mother Goose Way* (1921) Little Miss Muffet learns the importance of drinking milk and Jack Be Nimble the importance of exercise, all lessons easily taught by a nurse, teacher, or even an older child.[93] Fictional child characters gently try to educate doctors unsympathetic to preventive health work, and mock old-fashioned hygiene school textbooks "prepared by doctors who know little of pedagogy and nothing of modern methods of teaching."[94] In one 1925 story, Dr. Foster is overworked because children ignorant of good hygiene have been catching "measles, mumps and colds" from each other. When the children's health improves after Brownie health fairies teach them proper habits, he tells a sprite, "Cure them before they are sick! That sounds queer to me but [I] suppose that is the way Brownies talk."[95] In materials published in *Hygeia* but designed by child health organizers, the doctor and dentist were on occasion threatening figures whose knowledge was better gained from the classroom than an expensive office visit. As *Hygeia* readers learnt from one song in a 1927 health play *On Board the S.S. Health*:

Little Bo-Peep has lost her sleep
And can't tell where to find it.
If she were wise
She might realize
That coffee and tea are behind it.
Little Bo-Peep soon found her sleep
When told the reason behind it.
She paid a big price
For a doctor's advice
And had sense enough to mind it.[96]

Organizers did promote two linked pieces of technology: the height-weight chart and the scale. Based on developmental norms developed by child psychologists like Arnold Gesell, height-weight charts provided a scientific way to measure and compare health progress.[97] The scale was another recognizable tool of the child health movement; one of CHO's early slogans was "A scale for every school."[98] Children were encouraged to see gaining weight as a game, and to pressure their teachers to introduce scales and charts into the classroom. One 1924 textbook showed a teacher measuring students with the caption, "If you are not being weighed and measured at school, can't you find a way to do it? The greatest fun of all in playing the Health Game is getting weighed and seeing how fast you grow."[99] And a rhyme in *Better Health for Little Americans* (1926) read,

Eenie, meenie, minie, mo,
Catch a thin boy by the toe;
Put him on the scales to see
If he's as healthy as he should be.
If he's not what he should weigh,
Give him a quart of milk each day.[100]

The central roles of women in the child health movement also effectively distinguished the movement from mainstream medical professionals. While male doctors like pediatricians Emmett Holt and Philip Van Ingen were on the letterheads of the major health organizations, most of the work of the child health movement was done by women: professional health organizers, graduate teacher educators, public health physicians, child welfare and charity workers, members of women's clubs, schoolteachers, and public health nurses.[101] Indeed, the central professional figure in child health propaganda was the public health nurse with her scale, record sheets, and health rules. A rewritten version of "Little Orphan Annie" began:

> We got a bran' new health nurse t'come to our school today,
> To look us children up an' down an' watch us work and play.
> She weighs us an' she measures us, an' ef we're underweight
> She tells us what we orto eat an' makes us clean our plate.[102]

Drawing on the ideology of scientific motherhood, women were believed to give a softer, less dictatorial air to health work. Thus, a Maryland health official suggested that the Children's Bureau send a female doctor to ameliorate community tensions, for "she hobnobs better with the nurse, and presents no antagonism to the local doctors."[103] Mothers could also use child health messages to enhance their own authority. In a 1929 story, when her daughter Bettie refuses to drink enough milk and says she prefers cake and candy, Mother Squirrel refuses to let her go to the movies until she weighs as much as the other little squirrels in her class at school.[104]

Immunization was the only medical technique regularly mentioned in interwar child health work. In awkward rhyming, Red Riding Hood's mother tells her daughter,

> You'll surely outwit the old wolf called Disease
> By your doctor's advice after clear explanation
> We protected you early by immunization.
> So run on, Red Riding Hood, you need not fear
> Diphtheria, smallpox or typhoid, my dear.[105]

Immunization was presented as the sensible choice of a health-aware community, an area where health officials had clear powers buttressed by the 1922 Supreme Court decision *Zucht v. King*, which had approved the compulsory vaccination of school children without the threat of an epidemic. Although health organizers and local physicians might disagree about where immunization (the popular term for diphtheria anti-toxin and the typhoid and smallpox vaccines) should take place—whether health clinic or doctor's office—the worth of the technique itself was presented as undeniable. For a "Health Stunt," Virginia organizers suggested dressing two boys as knights on horseback wearing placards that listed the number of immunized children in the county; and an Indiana classroom held a parade of exposed vaccination scars.[106]

Immunization was not, however, easy to present playfully for, as educators admitted, it "suggests an unpleasant performance with serums and hypodermics," which a teacher might fear "as much as do her pupils."[107] Nonetheless, stories and plays produced by the AMA emphasized the wonder of this and other products of modern science when wielded by a medical expert.[108] AMA guides had warned physicians who ventured into the field of health propaganda to "make your doctors human beings. Don't transform them into shining knights in white armor [or]...let your doctors be smug, pompous, sententious or pedantic."[109] But in *The Magic Fluid*, an AMA play and film, the terrible Ogre Diph-Theria who threatens children in the Land of Youth is defeated by "a Prince called Science" clad in a white tunic. The prince declares, "I am sworn to the service of fighting the Ogre who steals your people away. I carry a magic fluid called Serum, which will put him to flight." The serum, the prince explains, was "cunningly contrived from the blood of a young horse, purified by a white flame, given into my hands in the kingdom of Wisdom." A grateful king awards the prince half the kingdom and the hand in marriage of Princess May.[110]

In contrast to the AMA's reductionist approach, child health organizers more often stressed the benefits of immunization as part of a broader goal of individual and civic health. In Santa Rosa County, Florida, a parade of school children dramatized "cleanliness, proper play, wholesome food, the city's responsibility to create the right environment, and immunization."[111] Educators proudly reported the numbers of children immunized during health weeks and child health days. Travelling clinics, of course, did not ensure a stable health infrastructure, but even with permanent institutions, the right people had to run them. Thus, the story of immunization could become a lesson in the superiority of American colonialism. Children reading the school text *Cleanliness and Health* (1926) learnt that when American troops took over the Philippines and made smallpox vaccination compulsory, the disease almost disappeared, but when Filipinos who did not enforce vaccination ran health organizations, 50,000 local people died in a "great epidemic" in 1918. Only one American was infected, and only "lightly."[112]

In child health fiction and textbooks, scientists made rare appearances, and scientific research was presented not as an exciting process but a method, largely standardized, that provided useful knowledge and products.[113] Robert Koch and Louis Pasteur were featured in the *Health Hero* series published by Metropolitan Life in the 1920s and 1930s, but they shared the spotlight with sanitary activists like Florence Nightingale and Edward Trudeau.[114] In a modernized Cinderella play, Prince Good Health has a herald named Research, but his only job is to present the prince with the missing slipper.[115] Popularized science was intended to be simple and accessible, far from elite laboratories in ivory towers. "No longer are medicine and physiology surrounded by mystery," Philip Van Ingen explained as he characterized the child health movement in 1921. "Today health is a game, a story, a place, or a 'movie.'"[116] Scientific researchers were difficult to turn into heroes. Listen to the defensive tone of a doctor in the 1931 history published by the Cleanliness Institute who tells a skeptical young boy, "Maybe you think Pasteur wasn't a hero because he worked in a laboratory with deadly germs instead of fighting Indians, but I tell you that what he learned about microbes has saved thousands and thousands of lives! And how about Dr Lazear who died for science?"[117]

Specialist groups like the AMA's Section on Diseases of Children and the American Pediatric Society had supported the Sheppard-Towner Act. Conservative general practitioners, by contrast, feared that the act, along with health insurance proposals and the expansion of the Veteran's Bureau, was part of a broader movement to socialize medicine. By the late 1920s the enthusiasm of these elite pediatricians had cooled, as many believed the act's agencies were competing with private practice. Organized medical groups managed to defuse its Congressional support, and the act ended in 1929.[118] Its demise showed that child health efforts to create a consensus as part of improving the nation's health had failed. Child health organizers urged children to embrace the products and discoveries of immunology, bacteriology, and nutritional biochemistry, but most of the movement's work kept its distance from medical science, the laboratory, and the scientist. Immunization, even in AMA propaganda, was explained as the "magic fluid." Organizers' "hands off" policy towards the medical establishment was reflected in their support of travelling clinics, and in the fictional characterization of medical practice and certain medical techniques—adenoid, tonsil, and tooth extraction—as crucial to a happy, healthy life. But these stories and plays simultaneously warned their participants and audiences that the doctor's and dentist's offices were places best avoided, and instead welcomed children into a largely feminized medical world featuring the public health nurse as a kind of happy substitute health teacher and simple technologies easily used by teachers and parents.

Pageants and Parades: The Colour of Civic Health

While CHO and ACHA focused on the schoolchild as a target in itself and as an individualized entry into the family and community, organizers still needed ways to bring the community into the school or to have children demonstrate their newly acquired health habits in a prominent place outside the school for all to admire. Hence the appeal of children's parades and pageants, designed to combine old and new forms of civic celebration.[119] As the NTA's Modern Health Crusade had shown, health reformers could build on civic traditions like the public parade, long associated with working-class and community pride. In 1924 ACHA

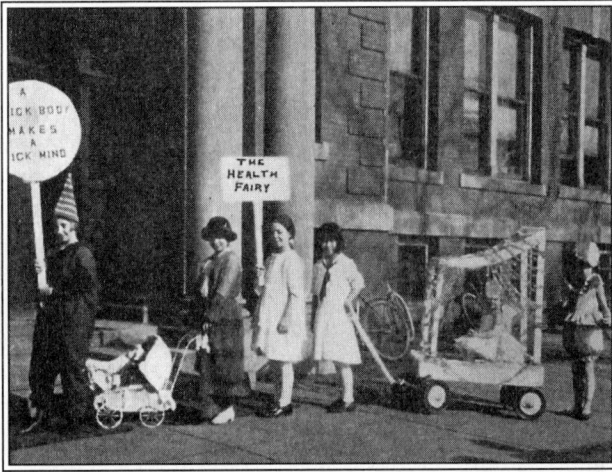

A children's health parade with signs that read "A Sick Body Makes a Sick Mind" and "The Health Fairy"; Charlotte Townsend Whitcomb and John H. Beveridge, *Our Health Habits: A Complete Course in Child Hygiene for the Grades* (Chicago: Rand McNally, 1926)

organizers created Child Health Day to replace May Day, a holiday already changing, as Alan Dawley has shown, from a radical labour celebration to a re-imagined "ancient Anglo-Saxon festival."[120] Merchants quickly gained control of Child Health Day and similar celebrations, and, with Macy's first Thanksgiving Day parade of 1924, to use the words of historian William Leach, "exploited them to the hilt."[121] Pageants, similarly, were no longer the artistic demonstrations familiar to pre-war generations but now a rather conventional civic genre produced by professional pageant companies. It was not surprising that Atlantic City businessmen in 1921 who wanted to make their new Miss America beauty contest respectable decided to call it a "pageant."[122]

Using parading children to inspire civic health responsibility was not new. In the 1890s George Waring, head of New York City's Department of Street Cleaning, had organized children's sanitary parades, and in 1915 a children's Spotless Town League, based on the famous advertising campaign by soap maker Sapolio, had marched through the streets of New Britain, Connecticut. Parades featuring children on floats carrying brooms, soap, bathtubs, garbage cans, flypaper, and chloride of lime were proposed by many public health guides of the 1910s.[123]

With the expansion of public schools and the enforcement of more stringent truancy laws, school plays became a new way to draw the public into the school. When he was in elementary school in the 1920s, public health historian John Duffy recalled recently, he had been the third germ in a health play.[124] Health educators hoped that this kind of experience would linger in the minds of their students, and Grace Hallock, editor of *Dramatizing Child Health*, believed that the health play could rise "out of the realm of propaganda into the realm of art."[125] Still, Louise Bache, an organizer of the Milbank Fund's health demonstration in Syracuse, New York, admitted in 1928, "I must confess that being a carrot or a tomato or a bottle of milk in a health play would never make me an enthusiast for any of these products." Nonetheless, child actors in plays, Bache assured other educators, could lure "fathers and mothers and older brothers and sisters" to the school. "Story telling, plays, pageants, parades will call forth a crowd," she reminded her audience, "when a lecture will draw only a handful."[126] Bache herself preferred pageants that, unlike school plays, could "put over the message of public health in a clear-cut and colorful manner" as "the larger cast creates greater community interest."[127]

Its reliance on the sentimental and comical appeal of festively costumed children helped to situate this movement far away from politically dangerous debates over the abolition of child labour or the reorganization of health care. The topic of food was especially popular. It was a subject that was easy to symbolize and a powerful way of inculcating the child health movement's central faith in health through education, in preventing disease through understanding and following simple health rules. Health activists made extravagant promises of the benefits children would gain from a good diet: energy, strength, mental ability, and a way to overcome the disadvantages of class, region, or family background.[128] To suggest the benefits of balancing sanitary regulation and individual control of diet, a Washington County, Florida, parade featured children wearing costumes of different fruits and vegetables, while other floats illustrated the value of hot lunches, milk, and healthy cows.[129] More pointedly, in a play written by a West Virginian health official, Jimmy, too sickly to study or play ball, is taken to Healthland by Sanitary Sam. There he is shown how to use "a silver dollar" to gain health by spending it entirely on food: vegetables, grains, sweets and fats, meat, fish and eggs, and milk. At first Jimmy is sullen and, at the suggestion that he is undernourished, says angrily, "You needn't laugh at me just because we haven't any money to buy expensive foods like some folks. We have a big family and it takes lots of money to buy candy and cake." "It is not the amount of money we spend for food," he learns finally, "but the wise way in which it is spent that counts."[130]

In these fictional portrayals of American life there was little place for class, race, or regional differences. Good nutrition was not recognized as requiring a redistribution of social or political resources; eating well and staying healthy, as the example of Jimmy made clear, was simply a matter of distributing one's money wisely. During Denver's Health Week, organizers prepared a list of "facts" to be used during Sunday sermons including: "That it is not poverty, inherited disease or vice, but ignorance which is responsible for most of the deaths among infants and children and that health education...is one of the most potent weapons in further lengthening the span of human life."[131] "Just square your shoulders to the world / You're not the sort to quit," concluded a children's "Ode to Posture," "It isn't the load that breaks us down, / It's the way we carry it."[132]

Most child health work was premised on the conservative notion that poor health was the result of individual choice rather than structural inequity, and the unequal distribution of wealth but not of knowledge. Indeed, ACHA leaders urged local organizers to work with as many politicians, chambers of commerce, service clubs, and religious leaders as possible. But it was difficult to strip this work of its broader implications or to avoid raising the public's awareness of other factors in American life that contributed to disease and disability: uncertain employment, low wages, poor food, inadequate housing and sanitation, costly and poorly distributed medical services, and racial segregation.[133] Nonetheless, most child health promoters resolutely avoided any radical political implications of their work.[134] In one health play, members of an imaginary children's Good Health Club of Wellville sing (to the tune of "Old Black Joe"), "Gone are the days when we were underweight / Gone are the days when our teeth did hurt and ache." Concerned about Paul Ailing, a widow's son who needs glasses and has toothache, the club members debate whether to give him some of the club money to pay for an eye examination. They decide against it for, as club president Jimmy Justice explains, "I wonder if he would accept our money as a gift and I doubt his mother would be willing for him to do so. Can we not think of some plan to help him which would not hurt his pride?" Instead the club members agree to lend Paul the money to get glasses through the State Association for the Blind—where, the audience is informed, anyone can get glasses for three dollars if they have a doctor's prescription and a certificate saying they are unable to pay—and to find Paul a job with the local dentist so he can earn the money to have his teeth fixed.[135]

Pragmatic and not naive about the ways race and religion did divide many communities, child health reformers practised a highly self-conscious politics of cautious pluralism. "Be sure to allay, if possible all [charge] of religious dissension. Court Jews, Catholics and Protestants assiduously," read one ACHA directive in 1924.[136] To avoid antagonizing Christian Scientists, organizers of a health program in San Francisco schools "stressed neither fear nor disease with the child."[137] Like the optimism of health reformers at the postwar meeting in Cannes, health was portrayed as a neutral good beyond partisanship. In the NTA's children's "Crusader's Creed," colourful patriotic images were linked to a healthy body and nation:

I love my country's Flag. To me its bright red stands for bright red blood, which means energy and power, cheerfulness and hope, human kindness and the joy of living. Its pure white stands for clean bodies which house clean minds. Its blue stands for the clear sky, the sunshine, fresh air, play and exercise. As an American I will be a faithful solder in the children's army of peace, the Modern Health Crusade.[138]

Oaths like these bore a strong resemblance to the rituals of the Junior Klan for boys and the Tri-K Klub for girls developed in the 1920s.[139] The shift from the healthy American body to the purified Aryan body was not a difficult one, and while eugenics, nativism, and racism were not promoted by most child health interwar groups, they were not challenged either.

Like many pre-war Progressive reformers, child health organizers accepted the racial segregation of the communities they sought to inspire. Always aware that child health agents could be seen as "those people from New York," the ACHA warned its organizers to "tactfully try to get the people of the South to extend the observance among the colored children. But let [white] Southerners handle the situation and don't intrude upon local problems."[140] The Children's Bureau encouraged health departments to hire African-American public health nurses, and included black communities in most of its studies of rural child health. But its agents continued to work with all-white women's groups like the General Federation of Women's Clubs, and did not object when Georgia's state board of health refused to hire a black nurse because the bureau's proposed salary was "too much for any negro."[141]

The fear that child health programs run by Northerners could disrupt the segregated system of race relations did disturb many white Southern officials. During the 1920s Samuel Wallace Welch, Alabama's state health officer, had successfully used the state's war record—from February to July 1918 Alabama had the highest percentage of draft rejections—to expand the state board of health with new bureaus of child health and venereal disease control, and more public health nurses.[142] In 1923, however, Welch refused to cooperate with the ACHA, whose members, he believed, were "thoroughly unacquainted with Southern customs and habits of thought." ACHA programs, Welch feared, would disturb the delicate balance between state public health officials and local communities, for the ACHA could simply ignore any directives made by state and county boards of health or education. "Our problems in Alabama are entirely different from the problems of New York and

Boston and other cities of the East," Welch explained to a local legislator; "people coming here from the East knowing exactly what ought to be done to reform Alabama succeed only in demoralizing things and making public health administration unpopular."[143] Unorthodox groups like Christian Scientists, similarly, were not convinced by the ACHA's tactful efforts to build consensus. Long suspicious of state-sponsored orthodox medicine, Christian Scientists had developed significant political influence in a number of Western states, as Children's Bureau director Grace Abbott discovered when her agents reported on the difficulties of getting state legislators to renew the Sheppard-Towner Act. As one Colorado activist explained, Christian Scientists "who are so well organized and who are so strong in the Legislature" had employed a full-time lawyer "of high standing" to "watch over legislation." The lawyer had passionately attacked funding nursing services, and was trying to turn legislators against funding existing health services.[144]

As historians have shown, many African Americans were willing to use elements of the gospel of germs to improve the health of their families and communities, efforts that were formalized into the Negro Health Movement of the 1920s. Public health nurses working in black schools and other African-American educators were "receptive to the promotion of child health," a white ACHA organizer reported happily in 1923.[145] During National Negro Health Week, officials in Tuskegee organized children's parades on Child Health Day, and in Virginia, according to the state's Child Health Bureau, Child Health Day was "used to especial advantage in our Negro schools."[146] Nancy Tomes has described the children who participated in National Negro Health Weeks in the early 1920s and coloured the faces of good health in child health posters to "look like their own."[147] But, as Tomes has also pointed out, national health campaigns frequently featured pictures of people of colour as "dangerous disease carriers" contrasted with "images of little blonde crusaders dressed in white" showing that "whiteness and cleanliness were one and the same."[148]

Their faith in the consensus appeal of the child health message led organizers to believe that the movement could rise above racial and cultural barriers. Organizers reported proudly on the ways that child health methods were integrated into other cultures. At the San Juan Pueblo in New Mexico, Indian schoolchildren performing a child health play in 1929 wore red bands and feathers in their hair, and sang to the accompaniment of a big drum brought from the pueblo.[149] A prizewinning health play written in 1926 by a Native-American high school girl, however, made the subtle child health message about non-white cultures more obvious. *Nelagony, or Good Water*, written by Anemone Pemberton, an Osage Indian from Pawhuska, Oklahoma, won one hundred dollars in the NTA's play competition for high school students. In Pemberton's play a white doctor discovers contaminated water that is causing a typhoid epidemic. With difficulty he overcomes the local Indian tribe's "super-stitions" and finally vaccinates them all. "The Indian beliefs regarding sickness are not wholly peculiar to that people," an NTA organizer assured other health workers, "so the health message is applicable to all towns and cities in which infected water is a danger to life and in which the citizens need to be convinced that vaccination is a protection against typhoid."[150] At the play's original performance, about twenty-five Native American men, women, and children took part. During the dance of the "medicine men," one boy, a "half-breed Indian," danced while his father beat a drum and sang.[151] Just what messages this performance conveyed to its participants or to the Native Americans in the audience is hard to assess, but certainly child health reformers' optimistic faith in the sim-plicity of health conversion seems naive and ill-founded.

Indeed, it was rare to find any explicit discussion of race, class, or region in child health stories and plays. Yet surely the dissonance between the ways most children lived and the health characters they performed was often striking. What, for example, did the school-age sons and daughters of South Carolina mill workers and tenant farmers think about the domestic relations reflected in their "Health Pageant" that featured Fly (in black suit with grey wings) and his maid Typhoid (dressed in black and red)?[152] The health games of the ACHA and the Junior Red Cross, historian Katherine McCuaig has argued, were "a very effec-tive means of inculcating middle class standards and values in all school children," who were "being trained to be healthy, responsible citizens and, possibly more importantly, future members of service clubs and volun-tary associations."[153] But how effective these methods were is hard to say. Parades, pageants, and plays that featured child health crusaders were fun to participate in and fun to watch. A number of schools, even in the rural South, began to build toilets, washbasins, and water fountains, and raise money to buy soap and tissue paper. But how much did the meth-ods of the child health movement change the habits of the child, other than in a classroom papered with ACHA posters? And did the child's new-found sanitary consciousness alter the behaviour of his or her family? Organizers could threaten children with disease and disability, with aca-demic failure and social ostracism. But adults were more likely to recog-nize the shared necessity of preventive health work during an epidemic when disability and death could result from the fact that "germs have no color line." Junior health crusaders, however colourful, were designed to reflect a community's status quo, not challenge it.

Ikey Ain't No Rose: A
Crusade Era Ends

By the early 1930s, CHO-style health propaganda had become an integral part of public health work. Private publishers found it profitable to produce standardized guides for the production of plays, pageants, and parades for child health days and weeks.[154] Some health work began to show a lighter and more satirical side, suggesting that certain child health styles were familiar enough to mock. *When Germs Get Together*, a play produced by West Virginia's state health department, is set during a meeting of a "disease" committee. The committee, chaired by Fly, is made up of various characters—Typhoid, Diphtheria, Whooping Cough, Measles, Smallpox, and Scarlet Fever—who complain about officials who have made the local health department too activist. Poking fun at personalities often found on civic boards, these characters are supposed to sound, according to stage directions, annoyed, cocky, smug, and petty. At the play's dramatic conclusion a doctor, two nurses, and a sanitarian (armed with, respectively, a smallpox needle, a typhoid vaccine tube and a hypodermic needle, and a handkerchief and fly swatter) appear and kill all committee members.[155]

Despite the wide distribution of scales and height–weight charts, child health promoters acknowledged privately that it was difficult, perhaps impossible, to measure the impact of the movement in any quantified way. In a letter "not for public statement," Clair Elsmere Turner, a prominent health educator at MIT's Department of Biology and Public Health, admitted to Thomas Wood that although there was "no yardstick to completely measure the results," he felt that "the contribution has been partly spiritual. (I think you will understand the term, although I doubt if it would be understood in a published statement going to the general public.)" Cities, Turner believed, were "full of happier teachers and happier children," the result of "this movement like a religious movement." "We must not forget," he told Wood, "that Child Health is in some respects a kind of gospel which changes habits, attitudes and human relationships. It would be [as] foolish to try to measure this completely as to ask the preacher to measure his work in the units of the metric system."[156]

The most difficult part of this story to ascertain is the response of both children and parents to the movement's simple, bright messages. Few parents could have missed the patronizing edge in textbooks that told children to "talk to your mother about mold. Find out what she does to keep her pantry free from it. Bring your information into class for discussion."[157] It was clear to many parents, if not also to their children, how few public clinics their community supported and how prohibitive the cost of private medical, dental, and nursing services. Child health stories and plays dealt with these issues by easy optimism; faced with the ill health of Paul Ailing, a fatherless child living in poverty, the fictional members of the Wellville Club, after all, blithely assume that a part-time job will enable Paul to fix his teeth and maintain his health.

Although child health activists presented themselves as safely neutral agents of the state-approved health work, some families were not convinced. In Rutherford County, Tennessee, organizers of the Commonwealth Fund's Health Demonstration Project noted the reluctance of poor white sharecroppers like the woman who asked anxiously, after hearing her husband agree to let their children attend a clinic, "Now, tell me the truth—will they take the children away from us, if we bring 'em?"[158] In 1924, similarly, sociologists Robert and Helen Lynd were unable to explain the responsive crowd gathered at Muncie's high school to hear a speaker from the State Society for Medical Freedom. Dramatically, the man presented child health work as part of a fearful entangling network of the medicalization of everyday life. Public money, he asserted, should not be used for vaccinating school children, school medical examinations, or public health nurses, for:

Preventive medicine is just another excuse of the doctors for getting work. It's ridiculous to frighten people by talking about millions of germs in our food, air, and water. I went to school in a small room with lots of other children, and we were all rosy-cheeked and healthy and didn't know a thing about germs. There wasn't any of this other foolishness of weighing children and frightening them to death because they may be underweight.[159]

Health organizers tended to see this resistance as mildly annoying or humorous. Josephine Baker used to entertain her public health audiences by repeating one response from an immigrant mother in New York whose son was sent home from school because he needed a bath. The mother replied in a note to the teacher, which read, "Dear Teacher, Ikey aint no rose. Don't smell him—learn him." Baker also liked the note from another parent to the school nurse: "Dear Nurse: As for his nose, it don't need it. As for his tonsils, he was born with them. As for his teeth, he'll get new ones. Please mind your own business."[160] Here, parents' clearly articulated expectations of the content of public education—and the extent to which teachers and other public officials had the right to intervene in family affairs—conflicted starkly with health reformers' efforts to remake children's bodies and minds into a hygienic whole.

When Herbert Hoover was elected in 1928 to the White House, he was hailed by health activists as the "children's president." But during the early years of the Depression, his political fortunes worsened as he refused to jettison his faith in voluntarism. In Hoover's view, improving health habits could solve the problem of hungry, sick children who appeared with greater frequency in Children's Bureau reports.[161] Hadn't that been the primary message of child health work throughout the 1920s? When officials at the Children's Bureau continued to argue that poverty, not ignorance, was the leading cause, Hoover threatened to transfer much of the bureau's work to the Public Health Service, and he spoke vaguely and unconvincingly about federal action to replace the dying Sheppard-Towner Act.[162] At a 1930 White House Conference on Child Health, Hoover proclaimed in his opening speech: "If we could have but one generation of properly born, trained, educated, and healthy children, a thousand other problems of government would vanish." Words like this, historian Kriste Lindenmeyer has concluded, were just "romantic cliches."[163]

The argument that improving child health did not require redistributed resources but simply a change of mind and behaviour became even less convincing as the Depression deepened. Hoover's defeat by Franklin Roosevelt led to a newly active federal government that began to set up a welfare system. Children were a central feature of the 1935 Social Security Act. Title V of the act provided federal funding for disabled and dependent children and for child welfare services, an achievement that historians have considered the culmination of child health activism of the prewar Progressive Era. Methods from the child health movement were immediately used to popularize these new government services. Health plays now tried to teach the public how to apply to government clinics and for welfare assistance, and spent less time teaching audiences health habits.[164] Both plays and posters were taken up by federal agencies, especially the Works Progress Administration, as ways of gaining community participation in public theatre, and in posters whimsy was replaced by bold realism. In 1935 the symbolic end of the child health movement occurred when, under financial pressure, the ACHA disbanded.[165] Yet the faith in children as the ideal health education recipients lingered. In 1939 a South Carolina doctor treating adults who were children during the hookworm campaign of 1910 was gratified to find his patients recalled his lectures and his old projection machine, and were putting his "pertinent points…to practical use in regards to health measures and sanitation." For him, this was evidence of the worth of child health education: "These young people would carry the message home to the older ones" for "any proved scientific fact that conflicts with local time-worn traditions must be 'put over' by intensive education of the children."[166]

From 1918 to 1935 the child health movement had fought its battle on two fronts: seeking the extension of government-funded protective services, and trying to change the public's behaviour and beliefs through voluntary propaganda work. Members of the ACHA saw themselves as social instructors, providing useful and new ways of thinking for the good of society. It was a pragmatic and optimistic program, far less naive and idealistic than the work of its Progressive predecessors, but it had, I think, a softer centre. The movement's consciously apolitical tone, while not allaying the fears of antagonistic physicians, did, however, appeal to many businessmen otherwise suspicious of do-gooders, and various proprietors found opportunities for commercial promotion by combining health messages with health products.

The work of child health activists in the 1920s and 1930s reflected profound changes in American society and in family life in particular. With the enforcement of school attendance and child labour laws, the public school was becoming more central in the lives of children and their families. Dealing with difference, especially over the so-called immigrant problem, had become a less intense public issue with federal restriction of Southern and Eastern European immigration in the early 1920s, and the propagation of a more homogenized American culture through radio and movies. The rising power of the commercial media, as well as the influence of the advertising industry, provided vocabulary and model for child health activists. Both reformers and retailers were intent on "selling" health and science. In their efforts to instruct and inspire, child health organizers turned to whatever contemporary popular appeals would grab the attention of their audience.

To explore the diverse constituencies that made up this movement, we need more studies of the men and women such as Sally Lucas Jean, Thomas Wood, Emmett Holt, Philip Van Ingen, and Josephine Baker, whose work bridged so many audiences. The movement they led was part of an ambitious effort to change the behaviour of children, families, and the whole nation.[167] But its narrow focus on individuals as a central motivating force was clearly part of the New Public Health movement, combining social reform, faith in reductionist science, and expansive regulatory powers of government officials. How reductionist this new ideology was remains a topic of debate among medical historians. Certainly child health work increasingly focused on smaller units: not the community and the workplace, but the classroom and the home, the bathroom and the kitchen, the parent and child. Still, as all schoolteachers recognize, children are at best incomplete messengers. It is a long journey from the classroom to the home. Nonetheless, as we try to assess the complex legacy of the interwar child health movement, we should acknowledge the significant role its proponents may have played in contributing to the American public's growing esteem for scientific medicine, especially its life-enhancing technologies. Perhaps one unexpected result of reiterated warnings against "defects" was the eager embrace by many families of government health services established during the New Deal, suggesting a belief that access to the products of medical science was a necessary requirement of modern life.

As some of the movement's populist critics warned, the interwar child health campaign reflected the growing medicalization of American life. Reformers hoped to inspire children with health ideals that would not only shape their own behaviour but also make them aware of the responsibility for fostering and monitoring a hygienic society. Parades, plays, contests, and other activities would help keep children healthy, counter improper habits learnt at home, change the behaviour of their parents, and knit together divided communities. As "vegetables on parade," children were to be a vehicle for the broader hygienic transformation of their community.

At the heart of these efforts, however, was a disturbing and unresolved conflict over the relations between health, the individual, and the state. Child health promoters did teach children the importance of *public* health work—sanitation, sewers, food and factory inspection, quarantine—but suggested that (apart from in some rural communities) this infrastructure was already largely established, and the place of health officials appropriately carved out. The responsibility of the state was to maintain these services and provide the basis for environmental sanitation and disease prevention; the rest was up to individuals. Nutrition, satisfying the programmatic and political goals of the child health movement, became its premier science, permeating every health text, play, and parade. This was a movement infused with the faith that transformation would occur through individual determination and group persuassion. But the Depression shook this complacency. The rise of fascism abroad and right-wing populism at home suggested that the idealism of the internationalist branch of the public health movement had not and could not achieve its postwar dream of stable health infrastructures as a vaccine against militarism and nationalism. No longer seen as simple, neutral reformist tools, parades and pageants now seemed closer to the hallmarks of state-sponsored fascism. With the end of the Sheppard-Towner Act, the defeat of Hoover's presidency, and the establishment of a Democratic administration and its new welfare system, CHO's techniques of inspiration, shame, competition, and consumerism became remnants of an earlier, foolish age.

Notes

1 Jesse Feiring Williams, *Personal Hygiene Applied* (Philadelphia: W. B. Saunders, 1922), 23; and Harry H. Moore, *Public Health in the United States: An Outline with Statistical Data* (New York: Harper and Brothers, 1923), 50.

2 Sally Lucas Jean, "Creating a Demand for Health," *Proceedings of the National Conference of Social Work at the Forty-Seventh Annual Session Held in New Orleans, Louisiana, April 14–21, 1920* (Chicago: University of Chicago Press, 1920), 13.

3 For England, see Deborah Dwork, *War Is Good for Babies and Other Young Children: A History of the Infant and Child Welfare Movement in England 1898–1918* (London: Tavistock, 1987); and on the rejection rate among New Zealand army recruits and its political consequences, see Margaret Tennant, "Complicating Childhood: Gender, Ethnicity, and 'Disadvantage' within the New Zealand Children's Health Camps Movement," in this volume.

4 For the national picture, see Martin V. Melosi, *The Sanitary City: Urban Infrastructure in America from Colonial Times to the Present* (Baltimore: Johns Hopkins University Press, 2000); and for an important case study, see Barbara Gutmann Rosenkrantz, *Public Health and the State: Changing Views in Massachusetts, 1842–1936* (Cambridge: Harvard University Press, 1972).

5 James A. Hayne, quoted in Edward H. Beardsley, *A History of Neglect: Health Care for Blacks and Mill Workers in the Twentieth-Century South* (Knoxville: University of Tennessee Press, 1987), 136–37. On the history of venereal disease, Progressive reform, and the First World War, see Allan M. Brandt, *No Magic Bullet: A Social History of Venereal Disease in the United States Science 1880* (New York: Oxford University Press, 1987), 52–121.

6 S. Josephine Baker, *Child Hygiene* (New York: Harper and Brothers, 1925), 58, 38. On children and the need for "a sanitary conscience," see Charles-Edward Amory Winslow and Pauline Brooks Williamson, *The Laws of Health and How To Teach Them* (New York: Charles E. Merrill, 1925), 169.

7 C. J. Fagan quoted in Katherine McCuaig, *The Weariness, the Fever, and the Fret: The Campaign against Tuberculosis in Canada, 1900–1950* (Montreal: McGill-Queen's University Press, 1999), 165. On the creation of the newly "priceless" child of the twentieth century, see Viviana Zelizer, *Pricing the Priceless Child: The Changing Social Value of Children* (New York: Basic Books, 1985).

8 For important studies of maternal and child health reform in this period, see Kriste Lindenmeyer, *"A Right to Childhood": The U.S. Children's Bureau and Child Welfare, 1912–1946* (Urbana: University of Illinois Press, 1997); Molly Ladd-Taylor, *Mother-Work: Women, Child Welfare, and the State, 1890–1930* (Urbana: University of Illinois Press, 1994); and Robyn Muncy, *Creating a Female Dominion in American Reform 1890–1935* (New York: Oxford University Press, 1991; Alisa Klaus, *Every Child a Lion: The Origins of Maternal and Infant Health Policy in the United States and France* (Ithaca: Cornell University Press, 1993); Richard A. Meckel, *Save the Babies: American Public Health Reform and the Prevention of Infant Mortality, 1850–1929* (Baltimore: Johns Hopkins University Press, 1990); and Susan Tiffin, *In Whose Best Interest: Child Welfare Reform in the Progressive Era* (Westport, CT: Greenwood Press, 1982). For insightful studies of health education, see Nancy Tomes, *The Gospel of Germs: Men, Women, and the Microbe in American Life* (Cambridge: Harvard University Press, 1998); and Elizabeth Toon, "Managing the Conduct of the Individual Life: Public Health Education and American Public Health, 1910–1940" (PhD dissertation, University of Pennsylvania, 1998).

9 For exceptions to this, see Margaret Tennant, "'Missionaries of Health': The School Medical Service during the Inter-War Period," in *A Healthy Country: Essays*

on the Social History of Medicine in New Zealand, ed. Linda Bryder (Wellington: Bridget Williams Books, 1991), 128–37; and Linda Bryder, "'Wonderlands of Buttercup, Clover and Daisies': Tuberculosis and the Open-Air School Movement in Britain, 1907–39," in *In the Name of the Child: Health and Welfare, 1880–1940*, ed. Roger Cooter, 72–95 (London: Routledge, 1992).

10 For a very critical view of the "health habits" approach in popularizing science and health, see John C. Burnham, *How Superstition Won and Science Lost: Popularizing Science and Health in the United States* (New Brunswick: Rutgers University Press, 1987), 56–62.

11 The focus of this paper is on the perspectives of the organizers, not their subjects. For recent calls that urge historians to seek out the perspectives of children, see Russell Viner and Janet Golden, "Children's Experiences of Illness," in *Medicine in the Twentieth Century*, ed. Roger Cooter and John Pickstone (London: Harwood Academic, 2000), 575–78; and this volume's introduction.

12 On the development of a distinctive aesthetic based on the gospel of germs that shaped domestic design, see Tomes, *Gospel of Germs*, 159–71; see also Nancy Tomes, "Merchants of Health: Medicine and Consumer Culture in the United States, 1900–1940," *Journal of American History* 88 (2001): 519–47.

13 Louise Franklin Bache, *Health Education in an American City: An Account of a Five-Year Program in Syracuse, New York* (Garden City: Doubleday, Doran, 1934), opposite 62.

14 Anonymous, "Thanksgiving à la Hoover (as Recorded the Day After)," *St. Nicholas* 45 (November 1917): 26. On the sensationalism used by the Red Cross during and after the war, including "heart rending scenes of dying infants," see Patricia T. Rooke and Rudy L. Schnell, "'Uncramping Child Life': International Children's Organizations, 1914–1939," in *International Health Organisations and Movements, 1918–1939*, ed. Paul Weindling (Cambridge: Cambridge University Press, 1995), 180.

15 See James N. Giglio, "Voluntarism and Public Policy between World War I and the New Deal: Herbert Hoover and the American Child Health Association," *Presidential Studies Quarterly* 13 (1983): 431.

16 Henry Noble MacCracken, "The Junior Red Cross," *Delineator* 91 (December 1917), 1; Anonymous, "The Junior Red Cross," *St. Nicholas* 45 (November 1917): 26.

17 Junior Red Cross, *Common Sense in Health* (1919), quoted in John F. Hutchinson, "The Junior Red Cross Goes to Healthland" (unpublished paper in author's possession), 11; see also Hutchinson, "The Junior Red Cross Goes to Healthland," *American Journal of Public Health* 87 (1997): 1816–23. By 1920, some twelve million American school children in 83,000 schools were members of the Junior Red Cross; Anonymous, "The Work of the Junior Red Cross," *Literary Digest* 66 (August 28, 1920): 35.

18 Rheeta Childe Dorr, "The Children's Crusade for Peace," *Ladies Home Journal* 41 (March 1924): 168. On the parallel movement to teach children "peace habits," see Imogene M. McPherson, *Educating Children for Peace* (New York: Abingdon Press, 1936).

19 This description is based on the analysis by Lindenmeyer, *"A Right to Childhood,"* 71–75; quote 71. See also Klaus, *Every Child a Lion*, 162–71, 258–59; and Meckel, *Save the Babies*, 147–48, 200–201.

20 Sheila Rothman, *Woman's Proper Place: A History of Changing Ideas, 1870 to the Present* (New York: Basic Books, 1978), 136–53; quote Lindenmeyer *"A Right to Childhood,"* 74.

21 See also Lela B. Costin, *Two Sisters of Social Justice: A Biography of Grace and Edith Abbott* (Urbana: University of Illinois Press, 1983); Nancy Pottisham Weiss, "Save the Children: A History of the Children's Bureau, 1903–1918" (PhD dissertation, University of California at Los Angeles, 1974); Ladd-Taylor, *Mother-Work*; and Muncy, *Creating a Female Dominion*.

22 Philip Van Ingen, "The History of Child Welfare Work in the United States," in *A Half Century of Public Health: Jubilee Historical Volume of the American Public Health Association*, ed. Mazyck P. Ravenel (New York: American Public Health Association, 1921), 301; R. L. Duffus and L. Emmett Holt, Jr., *L. Emmett Holt: Pioneer of a Children's Century* (New York: D. Appleton-Century, 1940), 214–16, 225. Luther Emmett Holt (1855–1924) received his MD in 1880 from New York's College of Physicians and Surgeons, and published *The Care and Feeding of Children: A Catechism for the Use of Mothers and Children's Nurses* (1894) and *Diseases of Infancy and Childhood* (1897). He was a member of the Rockefeller Institute's Board of Directors, president of the American Pediatrics Society in 1897, professor of pediatrics at the College of Physicians and Surgeons 1901–21, on the board of directors of the Henry Street Settlement, and founding editor of *Archives of Pediatrics* (f. 1884) and *American Journal of Diseases of Children* (f. 1911); see Edwards A. Park and Howard H. Mason, "Luther Emmett Holt (1855–1924)," in *Pediatric Profiles*, ed. Borden S. Veeder (St. Louis: C. V. Mosby, 1957), 33–60; and see Rima D. Apple, *Mothers and Medicine: A Social History of Infant Feeding, 1890–1950* (Madison: University of Wisconsin Press, 1987).

23 On Jean, see Toon, "Managing the Conduct," 133–35; and Richard K. Means, *A History of Health Education in the United States* (Philadelphia: Lea and Febiger, 1962), 183–84, 216–17.

24 For important studies on public health, the Red Cross, and the League of Nations, see John F. Hutchinson, *Champions of Charity: War and the Rise of the Red Cross* (Boulder: Westview Press, 1996); Norman Howard-Jones, *International Public Health between the Two World Wars: The Organization Problems* (Geneva: World Health Organization, 1978); and Paul Weindling, ed., *International Organizations and Movements 1918–1939* (Cambridge: Cambridge University Press, 1995), especially John F. Hutchinson, "'Custodians of the Sacred Fire': The ICRC and the Postwar Reorganization of the International Red Cross," 17–35, quote 24. See also Bridget Towers, "Red Cross Organizational Politics, 1918–1922: Relations of Dominance and the Influence of the United States," in *International Organizations*, ed. Weindling, 43,.

25 Holt on the *S.S. Leviathan*, March 21, 1919, quoted in Duffus and Holt, *L. Emmett Holt*, 237; Holt in Cannes, April 8, 1919, quoted in Duffus and Holt, *L. Emmett Holt*, 251–52.

26 Hutchinson, "'Custodians of the Sacred Fire,'" 25.

27 Paul Weindling, "Social Medicine at the League of Nations Health Organisation and the International Labor Office Compared," in *International Organizations*, ed. Weindling, 134; and on child health on the international scale, see Rooke and Schnell, "Uncramping Child Life," 176–202.

28 Hutchinson, "Junior Red Cross," 1817. Winslow was also president of the American Public Health Association in 1925, a member of the League of Nations' National Health Care Committee 1927–30, and chair of the executive committee of the Committee on Costs of Medical Care; see Arthur Viseltear, "C-E. A. Winslow and the Early Years of Public Health at Yale, 1915–1925," *Yale Journal of Biology and Medicine* 55 (1982): 137–151. Before joining the public health department at Yale's medical school, Winslow had organized several public

health exhibits at the American Museum of Natural History, and edited the New York City public health department's "Health Hints," published in daily newspapers.

29 Martin David Dubin, "The League of Nations Health Organization," in *International Organizations*, ed. Weindling, 58.

30 Grace T. Hallock and C.-E. A. Winslow, *The Land of Health: Children May Become Citizens of the Land of Health by Learning and Obeying Its Laws* (New York: Charles E. Merrill, 1922); and Hutchinson, "The Junior Red Cross Goes to Healthland."

31 See Richard Wightman Fox and T. J. Jackson Lears, eds., *The Culture of Consumption: Critical Essays in American History 1880–1980* (New York: Pantheon, 1983); and Roland Marchand, *Advertising the American Dream: Making Way for Modernity, 1920–1940* (Berkeley: University of California Press, 1985).

32 "Health Songs," [enclosed in] B. B. Bagby [director, Bureau of Child Health, Virginia State Department of Health] to Martha E. Eliot [acting chief, Children's Bureau], June 18, 1936, folder 4-9-0-5 "Baby Campaigns (Saving)," box 511, Children's Bureau central file 1933–1936, Record Group 102, United States National Archives and Records Administration, College Park, MD.

33 Elizabeth Cole, "Playing for Health: By Means of a Health Play Contest," *Hygeia* 4 (1926): 649.

34 Nathalie Forbes Moulton, *The Brownies' Health Book: A Supplementary Reader for the Second School Year* (Boston: Little, Brown and Company, 1925), 67. On the songs, rituals, and creeds used in hookworm and midwifery programs, see John Ettling, *The Germ of Laziness: Rockefeller Philanthropy and Public Health in the New South* (Cambridge: Harvard University Press, 1981); and Susan L. Smith, *Sick and Tired of Being Sick and Tired: Black Women's Health Activism in America, 1890–1950* (Philadelphia: University of Pennsylvania Press, 1995), 129. Perhaps the focus by Northern middle-class white reformers on poor rural white Southerners and on African-American midwives made infantilizing education methods seems more appropriate.

35 On child health education and the NTA, see Cynthia A. Connolly, "Prevention through Detention: The Pediatric Tuberculosis Preventorium Movement in the United States, 1909–1951" (PhD dissertation, University of Pennsylvania, 1999). For an important analysis of tuberculosis in relation to public health policy, see Georgina D. Feldberg, *Disease and Class: Tuberculosis and the Shaping of Modern American Society* (New Brunswick: Rutgers University Press, 1995).

36 Tomes, *Gospel of Germs*, 122–23; see also Barbara Bates, *Bargaining for Life: A Social History of Tuberculosis, 1876–1938* (Philadelphia: University of Pennsylvania Press, 1992), 254–57, 274–78; Michael E. Teller, *The Tuberculosis Movement: A Public Health Campaign in the Progressive Era* (Westport: Greenwood Press, 1988), 112–17; and Toon, "Managing the Conduct," 71–74. In 1919, three million American school children qualified as Modern Health Crusaders; Anonymous, "Modern Health Crusaders," *Outlook* 122 (June 18, 1919), 276.

37 Feldberg, *Disease and Class*, 111–14; see also Van Ingen, "History of Child Welfare," 304; and Means, *Health Education*, 115–25.

38 Sally Lucas Jean, "Instruction of School Children in Health Habits and Ideals," *Proceedings of the National Conference of Social Work at the Fiftieth Anniversary Session Held in Washington, D.C., May 16–23, 1923* (Chicago: University of Chicago Press, 1923), 379.

39 Jean, "Creating a Demand for Health," 13. On a health cartoon series used by Rockefeller Foundation health officials in France after the war for anti-tubercu-

losis work and then reprinted in the United States, see Tomes, *Gospel of Germs*, 120, 302n21.

40 Duffus and Holt, Jr., *L. Emmett Holt*, 225.

41 The best history of this organization is Meckel, *Save the Babies*; for this statistic, see Meckel, *Save the Babies*, 113.

42 S. Josephine Baker, *Fighting for Life* (New York: Macmillan, 1939), 170; Meckel, *Save the Babies*, 134–46. During the war, the Public Health Service had refused to allow Baker to go to France to direct "a large international organization" to help refugee and homeless children, explaining that she was "needed at home more"; Baker had so yearned to take on this "huge and important and intoxicatingly useful job" that she had travelled to Washington to protest that she would look "both impolite and yellow" if she turned the position down; Baker, *Fighting for Life*, 168–70.

43 According to Baker, Boston's mayor told her "the name of your society" was the reason she found it hard to raise money, for "nobody is going to write anything as long as that on a check. By the time they get halfway through, they will change their minds"; *Fighting for Life*, 143. See also Duffus and Holt, Jr., *L. Emmett Holt*, 229; and Meckel, *Save the Babies*, 200–202.

44 Holt, now sixty-eight, had sought in vain for a "younger man" to replace him as head of CHO and become frustrated as the CHO presidency became primarily a fund-raising job; Duffus and Holt, Jr., *L. Emmett Holt*, 228–29, 259.

45 American Child Health Association, "To Learn To Live Together" [1923], folder 23, box 38, series III, Charles-Edward Amory Winslow papers #749, Manuscripts and Archives, Yale University Library, New Haven, CT.

46 Charles H. Keene [director, Department of Public Instruction, Commonwealth of Pennsylvania, Harrisburg] to C. E. A. Winslow, September 20, 1922, folder 28, box 39, series III, Winslow #749, Yale University Archives. On the continuing debate among health organizers over the value of health habits and the danger of their separation from scientific understanding, see Burnham, *Superstition Won*, chapter 2.

47 See letterhead on reverse of letter, Emma Dolfinger [director, Health Education Division, ACHA] to Grace Abbott [Children's Bureau], November 1, 1924, folder 4-12-1-2, box 198, Children's Bureau central file 1921–24, Record Group 102, National Archives.

48 Quoted in Duffus and Holt, Jr., *L. Emmett Holt*, 227; see also Park and Mason, "Luther Emmett Holt," 40–41. Park and Mason noted that Holt had always liked parlour games.

49 On the "various squabbles" within ACHA and between the ACHA and other agencies that later led the Commonwealth Fund to retreat from joint cooperation of child health demonstrations, see Peter Buck, "Why Not the Best? Some Reasons and Examples from Child Health and Rural Hospitals," *Journal of Social History* 18 (1985): 413–31. For examples of health demonstrations, see also Bache, *Health Education in Syracuse*; Maud A. Brown, *Teaching Health in Fargo* (New York: Commonwealth Fund, 1929) and *A Chapter of Child Health: Report of the Commonwealth Fund Child Health Demonstration in Clarke County and Athens, Georgia 1924–1928* (New York: Commonwealth Fund, 1930).

50 Means, *History of Health Education*, 140–47, 218–25.

51 The WCTU also organized "bands of mercy" where children pledged to be kind to animals, which inspired the Boy Scouts merit badge for first aid to animals; see Means, *History of Health Education*, 50–56; Susan E. Lederer, *Subjected to Science: Human Experimentation in America before the Second World War* (Baltimore:

Johns Hopkins University Press, 1995), 39–40; Philip J. Pauly, "The Struggle for Ignorance over Alcohol: American Physiologists, Wilbur Olin Atwater, and the Woman's Christian Temperance Union," *Bulletin of the History of Medicine* 64 (Winter 1990): 366–92; and Jonathan Zimmerman, "'The Queen of Lobby': Mary Hunt, Scientific Temperance, and the Dilemma of Democratic Education in America, 1879–1906," *History of Education Quarterly* 32 (Spring 1992): 1–30.

52 For an argument that these earlier texts provided children with greater knowledge of physiology and anatomy and the workings of the body than later "health habits" books, see Burnham, *Superstition Won*, 55.

53 Eleanor Glendower Griffith, "The House the Children Built," in *Dramatizing Child Health: A New Book of Health Plays*, ed. Grace T. Hallock (New York: American Child Health Association, 1925), 206.

54 Research Division of the American Child Health Association, *A Health Survey of 86 Cities* (New York: American Child Health Association, 1925), 146.

55 American Child Health Association, "Scholarships and Fellowships Offered by American Child Health Association Health Education Division" (New York: American Child Health Association, 1923).

56 "Report by Lucy Wood Collier, Committee on Health Education of the American Child Health Association held at 163 East 78th Street, New York, 22 October 1923, 7.30 P.M.," folder 19, box 38, series III, Winslow #749, Yale University Archives.

57 Ernest Bryant Hoag and Lewis M. Terman, *Health Work in Schools* (Boston: Houghton Mifflin, 1914), cited in Means, *History of Health Education*, 82.

58 Cited in Kathleen W. Jones, *Taming the Troublesome Child: American Families, Child Guidance, and the Limits of Psychiatric Authority* (Cambridge: Harvard University Press, 1999), 94. See also Jones, *Taming the Troublesome Child*, chapter 4, "Popularizing Child Guidance," 91–119.

59 Jean Broadhurst, *Home and Community Hygiene: A Textbook of Personal and Public Health* (Philadelphia: J. B. Lippincott, 1918), 265. On schools and the mental hygiene movement, see Margo Horn, *Before It's Too Late: The Child Guidance Movement in the United States, 1922–1945* (Philadelphia: Temple University Press, 1989); and Sol Cohen, "The Mental Hygiene Movement, the Development of Personality and the School: The Medicalization of American Education," *History of Education Quarterly* 23 (Summer 1983): 123–49.

60 Jessie I. Lummis [secretary, Denver Public Health Council], "Report of Health Week in Denver, Colorado 24 April–1 May 1927," folder 4-12-0-5, box 279, Children's Bureau central file 1925–1928, Record Group 102, National Archives, 4–5.

61 See Martin S. Pernick, *The Black Stork: Eugenics and the Death of "Defective" Babies in American Medicine and Motion Pictures since 1915* (New York: Oxford University Press, 1996); Pernick, "The Ethics of Preventive Medicine: Thomas Edison's Tuberculosis Films: Mass Media and Health Propaganda," *Hastings Center Report* 8 (1978), 21–27; and Susan Lederer and Naomi Rogers, "Media," in *Medicine in the Twentieth Century*, ed. Roger Cooter and John Pickstone (London: Harwood Academic, 2000), 487–502. The ACHA urged local organizers of Child Health Days and May Days to get camera-men to cover larger May Day celebrations, as well as to seek the endorsement of Will Hays, postmaster-general and film censor. Its national directors also contacted five motion picture news weeklies to interest them in child health activities; "Minutes of a Regular Meeting of the Executive Committee of the American Child Health Association, held at 10 A.M. Saturday, 16 February 1924, in Room 1722 Penn Terminal Building, New York N.Y.," folder 17, box 38, series III, Winslow #749, Yale University Archives.

62　Lummis, "Health Week in Denver, 1927," 6–7; "List of Material Available from: American Dental Association, Bureau of Dental Health Education, 58 E. Washington St., Chicago, Illinois" [1929], folder 4-8-6-2, box 383, Children's Bureau central file 1929–32, Record Group 102, National Archives. For a list of AMA child health plays, including *The Magic Fluid* [diphtheria antitoxin], *The School Luncheon, The Medicine Man*, and *The Trial of Jimmy the Germ*, see J. W. Studebaker [Commissioner of Education, U.S. Department of Interior, Office of Education], "Inventory of School Conditions and Activities Affecting Health and Safety," in "May Day—Child Health Day, May First, 1938," "Bulletins," folder 4, box 1, Record Group 894, series 258 [State Board of Health], State Library and Archives of Florida, Tallahassee, FL.

63　American Child Health Association, "Suggestions for Celebrating May Day" [1930], folder 27, box 39, series III, Winslow #749, Yale University Archives. Happy was also asked to redesign it as a permanent exhibit for the Smithsonian Museum; Committee on Health Education of ACHA, February 1, 1923, New York City, folder 19, box 38, series III, Winslow #749, Yale University Archives.

64　See Lummis, "Health Week in Denver, 1927," 6–7; and Suellen Hoy, *Chasing Dirt: The American Pursuit of Cleanliness* (New York: Oxford University Press, 1995), 134, 228n37. On *Working for Dear Life* and *Our Children*, Children's Bureau movies in the 1920s, see Lindenmeyer, *"A Right to Childhood,"* 97–98.

65　Brown, *Teaching Health in Fargo*, 79.

66　Jean, "Instruction of School Children," 381.

67　Holt, undated letter, quoted in Duffus and Holt, Jr., *L. Emmett Holt*, 227.

68　American Child Health Association, "To Learn To Live Together."

69　American Child Health Association, *Celebrating May Day in 1929* (New York: American Child Health Association, 1929), 37.

70　American Child Health Association, "Suggestions for Celebrating May Day."

71　Jean, "Instruction of School Children," 380.

72　Ethel M. Watters [Hutchinson, KS] to Doctor [Anna E.] Rude [chief, Division of Maternity and Infant Hygiene, Children's Bureau], 12 November 1922, folder 11-18-1, box 247, Children's Bureau central file 1921–24, Record Group 102, National Archives.

73　Annette K. Vance Dorey, *Better Baby Contests: The Scientific Quest for Perfect Childhood Health in the Early Twentieth Century* (Jefferson, NC: McFarland, 1999), 186–88; and see Anna T. McNulty [correspondence clerk, Children's Bureau] to William Wiseman [secretary, Toe River Fair, NC] 13 September 1927, folder 4-11-0-5-1, box 275, Children's Bureau central file 1925–1928, Record Group 102, National Archives.

74　Wendy Kline, *Building a Better Race: Gender, Sexuality, and Eugenics from the Turn of the Century to the Baby Boom* (Berkeley: University of California Press, 2001). I have seen few explicit attacks by child health organizers on Fitter Family contests, but, unlike the intensifying eugenic messages in maternal health education, the "eugenic" sections of child health texts are surprisingly muted. On Emmett Holt's explicit rejection of eugenics during his presidency of AASPIM in 1913, see Meckel, *Save the Babies*, 117–18.

75　Alma Overholt, "Summer Healthy Schools: As Inaugurated in Los Angeles County," *Hygeia* 9 (1931): 547–50, quote 550.

76　Woods Hutchinson, *The Child's Day* (Boston: Houghton Mifflin, 1912), 86–87. On the connection between ill-health and social ostracism made by many advertising campaigns in the 1920s, see T. J. Jackson Lears, "From Salvation to Self-

Realization: Advertising and the Therapeutic Roots of the Consumer Culture, 1880–1930," in *The Culture of Consumption*, ed. Fox and Lears, 24–27.

77 Duffus and Holt, Jr., *L. Emmett Holt*, 223–24.

78 Giglio, "Voluntarism and Public Policy," 435.

79 Sinclair Lewis, *Arrowsmith* (New York: New American Library, 1961), 189, 215–16. See Thomas Neville Bonner, *The Kansas Doctor: A Century of Pioneering* (Lawrence: University of Kansas Press, 1959), 120–71; Samuel J. Crumbine, *Frontier Doctor: The Autobiography of a Pioneer on the Frontier of Public Health* (Philadelphia: Dorrance, 1948), 260–61; Naomi Rogers, "Germs with Legs: Flies, Disease and the New Public Health," *Bulletin of the History of Medicine* 63 (1989): 599–617; William C. Summers, "Microbe Hunters Revisited," *International Microbiology* 1 (1998): 65–68; and Tomes, *Gospel of Germs*, 240–41.

80 Giglio, "Voluntarism and Public Policy," 430–52.

81 Vincent Vinikas, *Soft Soap, Hard Sell: American Hygiene in an Age of Advertisement* (Ames: Iowa State University Press, 1992), 140n15, 86–89, quote 86–87. The association represented manufacturers such as Colgate, Lever Brothers, and Palmolive who produced approximately 80 per cent of the nation's soap.

82 See Vinikas, *Soft Soap, Hard Sell*, 141n20; and Vinikas, "Lustrum of the Cleanliness Institute, 1927–1932," *Journal of Social History* 22 (1989): 618–20, and 627–28n20, 21.

83 Alice Mary Kimball and Mary Alden Hopkins, *The Judd Family: A Story of Cleanliness in Three Centuries* (New York: Cleanliness Institute School Service, 1931), 92.

84 Robert S. Lynd and Helen Merrell Lynd, *Middletown: A Study in American Culture* (1929: reprinted San Diego: Harvest/HBJ Books, 1986), 443, 451. For a 1921 survey that found tuberculosis clinics in seventy-six cities (thirty-eight government funded) and venereal disease clinics in eighty-two cities (forty-two government funded), see Moore, *Public Health in the United States*, 223, 230. On the need to prepare literature to encourage medical men to develop "sympathy with child health work in relation to their practice," see "Abstraction from Minutes of Meeting of Medical Committee [of ACHA] held at Detroit, Michigan, 15 October 1923," folder 13, box 38, series III, Winslow #749, Yale University Archives.

85 Mrs. Douglas, "our supervisor of nurses," quoted in Estelle N. Mathews [special agent, U.S. Children's Bureau, Colorado Child Welfare Bureau, Denver] to Grace Abbott, 8 May 1929, folder 4-9-0-7-4 (7), "Colorado," box 384, Children's Bureau central file 1929–1932, Record Group 102, National Archives. For an example of antagonism by Massachusetts physicians, see Rosenkrantz, *Public Health and the State*, 154–59.

86 S. J. Crumbine [executive secretary, ACHA] to Grace Abbott, 22 December 1926, folder 4-11-0-4, box 275, Children's Bureau central file 1925–1928, Record Group 102, National Archives. See also Frances Fitzgerald, *America Revised: History Schoolbooks in the Twentieth Century* (Boston: Little, Brown, 1979).

87 Louise Franklin Bache, "Health with the Aid of the Footlights," *Hygeia* 6 (1928): 40.

88 Ettling, *A Chapter of Child Health*, 11, 10. On the "gratifying increase" in one physician's general pediatric practice in Marion County, OR, see Courtenay Dinwiddie, *Child Health and the Community: An Interpretation of Cooperative Effort in Public Health* (New York: Commonwealth Fund, 1931), 39. In Muncie, ID, children were inspected at school, and then their parents were sent a card identifying the child's defects, urging them to consult a private practitioner; Lynd and Lynd, *Middletown*, 449.

89 See, for example, *A Chapter of Child Health*, 65–66; *Virginia Health Bulletin* 20 (April 1928): 4–5; and American Child Health Association, *Celebrating May Day in 1929*, (Indiana) 42, (Missouri) 63, (Ohio) 73, and (Kentucky) 80; Mary S. Hoff-schwelle, "Organizing Rural Communities for Change: Commonwealth Fund Child Health Demonstration in Rutherford County, 1923–1927," *Tennessee Historical Quarterly* 53 (Fall 1994): 157; and see organizers' delight when Mansfield, Ohio, decided its town slogan would be "Mansfield: The Home of Blue Ribbon Children," in American Child Health Association, *Child Health Demonstration: Mansfield and Richland County, Ohio, 1922–1925* (New York: American Child Health Association, [1926]), 28. Inspections of schoolchildren by a doctor or nurse initially sought to identify and exclude children with contagious diseases but gradually expanded in scope to include the detection of physical defects; see Van Ingen, "History of Child Welfare," 296–99; and S. Josephine Baker, "Child Hygiene," in *Public Health and Hygiene*, ed. William Hallock Park, 685–89, 2nd ed. (Philadelphia: Lea and Febiger, 1928).

90 The ADA distributed plays such as *The Bad Baby Molar* (1924) and *Stepping Stones to Health* (1925), both written by dentist Lon W. Morrey, as well as *Toothsome Stories*, and guides such as "Mouth Health Week in Mississippi" (1926) by Gladys Eyrich; see "List of Material Available." For a two-page list of child health songs, plays, poems, and games distributed by professional groups, see Charles-Edward Amory Winslow and Pauline Brooks Williamson, *The Laws of Health and How To Teach Them* (New York: Charles E. Merrill, 1925), 375–76.

91 Means, *History of Health Education*, 91–96, 178.

92 See, for example, Ethel M. Dox, "Playing the Game of Health," *Hygeia* 8 (1930): 663–65; Anonymous, "The Vegetable Parade in Healthville," *Hygeia* 9 (1931): 152–54; and Katherine L. Carber, "A Parade of Clean Children," *Hygeia* 4 (1926): 149.

93 Jean Broadhurst, *All through the Day the Mother Goose Way: Mother Goose's Children of Long Ago; What Gave Them Pains and Aches and What Made Them Grow* (Philadelphia: J. B. Lippincott, 1921).

94 Jean, "Instruction of School Children," 379.

95 Moulton, *Brownies' Health Book*, 154.

96 Lucille Sissman, "On Board the S.S. *Health*: A Short Play for Children," *Hygeia* 5 (1927): 154.

97 Klaus, *Every Child a Lion*, 274–76; and Jeffrey P. Brosco, "Weight Charts and Well Child Care: When the Pediatrician Became the Expert in Child Health," in *Formative Years: Children's Health in the United States, 1880–2000*, ed. Alexandra Minna Stern and Howard Markel (Ann Arbor: University of Michigan Press, 2002), 91–120.

98 Baker, *Child Hygiene*, 52. On the "weighing and measuring ritual," see Viner and Golden, "Children's Experiences of Illness," 582–83.

99 C. E. Turner and George B. Collins, *Health* (New York: D.C. Heath, 1924), 14–15.

100 Edith Wilhelmina Lawson, *Better Health for Little Americans* (Chicago: Beckley-Cardy Company, 1926), 19.

101 See Muncy, *Creating a Female Dominion*, 38–65; Borden S. Veeder, "Philip Van Ingen (1875–1952)," in *Pediatric Profiles*, ed. Borden S. Veeder (St. Louis: C. V. Mosby, 1957), 182–88. On the primary position of female nurses and health teachers in public health photography, see Janet Golden, "The Iconography of Child Public Health: Between Medicine and Reform," *Caduceus* 12 (Winter 1996): 67–68 and in this volume. On the prominence of women in civic and sanitary reform movements in the Progressive Era, see Suellen Hoy, "Municipal

Housekeepers: The Role of Women in Improving Urban Sanitation Practices, 1880–1917," in *Pollution and Reform in American Cities*, ed. Martin Melosi (Austin: University of Texas Press, 1980), 173–98.

102 Louise F. Brand, "Ef You Don't Watch Out," [enclosed in] West Virginia State Department of Health, Bureau of Public Health Education [Child Health Day 1936], folder 4-9-0-5-3, box 511, Children's Bureau central file 1933–1936, Record Group 102, National Archives.

103 J. H. Mason Knox, Jr. [chief, Bureau of Child Hygiene, Maryland State Department of Health] to Grace Abbott, 15 April 1925, folder 4-11-0-2, box 275, Children's Bureau central file 1925–1928, Record Group 102, National Archives.

104 Emma Serl, *Everyday Doings in Healthville: A Health Reader* (New York: Silver, Burdett and Co., 1929), 29–30. On the broader cultural interest in body image and the dangers of an underweight child, see Joan Jacobs Brumberg, *The Body Project: An Intimate History of American Girls* (New York: Random House, 1997).

105 Ada E. Schweitzer [Child Health Division, Indiana State Board of Health], "Indiana Child Health Day Plans—1929," folder 4-9-0-5-3 "Baby Saving Campaigns (1929)," box 383, Children's Bureau central file 1929–1932, Record Group 102, National Archives.

106 *Virginia Health Bulletin* 20 (April 1928), 9; Indiana State Board of Health, Division of Infant and Child Hygiene, "Indiana White House Conference Anniversary. Children's Charter Day—15 January 1932," folder 4-8-6-2, box 383, Children's Bureau central file 1929–1932, Record Group 102, National Archives.

107 Sally Lucas Jean, "Health Education Source Material and Criterion by Which It Can Be Judged," *American Journal of Public Health* 16 (1926): 1096.

108 Unlike the games of CHO, NTA, or ACHA, the set of child health rules developed by the Joint Committee listed diphtheria protection and a regular examination by doctor and dentist; see Joint Committee on Health Problems in Education, "A Child's Rules of Health," in Thomas D. Wood and Anette M. Phelan, *Growing Up* (New York: Teacher's College, Bureau of Publications, n.d.) [enclosed in] Ella Oppenheimer [Children's Bureau] to Thomas D. Wood [chairman, Joint Committee] November 22 1933, folder 4-9-0-5-(0) "General," box 503, Children's Bureau central file 1933–1936, Record Group 102, National Archives.

109 Bauer and Edgely, *Your Health Dramatized*, cited in Toon, "Managing the Conduct," 325.

110 Harry C. Phibbs, "The Magic Fluid," *Hygeia* 4 (1926): 275–78.

111 American Child Health Association, *Celebrating May Day in 1929*, 31.

112 C. E. Turner and George B. Collins, *Cleanliness and Health* (Boston: D. C. Heath, 1926), 155.

113 Burnham, *Superstition Won*, 247–50, 257–59.

114 See Means, *History of Health Education*, 184; Toon, "Managing the Conduct," 256–61.

115 In *Cinderella at the Race*, the Good Health Prince selects a bride by holding games and races. The stepmother Mrs. Stale Air and her daughters Fidgets and Languor are too sickly to win; other prospective brides wear signs such as "Unbrushed Teeth" and "Miss Hate Vegetables"; and Cinderella's godmother tells her to get more rest and exercise in the open air, brush her teeth, keep her body very clean, then gives her slippers marked "Regular Meals" and "Balanced Diet"; Ethel T. Wolverton [National Food Bureau, Chicago], *Cinderella at the Race*, [enclosed in] State Department of Health, West Virginia 1936, folder 4-9-0-5-3, box 511, Children's Bureau central file 1933–1936, Record Group 102, National Archives.

116 Van Ingen, "History of Child Welfare," 302.

117 Van Ingen, "History of Child Welfare," 302.

118 Sydney A. Halpern, *American Pediatrics: The Social Dynamics of Professionalism 1880–1980* (Berkeley: University of California Press, 1988), 84, 98–101; see Meckel, *Save the Babies*; Ladd-Taylor, *Mother-Work*. Note, however, that during this period critics of the Left, like physician-economist Isaac M. Rubinow and welfare activist Michael M. Davis, argued that the country's pervasive health problems were not under the control of individuals but required pervasive structural change of the health care system; see Ronald L. Numbers, *Almost Persuaded: American Physicians and Compulsory Health Insurance, 1912–1920* (Baltimore; Johns Hopkins University Press, 1978); and Elizabeth Fee and Theodore Brown, eds., *Making Medical History: The Life and Times of Henry E. Sigerist* (Baltimore: Johns Hopkins University Press, 1997).

119 On the broader history of parades as civic celebrations, see Mary P. Ryan, "The American Parade: Representations of the Nineteenth-Century Social Order," in *The New Cultural History*, ed. Lynn Hunt (Berkeley: University of California Press, 1989), 131–53. See also Ryan, *Women in Public: Between Banners and Ballots, 1825–1880* (Baltimore: Johns Hopkins University Press, 1990); and Susan G. Davis, *Parades and Power: Street Theater in Nineteenth-Century Philadelphia* (Philadelphia: Temple University Press, 1986).

120 Alan Dawley, *Struggles for Justice: Social Responsibility and the Liberal State* (Cambridge: Belknap Press of Harvard University Press, 1991), 309; on Child Health Day, see Giglio, "Voluntarism and Public Policy," 441–42.

121 William Leach, *Land of Desire: Merchants, Power and the Rise of a New American Culture* (New York: Pantheon Books, 1993), 180–82, 328–38, quote 182; see also Tomes, *Gospel of Germs*, 130.

122 David Glassberg, *American Historical Pageantry: The Uses of Tradition in the Early Twentieth Century* (Chapel Hill: University of North Carolina Press, 1990), 230–68.

123 See Martin Melosi, *Garbage in the Cities: Refuse, Reform, and the Environment, 1800–1980* (College Station, Texas A&M Press, 1981), 74–76, 130–31; Frances Williston Burks and Jesse D. Burks, *Health and the School: A Round Table* (New York: D. Appleton, 1913), 137; and Harold Bacon Wood, *Sanitation Practically Applied* (New York: John Wiley and Sons, 1917), 455.

124 John Duffy, *The Sanitarians: A History of American Public Health* (Urbana: University of Illinois Press, 1990), 210. Many readers will also vividly recall the health play in Harper Lee's *To Kill a Mockingbird* (Philadelphia: Lippincott, 1960) set in Alabama in the 1930s.

125 Hallock, "On Health Plays," in *Dramatizing Child Health*, ed. Hallock, 4.

126 Bache, "Health with the Aid of the Footlights," 40, 39.

127 Bache, "Health with the Aid of the Footlights," 40. While the participants were children, the design and staging was directed largely by adults, usually authority figures like teachers or health officials. My caveat here is to reinforce the often-unrecognized problem in applying some of the techniques of social history to child-oriented topics. It is difficult, perhaps impossible, to seek out the child's perspective, for, other than in adult memory, it is rarely available. Nonetheless, analysis of performances in which children took part can tell us something about popular expectations of school and family life, relations between the lay public and health authorities, and relations among teachers, reformers, and health professionals.

128 Moore, *Public Health in the United States*, 256.

129 American Child Health Association, *Celebrating May Day in 1929*, 32.

130 Dorothea Campbell [director, Bureau of Public Health Education, State Department of Health, Charleston, WV], *Sanitary Sam Visits Healthland* [1936], folder 4-9-0-5-3, box 511, Children's Bureau central file 1933–1936, Record Group 102, National Archives.

131 Lummis, "Health Week in Denver, 1927," 5.

132 Lillian Curtis Drew, "Ode to Posture," in Schweitzer, "Indiana Child Health Day Plans–1929."

133 Bache, *Health Education in Syracuse*, 57; "Minutes of a Regular Meeting of the Executive Committee" of the ACHA, 16 February 1924.

134 On this point, see also Tomes, *Gospel of Germs*, 131.

135 Virginia State Department of Health, *The Good Health Club of Wellville* [enclosed in] Bagby to Eliot, 18 June 1936.

136 "Minutes of a Regular Meeting of the ACHA Executive Committee, 16 February 1924."

137 "Report by Lucy Wood Collier" to ACHA, 22 October 1923.

138 The National Tuberculosis Association, "The Modern Health Crusade," [enclosed in] Dr Linsley R. Williams [managing director, NTA] to Grace Abbott, 31 October 1925, folder 4-11-6-0, box 277, Children's Bureau central file 1925–28, Record Group 102, National Archives. For another creed, repeated daily by school children during the 1916 Baby Week, see Klaus, *Every Child a Lion*, 167–68.

139 Kathleen M. Blee, *Women of the Klan: Racism and Gender in the 1920s* (Berkeley: University of California Press, 1991), 158–65.

140 "Minutes of a Regular Meeting of the ACHA Executive Committee, 16 February 1924."

141 Klaus, *Every Child a Lion*, 161. Note that no black doctor was ever employed by the Rockefeller Foundation's Hookworm Commission; Ettling, *Germ of Laziness*, 174.

142 Howard L. Holley, *A History of Medicine in Alabama* (Birmingham: University of Alabama School of Medicine, 1982), 285–88. Welch was health officer from 1917 to 1928.

143 S. W. Welch [state health officer, Alabama State Board of Health] to Hon. W. W. Brandon, 26 May 1923, Record Group 2-G165, Brandon Administration Records, State Board of Health, Alabama Department of Archives and History, Montgomery, AL. Despite Welch's opposition, during the mid-1920s fifty thousand children from every Alabama county enrolled in the Modern Health Crusade, and Cho-Cho visited Alabama twice in 1926; Holley, *History of Medicine in Alabama*, 303–304.

144 Estelle N. Mathews to Grace Abbott, 19 March 1929, folder 4-9-0-7-4 (7) "Colorado," box 384, Children's Bureau central file 1929–32, Record Group 102, National Archives; see also Rennie B. Schoeoflin, *Christian Science on Trial: Religious Healing in America* (Baltimore: Johns Hopkins University Press, 2003).

145 American Child Health Association Committee on Health Education, 1 February 1923, New York City, folder 19, box 38, series III, Winslow #749, Yale University Archives.

146 "National Negro Health Week," [press release, enclosed in] Robert R. Moton, [principal, Tuskegee Institute] to Grace Abbott, 4 March 1922, folder 4-12-0-5 Investigations, box 198, Children's Bureau central file 1921–24, Record Group 102, National Archives. See also Smith, *Sick and Tired*, 32–57; Tomes, *Gospel of Germs*, 220–33; and Mildred M. Williams, Kara Vaughn Jackson, and National Association of Supervisors and Consultants Interim History Writing Committee,

The Jeanes Story: A Chapter in the History of American Education 1908–1968 (Jackson: Southern Education Foundation Inc., 1979). On a big health fête organized by the black community in Arkansas for Child Health Day, see American Child Health Association, *Celebrating May Day in 1929*, 24; and on the receptivity of black communities in Tennessee, see Hoffschwelle, "Organizing Rural Communities," 162.

147 Tomes, *Gospel of Germs*, 232.

148 Tomes, *Gospel of Germs*, 232, 213.

149 American Child Health Association, *Celebrating May Day in 1929*, 69. Similar events were held at the Blackfoot Indian School on Montana's Bighorn Reservation, the Onondaga Indiana Reservation in New York, and the Kiowa Indian Agency in Lawton, Oklahoma.

150 Cole, "Playing for Health," 646.

151 Cole, "Playing for Health," 347. Many of the play's costumes as well as its wigwam had been loaned by local Indians. On the NTA's health playwriting contest for high school students from 1924 to 1928, see Means, *History of Health Education*, 203.

152 *A Health Pageant* by Mrs. M. P.C. Youmans, Jonesville, SC, in Bagby to Eliot, 18 June 1936.

153 McCuaig, *The Weariness, the Fever, and the Fret*, 172–75.

154 "Some Suggestions for May Day—Child Health Day Celebrations in the Schools: Some References," in Anne Whitney [director, School Health Education Service, Joint Committee on Health Problems in Education] to Edith Rockwood [Children's Bureau] 12 May 1936, folder 4-9-0-5-3 "Baby Saving Campaigns," box 511, Children's Bureau central file 1933–36, Record Group 102, National Archives.

155 Annette King [Bureau of Public Health Education, West Virginia State Department of Health], *When Germs Get Together*, 1936, folder 4-9-0-5-3, box 511, Children's Bureau central file 1933–36, Record Group 102, National Archives.

156 C. E. Turner to Thomas Wood, 9 November 1923, folder 7, box 38, series III, Winslow #749, Yale University Archives.

157 Turner and Collins, *Cleanliness and Health*, 57. For an important analysis of mothers' responses to aspects of the scientific motherhood movement, see Julia Dent Grant, *Raising Baby by the Book: The Education of American Mothers* (New Haven: Yale University Press, 1998), 137–60.

158 Hoffschwelle, "Organizing Rural Communities," 158. On anti-government attitudes by New Zealand parents who resisted school medical and dental inspection, see Tennant, "Missionaries of Health," 144.

159 Lynd and Lynd, *Middletown*, 454n24. On the fear of federal usurpation of states rights by lay groups in Massachusetts, see Rosenkrantz, *Public Health and the State*, 154–55; and for the broader picture of medical populism, see Robert Johnston, ed., *The Politics of Healing: Essays in Twentieth-Century North American Alternative Medicine* (New York: Routledge, 2003).

160 Baker, *Fighting for Life*, 147.

161 Giglio, "Voluntarism and Public Policy," 432.

162 On "a President who stood by while Congress killed the Sheppard-Towner law," see "Mr. Hoover and the Children," *The New Republic* 65 (December 1930): 59; and "Hoover's Fight for the Children," *Literary Digest* 107 (December 1930): 58.

163 Lindenmeyer, *"A Right to Childhood,"* 163–75, quote 170.

164 See "Suggestive Material for Cooperative Programs with Health and Education Officials," State Health Officer, SG-7067, Department of Public Health, Bureau

of Hygiene and Nursing 1935–36, Administrative Files, Alabama Department of Archives and History.

165 Giglio, "Voluntarism and Public Policy," 434.

166 Ettling, *Germ of Laziness*, 215.

167 The popularity of the health play continued into the 1980s and 1990s; see, for example, Calvin's experience as an onion in his school play in the newspaper cartoon *Calvin and Hobbes*. I thank Hughes Evans for pointing this out to me.

No More Surprising Than a Broken Pitcher?

Maternal and Child Health in the Early Years of the Pan American Sanitary Bureau

CR

Anne-Emanuelle Birn

Historically, the priorities and activities of international health organizations have been determined at the metropolitan level or through a confluence of central and local interests. Early twentieth-century campaigns against epidemic diseases were prototypes of this arrangement, whereby the threat to international commerce was of greater importance in guiding actions than was the local epidemiological reality. For example, the 1920 outbreak of yellow fever in Mexico elicited a four-year multi-million-dollar eradication campaign by the Rockefeller Foundation (RF), but the disease resulted in only a few hundred deaths, compared to some fifty thousand annual deaths from gastroenteritis. Even when countries requested and received assistance, local demand was arguably generated or guided by central organizational interests.

The case of maternal and child health and the Pan American Sanitary Bureau (PASB)[1] during the first half of the twentieth century demonstrates a different phenomenon. Rather than sparking interest and actions in maternal and child health in Latin America, the PASB ignored this area, even though the agency was repeatedly urged over several decades by numerous countries in the region to provide support. Only in the 1940s, when maternal and child health was squarely on the international agenda, did the PASB respond to these demands.

Founded in 1902, during its early years the PASB was devoted to the establishment of region-wide protocols on the reporting and control of epidemic diseases, including yellow fever, plague, and cholera. The bureau was headed by a succession of U.S. surgeons-general until 1947, when long-time RF officer Fred Soper became its director. In its leadership and sphere of activities, the bureau clearly reflected U.S. hegemonic interests in Latin America in the early twentieth century. Burgeoning U.S. investment in Latin American oil, fruiticulture, mining and metallurgy, real estate, railroads, banking, and other industries, coupled with the explosion of trade resulting from the Panama Canal's new shipping routes, meant that any interruption in commerce would have dire economic consequences. The United States was particularly concerned that Latin American countries participate in the drafting of, and thus comply with, enforceable sanitary codes. By the early 1920s these concerns began to shift. Legislative, medico-sanitary, and engineering efforts helped to lessen the menace of epidemics. Also, the potential of an international health organization to provide technical assistance on other matters, such as maternal and child health, became evident to the PASB's member countries.

Almost without exception, the PASB's past has been documented from a central and bureaucratic perspective, with historically minded functionaries recounting the great moments and men in the organization's founding, evolution, and name-changing parade.[2] Norman Howard Jones has argued that in its first decades the organization was virtually dormant. This assertion is based on U.S. Surgeon-General Hugh Cumming's rather immodest declaration in 1934: "Fourteen years ago, when the Pan American Sanitary Conference did me the honor of electing me as Director of the Pan American Sanitary Bureau, it existed in name only."[3]

While it is true that the PASB operated without a separate office, staff, or programs in its first two decades, relying on the surgeon-general's headquarters for these functions, the first seven International Sanitary Conferences organized by the bureau between 1902 and 1924 generated considerable activity. In offering a venue for the region's health officials to meet periodically, the conferences stimulated country-to-country interactions, continent-wide exchanges, and informal networking by policymakers, health officers, and government authorities. Country delegates also utilized the conferences to press their own governments to support measures that had been discussed in these forums or that were already in force elsewhere. It was these exchanges that helped frame the regional pressure for a Pan American promotion of maternal and child health.

This paper begins with a brief examination of the international emergence of maternal and child health, emphasizing the different cultural contexts and exigencies that shaped this concern circa 1900 in Europe, North America, and Latin America (with special emphasis on Mexico and Uruguay). I then turn to the PASB's early history and modus operandi, the pressure exerted by Latin American countries upon the PASB to pay attention to maternal and child health matters, and the bureau's unwillingness to work in this area. Next I explore concomitant developments in maternal and child health and eugenics within Latin America in the 1920s and 1930s, and the PASB's first steps in this area. Finally, I discuss the conflict over the PASB's role in maternal and child health on several dimensions: first, as a manifestation of differing cultural priorities in the United States and Latin America; second, as a struggle for organizational power within the PASB; and third, as part of a richer understanding of the diffusion of early twentieth-century public health and medical practices.

The Emergence of Maternal and Child Health Concerns

Philippe Ariès and other social historians of the family and childhood in Europe have argued that the idea of childhood was only "discovered" at the end of the Middle Ages, when these previous "miniature adults" began to be educated, and the family emerged at the expense of communal life.[4] By the nineteenth century, urbanization, industrialization, a decline in fertility, and the transformation of the family into nuclear units made the survival of children more important in economic terms to the working family, which relied on the industrial wages of each surviving child far more than their agrarian predecessors had upon the marginal field work provided by each extra child, and to the industrial sector, which required an ever-growing pool of persons fit to work in factories. Urban social conditions did not comply with these exigencies. In Britain, for example, mortality, particularly infant mortality, appears to have risen in the first half of the nineteenth century before beginning its steady but bumpy decline.[5] Had fertility remained consistently high in this period, elevated and even increasing infant mortality would have posed a lesser problem. Because urbanization and industrialization tended to be accompanied by decreases in fertility, infant mortality could not be ignored.

By the early twentieth century, most European countries embraced a mix of measures in reaction to these problems, including ideological campaigns, voluntary initiatives, and large-scale state activities to improve infant and maternal health and welfare. France experienced the fertility and infant mortality crunch more than its neighbours, the result, in part, of high female participation in the labour force. It responded with an early and extensive array of protective legislation from the Roussel Law of 1874, which promised breastfeeding for abandoned infants, as well as a range of maternal pensions, leave, and child-health programs. Many of these ideas and directives drew from the field of puericulture—French obstetrician Adolphe Pinard's notion of the scientific cultivation of childhood and the improvement of child health and welfare through better conditions of child rearing.[6] France's early commitment to universally implemented state measures, which were at once medically recommended and socially oriented, set it apart from many countries, which took more tentative steps to address maternal and child health.[7]

In the United States, fire-and-brimstone Boston preacher Cotton Mather's eighteenth-century observation that the death of a child was "no more surprising than a broken pitcher" continued to hold true for the early nineteenth century. By the 1850s, however, infant mortality was discovered as a problem in need of amelioration, and a series of reforms were instituted, beginning with attempts to sanitize the general environment and then to improve infant feeding and the quality of milk supplies, starting in the 1880s. There is some evidence that nineteenth-century parents were motivated to improve the chances of survival for their children, but they had few tools available other than extending the breastfeeding period.[8] By the early twentieth century, a focus on mothers' child-bearing and child-raising abilities emerged, based on bacteriological advances and social reform campaigns.[9]

This growing medical and social expertise translated into fits and starts of activity in a mix of voluntary and government venues: Josephine Baker's Bureau of Child Hygiene in New York begun in 1908, Jane Addams's Hull House in Chicago, and the U.S. Children's Bureau founded in 1912 by Julia Lathrop. Likewise in Canada, infant health became a leading public-health concern after 1900 and was addressed through a mix of government and private initiatives; for example, through the creation of a federal child-welfare division, headed by Helen MacMurchy in 1920 and the Canadian Council on Child Welfare.[10]

Although U.S. social reformers, particularly women, pioneered many new approaches that were emulated around the world, they did not succeed in making maternal and child health a government priority or a universal commitment. The rise and fall of the short-lived federal Sheppard-Towner Act (1921–29) providing federal funding for state maternal and child health initiatives typifies the ambiguous backing for these services in the U.S. cultural context. Sheppard-Towner was passed the year after women obtained the right to vote, in a highly politicized bid by the U.S. Congress to meet women's claims on the state. But right-wing hysteria about growing socialism, buoyed by the jealousy of private practice doctors, led to polemics about the appropriate role of government in the provision of health services. By the late 1920s, organized medicine's promise that doctors would meet maternal and child health needs through routine and charity care, coupled with the now diminished menace of the "women's vote," doomed Sheppard-Towner, and the legislation was not renewed.[11]

While European and North American maternal and child health efforts differed in style and organizational aspects, the countries in these regions shared similar problems of urbanization, industrialization, dropping fertility rates, and the concomitant economic importance of the survival of children. These circumstances coupled with vociferous social-reform movements and medicine's and public health's growing armamentaria of specific interventions, provided the principal stimuli for the field of maternal and child health.

At the turn of the century Latin American countries were, for the most part, not undergoing the same demographic, social, and economic trends as Europe and North America, but many countries in the region shared a concern for maternal and child health. While long-time French influence upon Latin American medicine undoubtedly fed this interest, the Latin American commitment to maternal and child health had deeper cultural roots than did Aries's child-ignoring Europe.

Anthropological research on pre-Colombian societies suggests that pregnancy and childbirth were community events and that reproduction was closely tied to social and religious prestige. Mayans in particular considered children to be a sign of wealth and good fortune, and paid special attention to infant health.[12] Pre-Colombian cultures are also known for their adherence to hygienic precepts, such as bathing rituals following childbirth, testing the milk of wet nurses, monitoring the nursing mother's diet, as well as treating ailments with a combination of magic and empiricism. Concern for maternal and child health formed part of larger public hygiene routines. The Aztecs, for example, had a highly developed practice of sanitation, keeping the streets and plazas of Tenochtitlan (razed by conquering Spaniards in order to build Mexico City) conspicuously clean through regular refuse collection and market and street sanitation. Lake Texcoco, which surrounded the city, was divided into clean and waste-water lagoons through the construction of causeways.[13]

The early ethical education children received, the joy surrounding procreation, and, given contemporaneous rituals, the sacrifice of five- to ten-year-olds all reflected the high value pre-Colombian societies placed on children. Aztec children even had their own medical god, Ixtlilton, unknown elsewhere in the world.[14] In sum, the cultural importance of children and child health may explain in part why ideas about puericulture were adopted so readily in Latin America.

While the influence of pre-Colombian practices on the receptivity of modern attention to maternal and child health may appear to be a leap, there is significant recent anthropological evidence, from Oscar Lewis to Kaja Finkler, that twentieth-century midwifery in *mestizo* Mexico was based upon ancient practices of herb baths, massages, and spiritual counselling.[15] Moreover, the Mexican Department of Public Health itself was receptive to indigenous practices. In the late 1920s, the department sponsored research on a lactogenous plant known in maya as *ixbut* (*Euphorbia lancifolia*), used to stimulate milk production in new mothers and wet nurses in indigenous Central American communities. Mexican agricultural researchers were sent to El Salvador to carry out experiments with *ixbut* on cows, finding that the test group of cows fed milky secretions from the *ixbut* plant experienced a threefold increase in daily milk production.[16]

Following the imposition of Spanish colonial rule, pre-Colombian childhood culture survived unevenly. The introduction of formalized primary education, for example, led to the removal of children from the purview of the traditional community, while colonial authorities barred many indigenous child-rearing practices.[17] At the same time, private-practice physicians governed by *protomedicatos* (early medical boards) and Catholic charity hospitals and orphanages began to introduce European medicine to the very rich and the very poor in the Iberian colonies. Perhaps the most prominent official activity in these years was the Bourbon monarchy's sponsorship of mandatory smallpox vaccination for children, leading to the creation of scattered local, public-health organizations active in the care of foundlings and other matters relating to children's health.[18]

After achieving independence from Spain and Portugal in the nineteenth century, some Latin American countries began to organize health and social-welfare institutions specifically for women and children; however, state involvement was minimal, and the reach of these institutions remained limited.[19] The ranks of trained physicians increased as Latin American medical schools followed the French model of medical education. Still, as during the colonial period, indigenous and *mestizo* populations continued to rely upon traditional healers, midwives, and community leaders.

Towards the end of the nineteenth century, however, this situation began to change on a number of fronts. Growing foreign investment in the region disrupted subsistence farming, displaced populations, and generated new problems of ill health and child abandonment. At the same time, the improvement of transportation networks, the expansion of national bureaucracies, the emergence of a professional class, and the medicalization of the poor[20] made both old and new health problems more visible. The high infant mortality rates "discovered" in this period became a vital concern to nations seeking to modernize and grow. Together, these circumstances made Latin American countries particularly amenable to the French puericulture movement.[21] As in France but in contrast to the situation in the United States, many Latin American physicians supported a state role in the provision of health services, and physicians provided vital leadership in the regional movement for maternal and child health.

Feminism in Latin America at this time also influenced the development of maternal and child health concerns. Movements for women's equality in Latin America typically did not deny femininity and motherhood but rather embraced these roles. Mother-feminism, based in part on Catholic spirituality, protested "laws and conditions which threaten[ed women's] ability" to bear children and nurture their families, including war, drugs, prostitution, urban misery, adultery, and exclusion from suffrage and property ownership.[22] In Mexico, for example, a feminist agenda emerged in the context of the Mexican Revolution, spurring regulation of wet-nursing and adoption, assessment of maternal fitness by the welfare system, and other maternal and child health reforms.[23] As in other countries, these movements were most influential in urban settings, where middle-class women made social issues part of public policy and mobilized to improve and regulate social conditions for poor women.

The "mother-feminism" movement deftly turned to Pan-Americanism to gain support, meeting at the same or parallel sessions of the Latin American Scientific Congresses, International Congresses of American States, and other meetings. Soon, feminists began to set up their own regional conferences where Latin American women were able to share their ideas and activities with their North American counterparts, focusing on juridical protection for working women, civil and political equality of women throughout the continent, and the well-being of children.[24] Most notably, the Pan American Child Congresses, first organized by Latin American feminists in 1916, attracted the support of male physicians and lawyers across the region. Usually in agreement, these groups joined forces in crafting pioneering legislation to protect children.[25]

This combination of factors—cultural predisposition to protecting mothers and children, the nature and projects of Latin American feminism, the French medical influence, physician leadership, and nation-building imperatives in an earlier era of globalization—shaped Latin Americans' advocacy of maternal and child health. If economic preoccupations sparked the maternal and child health movements of Europe and North America, it was moral and cultural concerns that enlivened these movements in Latin America.

Maternal and Child Health without and with the Pan American Sanitary Bureau

A series of international sanitary conferences beginning in 1851 attempted to establish systems of disease notification, ship inspection, and port sanitation, principally in European countries, but these efforts were initially fruitless, since national sovereignty superseded such international economic concerns. North and South Americans rarely participated, except in 1881, when the International Sanitary Conference was held in Wash-

ington, DC.[26] There were two South American efforts at sanitary cooperation in the 1880s, one among the Southern Cone countries of
Argentina, Brazil, and Uruguay (the Rio Sanitary Convention of 1887),
and the second among the Andean countries of Bolivia, Chile, Ecuador,
and Peru (the Lima Convention of 1888). However, as with the international conferences, recommended measures were not enforceable.

Soon after 1900 the commercial and epidemic prospects associated
with resumed construction of the Panama Canal made the need for
international sanitary cooperation in the Americas more pressing. In
addition, the U.S. economic and political dominance over most of Latin
America, most freshly demonstrated in the U.S. victory over Spain and
occupation of Cuba, enabled cooperation in the Americas well before
European powers were able to agree on the substance of a potential sanitary treaty.

The first so-called International Sanitary Convention (really a regional
meeting for the Americas) was organized in December 1902 in Washington, DC, at the behest of the Second International Conference of the
American States (the precursor to the Organization of American States)
held in Mexico City earlier that year. At the opening of the convention
in Washington, DC, U.S. Surgeon-General Walter Wyman remarked to the
representatives of eleven republics, "Health, cleanliness, intellect, and
morals might well be the motto of this conference."[27] Discussion topics
included the sharing of scientific information, the enforcement of quar-
antines, port sanitation, and scientific investigation. Wyman optimistically
noted that, if successful, the "young Republics of the Western Hemi-
sphere" would be in a position to influence other continents.

The first three International Sanitary Conventions focused attention
on organizational issues and the control of epidemic diseases. At the
first conference, it was decided that an International Sanitary Bureau,
consisting of seven members under the presidency of the U.S. surgeon-
general, would serve as a governing committee in charge of receiving
reports on sanitary conditions in the ports of the Americas and organizing quadrennial conferences.

The conferences themselves were divided into two sections, as were
the conference *Transactions*. In the first section, a central agenda was
formally presented and discussed point by point. Devised by the surgeon-
general, the agenda was based on interests expressed at the previous
conference, advice of the governing committee, and particularly, priorities determined by the surgeon-general himself. During the second
section, each country representative presented a report on national sanitary conditions, typically making reference to the themes of the main
agenda. While the country reports were a vehicle for spirited debate
and often put forward important new health matters, the final resolutions

of each conference related only to the points made during discussion of the official agenda in the first section. It was in the country reports, appended to the minutes of each conference, that discussions of maternal and child health first appeared.

Women and children were neither seen nor mentioned until the fourth International Sanitary Conference held in Costa Rica in 1909.[28] The photograph commemorating that meeting appears to be the only portrayal of women alongside the male delegates until the late 1930s. What remains unclear is whether these were wives, daughters, amanuenses, or local gals. The female presence may be in part explained by the conference dates—December 25, 1909 to January 3, 1910—and these ladies were certainly wearing their party hats![29]

Notwithstanding the official invisibility of women and children in the conference agenda and resolutions, Latin American authorities clearly expressed maternal and child health as an early priority for the PASB. In 1909 host country Costa Rica offered a detailed analysis of sanitary conditions that made extensive reference to child health. The report began by proudly recounting the country's success with compulsory smallpox vaccination, which was "practiced with due frequency, especially among school children."[30] It then quickly turned to more disagreeable topics such as the excessive death rate among children in the Caribbean port of Limón. "But what really causes horror," the report continued, "is the [national] mortality rate in children. *Fourteen* children die every day [of a total population of 400,000], that is to say, one every two hours; or 5,000 per year, on account of the ignorance of the quack, the poor quality of water in small towns, poor food, and the carelessness in properly attiring the children....Infantile mortality is the gravest of problems that the country has to confront;...the constant and awe-inspiring danger of infantile mortality, which, hour after hour, snatches away from the country precious energies, incessantly shatters to pieces our hopes for the future."[31] The Costa Rican delegate argued that hospitals and asylums for children and improvements in general sanitary conditions would provide part of the solution; he also called for the application of strategies developed in England, which was seen as the pioneer in sanitation.

The Costa Rica report fuelled a lively discussion about maternal and child health needs and served as a springboard for sustained debate among conference delegates, many of whom continued to recount their woes and activities through inter-conference correspondence. Upon returning home, delegates also shared the lessons learned from other countries with Ministry of Health colleagues and government officials.

Maternal and child health issues were framed variously in terms of pessimism about the magnitude of the task of helping children survive infancy, more positively in terms of the importance of children to nation-building and progress, and even in terms of religious salvation. Colombian delegate Dr. Amador remarked that it was especially appropriate that the Costa Rica conference had opened on Christmas, the day of birth of the infant saviour, who survived despite his family's poverty and homelessness.[32] These assorted perspectives on the problem of child mortality were unified by calls for government action to resolve child mortality. But discussions of maternal and child health were not reflected in the crucial first section of the *Transactions*, nor in the resolutions passed at the conference.

By the time of the Sixth International Sanitary Conference held in Montevideo in 1920, delegates had moved from documenting maternal and child health problems in the country reports to demanding their insertion into the official agenda. While the majority of the conference's forty-six resolutions related to tropical disease control, delegates asked that school health be included as a topic for the next conference and that schools establish educational programs covering basic hygiene and prevention of transmissible diseases.[33] Despite this plea, school health was not part of the agenda at the Seventh Pan American Sanitary Conference, held in Havana in 1924. There, once again, Latin American delegates voted for resolutions favouring the development of families and calling "the attention of all the American Governments to the urgent necessity of undertaking...an energetic child-welfare campaign, from the point of view of hygienic environment, eugenics, and homiculture; to recommend to all American countries the creation of the guardianship of the State over infancy; to fix as one of the principal topics for the next Conference, the study of infant morbidity and mortality."[34] Indeed, at every conference of the 1920s Latin American delegates asked that infant mortality and morbidity be incorporated into the main agenda, but these topics were repeatedly left out.

At the 1920 Sanitary Conference U.S. Surgeon-General Hugh Cumming was elected director of the PASB, a position he held for twenty-seven years, extending to more than a decade after he retired from the Public Health Service. Cummings's reign transformed the PASB. He reorganized the governing structure, launched a major fund-raising effort, established regional offices and a permanent home for the bureau in Washington, and in the 1940s instituted country-level, public-health programs. In the 1920s, the bureau began to provide technical assistance in response to country requests via its one-man peregrinator Public Health Service John Long. Over several decades, Long advised the development of health legislation in Chile, helped stamp out bubonic plague in Peru and Argentina, and assisted the reorganization of Argentina's federal health service.[35] But given its staff size of one, the PASB's direct assistance was highly limited.

It might be argued that the early potential of the PASB to provide targeted technical assistance and to run public-health programs in individual member countries was displaced by a new actor on the international health stage. Beginning in 1916, the United States–based Rockefeller Foundation and its International Health Board (renamed the International Health Division in 1927) launched a series of campaigns against hookworm, yellow fever, and malaria in almost every country in Latin America and the Caribbean and throughout the tropical world.[36] Aimed at social advancement, strengthening public health and medical institutions, fostering goodwill, improving trade, productivity, and political stability, and showcasing U.S. scientific expertise, these programs were not the fruition of regional claims but, rather, were negotiated and moulded country by country. Anxious to limit the scope and length of its commitment and to demonstrate public health's technical capacity over its social aspects, the International Health Board distanced itself from problems such as infant diarrhea or tuberculosis.[37] In the course of developing permanent local health units in Mexico, the board stumbled upon maternal and child health problems. It addressed them as a technical question of better training for midwives and nurses, without including questions of state responsibility, living conditions, and social rights as had been delineated by many Latin American advocates of maternal and child health.[38] Thus, although the RF overshadowed the PASB in the area of cooperative, large-scale disease campaigns within particular countries, it left maternal and child health as a wide-open area of action. Given the importance of maternal and child health to public health officials across Latin America, it might have been a natural area for PASB attention and one that would not have competed with the RF.

The PASB under Cumming did not pursue a wider role in regional technical assistance, and Cumming appears to have been little interested in Latin-style state-run maternal and child health services. Like many of his compatriots, Cumming believed that private, voluntary, and local efforts in health and welfare should not be dislodged by new government activities but rather complemented by them. The PASB might foster administrative development and regulatory oversight, for example, but not support government-run prenatal care or daycare centres and milk depots.

Cumming also attempted to sideline prospects for European collaboration in Latin American maternal and child health. At the same time as the PASB was expanding, the League of Nations Health Organization promoted health cooperation in interwar Europe. It collected detailed health statistics, helped war-torn nations build and reorganize their health bureaucracies, laboratory capacity, and epidemiological services, stimulated health legislation and standardization, and responded to a variety of disease problems.[39] Led by Polish hygienist Ludwik Rajchman,[40] who later founded UNICEF, the health organization was particularly concerned with improving the health and welfare of children. Jealous of this potential competitor (despite his designation by the State Department as its U.S. member) and suspicious of Soviet influence in the league, Cumming viewed official league visits to Latin America as "a quite evident effort to lessen the prestige of the Pan American Sanitary Bureau."[41]

While the struggle over the main agenda and activities of the PASB continued, other developments point to the growing importance of maternal and child health within the medical community in the United States and Latin America alike. At the 1920 Montevideo meeting, PASB delegates approved the establishment of an international journal for the collection of national health statistics and the publication of scientific articles. Originally conceived as a way for Latin American physicians and public-health workers to be exposed to the latest U.S. research through the translation into Spanish and Portuguese of previously published articles and medical guidelines, the *Boletín de la Oficina Sanitaria Internacional* became an extremely important means of information dissemination. Virtually all local, regional, and national health departments in small towns and large cities received the *Boletín*, and each year the main office sent out hundreds of reprints and technical letters to its readers. In the 1930s the editors reached their goal of distributing each issue free to every community with a population over 2000 (by 1938 it reached 3,590 communities) and the *Boletín* rapidly became the most widely known publication in health and medicine in Latin America.[42] In providing administrative guidelines, research results, international news, and direct advice, the *Boletín* substituted for direct technical cooperation and, together with the sanitary conferences, enabled the PASB to influence health developments throughout Latin America efficiently and effectively.

By the late 1920s the *Boletín* began to cover maternal and child health issues, with dozens of articles on child hygiene, maternology (the science of motherhood), the role of visiting nurses and social workers, school health, nutrition, news of conferences, and national examples of maternal and child health care organization. Sections on puericulture offered a roundup of relevant news items published in journals from around the world, detailing the latest developments on milk stations, the average weight of newborns in Bogotá and Lima, mandatory vaccination recommendations, new treatment modalities in Baltimore, the success of DDT in reducing school absenteeism thanks to the elimination of head lice, and infant mortality trends in Latin America.[43]

Articles and pamphlets on maternal and child health published by the *Boletín* in its first decades typically presented U.S. dictates. A letter to pregnant women recommended a diet low in sugar and fat, high in fruits, vegetables, cereals, and protein, baths three times a week, loose clothing, and attention to mental health.[44] "Guidelines for Infant Health Centers" detailed everything from the type of furniture necessary, the appropriate number of visits per day, to the contents of each child health exam. In the late 1920s, the PASB published a series of pamphlets by U.S. Public Health Service Dr. E. Blanche Sterling on prenatal, infant, and pre-school health.[45] Latin American contributions, while not ignored in this period, generally consisted of compilations of national or regional declarations, such as a 1930 pamphlet, "The Rights of Children,"[46] rather than original scientific articles. As with the Pan American Sanitary Conferences, then, the *Boletín* furthered U.S. experience and interests more than it showcased efforts throughout the region.

Until the 1940s, the PASB marginalized Latin American support for maternal and child health when an overlapping regional effort was marshalled by Latin Americans. As Donna Guy has shown, the Pan American Child Congresses served for almost half a century as an influential hemispheric forum for pediatricians, nurses, policy-makers, sociologists, lawyers, reformers, and others to discuss medical and social problems affecting children.[47] The eight congresses that met between 1916 and 1942 resulted in dozens of laws protecting children and their mothers and delineating children's rights in such areas as adoption, infant health, and child labour. The initial efforts by South American feminists and doctors to press for the state's role in child protection were joined by those of North American feminists affiliated with the U.S. Children's Bureau, who "eventually encourag[ed] the Pan American Child Congresses to attenuate their insistence on using the welfare state," instead turning to a mix of public and private solutions.[48]

In 1927 the child congress organizers' decade-long dream of founding a permanent Instituto Internacional Americano de Protección a la Infancia (International Institute for the Protection of Childhood) was realized in Montevideo. The first of its kind in the world, the institute collected and disseminated research and policy information pertaining to the care and protection of mothers and children. Its *Boletín*, library, health education materials, and the child congresses it organized rapidly established a strong reputation for the institute and generated a large network of informants and collaborators throughout the region and the world.[49] While the PASB participated in the founding of the institute, the two organizations had little to do with one another. In the 1920s and 1930s, under the leadership of Gregorio Aráoz Alfaro, Luis Morquio, and others, the institute pioneered social legislation relating to the health and welfare of children.[50] Dr. Morquio and his colleagues at the institute were frequently invited to share their research and knowledge with Europeans, serving as exporters, as well as importers, of childhood-related scientific theory and practice.

Influenced by the child congresses and the institute, many countries began to hold national child conferences and set aside a day or week of the child (Día del Niño) to draw attention to matters of child health and social welfare. These efforts reflected an era of burgeoning social action in the 1920s and 1930s in Latin America, including the development of social security legislation, health systems, local and national health services for the indigent, and protective legislation for pregnant mothers and children.[51]

Another important ingredient in the region's support for maternal and child health, and a source of antagonism between North American and Latin American social policy, was the response to eugenics in the late nineteenth and early twentieth centuries. Anglo-Saxon eugenics was principally informed by Mendelian genetics. Improving society's genetic stock entailed the breeding out of bad genes through sterilization and prohibitions on procreation ("negative eugenics"). While such ideas generated tremendous divisions among researchers within the United States, the precepts of "negative eugenics" were successfully translated into policy, with thirty-one of forty-eight states passing compulsory sterilization laws between 1907 and 1937.[52]

Eugenics in Latin American countries, by contrast, reflected French influences. As Nancy Stepan has demonstrated, Latin American eugenics was interpreted through attention to neo-Lamarckian ideas about the inheritance of acquired characteristics and to homiculture (a Cuban-coined expansion of Pinard's concept of puericulture, which includes cultivation of the child from pre-birth to adulthood). Latin eugenics stressed reforming the social and moral environment of prospective parents and children instead of blocking reproduction. Children raised would not only overcome an unfavourable genetic background, they would also pass on these new traits to future generations, improving the larger society. This "positive eugenics" movement, with its emphasis on sanitation and the scientific improvement of the circumstances surrounding conception and childhood, overlapped with the concerns over maternal and child health.[53]

The differing approaches to eugenics, and to maternal and child health generally, stems from distinct cultural milieus. Notwithstanding U.S. economic domination of much of Latin America, the region was far more influenced by France and Southern Europe than by North America in areas such as science, the role of the state versus private and voluntary sectors, social rights, and religion. While there were some Latin American physicians who advocated "negative eugenics," the majority held to the Catholic prohibition on interference with reproduction.

Adherence to homiculture, too, was consistent with values surrounding family and children. The local social order, however, played an important role in the reception and transformation of positive eugenics. Stepan suggests that in Mexico, for example, eugenics was used in the development of a national identity amidst the large *mestizo* (mixed European and indigenous heritage) population; here the mixing of peoples was dubbed to have a desirable, synergistic effect. In Argentina eugenics helped mediate immigration policy with arguments about how the proportion of migrants from particular places settling in the Argentinean environment could make or break the nation's prospects for the future.

Eugenics was also taken up as a Pan-American concern. Tremendous tensions arose between negative eugenicists from the United States, typified by Eugenics Records Office Director Charles Davenport's advocacy of sterilizing all unfit parents, and Latin American neo-Lamarckians, who viewed such policies as racist and reductionist. Davenport, in turn, opposed the Latin American puericultural outlook. These differences reached a climax at both the First and Second Pan American Conferences of Eugenics and Homiculture, the former held several weeks after the Fifth Pan American Child Congress in Havana in 1927, and the latter held in conjunction with the Ninth Pan American Sanitary Conference in Buenos Aires in 1934. At the Havana conference, delegates refused to support a dogmatic code that would have classified citizenry according to their genetic fitness and would have determined eligibility standards for marriage, procreation, and migration. Instead most delegates advocated the less racist approach favoured by the child congresses of improving home environments and increasing the state's role in social welfare.[54]

At the joint Buenos Aires conference, a rounding endorsement of the socially oriented Uruguay's Children's Code (further discussed below), aimed at protecting the health and welfare of children in a non-coercive manner, marked an outright rejection of the U.S. approach on sterilization and the "improvement" of heredity. The outvoted Americans could find little ground for agreement, for U.S. eugenicists "deliberately excluded public-health and social welfare measures from consideration."[55]

It was at this 1934 joint eugenics and sanitary conference[56] that a session devoted to the "Protection of Infancy and Motherhood" was finally on the official Pan American Sanitary Conference agenda, following many years of repeated requests by delegates. This session was organized, at least in part, to counter the "negative eugenics" sessions organized by U.S. eugenicists. Overall, three of thirty-two thematic areas discussed at the conference related to maternal and child health issues: the promotion of the campaign against infant mortality, the protection of maternity and infancy, and the protection of pre-schoolers and the promotion of school health.

Country delegates entered into a series of lively debates over the causes of and solutions to infant mortality. Uruguayan delegate Javier Gomensoro noted that, despite his country's racial and climatic unity, the presence of few of the major causes of infant mortality of other countries in the region, and tremendous technical efforts, the infant mortality rate had remained stuck at 110–112/1000. He postulated two major reasons for continued high rates: lack of health education, and poor living conditions. Gomensoro explained that the Ministry of Public Health was attempting to coordinate the construction of new houses as a preventive measure against tuberculosis and infant mortality in general.

Uruguay's major governmental effort that year was the development of a "Código del Niño" or Children's Code that spelled out children's rights to health, welfare, education, and decent living conditions, and created specific institutions to both run and oversee child and maternal aid programs.[57] While several other countries had previously enacted children's codes, it was Uruguay, with its well-developed welfare state, close links to the Instituto Internacional Americano de Protección a la Infancia, and extreme anxiety about infant mortality stagnation,[58] that served as a model in this area.

Other country representatives responded to Uruguay's experiences by recounting their own developments. Chilean delegate Dr. Coutts explained that since 1931, state law in his country also "defended" both mother and child through a variety of mechanisms. Mother's milk "is the exclusive property of the child, and, barring medical problems or the birth of her own second child, the mother is prohibited from providing wet nurse services until her child is five years old."[59] Expectant mothers were also guaranteed fully paid maternity leave for one month before and one month after childbirth, and infants in Chile were provided an allowance for one year of proper nutrition and physician visits. Uruguayan delegate Gomensoro countered that these laws were insufficient to reduce infant mortality, for his country had already enforced a policy of mandatory breastfeeding for the first six months of life; consequently further social measures were still needed to combat high rates of infant mortality.[60]

Then president of the Instituto Internacional Americano de Protección a la Infancia, Gregorio Aráoz Alfaro, noted that Argentina had seen a steady decline in its infant mortality rate from 143 per 1000 in 1912, to 88 per 1000 in 1932 (excluding the two provinces that had missing data). Particularly striking was the lower rate in the capital (63.8/1000) compared to that in the provinces. Aráoz Alfaro asserted that this difference was attributable to the greater severity of malaria and gastrointestinal diseases in tropical regions, and particularly to the absence or slow appearance of organizations to protect infancy, which abounded in Buenos Aires. He restated and added to Gomensoro's explanation for persistent high rates of infant mortality as (1) ignorance and lack of general culture and sanitary education, (2) poverty, which led to problems of nutrition, housing, general hygiene, and well-being, and (3) the lack of well-organized medical and social services, such as prenatal care. Accordingly, he argued, there existed a strong need for the centralization of services.[61]

More delegates chimed in. Dr. Bejarano of Colombia described the help his country had received from the Red Cross in establishing milk stations (*gotas de leche*), infant orphanages, and public dining halls for pregnant women. Cuba, too, could cite its efforts in homiculture, the creation of maternal and child health divisions within the Ministry of Health, and the development of community-run clinics.[62]

Several delegates championed regulations mandating the reporting of pregnancy so that the state could better meet the needs of poor women. The Argentinean delegate took this one step further, stressing that pregnant women should be divided into two groups, those who "expend energies" and those who did not. Those who expended energies required greater "maternal security."[63] While many of the proposed and existing activities bore the imprint of eugenic measures, with the state seeking to control the weakest in society, they invariably entailed "positive eugenic" measures, that is, improving conditions for mothers and children rather than, for example, prohibiting marriage or reproduction.

At the end of the 1934 conference four resolutions related to maternal and child health were approved: (1) the mandatory early declaration of pregnancy, (2) the intensification of infant mortality campaigns by member governments (especially in rural areas, with provisions to be made for infant protection centres, free medical services, and visiting nurses and midwives), (3) preschool health services (including the organization of parents' associations, which would be charged with disseminating modern scientific knowledge about the care and education of preschoolers), and (4) school health services, encompassing health education, periodic medical exams, and the prevention and early treatment of diseases. In addition, Uruguay was given a vote of applause for having established its Children's Code.[64] The Tenth Pan American Sanitary Conference, held in Bogotá in 1938, marked the presence of a woman delegate for the first time. Marion Crane, of the United States, received a special homage for her participation. Dr. Crane's presence may have been largely symbolic; however, at the level of the individual country substantive changes had taken place. Venezuela, for example, had established a National Puericulture Service in 1936 sponsoring prenatal and child visits, educational milk stations, dietary laboratories, foundling homes, mandatory birth certificates, maternal education, and licensing for nurses and midwives[65]. In his "Developments Related to the Protection of Infancy and Maternity in the American Republics since the IX Panamerican Sanitary Conference (1934),"[66] Aristides Moll reported that most republics now had bureaus dedicated to maternal and child health protection. These included new institutions in Argentina (which included a division of child cinematography), Bolivia, Brazil, Chile, Colombia, Costa Rica, Cuba, Ecuador, Mexico (which created a separate Departamento de Asistencia Social Infantil in 1937), Nicaragua, Paraguay, the United States, and Venezuela.[67]

Growing attention to maternal and child health through the first half of the twentieth century culminated in the development of a region-wide Children's Sanitary Code co-authored by the Instituto Internacional Americano de Protección a la Infancia, the PASB, and the U.S. Children's Bureau. Signed at the Ninth Pan American Child Congress held in Caracas in 1948, the code stipulated that:

all measures necessary must be taken in order to assure that all children, regardless of race, color, or creed, enjoy the best health conditions, based on adequate hygiene, together with the necessary good housing, sun, air, cleanliness, and clothing in order that they may benefit from the opportunity to live healthy, happy, and peaceful lives.[68]

Ironically, by the time the PASB had endorsed the Children's Sanitary Code, another international actor had appeared that would dislodge its short-lived advocacy of maternal and child health. The creation of UNICEF in 1946, initially designed to provide refugee and relief services to children in war-torn Europe, had important consequences for the PASB. It led to a large influx of maternal and child health resources to Latin America beginning in the 1950s, to an opportunity for collaboration with the PASB, and to the emergence of a strong competitor.[69] The appearance of UNICEF also marked the decline of the leadership provided by the Pan American Child Congresses, the disappearance of informal groupings of Latin American physicians and puericulturalists, and the placement of maternal and child health squarely on the international health agenda. It may well have been UNICEF that prompted the PASB to finally appoint its own regional consultant in maternal and child health. In 1950, Federico Gómez (former director of the Hospital Infantil in Mexico City) was sent on an extensive trip around the region to gather the necessary information to launch a campaign to reduce infant mortality.[70]

Conclusions

The fate of maternal and child health in the Pan American Sanitary Bureau illuminates several stories about the practice of international health in the early twentieth century. The first story covers the emergence of maternal and child health concerns in Latin America, tracing the cultural, scientific, and ideological differences with the U.S. context. This leads to the second story, which has to do with the interaction of the advocacy for maternal and child health with the structures of power within the PASB. The third story takes a broader look at the international development and diffusion of health priorities in the early twentieth century.

Latin Americans recognized the societal importance of maternal and child health almost at the same time as Europeans and North Americans did, but the impetus differed markedly. While industrializing and urbanizing countries typically faced a decline in fertility at the same time as the demand for labour was increasing, making infant, child, and maternal mortality a pressing public problem, Latin American countries made maternal and child health a priority in the absence of these economic pressures. Concern for the health of mothers and children was rooted in the region's indigenous cultures; by 1900 this concern began to resonate with state-building efforts and burgeoning nationalism. The receptiveness of physicians and feminists to French puericultural ideas and practices created an inviting environment for a modern maternal and child health movement.

It was not only the circumstances framing the emergence of maternal and child health that differed. The contrasting political contexts and cultural milieus in the United States and Latin America meant that the advocates for and organizational visions of maternal and child health also differed. The United States, a relatively weak state in the early twentieth century, enabled women to fill the social policy vacuum and become pioneers in the organization of maternal and child health services.[71] However, they never succeeded in converting these needs into a government responsibility or a universal right, nor were these women able to fend off the opposition of organized medicine, for the ideology of the private and voluntary provision of social services predominated in the United States.

A strong state—or even, as in the case of Uruguay, an early welfare state—characterized many Latin American countries in this period. Here maternal and child health services found a far more supportive home than in the United States. At the same time, many Latin physicians, rather than opposing the government's involvement, became leading advocates of maternal and child health and worked hand in hand with feminists.

This brings us to the second story of how these differences played out in the PASB's reluctant backing of maternal and child health. On one level, maternal and child health held little interest for the PASB's U.S. patron and its powerful directors who, at least in the bureau's early years, were far more concerned with controlling diseases that might interrupt trade than with other activities. The PASB gained consensus for these priorities at its international conferences and through the *Boletín de la Oficina Sanitaria Internacional*, which together served as an efficient means of influencing regional developments in public health. It was in the *Boletín* that the PASB first incorporated maternal and child health concerns, and it was here that the contrasting U.S. and Latin American positions became evident.

Gauging who influenced whom in the development of a maternal and child health agenda at the PASB remains a complicated question. Donna Guy has argued that regional and international activities surrounding maternal and child health and welfare, such as the Pan American Child Congresses and the *Boletín del Instituto Internacional Americano de Protección a la Infancia*, helped spur the development of local and national puericulture societies and journals. According to this argument, international scientific meetings and publications enabled national legislators (particularly in the host country) to develop laws protecting maternal and child health and welfare.[72]

The influence can also be argued in the other direction, however, with participating countries shaping one another and international organizations and journals. In the case of the PASB, it was member countries, rather than the U.S.-dominated governing committee, that insisted upon the placement of maternal and child health on the organizational agenda. This insistence was facilitated through correspondence and visits that took place among Latin American countries in non-conference years and through the existence of parallel Latin American organizations—such as the Instituto Internacional Americano de Protección a la Infancia. Developments in tiny Uruguay, for example, became a model for all of Latin America and helped shape maternal and child health policy throughout the region, if not the world. Thus the cultural and ideological differences over maternal and child health between the United States and Latin America did not hinder the field's development and diffusion.

Still, maternal and child health never became a cornerstone of PASB activities, as envisioned by its early advocates. A study of the PASB's governing board resolutions from 1942 to 1982 found that maternal and child health received the attention of just 2.4 per cent of all resolutions, the second lowest of all programmatic areas.[73] At the beginning of 1995, the special maternal and child health program was disbanded altogether, leaving it to be incompletely absorbed by the offices of communicable diseases and health promotion. This lack of attention might be partially explained by the presence of first the Instituto and then UNICEF, which allowed the organization to limit its activities in this area, given this presence of other actors.

The PASB's lack of appreciation for the importance of maternal and child health leads us to the third story of internationalism and the diffusion of public health ideas and practice. The Pan-American sanitary and eugenics congresses were among dozens of regional meetings held in the first decades of the twentieth century. Beginning in 1889, with the first International American Conference held in Washington, DC, Pan-American meetings were held on topics ranging from housing to sociology, commerce, crime, children, literature, Jews, coffee, highways, electricity, and democracy. Many of these meetings engendered active organizations at both the national and regional level, but few of them led to government decision-making. The Pan American Sanitary Conferences, by contrast, were attended by high-ranking government officials in a position to negotiate legally binding international agreements. Indeed, the Pan American Sanitary Code of 1924 was the first treaty of any kind to be signed by all American republics and remains in force today.

On one level, then, maternal and child health was not of sufficient legal importance to matter to the PASB. On another level, the development of maternal and child health in Latin America might be interpreted as a realm of inter-imperialist competition between French and U.S. public health models in which the United States lost. The U.S. model was technically oriented, with public-health problems addressed principally by the curative and preventive interventions of the medical profession under the aegis of voluntary agencies or local-level government. The French public health model, while still guided by medical experts, was far more socially oriented, with protective measures, such as maternal leave and mandatory breastfeeding for abandoned infants, designed by the state and implemented universally. If Latin Americans admired U.S. technical expertise, they were also skeptical of the country's public policies, ranging from eugenic sterilization laws to the lack of government commitment to maternal and child health needs, and were far more comfortable hosting French social policy ideas. But Latin Americans did far more than adapt French thinking to local conditions. Instead, the region's maternal and child health advocates used their own regional organizing capacity to further research, disseminate theory and practice, pioneer a children's code, and ultimately influence developments throughout the world. These forces insisted that the glue for the "broken pitcher" of infant mortality become a leading public health preoccupation for the Americas, with or without the Pan American Sanitary Bureau.

Notes

1 From 1902 to 1923 it was known as the International Sanitary Bureau (ISB), from 1923 to 1958 as the Pan American Sanitary Bureau (PASB), and since 1958 as the Pan American Health Organization (PAHO). This article will mainly employ the name Pan American Sanitary Bureau, because it was used during most of the period under investigation, but the other names will be employed when appropriate.

2 See "PAHO. In the beginning: 1920–20," *Boletín de la Oficina Sanitaria Panamericana* 113 (1992): 381–85; "PAHO. The Office in Expansion: 1920–1946, *Boletín de la Oficina Sanitaria Panamericana* 113 (1992): 386–95; and "Response to the Health Needs of Mothers and Children," *Boletín de la Oficina Sanitaria Panamericana* 113 (1992): 511–17. PAHO calls itself the historian of public health in the Americas (see *Pro Salute Novi Mundi: A History of the Pan American Health Organization* [Washington, DC: Pan American Health Organization, 1992], 268), but it has retained almost no primary, unpublished documents from before 1950. Many of the organization's own publications are more complete and in better condition in the medical libraries of towns in Latin America than they are at the central office in Washington. Fortunately, records of the Pan American Sanitary Conferences were preserved, and these documents, together with more abundant records available in the countries of the region, form the basis of this paper.

3 *Actas de la Novena Conferencia Sanitaria Panamericana* (Washington, DC: Oficina Sanitaria Panamericana, 100, 1935), 47. See also Norman Howard Jones, *The Pan American Health Organization: Origins and Evolution* (Geneva: World Health Organization, 1981), 7–12.

4 Philippe Ariès, *Centuries of Childhood* (New York: Vintage Books, 1962). Ariès's theory has been challenged, reinforced, and modified by a number of successors. See, for example, Peter Laslett, *The World We Have Lost* (London: Methuen, 1971); Lawrence Stone, *The Family, Sex and Marriage in England, 1500–1800* (New York: Harper Torchbooks, 1979); Edward Shorter, *The Making of the Modern Family* (New York: Basic Books, 1977); John Boswell, *The Kindness of Strangers: The Abandonment of Children in Western Europe from Late Antiquity to the Renaissance* (New York: Pantheon Books, 1988); Michael Anderson, *Approaches to the History of the Western Family, 1500–1914* (London: Macmillan, 1980); Rosemary O'Day, *The Family and Family Relationships, 1500–1900: England, France, and the United States of America* (London: Macmillan, 1994); and Linda Pollock, *Forgotten Children: Parent–Child Relations from 1500 to 1900* (Cambridge: Cambridge University Press, 1983).

5 E. A. Wrigley, *Population and History* (New York: McGraw-Hill, 1969); Simon Szreter, *Fertility, Class and Gender in Britain, 1860–1940* (Cambridge: Cambridge University Press, 1995); T. McKeown, *The Modern Rise of Population* (New York: Academic Press, 1976); T. McKeown and R. G. Record, "The Reason for the Decline of Mortality in England and Wales during the Nineteenth Century," *Population Studies* 16 (1962): 94–122. The McKeown thesis has been extensively analyzed by Simon Szreter in "The Importance of Social Intervention in Britain's Mortality Decline, 1850–1914: A Reinterpretation of the Role of Public Health," *Social History of Medicine* 1 (1988): 1–37; and in a debate with Sumit Guha in *Social History of Medicine* 7 (1994): 89–113, 269–82. See also Anne Hardy, *The Epidemic Streets: Infectious Disease and the Rise of Preventive Medicine* (Oxford: Clarendon Press, 1993); and Peter Razzell, *Essays in English Population History* (London: Caliban Books, 1994).

6 Nadine Lefaucheur, "La puériculture d'Adolphe Pinard," in *Darwinisme et Société*, edited by Patrick Tort (Paris: Presses Universitaires de France, 1992), 413–36;

and William H. Schneider, "Puericulture and the Style of French Eugenics," *History and Philosophy of the Life Sciences* 8 (1986): 265–77.

7 Several volumes comparing the history of maternal and child health and welfare movements in the West have appeared in the last few years, but little has been written about less industrialized cultures. A notable exception is Donna J. Guy, "The Pan American Child Congresses, 1916 to 1942: Pan Americanism, Child Reform, and the Welfare State in Latin America," *Journal of Family History* 23 (1998): 272–91.

See Seth Koven and Sonya Michel, eds., *Mothers of a New World: Maternalist Politics and the Origins of Welfare States* (New York: Routledge, 1993); Valerie Fildes, Lara Marks, and Hilary Marland, eds., *Women and Children First: International Maternal and Infant Welfare, 1870–1945* (London: Routledge,1992); Gisela Bock and Pat Thane, eds., *Maternity & Gender Policies: Women and the Rise of the European Welfare States 1880s–1950s* (New York: Routledge, 1991); and Diane Sainsbury, *Gender Equality and Welfare States* (London: Cambridge University Press, 1996).

Alisa Klaus has argued that "making maternity compatible with wage labor was a primary focus of many French maternal-and infant-health programs," in "Depopulation and Race Suicide: Maternalism and Pronatalist Ideologies in France and the United States," in *Mothers*, ed. Koven and Michel, 195. In the French case, concern about babies dying when mothers gave up breastfeeding to return to work, and low fertility because working-class women did not want to undergo the physical and financial suffering of pregnancy and motherhood, led to protective maternalist legislation. Such legislation served multiple interests: nationalism, women's rights, and the quelling of working-class strife.

In the United States, a female movement for maternal and child health was shaped by women in prominent positions who collaborated with the public health system in a key provision role. Strong women's leadership, however, did not translate into redistributive infant and maternal welfare laws in the United States. See Koven and Michel, *Mothers*, 20.

8 Samuel H. Preston and Michael R. Haines, *Fatal Years: Child Mortality in Late Nineteenth-Century America* (Princeton: Princeton University Press, 1991), 3–48.

9 Richard A. Meckel, *Save the Babies: American Public Health Reform and the Prevention of Infant Mortality, 1850–1929* (Baltimore: Johns Hopkins University Press, 1990), 5–6. See also Charles R. King, *Children's Health in America: A History* (New York: Twayne Publishers, 1993); Rima D. Apple, *Mothers and Medicine: A Social History of Infant Feeding, 1890–1950* (Madison: University of Wisconsin, 1987); and Janet Golden, *A Social History of Wet-nursing in America: From Breast to Bottle* (Cambridge: Cambridge University Press, 1996). For further examination of the family in the United States, see John Demos, *Past, Present, and Personal: The Family and the Life Course in American History* (New York: Oxford University Press, 1986); and Herbert Gutman, *The Black Family in Slavery and Freedom* (New York: Pantheon, 1976). For further examination of maternal and infant welfare in Europe and the commonwealth countries, see Deborah Dwork, *War Is Good for Babies and Other Children: A History of the Infant and Child Welfare Movement in England, 1898–1918* (London: Tavistock, 1987); Rachel G. Fuchs, *Poor and Pregnant in Paris: Strategies for Survival in the Nineteenth Century* (New Brunswick: Rutgers University Press, 1992); George D. Sussman, *Selling Mother's Milk: The Wet-nursing Business in France, 1715–1914* (Urbana: University of Illinois Press, 1982); Jane Lewis, *The Politics of Motherhood: Child and Maternal Welfare in England, 1900–1939* (London: Croom Helm; Montreal: McGill-Queen's University Press, 1980); Philippa Mein Smith, *Mothers and King Baby: Infant Survival and Welfare in an Imperial World:*

Australia 1880–1950 (Basingstoke: Macmillan, 1997); and Cynthia R. Comacchio, *"Nations Are Built of Babies": Saving Ontario's Mothers and Children 1900–1940* (Montreal: McGill-Queen's University Press, 1998).

10 See Comacchio, "Nations Are Built of Babies," and Katherine Arnup, *Education for Motherhood: Advice for Mothers in Twentieth-Century Canada* (Toronto: University of Toronto Press, 1994).

11 See Meckel, *Save*; Molly Ladd-Taylor, ed., *Raising a Baby the Government Way: Mothers' Letters to the Children's Bureau, 1915–1932* (New Brunswick: Rutgers University Press, 1986); and Molly Ladd-Taylor, "'Why does Congress wish Women and children to die?': The Rise and Fall of Public Maternal and Infant Health Care in the United States, 1921–1929," in *Women and Children First*, ed. Fides, Marks, and Marland, 121–32. See also Arthur Lesser, "The Origin and Development of Maternal and Child Health Programs in the United States," *American Journal of Public Health* 75 (1985): 590–98; and Barbara Starfield, "Giant Steps and Baby Steps: Toward Child Health," *American Journal of Public Health* 75 (1985): 599–604.

12 Max Shein, *El Niño Precolombino* (Mexico, D.F.: Editorial Villicaña S.A., 1986).

13 Donald B. Cooper, *Epidemic Disease in Mexico City, 1716–1813: An Administrative, Social, and Medical Study* (Austin: Institute of Latin American Studies, University of Texas Press, 1965).

14 Shein, *El Nino*, 91.

15 Oscar Lewis, *Life in a Mexican Village: Tepoztlán Restudied* (Urbana: University of Illinois Press, 1963); Kaja Finkler, *Women in Pain: Gender and Morbidity in Mexico* (Philadelphia: University of Pennsylvania Press, 1994). For more on midwifery practices in Mexico in the 1930s and 1940s, see Anne-Emanuelle Birn, "Skirting the Issue: Women and International Health in Historical Perspective," *American Journal of Public Health* 89 (1999): 399–407; and Anne-Emanuelle Birn, "Local Health and Foreign Wealth: The Rockefeller Foundation and Public Health in Mexico, 1924–1951" (PhD dissertation, Johns Hopkins University, 1993), especially chapter 3.

16 G. Gándara, "La Hierba de Leche o Ixbut, para la sesión del 7 de octubre de 1929 de la sociedad científica AAntonio Alzate," folder 10, box 7, Sección Higiene Infantil, Fondo Salubridad Pública, Archivo Histórico de la SSA, Mexico City.

17 Angela Thompson, "Children and Schooling in Guanajuato, Mexico, 1790–1840," *Secolas Annals* 23 (1992): 36–52. See also Alejandro Solís Matías, "Familia y Trabajadores en la Ciudad y el Campo en el Siglo XIX," in *Familia, Salud y Sociedad: Experiencias de Investigación en México*, ed. Francisco Javier Mercado, Catalina A. Denman, Agustin Escobar and Leticia Robles (Guadalajara: Universidad de Guadalajara, 1993), 209–19. In the same volume, see Carmen Castañeda, La Investigación Histórica sobre la Familia," 19–26. See also Alida Metcalf, *Family and Frontier in Colonial Brazil: Santana de Parniba, 1580–1822* (Berkeley: University of California Press, 1992).

18 Angela Thompson, "To Save the Children: Smallpox Inoculation, Vaccination, and Public Health in Guanajuato, Mexico, 1797–1840," *The Americas* 49 (1993): 431–55. For an interesting analysis of nineteenth-century infant mortality, see Lilia Oliver Sánchez, "La Mortalidad Infantil de Guadalajara Hacia 1887–1896, Analizada por el Doctor Miguel Mendoza López," *Quipu* 3 (1986): 177–88.

19 See Margarito Crispín Castellanos, "Hospital de Maternidad e Infancia: Una Perspectiva Histórica de un Centro de Beneficencia Pública de Fines del Siglo XIX," in, México, Secretaría de Salud. Dirección General de Atención Materno Infantil, *La Atención Materno Infantil: Apuntes para su Historia* (México, D.F.: Secretaría de Salud, 1993), 95–115.

20 See Ann S. Blum, "Public Welfare and Child Circulation, Mexico City, 1877 to 1925," *Journal of Family History* 23 (1998): 240–71; and José Pedro Barrán, *La Ortopedia de los Pobres: Medicina y Sociedad en el Uruguay del Novecientos.* Vol. 2 (Montevideo: Ediciones de la Banda Oriental, 1994).

21 See Alexandra Stern, "Responsible Mothers and Normal Children: Eugenics, Nationalism, and Welfare in Post-Revolutionary Mexico, 1920–1940," *Journal of Historical Sociology* 12 (1999): 369–97; and Nancy Leys Stepan, *"The Hour of Eugenics": Race, Gender, and Nation in Latin America* (Ithaca: Cornell University Press, 1991).

22 Francesca Miller, *Latin American Women and the Search for Social Justice* (Hanover: University Press of New England, 1991). See especially chapter 4, "Feminism and Social Motherhood, 1890–1938," 68–109. Also see Asunción Lavrin, *Women, Feminism, and Social Change in Argentina, Chile, and Uruguay* (Lincoln: University of Nebraska Press, 1995); and Maxine Molyneux, *Women's Movements in International Perspective: Latin America and Beyond* (New York: Palgrave, 2001).

23 See Katherine Elaine Bliss, "Prostitution, Revolution and Social Reform in Mexico City, 1918–1940" (PhD dissertation, University of Chicago, 1996); and Ann S. Blum, "Children without Parents: Law, Charity, and Social Practice, Mexico City, 1870–1940" (PhD dissertation, University of California, Berkeley, 1997). For more on the development of women's rights in Mexico, see Anna Macías, *Against All Odds: The Feminist Movement in Mexico to 1940* (Westport, CT: Greenwood Press, 1982).

24 *Conferencias Internacionales Americanas 1889–1936* (Washington, DC: Carnegie Endowment for International Peace, 1938), 425–26. Accused of fostering divisiveness, the Inter-American Commission of Women received front-page coverage on its 1947 congress, shortly before the commission's independence was removed. See Francesca Miller, "Latin American Feminism and the Transnational Arena," in *Women, Culture, and Politics in Latin America,* ed. Emilie Bergmann (Berkeley: University of California Press, 1990), 10–25.

25 Guy, "Pan American Child Congresses."

26 Carlos Finlay, the representative for Spain's colonies in the Caribbean, announced his discovery that the transmission of yellow fever was based upon an intermediate agent.

27 *Transactions of the First General International Sanitary Convention of the American Republics, Held at the New Willard Hotel, Washington, D.C., December 2, 3, and 4, 1902, under the Auspices of the Governing Board of the International Union of the American Republics* (Washington, DC: Government Printing Office, 1903), 9.

28 The sole exception was Uruguay's 1907 report on the problem of the transmission of measles and whooping cough in the schools.

29 A detailed description of the exquisite holiday festivities, together with photographs, held a prominent place in the meeting's *Transactions.* Elaborately detailed reports of the social activities held in conjunction with the conferences were included until the 1920s.

30 Juan J. Ulloa, Carlos Duran, Elias Rojas, and José M. Soto, "Report Presented by the Delegation of the Republic of Costa Rica," *Transactions of the Fourth International Sanitary Conference of the American Republics, Held in San José, Costa Rica, December 25, 1909 to January 3, 1910* (Washington, DC: Pan American Union, 1910), 133.

31 Ulloa, Duran, Rojas, and Soto, "Report," 138.

32 Ulloa, Duran, Rojas, and Soto, "Report," 23.

33 *Actas de la Sexta Conferencia Sanitaria Internacional de las Repúblicas Americanas Celebrada en Montevideo del 12 al 20 de Diciembre de 1920* (Washington, DC: Pan American Union, 1921), 156–61.

34 *Transactions of the Seventh Pan American Sanitary Conference of the American Republics, Held in Havana, Cuba, November 5 to 15, 1924* (Washington, DC: Pan American Sanitary Bureau, 1924), 128.

35 *Memoirs of Hugh Smith Cumming, Sr.*, passim, RG Cumming family papers, box 5, folder 6922, Manuscripts Department, University of Virginia Library.

36 Recent scholarship about the RF includes Marcos Cueto, ed., *Missionaries of Science: The Rockefeller Foundation and Latin America* (Bloomington: Indiana University Press, 1994); Ilana Löwy, "What/Who Should be Controlled: Opposition to Yellow Fever Campaigns in Brazil, 1900–1939," in *Contested Knowledge: Reactions to Western Medicine in the Modern Period*, ed. Andrew Cunningham and Bridie Andrews (Manchester: Manchester University Press, 1997); Steven Palmer, "Central American Encounters with Rockefeller Public Health, 1914–1921," in *Close Encounters of Empire: Writing the Cultural History of U.S.–Latin American Relations*, ed. Gilbert Joseph, Catherine LeGrand, and Ricardo Salvatore (Durham: Duke University Press, 1998), 311–32; Luis Castro-Santos, "A fundacaõ Rockefeller e o estado nacional (historia e politica de uma missao medica e sanitaria no brasil)," *Revista Brasileira de Estudos de Populacaõ* 6 (1989): 105–10; Paulo Gadelha, "Conforming Strategies of Public Health Campaigns to Disease Specificity and National Contexts: Rockefeller Foundation's Early Campaigns against Hookworm and Malaria in Brazil," *Parassitologia* 40 (1998): 159–75; Soma Hewa, *Colonialism, Tropical Disease and Imperial Medicine: Rockefeller Philanthropy in Sri Lanka* (Lanham, MD: University Press of America, 1995); and Anne-Emanuelle Birn, "A Revolution in Rural Health? The Struggle over Local Health Units in Mexico, 1928–1940," *Journal of the History of Medicine and Allied Sciences* 53 (1998): 43–76.

37 Anne-Emanuelle Birn, "Wa(i)ves of Influence: Rockefeller Public Health in Mexico, 1920–1950," *Studies in History and Philosophy of Biological and Biomedical Sciences* 31 (2000): 381–95.

38 Birn, "Skirting the Issue."

39 See Paul Weindling, ed. *International Health Organisations and Movements, 1918–1939* (Cambridge: Cambridge University Press, 1995), especially chapter by Martin Dubin.

40 Marta Balinska, *Une vie pour l'humanitaire : Ludwik Rajchman 1881–1965* (Paris: Éditions la découverte, 1995).

41 *Memoirs.*

42 N.a. *Pro Salute Novi Mundi: A History of the Pan American Health Organization* (Washington, DC: Pan American Health Organization, 1992), 118–26. In 1966, an English version of the *Bulletin of the Pan American Health Organization* began publication.

43 N.a. "Puericultura," *Boletín de la Oficina Sanitaria Panamericana* 27 (1948): 557–64; 18, 6 (1939); 14, 1 and 11 (1935); 11, 9 (1932).

44 N.a. "A Las Madres," *Boletín de la Oficina Sanitaria Panamericana* 19 (1940): 345–46.

45 See, for example, E. Blanche Sterling, *Higiene Prenatal*, Publicación 3 (1928), *Higiene de la Infancia* Publicación 11 (1929); and *Higiene Pre-Escolar* Publicación 16 (1929), Oficina Sanitaria Panamericana (Washington, DC: Unión Panamericana, 1928); E. Blanche Sterling, *Higiene de la Infancia* (1929); E. Blanche Sterling, *Higiene Pre-Escolar* (1929).).

46 N.a. *Los Derechos del Niño*, Publicación 24, Oficina Sanitaria Panamericana (Washington, DC: Unión Panamericana, 1930).

47 Early congresses focused on legislative issues; for example, prohibiting the consideration of children as criminals, laws relating to immigration, mandatory

schooling, health protection of school children. Subsequent congresses examined issues from a social perspective, such as eugenics, the causes of family disintegration, children in the workplace, care and education of indigenous children, and the fight against poverty. Later congresses focused more precisely on the role of government in the well-being of children through social security schemes, social and economic services for poor families, and postwar plans for children, such as libraries, savings institutions, and recreation centres. *Conferencias Internacionales Americanas, Primer Suplemento 1938–1942* (Washington, DC: Carnegie Endowment for International Peace, 1943).

48 Guy, "Pan American Child Congresses," 274.

49 Each country wishing to participate was asked to designate two representatives to be associated with the institute. One representative resided in Montevideo and could be a diplomat already posted there. The second was a technical representative who would be based in his or her own country. See Victor Escardó y Anaya, "Veniticinco anos del Consejo Directivo y de la Direccidn General," *Boletín del Instituto Internacional Americano de Protección a la Infancia* 26 (1952): 91–105; *Conferencias Internacionales Americanas 1889–1936*, 499; and *Conferencias Internacionales Americanas Primer Suplemento 1938–1942*, 449–50.

50 Luis Morquio's work ranged from the identification of skeletal muscular dystrophy to the importance of a mixed diet to the growth and development of the child. See Luis Morquio, "Sobre Alimentación Mixta," *Boletín del Instituto Internacional Americano de Protección de la Infancia* 9 (1935): 230–40.

51 See, for example, Juan Cesar García, "La Medicina Estatal en América Latina, 1880–1930," *Revista Latinoamericana de Salud* 1 (1981): 73–104; Patricio Márquez and Daniel Joly, "A Historical Overview of the Ministries of Public Health and the Medical Programs of the Social Security Systems in Latin America," *Journal of Public Health Policy* 7 (1986): 378–94; Carmelo Mesa-Lago, *El Desarrollo de la Seguridad Social en América Latina* (Santiago: United Nations, 1985); and *Pro Salute Novi Mundi*, 206–15.

52 *Eugenic News* 22 (1937): 94.

53 Stepan, *"The Hour of Eugenics."* For more on the eugenics-influenced maternal and child health movement in Mexico, see Stern, "Responsible Mothers."

54 Guy, "Pan American Child Congresses."

55 Stepan, *"The Hour of Eugenics,"* 187. See chapter 6, "U.S., Pan American, and Latin Visions of Eugenics," 171–95. When the eugenic horrors of Nazi Germany came to light, Latin Americans could easily substitute their positive eugenics measures with puericulture, denying any attachment to racist Anglo-Saxon eugenics.

56 *Actas Generales de la Novena Conferencia Sanitaria Panamericana celebrada en Buenos Aires del 12 al 22 de Noviembre de 1934* (Washington, DC: Pan American Sanitary Bureau, 1934), 328–29.

57 *Actas Generales*, 328–53, passim.

58 Anne-Emanuelle Birn, "Diarrhea, Donkeys, and Delmonicos: The Infant Mortality Conundrum in Uruguay, 1895–1943" (paper presented at the 73rd Annual Meeting of the American Association for the History of Medicine, Bethesda, MD, May 2000).

59 *Actas Generales*, 330.

60 *Actas Generales*, 331.

61 This had been declared at the Second Panamerican Children's Congress held in Montevideo in 1918. *Actas Generales*, 332–35.

62 *Actas Generales*, 337–38.

63 *Actas Generales*, 338–41.

64 *Actas Generales*, 418–19.

65 *Actas de la Décima Conferencia Sanitaria Panamericana, Bogotá, Septiembre 4–14, 1938* (Washington, DC: Pan American Sanitary Bureau, 1938), 772, 727–28.

66 *Actas de la Décima Conferencia*, 895–99.

67 While these developments continued at the country level through the 1940s, the response of the Pan American Sanitary Bureau was limited by wartime demands. The 11th Pan American Sanitary Conference held in Rio de Janeiro in 1942 focused on war sanitation and degenerative diseases. The twelfth conference held in Caracas in 1947 focused largely on the development of a draft agreement establishing formal ties with the new World Health Organization.

68 N.a. "Puericultura," *Boletín de la Oficina Sanitaria Panamericana* 27 (1948): 557–58.

69 Maggie Black, *Children First: The Story of UNICEF, Past and Present* (New York: Oxford University Press, 1996); "UNICEF en América Latina," *Boletín de la Oficina Sanitaria Panamericana* 29 (1950): 685; and Jorge Rosselot V., "UNICEF y la Protección de la Infancia 1946–1990," *Revista de Pediatría* (Santiago) 33 (1990): 165–77.

70 N.a. "Higiene Maternoinfantil," *Boletín de la Oficina Sanitaria Panamericana* 29 (1950): 686.

71 Kathryn Kish Sklar, "The Historical Foundations of Women's Power in the Creation of the American Welfare State, 1830–1930," in *Mothers*, ed. Koven and Michel. Also see Theda Skocpol, *Protecting Soldiers and Mothers: The Political Origins of Social Policy in the United States* (Cambridge: Belknap Press, 1992), especially 311–539, for a discussion of how means-tested New Deal programs displaced the maternalist social policies of the "woman movement."

72 Guy, "Pan American Child Congresses." Also see Victor Espinosa de los Reyes, "El Doctor Isidro Espinosa de los Reyes y los Inicios de la Atención Materno-Infantil en México," *Gaceta Médica de México* 117 (1991): 81–87.

73 "Estudio Sobre las Resoluciones de los Cuerpos Directivos de la OPS, 1942–82" (unpublished document, Pan American Health Organization, May 1985).

Entre la «Revanche» et la «Veillée» des berceaux

Les médecins québécois francophones, la mortalité infantile, et la question nationale, 1910–1940

❧

Denyse Baillargeon

> Une conférence retentissante du Père Louis Lalande a ramené notre attention sur le grave problème de notre natalité. D'elle-même la «Revanche des berceaux» devrait faire songer à la «Veillée des berceaux». Cette «Veillée», l'on nous a dit éloquemment ce qu'elle exige.
> — Lionel Groulx[1]

Au Québec, les questions démographiques ont toujours été scrutées et commentées à travers le prisme de la question nationale. Pour s'en convaincre, il suffit d'évoquer les déclarations alarmistes de nombreux observateurs au sujet de la diminution de la fécondité des Québécoises francophones depuis les années 1960 et les différentes législations linguistiques adoptées dans le but de «franciser» les immigrants en réponse à cette baisse. Le phénomène de la mortalité infantile, dont la société québécoise a commencé à s'inquiéter au tournant du XXᵉ siècle, ne fait pas exception à cette règle : tous ceux et celles – médecins, hommes politiques, intellectuels, membres du clergé et de groupes de femmes – qui sont intervenus sur ce sujet n'ont pas manqué de souligner les liens entre la survie des enfants et celle de la nation. Mais le nationalisme a fait plus que simplement alimenter ou exacerber les angoisses des élites franco-québécoises devant les décès infantiles. En fait, un examen attentif du discours médical pour les premières décennies du XXᵉ siècle montre que l'idéologie nationaliste a servi de cadre général d'interprétation pour appréhender ce «nouveau» problème social.

Le dépouillement des principales revues professionnelles destinées aux médecins et aux hygiénistes (*L'Union médicale du Canada*, le *Bulletin sanitaire* et le *Canadian Public Health Journal*) de même que d'autres publications à diffusion plus large (comme la revue féministe *La Bonne parole*, les brochures de l'École sociale populaire et la revue populaire *La Santé*) et les rapports annuels du Conseil d'hygiène de la province de Québec

(CHPQ) et du Service provincial d'hygiène (SPH) pour la période 1900–1940, permet en effet de constater que les médecins, hygiénistes et pédiatres, qui ont alimenté les débats publics autour de la mortalité infantile par leurs écrits et façonné l'opinion à ce sujet l'envisageaient dans les mêmes termes que la question nationale. De fait, cette élite médicale qui occupait des postes de pouvoir dans l'administration de la santé publique ou qui enseignait dans les universités francophones, entretenait des liens souvent étroits avec les cercles nationalistes, notamment le groupe de *L'Action française* et la Société Saint-Jean-Baptiste[2], et pouvait difficilement faire abstraction de ses convictions politiques lorsqu'elle se prononçait sur une question aussi délicate que la mort de milliers d'enfants. C'est donc en se référant à la destinée historique tragique des Canadiens français, à leur domination économique et politique et à leurs traits identitaires distinctifs que ces médecins ont tenté de comprendre et d'expliquer les taux particulièrement élevés de mortalité infantile qui sévissaient au Québec, comparativement au Canada anglais. Il en a résulté une certaine ambiguïté dans leur manière de considérer les décès d'enfants car le nationalisme qui les incitait à se scandaliser de la mort de tant de petits Québécois francophones, leur fournissait en même temps des arguments pour justifier, au moins partiellement, cette situation. Jusqu'aux années 1930, la mortalité infantile, perçue comme une marque «d'infériorité» a même souvent été mise en parallèle avec la «proverbiale» fécondité des mères canadiennes-françaises, un signe de supériorité qui lui faisait contrepoids et expliquait, aux dires de plusieurs, le nombre catastrophique des décès infantiles. Suivant le discours médico-nationaliste, la «Revanche» des berceaux devenait donc, en elle-même, un obstacle à leur «Veillée». La natalité légendaire des Québécoises francophones, élevée au rang de mythe par les nationalistes, pourrait ainsi expliquer, du moins en partie, le fait que les mesures de santé publique adoptées au Québec au cours de cette période aient été moins vigoureuses qu'en Ontario, la «province sœur» qui servait pourtant de point de référence à ces médecins.

La mortalité infantile au Québec

La fragilité des nourrissons face à la maladie et la mort n'était certes pas un phénomène nouveau à la fin du XIXe siècle, mais c'est à cette époque qu'elle est devenue une source de préoccupations pour les élites québécoises. La mise en place, en 1893, d'un système de collecte des statistiques démographiques couvrant toute la province et permettant d'obtenir des données plus globales et plus fiables[3] a probablement contribué à cette prise de conscience, mais celle-ci s'inscrivait également dans une mouvance occidentale. Les nombreux bouleversements socio-économiques engendrés par l'industrialisation et l'urbanisation, conjugués à une forte poussée de fièvre nationaliste, suscitaient en effet de graves inquiétudes au sujet de l'avenir dans les pays industrialisés, ce qui a favorisé la montée d'un vaste mouvement en faveur de la sauvegarde de l'enfance. Autant en Europe de l'Ouest qu'en Amérique du Nord, la préservation de la vie des nouveau-nés est alors apparue comme la solution la plus évidente pour résoudre un ensemble de problèmes sociaux réels ou appréhendés[4]. Que ce soit pour combler les besoins en main-d'œuvre du capitalisme industriel alors en pleine expansion, contrer la baisse de la natalité et ainsi assurer la sécurité des frontières face à un ennemi redouté, comme ce fut le cas en France, préserver la prédominance des populations blanches face à l'arrivée d'immigrants, ou même la suprématie d'un Empire, comme dans le cas britannique, les sociétés occidentales avaient des raisons très diverses de s'inquiéter[5]. S'appuyant sur la révolution pasteurienne qui avait permis de mieux comprendre l'origine des maladies diarrhéiques responsables de la plus grande proportion des décès de nourrissons, des groupes réformistes, que les médecins n'ont pas tardé à dominer, ont alors entrepris de combattre ce «fléau» qui risquait d'entraver le «progrès, l'existence, et la suprématie des diverses collectivités»[6]. La mise en place de dépôts de lait puis de cliniques de puériculture, l'adoption de législations pour rendre la pasteurisation du lait obligatoire, la publication de brochures à l'intention des mères sur l'hygiène du nourrisson, la création de structures gouvernementales et d'organismes privés voués au bien-être de l'enfance ont fait partie de l'arsenal de mesures déployées dans la plupart de ces pays pour mettre un terme à ce qui prenait figure d'hécatombe.

La mobilisation autour de la cause des enfants qui s'est amorcée au Québec dans les années 1890 pour s'amplifier dans les premières décennies du XXe siècle, s'inscrivait donc dans un courant qui débordait largement ses frontières. Les médecins québécois francophones qui se sont hissés à l'avant-garde de ce mouvement se trouvaient néanmoins confrontés à une situation presque sans équivalent parmi les grandes puissances occidentales car les décès d'enfants atteignaient ici des niveaux records[7] et survenaient principalement au sein du groupe ethnique auquel ils appartenaient. De fait, comme le montre le premier tableau présenté en annexe, pour l'ensemble de la période où il est possible d'établir une comparaison, le taux de mortalité des enfants québécois a constamment dépassé la moyenne canadienne, alors qu'il était entre 53 % et 66 % plus élevé qu'en Ontario[8]. L'écart était tel que lorsque le Québec a finalement adhéré au système national de la statistique de l'état civil en 1926, le Conseil canadien pour le bien-être de l'enfance et de la famille (*Canadian Council on Child and Family Welfare*) n'avait pu s'empêcher de faire remarquer, de manière plutôt sarcastique, que son inclusion avait eu un effet désastreux sur le taux canadien :

In her Confederation memorial year, Canada enjoys the apparently unenviable distinction of attaining the highest infant mortality rate recorded in recent years [...] In 1926, Quebec province entered the Registration Area. This province, for years has recorded the highest infant mortality rate in the Dominion. Consequently, its inclusion in the national statistics has sent the national rate from 78.6 to 101.9 per 1000 living birth. The rate for the former Registration Area, had Quebec not been included, would have stood at 80. The Quebec rate of 142 is therefore some 75% higher then the rate for the other eight provinces, but this rate in itself is an improvement over what has prevailed in Quebec in some recent years9.

Que cette mauvaise performance québécoise était due essentiellement aux francophones ne faisait non plus aucun doute : à l'échelle même du Québec, c'était surtout dans les comtés où ils étaient majoritaires que les taux de mortalité infantile atteignaient des sommets, alors qu'ils étaient les moins élevés – souvent deux et trois fois moins élevés – dans les comtés à prédominance anglophone[10]. En 1926, par exemple, le rapport du Service provincial d'hygiène[11] spécifiait :

Le comté à avoir le plus bas taux de mortalité infantile est Vaudreuil avec 48.4 par mille naissances vivantes, suivi par Châteauguay, 84.7, Brome, 92.2 et Huntingdon, 96.2, tous comtés en partie de population anglaise. Les comtés à avoir un taux considérable sont : Québec, 178.8; Montcalm, 174.7; Labelle, 170.0 et Saint-Maurice, 168.3, tous comtés à forts groupes français. Nous trouvons donc dans notre province même le terme de la comparaison entre comtés anglais et comtés français de même qu'entre les provinces du Canada12.

La situation était tout aussi démarquée à Montréal où le Service de santé municipal[13] établissait des statistiques par groupe ethno-religieux : non seulement la mortalité des bébés franco-catholiques était la plus élevée – un phénomène qui remontait d'ailleurs au milieu du XIXe siècle[14] – , mais elle a mis plus de temps à diminuer au sein de cette communauté que chez les autres groupes comme le montre le tableau II, en annexe.

Des différences aussi appréciables entre les taux de mortalité infantile francophone et anglophone n'ont pas manqué de faire vibrer la corde nationaliste du clergé catholique, des intellectuels nationalistes, des groupes féministes, des hygiénistes et autres spécialistes de l'enfance. À l'instar de leurs collègues canadiens et étrangers, les médecins canadiens-français qui ont principalement alimenté les débats publics autour de cette question ont constamment fait référence à leur savoir scientifique pour justifier leurs prétentions à diriger la lutte contre la mortalité infantile et à s'affirmer comme de nouveaux «experts» auprès des mères et des pouvoirs publics, mais c'est aussi au nom de la sauvegarde nationale qu'ils ont cherché à asseoir leur autorité[15]. La science, qu'ils incarnaient, se plaçait au service de la nation pour mieux assurer sa défense, un argument qui leur a valu l'appui de certains leaders nationalistes «traditionalistes», membres du clergé et de la petite bourgeoisie, même quand ils prônaient une plus grande intervention de l'État dans le domaine socio-sanitaire[16]. De fait, comme l'ont déjà souligné plusieurs historiens, la santé publique a sans doute été un domaine où l'intervention étatique a été la plus soutenue grâce, notamment, à l'action et aux pressions exercées par une élite médicale animée par un fort sentiment nationaliste, mais aussi par une volonté d'accroître son prestige socioprofessionnel[17]. Dans une société où l'Église s'est opposée de manière souvent virulente à l'action étatique sous prétexte de préserver le caractère confessionnel des institutions sociales perçues comme un des piliers de la pérennité nationale, l'instauration d'un système d'unités sanitaires de comtés – un réseau qui fera la fierté des hygiénistes québécois et l'envie de leurs collègues des autres provinces – , ou encore la mise en place d'un système municipal de consultations pour nourrissons à Montréal[18], deviennent d'autant plus notables[19]. Comme le mentionne François Guérard, les historiens qui se sont penchés sur l'histoire de la santé au Québec ont largement contribué à déconstruire la thèse du «retard» québécois, attribué en bonne partie à la présence d'un clergé au conservatisme frileux et capable d'imposer son ordre du jour à un État aux convictions libérales chancelantes[20]. La réfutation de cette thèse en matière de santé publique notamment ne doit pas cependant faire oublier les spécificités qui ont caractérisé le développement de ces infrastructures. En invoquant le thème de la survivance, les médecins se trouvaient en effet à reprendre à leur compte les grands paramètres de la vision nationaliste de la société québécoise, ce qui n'a pas été sans conséquence sur le type et l'ampleur des services offerts à la population féminine et à leurs nourrissons. Un bref retour sur les débats et la rhétorique nationalistes des premières décennies du XXe siècle permettra de voir dans quelle mesure le discours médical en a été tributaire.

La nation en péril

À partir du dernier tiers du XIXe siècle et jusqu'aux années 1920, les rapports entre francophones et anglophones à l'intérieur du Canada sont devenus de plus en plus tendus. La création d'une nouvelle entité politique en 1867 avait fait miroiter la possibilité pour les Canadiens français de préserver leur identité grâce à l'action d'un gouvernement provincial nanti de nouvelles juridictions, et même d'étendre la présence française et catholique à travers le nouveau Dominion : le passage du temps leur avait plutôt démontré que l'élite politique et économique anglophone détenait les rênes du pouvoir bien en main et qu'elle était en mesure de façonner l'avenir du pays à son image. En fait, le «siècle du Canada» s'ouvrait sur une série de constats alarmants : les francophones étaient marginalisés politiquement au sein de la députation fédérale, dominés économiquement à l'intérieur même du territoire où ils étaient pourtant majoritaires, bafoués dans leurs droits constitutionnels dans les autres provinces et menacés dans leur identité et leur culture par le nouveau mode de vie urbain. Les immigrants qui débarquaient dans le port de Québec pour s'établir dans la province, ou plus souvent pour prendre le train en direction de l'Ouest canadien, allaient grossir les rangs des anglophones, tandis que les communautés françaises hors Québec luttaient contre l'assimilation. Pour faire bonne mesure, des milliers de Québécois francophones prenaient la direction des États-Unis, diminuant un peu plus le poids démographique, et donc politique, de leurs concitoyens laissés derrière. Pendant ce temps, les Canadiens anglais avaient commencé à afficher leur attachement à l'Empire de manière ostentatoire, proposant même que le Canada participe aux guerres impériales. Et d'autres malheurs étaient encore à venir, comme allaient le démontrer la crise de la conscription de 1917 et celle des écoles ontariennes qui s'est amplifiée à peu près au même moment, sans compter la montée du féminisme, une «importation» anglo-saxonne aux dires de plusieurs, qui incitait les femmes à réclamer le droit de vote et l'accès aux études supérieures, au risque de détruire la famille[21].

L'addition de ces événements, perçus comme autant d'attaques contre l'épanouissement et l'existence même de la collectivité francophone, avait de quoi alimenter un climat d'anxiété. Mais si la plupart des nationalistes s'entendaient pour dire que l'avenir de leur peuple était grandement menacé, les avis divergeaient sur les solutions à mettre en œuvre pour reprendre l'initiative. Entre le repli sur la terre et la conquête de nouveaux outils économiques, quelle était la meilleure manière de favoriser le développement économique et social des Canadiens français? Au tout début du siècle, Errol Bouchette affirmait qu'ils devaient «s'emparer de l'industrie», un mot d'ordre que plusieurs ont repris à sa suite. Pour beaucoup d'autres, cependant, cette stratégie comportait le risque de voir les hautes valeurs spirituelles des Franco-catholiques sombrer dans le matérialisme le plus abject : s'emparer du sol leur paraissait plus sûr car la vie rurale placerait les Canadiens français à l'abri des influences culturelles venues de l'étranger, et dont la ville faisait étalage. Conscients de leur incapacité à renverser des tendances aussi lourdes que l'industrialisation et l'urbanisation, un troisième groupe, dont la revue *L'Action française* s'est fait l'écho, en arrivait finalement à suggérer un développement plus mesuré et un équilibre plus harmonieux entre les divers secteurs de l'activité économique, dans lequel les francophones du Québec pourraient plus facilement trouver une place, tout en préservant leur identité[22].

Les débats qui ont agité les cercles nationalistes durant les premières décennies du XXe siècle laissent voir une certaine ambivalence face aux remèdes à appliquer pour assurer la perpétuation de la nation, car il ne s'agissait pas seulement de favoriser l'affirmation économique des francophones, mais d'y parvenir sans sacrifier leur «nature» profonde. Face aux dominants anglophones, souvent gratifiés d'un esprit matérialiste, rationaliste et individualiste et d'une capacité quasi naturelle à s'adapter au monde «moderne», les nationalistes ont en effet construit une identité francophone reposant sur le triptyque de la langue, de la foi et de la vocation rurale, et sur l'attachement des Canadiens français aux valeurs familiales et au souvenir des ancêtres. Cette «mentalité» proprement canadienne-française, imprégnée de hautes valeurs spirituelles, paraissait plus saine, supérieure à la mentalité anglophone, parce qu'elle refusait de bousculer hâtivement les traditions pour faire place à la nouveauté, un penchant typiquement anglais, et d'accorder trop d'importance aux biens de ce monde. Mais la loyauté envers des institutions séculaires, comme la paroisse et la famille, pouvait aussi s'avérer néfaste car elle abandonnait aux anglophones tout le champ de l'économie qui représentait le principal instrument de leur puissance[23]. Pour certains, il était faux de prétendre que les anglophones avaient des qualités innées qui leur conféraient une supériorité dans les affaires ou que les francophones ne pouvaient les égaler sur leur propre terrain sans trahir leurs spécificités culturelles et nationales[24] : ces spécificités n'ont cependant jamais été remises en question.

Formant un groupe hétérogène composé de laïcs et de membres du clergé, d'hommes et de femmes, de partisans de l'idéologie libérale et cléricale, les nationalistes ont donc formulé de multiples réponses à la question de l'affirmation nationale des Canadiens français. Dans l'ensemble cependant, leur discours était empreint d'un sentiment d'infériorité face au groupe économiquement et politiquement dominant, compensé par la certitude d'appartenir à une collectivité moralement supérieure. Comme l'a déjà fait remarquer Susan Mann, les traits culturels que les nationalistes attribuaient aux Francophones et aux Anglophones ressemblaient aussi étrangement aux caractéristiques associées aux deux sexes[25]. Dans cette équation, la «féminité» du Québec s'exprimait par une «sensibilité» aux choses de l'esprit, mais aussi, pourrionsnous ajouter, par son «retard», par sa difficulté à «évoluer» sans trahir sa «nature» profonde et par son statut de victime : en imposant unilatéralement des changements majeurs qui bouleversaient les rapports sociaux, économiques et politiques, le Canada anglais menaçait l'intégrité du Canada français. Ceux qui préconisaient une plus grande participation des francophones aux domaines de la finance et de l'entreprise y voyaient d'ailleurs un moyen d'affirmer la «virilité ethnique» du peuple canadien-français, en d'autres termes de le «masculiniser» à l'égal des Canadiens anglais et des autres nations mieux affirmées[26].

La mortalité infantile faisait partie intégrante des angoisses des nationalistes car c'est avant tout par la force du nombre qu'ils comptaient raffermir la position de la collectivité francophone et assurer son plein épanouissement. «Notre premier capital, c'est le capital humain», affirmait Lionel Groulx, une déclaration maintes fois reprise par les leaders issus de tous les horizons, clérical, politique, économique, féministe, comme médical. Considérée sur le même plan que l'ensemble des «maux» qui affligeaient la collectivité francophone, la mort des enfants canadiens-français a ainsi fait l'objet d'un discours qui reprenait à son compte l'analyse nationaliste de la position des Canadiens français dans l'espace politique canadien. Hommes de «science», mais aussi hommes de leur époque, les médecins qui se sont prononcés publiquement sur cette question ne pouvaient sans doute pas plus échapper à la couleur du temps nationaliste qu'aux préjugés de classe ou de genre qui ont guidé leurs interventions en matière de sauvegarde de l'enfance[27]. De fait, comme on le verra dans la suite de ce texte, leur diagnostic au sujet de la mortalité infantile reflète les préoccupations d'une société incertaine de son statut, de son avenir et de sa capacité à relever les défis de la «modernité».

Une véritable saignée nationale

Les nationalistes de toutes allégeances, autant hommes que femmes, s'entendaient parfaitement au moins sur un point : les mères canadiennes-françaises, réputées pour leur nombreuse progéniture, constituaient le pilier de la survie des francophones en Amérique. Gardiennes de la langue et des traditions, elles assuraient la reproduction de la «race» dans tous les sens du terme, c'est-à-dire biologiquement, mais aussi culturellement. Chaque bébé qu'elles mettaient au monde représentait un actif inestimable pour la nation et chaque décès infantile, une perte irremplaçable. La mortalité infantile est une «véritable saignée nationale», disait le Dr C.-N. Valin, professeur d'hygiène à la Faculté de médecine de l'Université Laval à Montréal, en 1909, comme si ces décès constituaient une plaie béante par où s'échapperait le sang de la race. Saignée économique d'abord, puisque chaque enfant a une «valeur sociale» et «qu'il coûte à la famille une certaine somme d'argent et d'effort vital», somme dépensée en pure perte quand finalement la naissance se soldait par la mort. Saignée démographique surtout puisque, additionnée à l'émigration des Canadiens français aux États-Unis et à l'immigration en provenance de l'Europe, la mortalité infantile faisait perdre «du terrain [aux Canadiens français] dans le domaine des affaires et dans le domaine de la politique». Elle constituait, enfin, un véritable danger pour l'intégrité nationale, toujours aux dires du Dr Valin, car les enfants décédés étaient «remplacés» par des immigrants «de provenance douteuse» et «de santé physique et morale suspecte». Ceux-ci, ajoutait-il, «altèrent par leur diversité la physionomie de notre peuple et perturbent notre atmosphère sociale par l'introduction de leurs mœurs particulières»[28].

Ce genre de discours xénophobe, qui amalgamait la question de l'immigration et celle de la mortalité infantile, n'était pas unique aux francophones au début du siècle[29]. Partout au Canada, l'immigration suscitait des débats sociaux enflammés et une grande méfiance envers les nouveaux venus de plus en plus nombreux, réputés appartenir à des «races inférieures» et d'être porteurs de tares génétiques risquant de contaminer la population d'ascendance britannique (*british «stock»*)[30]. La peur de la «dégénérescence» de la race touchait d'autant plus les Anglo-canadiens qu'au même moment, la diminution de leur taux de natalité laissait également entrevoir son «suicide»[31]. Comme le faisait remarquer Mme «Jules» Tessier, fondatrice des Gouttes de lait de Québec, à un auditoire anglophone en 1917, le taux de natalité des Canadiennes françaises ne suscitait pas encore ce genre de craintes : «Be it as it stay [*sic*], there is no danger of race suicide on this part of the world»[32]. Du côté anglophone, cependant, certains groupes réformistes et religieux croyaient possible de «canadianiser» une partie des immigrants[33], tandis que chez les francophones, on considérait que ces «étrangers» présentaient des traits culturels trop différents pour qu'il soit possible d'espérer leur conversion aux valeurs de la société canadienne-française. Une immigration française aurait été acceptable parce que plus facilement assimilable croyait-on, mais il n'y avait guère à espérer de ce côté. Comme le soulignait le Dr Raoul Masson, professeur de pédiatrie et de clinique infantile à l'Université de Montréal, les Canadiens français avaient été laissés à eux-mêmes par leur ancienne mère patrie, au plan démographique à tout le moins, avec pour résultat qu'ils ne pouvaient compter que sur leurs propres moyens :

Éloignés de la France [...] par des conditions politiques et géographiques; encerclés par un puissant voisin [...] n'ayant ni notre idéal, ni notre mentalité, ni notre langue; faisant partie intégrante d'un Dominion composé de neuf provinces dont huit sont presque en totalité peuplées de compatriotes ne possédant ni notre langue, ni notre religion; dominés par une puissance qui n'a pas d'intérêt marqué à nous voir prospérer comme race ethnique; privés du secours que nous apporterait une immigration française [...] nous sommes réduits, pour assurer notre avenir national, à nos propres ressources, devrions-nous dire à notre natalité et à la survivance de nos enfants.[34]

Résumée de la sorte, la position des francophones était certainement inquiétante, presque désespérée : comme une forteresse assiégée par des ennemis qui se seraient ligués contre elle, les Canadiens français n'avaient d'autres alliés qu'eux-mêmes, d'autres armes que celle de la démographie. L'image de la victime, souvent véhiculée par les nationalistes du début du siècle quand ils débattaient des conséquences des bouleversements socio-économiques pour l'intégrité du Canada français, est ici manifeste : alimentée par le premier conflit mondial, la métaphore guerrière sera parfois poussée à l'extrême. Ainsi, le Père Bernier, o.m.i., curé de Hull et conférencier invité lors de la 8e convention des services sanitaires qui se tenait dans cette ville en 1920, affirmait que la mortalité infantile était «d'autant plus désastreuse que nous sommes dans la fournaise du combat, numériquement inférieurs à nos ennemis»[35]. Le Dr Édouard Laberge, médecin hygiéniste à la Ville de Montréal et un ardent promoteur des Gouttes de lait, n'osait pas, quant à lui, aller jusque là, mais il soutenait néanmoins que la campagne contre la mortalité infantile représentait, au plan national, «une question de vie ou de mort» car c'est uniquement par le nombre que les Canadiens français pouvaient espérer s'imposer. «Ne comptons pas sur la générosité, sur l'esprit de justice de nos *amis* d'autres nationalités: ce serait peine perdue», concluait-il[36]. Évidemment, avec des amis aussi peu accommodants, il n'était pas vraiment nécessaire d'invoquer un ennemi.

Tout comme le Dr Masson, cité plus haut, de même que plusieurs autres, le Dr Joseph Baudouin, sans doute l'un des hygiénistes les plus influents de son époque[37], considérait que la lutte contre la mortalité infantile représentait l'ultime recours pour les francophones qui n'avaient guère le choix de leurs stratégies de survivance : «Pour pourvoir à notre développement normal et pour en accélérer la marche, nous avons besoin d'une population plus nombreuse que ni l'immigration, ni l'augmentation des naissances ne peuvent nous fournir. Il ne nous reste donc d'autre alternative que de diminuer nos décès»[38]. Ainsi, c'est parce qu'elle était devenue la seule issue nationale possible que la survie des enfants faisait figure d'urgence et leur décès, de véritable désastre : l'enjeu se situait non pas au plan individuel, mais bien collectif. Au début du siècle, alors que les victimes infantiles québécoises, en grande majorité francophones, se chiffraient à plus de 10 000 chaque année, il n'y avait donc pas de mots assez forts pour décrire le phénomène. «Malheur irréparable», «massacre d'Hérode permanent», «atroce fléau», «calamité, saignée, catastrophe ou plaie nationales», le macabre décomptage annuel provoquait l'effroi et inspirait des métaphores des plus ima-gées.[39] Mais il suscitait aussi un profond malaise parmi les membres de l'élite car tout autant que le nombre, c'était la réputation des Canadiens français qui était en jeu, comme l'exprimait le Dr Joseph Gauvreau, registraire du Collège des Médecins et Chirurgiens de la province :

...tous les ans, le cortège des petits corbillards, s'en est allé grossissant à tel point qu'il nous a fallut (*sic*), un jour, subir l'humiliation de s'entendre dire, par une statistique étrangère, que seule l'insalubre et sale ville de Calcutta compte plus d'enfants morts que la nôtre, et un autre jour, par un journal soustrait depuis de la circulation, que les Canadiens-français (*sic*) ne sont vraiment supé-rieurs que sur un point, celui de la mortalité infantile[40].

En d'autres termes, la mortalité infantile, en plus de représenter une menace pour l'ensemble de la collectivité, mettait à nu une autre facette de l'état d'infériorité des Canadiens français et leur attirait un mépris quasi justifié. «La vérité cruelle et désolante», affirmait Marie Gérin-Lajoie, présidente de la Fédération nationale Saint-Jean Bap-tiste, la plus importante organisation féministe de l'époque, au début de la Première guerre, «est que nos bébés meurent dans des proportions qui nous rapprochent des barbares»[41]. Dans ce jugement lapidaire se trou-vent concentrées toute la honte et la frustration de voir que les franco-phones se comportaient de manière à s'exclure du nombre des nations civilisées, titre attribué à celles qui parvenaient à sauver leurs enfants de la mort[42]. La fierté nationale, déjà passablement amochée par l'infério-rité économique des Canadiens français, aussi bien que sa pérennité, exi-geaient «que la Canadienne étonne les autres races, non seulement par ses mœurs austères et sa capacité prolifique», mais aussi par son aptitude à élever «jusqu'à l'âge adulte les êtres qui ont été confiés à sa sollicitude maternelle»[43]. Celles qui savaient si bien donner l'exemple en matière de moralité sexuelle en produisant de nombreux enfants pouvaient, en fait devaient, relever le défi de leur sauvegarde. Premières responsables de la mortalité infantile, c'est à elles que revenait la tâche d'effacer le dés-honneur qui ternissait la renommée de toute la collectivité.

Le taux effarant de la mortalité infantile au Québec n'a effectivement pas manqué de soulever bien des critiques de la part de la communauté anglophone, que ce soit à l'intérieur ou à l'extérieur de la province, au point où, en 1921, le Dr E.-M. Savard, inspecteur général du CHPQ, s'est cru obligé de spécifier que le Québec n'était pas «la nécropole des bébés comme certains semblaient le croire»[44]. Comme on peut s'en douter, ce genre de dénégation n'a pas suffit à faire taire les critiques. Le laxisme des autorités publiques en matière de législation, sur la pasteurisation du lait notamment, et le peu d'effort et d'argent consentis pour mettre en place des structures socio-sanitaires efficaces étaient plus particulièrement pointés du doigt par des médecins anglophones, certains n'hésitant pas à taxer la province de *backwardness*[45]. Ainsi, dans son rapport pour l'année 1934–35, le directeur du SPH commentait : «On ne manque pas dans certains milieux de faire à notre désavantage des comparaisons entre la province de l'Ontario et la nôtre et, très souvent, on cite le taux de la mortalité infantile et celui de la mortalité par tuberculose dans la province voisine, et on ne manque pas de dire que nous faisons bien peu ici pour améliorer la santé publique»[46].

Devant l'opprobre que s'attiraient les Canadiens français, il s'est bien trouvé au moins un médecin pour prétendre qu'il valait mieux «taire la vérité […] parce que c'[était] injurieux pour la race»[47], mais cette position est demeurée marginale. La plupart des médecins et des hygiénistes étaient plutôt d'avis qu'il ne fallait pas hésiter à admettre les faits : «Quoique toujours il soit pénible de reconnaître un tort ou d'accuser une infériorité, il faut avoir le courage d'avouer le mal que l'on veut guérir» soutenait par exemple le Dr Raoul Masson au milieu des années 1920[48]. De toute façon, il aurait été bien difficile d'enterrer tous ces morts en secret ou de les faire disparaître des statistiques. Reconnaître le problème permettait au moins aux médecins d'expliquer la lenteur des progrès réalisés et, ainsi, de réhabiliter l'image quelque peu ternie des Canadiens français. À la décharge de leurs compatriotes ils ont invoqué diverses circonstances atténuantes qui plongeaient leurs racines dans l'histoire.

Ainsi, d'après le Dr Alphonse Lessard, directeur du SPH, si autant de bébés canadiens-français mouraient, c'était principalement parce que les francophones se retrouvaient dans une situation désavantageuse face aux anglophones collectivement plus riches et moins prolifiques :

Voyez-vous, nous subissons encore, et nous subirons encore longtemps les désavantages de nos origines. 'Pauvreté n'est pas vice,' c'est vrai, mais la richesse chez les peuples, est productrice d'œuvres philanthropiques dont la masse bénéficie. […] .Alors que l'immigration anglaise arrivait ici, peu chargée de famille, mais munie de capitaux, […], nos gens n'ayant rien, peu instruits, ayant peu ou pas de directions en ce qui concerne les nécessités de leurs nombreux enfants par rapport à l'hygiène, perdaient malheureusement une proportion trop considérable des grandes familles qui leur étaient données.[49]

L'état de pauvreté des francophones aurait donc représenté un frein au développement des initiatives privées nécessaires à la conservation des «grandes familles» et retardé la mise en place de services publics pour assurer l'encadrement de la population. De l'avis du Dr Gaston Lapierre, diplômé de l'École de puériculture de la faculté de médecine de l'Université de Paris et pédiatre à l'Hôpital Sainte-Justine, il ne faisait non plus aucun doute que «notre misérable abandon après la 'Cession'» avait privé les Canadiens français «des sources scientifiques toujours vigilantes et éclairées», ce qui avait contribué à «fausser leur mentalité»[50]. Pour lui, comme pour le Dr Lessard, les francophones étaient en quelque sorte victimes de leur histoire. Coupés de leurs racines et des enseignements de leur mère patrie française, handicapés par leur situation de minoritaires et de dominés, collectivement et individuellement pauvres, il était compréhensible que le bilan de santé de leurs enfants ne soit pas des plus reluisants.

Loin de la France et de ses enseignements, les Canadiens français n'en avaient pas moins préservé, selon d'autres observateurs, une mentalité typiquement française qui les rendait moins réceptifs aux conseils médicaux. Commentant les difficultés que rencontrait le CHPQ à faire appliquer certaines mesures sanitaires et à enseigner l'hygiène dans les campagnes, le Dr J. A. Beaudry, inspecteur général pour le Conseil, affirmait par exemple :

La population, tout en étant mieux disposée qu'autrefois, [...] reste encore [...] très indifférente aux choses qui intéressent la santé publique. [...] Sa mentalité particulière, son caractère ethnique, ses vieilles habitudes, son esprit bien français et généralement gouailleur, exigent de la part de nos inspecteurs, un certain tact et un certain doigté[51].

Selon le Dr Beaudry, il était plus facile d'imposer de nouveaux comportements à la ville, car ses habitants toléraient mieux «la compulsion». Le Dr Eugène Gagnon, surintendant de la division de l'Hygiène de l'enfance du Service de santé de la Ville de Montréal, était loin d'être convaincu : selon son expérience, les populations urbaines étaient tout aussi apathiques et, en même temps, tout aussi chicanières que celles des campagnes. Elles avaient la «manie de vouloir discuter tous les problèmes» et, en matière médicale, se cramponnaient à de «fausses théories» et à «des préjugés» qu'elles défendaient «avec une ténacité digne d'une meilleure cause». Elles étaient également dotées d'une «tournure d'esprit spéciale» qui les rendaient «méfiantes envers tout ce qui vient à l'encontre des notions acquises dans le milieu»[52], si bien qu'elles rejetaient les nouveaux comportements que les médecins souhaitaient les voir adopter.

Ces propos remontent à 1918, mais l'argument de la «mentalité particulière» des Canadiens français était promis à un bel avenir. Ainsi, lorsque, en 1940, le Dr Jean Grégoire, alors sous-ministre de la santé, prononça son allocution présidentielle devant les membres de la *Canadian Public Health Association*, il commença par déclarer qu'il interprétait sa présidence comme une reconnaissance du Canada anglais envers les «progrès éclatants accomplis par le Québec» en matière, notamment, de mortalité infantile, pour ensuite expliquer la lenteur des mêmes progrès «par l'attachement profond de notre âme aux choses du passé» :

Alors que chez nos voisins, on bâtit des choses nouvelles, nous cherchons à améliorer les nôtres, vieilles de trois cent ans. (…) Cette mentalité qui est bien nôtre, notre concitoyen de langue anglaise doit essayer de la comprendre comme nous nous efforçons de saisir la sienne dont les racines ne sont peut-être pas enfoncés aussi profondément que les nôtres dans le sol canadien.[53]

En d'autres termes, le «retard» des francophones en matière de santé publique s'expliquait par le poids de leurs traditions qui ralentissait leur marche, mais leur conférait aussi une sorte de stabilité sociale et une cohérence nationale supérieures aux anglophones. Tout comme l'argument de la «Cession» et de l'infériorité économique des Canadiens français évoqués par les Dr Lessard et Lapierre cités plus haut, on retrouve ici un thème cher aux nationalistes de la période.

D'esprit indépendant, contradicteur et traditionaliste, le Canadien français, et plus particulièrement la Canadienne française, ne se seraient donc pas laissés gagner facilement à la cause hygiénique, compliquant le travail des autorités sanitaires. Leur détermination à préserver leurs us et coutumes, qui en d'autres circonstances avait fait leur force et leur avait permis de surmonter l'adversité et de survivre, était tout à la fois à déplorer et à valoriser, dépendant de l'auditoire, comme d'ailleurs leur attachement à de «vieilles habitudes» qui les amenait à refuser d'entendre la voix de la raison et du progrès. Ces traits culturels, qui dans l'immédiat nuisaient considérablement à la baisse de la mortalité infantile, n'étaient pas immuables cependant et pouvaient être modifiés : l'enseignement de l'hygiène aux enfants dans les écoles, alors que «leur cerveau était encore malléable»[54], devait permettre de déraciner les préjugés et d'amener la génération suivante à adopter des comportements plus conformes aux préceptes de la médecine. Tout comme en matière économique, il y avait donc encore de l'espoir de voir les Canadiens français se «moderniser» et égaler leurs compatriotes canadiens-anglais qui, encore une fois, semblaient montrer la voie à suivre.

Ces jours meilleurs, où leurs enseignements seraient davantage écoutés et leurs conseils mis en pratique, tardaient cependant à se manifester et en attendant, les médecins étaient bien forcés de constater que le taux de mortalité infantile du Québec continuait de battre des records à l'échelle canadienne. Tout en s'alarmant et en se scandalisant de cette situation, ils ont donc appelé à la barre un autre élément d'explication : le taux de natalité des francophones, qui lui aussi atteignait des sommets. La «proverbiale fécondité» des Canadiennes françaises qui se trouvait au cœur même de la stratégie de survivance des nationalistes, leur fournissait un motif de réconfort et de fierté et, aux yeux de certains, une raison en apparence scientifique pour expliquer tant de morts d'enfants.

Jusqu'au début des années 1930, environ, les médecins constatent, en effet, avec une évidente satisfaction que le taux de natalité «qui tend à s'abaisser d'une façon inquiétante chez toutes les nations civilisées, se maintient encore chez nous assez favorable [*sic*]»[55]. Avec un taux supérieur à 35 pour mille à la fin des années 1920, il n'y avait pas de quoi trop s'alarmer de la faible baisse enregistrée durant les deux premières décennies du XXe siècle selon le Dr Émile Nadeau, directeur-adjoint du SPH, car la plupart des pays affichaient des taux ne dépassant pas les 25 pour mille[56]. Encore en 1930, le Père Ernest Savignac, président de la Fédération des œuvres sociales de santé, soulignait avec fierté que la race canadienne-française était «une des plus riche au monde» en raison de son taux de natalité élevé, un atout qui lui conférait une «incontestable supériorité» à travers le Canada[57]. L'exode rural était bien sûr à surveiller, car il entraînait généralement une réduction de la taille des familles, ce qui n'était pas sans en inquiétait plus d'un, mais au milieu des années 1920, ses effets semblaient encore limités : «notre natalité ne subit pas de fléchissement marqué, malgré l'augmentation de nos centres industriels et l'expansion de nos villes» affirmait avec optimisme le Dr Masson en 1925 qui ajoutait : «La pratique des vertus familiales, soutenue par la pratique des principes fondamentaux de la religion chrétienne et catholique qui est la nôtre a réussi jusqu'à présent à lutter avantageusement contre la tendance vers une aisance présumée plus grande et un confort plus marqué par la limitation volontaire de la famille»[58]. Mieux que les autres «races», les Canadiens français savaient résister aux tentations et au goût du luxe que la vie urbaine engendrait, une preuve incontestée de leur supériorité morale tant vantée par les nationalistes.

Comme de nombreuses études démographiques l'ont démontré, la fécondité des Québécoises francophones, si elle était toujours plus élevée que celle des autres Canadiennes, était néanmoins en nette décroissance au cours des premières décennies du XXe siècle, laissant deviner des comportements moins «orthodoxes» de la part des couples vis-à-vis la contraception, surtout dans les villes. Ainsi, le taux de fécondité générale[59] pour l'ensemble de la population féminine du Québec passe de 155 à 116 pour mille entre 1921 et 1931, tandis que les francophones nées en 1887 ont en moyenne 6,4 enfants contre 4,3 pour celles qui sont nées en 1913, ce qui représente une baisse de 2,1 enfants[60]. En comparaison, les mêmes générations de Canadiennes ont donné naissance à 4,3 et 3,1 enfants, soit une diminution de 1,2 enfant[61]. En outre, comme le souligne Marie Lavigne, les familles de 10 enfants et plus étaient en nette régression au début du siècle; alors qu'elles sont le fait d'un peu plus de 20% des femmes qui ont constitué leur famille à partir de 1907, seulement 13% de celles qui ont donné naissance à partir de 1923 ont eu autant d'enfants[62].

Par contre, les taux de natalité, une mesure plus limitée, mais à laquelle se référaient les médecins, n'ont guère varié avant le début des

années 1930, ce qui explique sans doute que c'est seulement vers le
milieu de cette décennie que les hygiénistes et le corps médical ont
commencé à véritablement s'alarmer du déclin de la natalité des francophones[63]. Encore là, ce fléchissement était essentiellement attribué
aux effets de la crise économique qui avait entraîné une baisse notable
de la nuptialité, et conséquemment du nombre des naissances, ce qui laissait présager un rétablissement prochain, une fois la prospérité revenue.
Ainsi, dans son rapport pour l'année 1934–35, le Dr Lessard commen-
çait par se demander si le Québec n'était pas en voie de s'acheminer vers
«une situation dont certains pays d'Europe souffrent depuis plusieurs
années et qui les force à regarder l'avenir avec appréhension», avant de
noter que les conditions économiques s'amélioraient, pour finalement
conclure sur une note plutôt encourageante : «l'année 1934 marque au
point de vue du nombre des unions matrimoniales, un avantage considérable sur les précédentes. [...] Nous avons lieu d'espérer que, comme
conséquence, la natalité de 1935 s'en ressentira et que nous pourrons l'an
prochain, en exposant les faits démographiques [...] marquer une reprise
de cette natalité qu'on a toujours dans le passé citée à notre honneur.»[64]
Ainsi, même au milieu de la crise, les autorités sanitaires se montraient
optimistes face à une situation qui leur paraissait nouvelle et conser-
vaient encore l'espoir de voir la natalité reprendre ses droits. Pour la plupart des nationalistes, la fécondité des Canadiennes françaises représentait un des traits distinctifs de leur peuple dont ils étaient le plus fiers,
en même temps que la meilleure garantie de sa survie. Malgré les craintes qu'ils exprimaient à son sujet, ils avaient, semble-t-il, beaucoup de
peine à imaginer un renversement radical et irréversible d'une tendance plusieurs fois séculaires.

Cette fécondité exemplaire des Canadiennes françaises, maintes
fois acclamée, perdait néanmoins de son lustre quand elle était mise en
parallèle avec les décès infantiles, ce que les médecins ne peuvaient
ignorer. Dès le début du siècle, il s'en trouve pour souligner cette
incongruité: «Il n'y a pas lieu de se glorifier de nos nombreuses progé-
nitures, de notre forte natalité, si nous ne savons ou ne voulons la sauvegarder.»[65], s'indignait, par exemple, le Dr Adélar Corsin en 1916.
Une certaine logique productiviste se profile derrière cette façon de
concevoir le problème : la natalité supérieure des francophones, loin
de donner le «rendement» espéré en terme de descendance, se tradui-
sait au contraire par un véritable «gaspillage» de ressources. Cette opinion a toujours cours dans les années 1930:

Pourquoi faut-il que notre race, si abondamment pourvue de ces richesses supérieures, soit en même temps si prodigue et si gaspilleuse? Pourquoi laissons-
nous notre capital humain s'évaporer en pure perte? Pourquoi ne tirons-nous pas
meilleur profit de notre forte natalité, nous surtout race minoritaire, qui ne

pouvons pas compter sur d'autres ressources pour contrebalancer l'immigration européenne, presque totalement anglaise?[66]

Pourquoi, effectivement? Les propos du Père Savignac donnent à penser que le «manque de sens des affaires» des francophones, souvent évoqué pour expliquer leur infériorité économique, en était arrivé à contaminer les dimensions les plus intimes de leur vie: «race» prolifique, les Canadiens français auraient été incapables de «capitaliser» sur un aussi précieux avantage. Renonçant à blâmer ne serait-ce qu'indirectement leurs contemporains, certains médecins affirment par ailleurs que la forte natalité était en elle-même génératrice de mortalité infantile élevée. Cette opinion n'était pas universellement partagée : à la fin des années 1920, le Dr Nadeau maintenait, par exemple, que la fécondité des francophones représentait une «explication partielle», mais ne pouvait totalement excuser le fait que plus de 300 000 enfants de moins de un an soient morts au Québec entre 1900 et 1925[67]. Il s'agissait là néanmoins d'un sentiment largement répandu jusque dans les hautes sphères de l'administration de la santé publique: ainsi, en 1926, Joseph-Wilfrid Bonnier, chef de la statistique démographique de la province, soutenait qu'il existait bel et bien un lien entre natalité et mortalité élevées puisque «dans les pays où la natalité est forte, le taux de la mortalité est presque toujours élevé»[68]. Encore en 1940, le sous-ministre Jean Grégoire prétendait que le Québec pourrait difficilement «diminuer la mortalité infantile au niveau des autres provinces», «car à natalité élevée correspond une mortalité infantile élevée.»[69]

La nature exacte de ce lien entre natalité et mortalité infantile élevées était cependant rarement explicitée, la plupart des médecins se contentant d'en affirmer péremptoirement l'existence. Seuls quelques-uns d'entre eux, avançaient, assez timidement d'ailleurs, une explication, à savoir qu'une famille nombreuse pouvait, à la limite, représenter un obstacle à la survie des enfants en raison de la charge de travail qu'elle imposait à la mère : «Une autre cause de mortalité plus rare, mais qu'il faut admettre, c'est le manque de soins. La mère qui a 5, 6, 7, 8, et 10 enfants, et même plus quelques fois, [...] malgré la meilleure volonté, ne peut pas longtemps ou toujours donner à son jeune enfant tous les soins dont il a besoin»[70], affirmait le Dr Laberge en 1930. Le Dr Gauvreau en était déjà arrivé à cette conclusion quelques années auparavant, tout comme le Dr Baudouin qui estimait cependant qu'il ne fallait pas «exagérer cette difficulté» comme en témoignait la baisse graduelle de la mortalité infantile, parallèlement au maintien d'une forte natalité[71]. Bien entendu, même s'ils reconnaissaient que les familles nombreuses représentaient un lourd fardeau pour les femmes, aucun de ces médecins n'a jamais envisagé de promouvoir une diminution de la taille de la famille pour soulager la mère et ainsi mieux assurer la survie des enfants : l'idéal de la famille nombreuse faisait partie intégrante de la vision nationaliste de la société québécoise francophone et, au reste, il ne pouvait être question de contredire les enseignements de l'Église sur un sujet aussi brûlant. À l'exception du Dr Grégoire, qui admettait, en 1941, que «les facteurs économiques [...] agissent au détriment des familles nombreuses»[72], aucun ne relevait non plus les liens entre le nombre d'enfants, la pauvreté des familles et leurs difficultés à les conserver tous vivants.

Aux yeux de plusieurs médecins, la «proverbiale» fécondité des Canadiennes françaises, signe évident de supériorité morale et particularité nationale à préserver à tout prix, est donc devenue en elle-même un obstacle à la diminution de la mortalité infantile, ce qui enfermait le problème dans une logique insoluble. Mais bien plus, aux dires même du directeur du SPH, cette natalité hors du commun aurait représenté un frein à l'implantation de mesures socio-sanitaires propres à contrer ces décès. Dans son rapport au secrétaire de la province pour l'année 1925–26, le Dr Lessard soutenait en effet que par le passé, le Québec avait mis du temps à se préoccuper des décès infantiles, ce qu'il mettait, explicitement, au compte d'une natalité «prodigue».

Il fut un temps, et cette période n'est pas très éloignée de nous, où tout ce qui touchait à l'hygiène [...] n'excitait que d'une manière bien secondaire l'intérêt public. Notre natalité était si forte que nous ressemblions au prodigue qui possesseur d'un bien qu'il s'imagine inépuisable, jette à pleines mains et sans compter ses trésors.[...].

Notre natalité est encore forte, oui, mais il nous faut déchanter. Comme dans tous les pays du monde, celle-ci décroît et d'année en année son taux suit une courbe descendante, légère peut-être, mais constante. Elle est encore de beaucoup supérieure à celle des autres provinces du pays, et il naît dans la province de Québec plus du tiers des enfants qui voient le jour dans tout le Canada, mais le temps s'en vient où nous devrons plutôt compter pour continuer nos progrès remarquables au point de vue de l'augmentation naturelle de la population, sur la sauvegarde des enfants qui nous naissent et la conservation de leur vie, que sur ces abondantes naissances qui autrefois faisaient notre gloire[73].

Cette longue citation fait clairement état d'une ambivalence de la société québécoise du début du siècle envers le sort des enfants. Tant que ceux-ci s'avèrent une «ressource abondante», tant que leur «production» se maintient, tant que les mères demeurent « des sources vives d'où jaillissent avec un si admirable élan, ces petits anges terrestres»[74], les décès de nourrissons inquiètent, et même scandalisent, mais cette angoisse, dirait-on, n'arrive pas tout à fait à contrebalancer le sentiment diffus qu'un nombre quand même respectable de bébés parviennent à survivre. Dans la comptabilité nationaliste, il y avait toujours place, bien sûr, pour un accroissement des effectifs, mais à tout prendre, le bilan n'était pas si mauvais, surtout lorsqu'il était comparé à celu˙ ⹁⹁˙ anglophones. Au milieu des années 1920, «le temps s'en venait» où il deviendrait crucial de préserver la vie des nouveau-nés, sans qu'il soit encore tout à fait arrivé semble-t-il car la natalité diminuait plus lentement au Québec que dans le reste du Canada. La «gloire» que conférait la «Revanche des berceaux» paraissait à peine ternie et leur «Veillée» encore à l'état de projet.

Bien sûr, les autorités sanitaires provinciales ne sont pas restées totalement inactives devant la mortalité des enfants : comparé aux timides interventions de l'État québécois en matière d'éducation ou d'assistance, on peut même affirmer qu'elles se sont particulièrement distinguées, comme en témoigne la création du CHPQ dès 1887 ou celle du réseau des Unités sanitaires de comtés à compter de 1926. Mais force est aussi de constater que les mesures mises en œuvre sont demeurées bien limitées face à l'ampleur du problème. Ainsi, la pasteurisation du lait a mis très longtemps avant de devenir obligatoire sur l'ensemble du territoire québécois, même si le lait cru était, de l'avis de tous les hygiénistes, le principal vecteur des diarrhées infantiles trop souvent mortelles. En 1938, alors que l'Ontario adoptait une législation pour imposer la pasteurisation à l'échelle de cette province[75], seules quelques villes québécoises, comme Montréal, avaient réglementé la vente du lait et mis en place un système d'inspection des troupeaux et des établissements de pasteurisation qui alimentaient les laiteries situées sur leur territoire. Avant l'entrée en vigueur de la loi ontarienne, le lait vendu dans plus du tiers des cités et villes de plus de 2 000 habitants de cette province était déjà entièrement pasteurisé et dans les trois quart de l'ensemble de ces villes, au moins 50 % du lait l'était. Au Québec, à la même époque, la vente de lait pasteurisé atteignait 100 % dans moins de 10 % des cités et villes, et plus de 50 % dans à peine plus du quart des agglomérations de plus de 2 000 habitants[76]. À l'exception de quelques villes, notamment Montréal, les municipalités, dont relevait en premier lieu la santé publique, ont généralement fait preuve de laxisme dans l'application des diverses mesures préventives recommandées par le CHPQ, puis le SPH[77]. Très peu possédaient un bureau de santé digne de ce nom et pratiquement aucune un service destiné spécifiquement au bien-être de l'enfance. Dans bien des cas, y compris à Sherbrooke et dans la Capitale où les taux de mortalité infantile sont demeurés supérieurs à 100 pour mille naissances vivantes jusque dans les années 1940, les cliniques de puériculture y avaient été fondées par des organisations philanthropiques qui ont été maintenues même après que des études aient souligné la qualité assez médiocre de leurs services[78]. À Montréal, les autorités sanitaires ont mis en place un réseau de consultations municipales à partir de 1919, mais chez les catholiques francophones, elles ont ouvert ces cliniques uniquement dans les paroisses où il n'existait pas de gouttes de lait privées. Fondées à partir de 1910, celles-ci sont demeurées actives jusqu'en 1953 car elles refusaient d'être intégrées au réseau municipal et la Ville n'a pas osé les y forcer[79]. En comparaison, soulignons que les grandes villes ontariennes ont municipalisé les cliniques de puériculture peu après la Première guerre mondiale.[80] Au niveau provincial, la première campagne de lutte contre la mortalité infantile, lancée en 1922 par le SPH après qu'un comité formé pour étudier ce problème en ait fortement recommandé le déclenchement, a finalement été jumelée à une compagne de lutte contre la tuberculose, une stratégie qui avait peut-être sa raison d'être puisque la «peste blanche» faisait également des ravages impressionnants parmi la population, mais un signe que les autorités sanitaires n'étaient pas encore prêtes à s'attaquer en priorité au problème de la mortalité des enfants et ce, principalement en raison des coûts que cela pouvait entraîner : effectivement, cette stratégie a été adoptée principalement parce qu'elle permettait «de réduire les dépenses d'un tiers»[81]. La mise en place du réseau des Unités sanitaires, à partir de 1926 témoigne aussi d'une stratégie globale en matière de santé publique car elles avaient été conçues dans le but de surveiller l'ensemble des conditions hygiéniques d'une population donnée et non pas uniquement la santé des mères et des bébés : jusqu'aux années 1950, la surveillance médicale des écoliers a d'ailleurs occupé le plus gros des énergies des infirmières[82]. Autre élément troublant, le CHPQ, le SPH, de même que le ministère de la Santé qui leur a succédé, ne comprenaient pas de Division spécifiquement attitrée à l'hygiène infantile et maternelle, comme c'était le cas aux ministères fédéral et ontarien de la Santé. Ce n'est qu'en 1954 que la Division de la nutrition du ministère québécois de la Santé, fondé en 1936, se verra finalement confier la charge de l'hygiène maternelle et infantile, devenant alors la Division de la Nutrition, Hygiène maternelle et infantile, et qu'un programme spécifique de prévention sera élaboré à l'intention des femmes enceintes et des nourrissons[83].

Conclusion

Le Québec n'a pas été la seule société à lier la sauvegarde de l'enfance à la question nationale. Au Canada également, tout comme en France et en Angleterre, la lutte contre la mortalité infantile a été étroitement associée à la préservation ou à la défense de la nation contre l'envahisseur, peuple ennemi ou immigrants indésirables. La position minoritaire des Canadiens français dans l'espace politique canadien a cependant engendré un discours nationaliste «victimisant» qui offrait toute une série d'arguments en apparence inébranlables aux médecins qui cherchaient à expliquer, sinon à justifier, la très forte mortalité infantile des Québécois francophones. Obsédés par la conservation des traits identitaires des Canadiens français, les nationalistes ont aussi élevé la famille nombreuse au rang de pilier de cette identité. Même si elle était en déclin durant la première moitié du XXe siècle, la «proverbiale fécondité» des Canadiennes françaises représentait un point de référence incontournable quand venait le temps d'aborder le problème de la mortalité infantile. Intimement liés l'un à l'autre, les deux phénomènes, mortalité infantile et natalité élevées, apparaissaient comme les deux faces d'une même médaille : dans la balance, ils s'annulaient, ce qui n'était pas de nature à accélérer le développement des mesures de santé publique.

Sans vouloir minimiser les interventions des autorités sanitaires de la province et de certaines municipalités, en particulier Montréal, force est, en effet, de reconnaître que les efforts consentis pour combattre la mortalité infantile n'ont pas été à la hauteur des inquiétudes exprimées à son sujet. Compte tenu des enjeux que représentait la survie des bébés canadiens-français pour la sauvegarde nationale et des propos souvent horrifiés des médecins et des ténors nationalistes sur la question, on aurait pu s'attendre à ce que le Québec soit à l'avant-garde des mesures de santé publique visant à contrer ce «fléau». Or il n'en fut rien. Si l'État québécois s'est montré plus interventionniste dans ce domaine que dans celui de l'éducation ou de l'assistance publique, il a aussi fait preuve de timidité face à des groupes qui s'opposaient à la pasteurisation du lait, ou face aux organisations bénévoles qui gravitaient autour de l'Église et qui avaient fondé des Gouttes de lait dans plusieurs grandes villes. Ce paradoxe ne devient compréhensible que dans la mesure où l'on considère l'autre versant de la rhétorique médico-nationaliste qui faisait tout aussi grand cas de la forte natalité des francophones. Le «capital humain» que représentaient les enfants était effectivement assimilé à du capital et même si les nationalistes déploraient les «pertes», ils ne pouvaient s'empêcher de lorgner du côté des «gains» qui étaient encore considérables et avec lesquels ils parvenaient à se consoler.

Tableau I. Taux quinquennal moyen de mortalité infantile (par mille naissances vivantes) Canada, Québec et Ontario, 1921–1940

Années	Canada	Québec	Ontario	Qc/Ont
1921–25	99.0	127.1	83.0	53 %
1926–30	93.4	127.1	76.1	67 %
1931–35	74.7	98.4	60.7	62 %
1936–40	64.4	82.7	49.7	66 %

Source: Rapports annuels du ministère de la Santé du Québec

Tableau II. Taux de mortalité infantile par mille naissances vivantes
selon les groupes ethno-religieux, Montréal, 1901–1940

Années	Canadiens français	Autres catholiques	Protestants	Juifs	Tous groupes
1901–05	289.4	273.6	186.2	—	275.0
1906–10	277.0	254.9	186.4	138.5	262.0
1911–15	237.6	224.6	173.8	113.8	209.0
1916–20	205.4	210.1	126.7	56.3	184.9
1921–25	164.1	159.9	79.5	39.6	141.7
1926–30	146.0	163.6	75.2	40.5	130.5
1931–35	109.9	103.1	62.9	37.3	98.9
1936–40	86.9	64.1	48.3	26.2	76.4

Source : Rapports annuels du Service de santé de la ville de Montréal

Note tableau II

Le recours ou non à l'allaitement maternel explique en grande partie les
différences constatées entre les taux de mortalité infantile des populations juive, anglo-protestante, anglo-catholique et franco-catholique de
Montréal. Comme plusieurs auteurs et contemporains l'ont souligné, la
pratique prolongée de l'allaitement était quasi universelle dans la communauté juive, mais beaucoup moins courante chez les mères canadiennes-françaises, ce qui avait des conséquences assez catastrophiques pour
leurs nourrissons. Il serait cependant hasardeux de comparer ces statistiques sans mentionner d'autres facteurs, notamment le sous-enregistre-
ment des naissances et des décès des enfants juifs et anglo-protestants
au début du siècle, mais aussi la plus grande propension, chez les catholiques, à faire entrer dans la catégorie des enfants «nés vivants» – catégorie qui servait à établir les statistiques de mortalité infantile – , des
enfants qui étaient mort-nés et qui auraient dû en être exclus. La croyance
que les enfants morts sans baptême étaient condamnés à errer pour
l'éternité dans les limbes, amenait en effet les médecins catholiques
(francophones comme anglophones), à interpréter très largement la
définition d'un «mort-né» afin de pouvoir ondoyer l'enfant. Ces deux facteurs ont généralement eu pour effet de gonfler le taux de mortalité
infantile des Franco-catholiques et des Anglo-catholiques et de faire
diminuer celui des Anglo-protestants et des Juifs, sans qu'il soit possible de déterminer précisément dans quelle proportion. Ajoutons à cela
que les enfants «illégitimes», chez les catholiques, étaient pris en charge
par des institutions dirigées par des communautés religieuses où leur
entassement produisait régulièrement des épidémies qui en fauchaient
un très grand nombre, alors que chez les Anglo-protestants et les Juifs,

beaucoup de ces enfants étaient pris en charge par des familles d'accueil ou placés en pension, des pratiques qui réduisaient considérablement les risques de décès. Sur la question de la construction sociale des données démographiques et des distorsions qu'elles comportent, voir George Emery, *Facts of Life. The Social Construction of Vital Statistics. Ontario 1869–1952* (Montréal et Kingston : McGill-Queens, 1993), en particulier le chapitre 5 qui s'intéresse à la comptabilisation des mort-nés au Québec et en Ontario, et François Guérard, «La santé publique dans deux villes du Québec de 1887 à 1939. Trois-Rivières et Shawinigan», Thèse de Phd. (Histoire), UQAM, 1993, p. 507–13.

Remerciements

Cette recherche a bénéficié du soutien financier du fonds FCAR du gouvernement du Québec et de l'Institut Hannah d'histoire de la médecine. Mes plus vifs remerciements à Marie-Josée Blais, Karine Hébert et Nathalie Pilon qui ont contribué à la recherche.

Notes

1 Extrait d'une conférence intitulée «Pour l'Action française», prononcée le 10 avril 1918, cité dans François Guérard, «La santé publique dans deux villes du Québec de 1887 à 1939. Trois-Rivières et Shawinigan», Thèse de Phd. (Histoire), UQAM, 1993, p. 247.

2 Comme l'illustrent les nécrologies publiées dans *L'Union médicale du Canada*.

3 Guérard, «La santé publique», p. 63–67.

4 Pour une perspective comparative au sujet de la lutte contre la mortalité infantile dans les pays européens et plus généralement du mouvement en faveur du bien-être infantile et maternel, voir Seth Koven et Sonya Michel, dir., *Mothers of a New World. Maternalist Politics and the Origins of Welfare States* (New York et Londres : Routledge, 1993); et Gisela Bock et Pat Thane, dir., *Maternity and Gender Policies. Women and the Rise of the European Welfare States 1880s-1950s* (Londres et New York : Routhledge, 1994). Sur la situation américaine, voir Molly Ladd-Taylor, *Mother-Work. Women, Child Welfare, and the State, 1890–1930* (Chicago : University of Illinois Press, 1994). Pour la France, Catherine Rollet-Échalier, *La politique à l'égard de la petite enfance sous la IIIᵉ République* (Paris : INED, 1990). Pour le Canada anglais, Cynthia R. Comacchio, *Nations Are Built of Babies. Saving Ontario's Mothers and Children 1900–1940* (Montréal et Kingston : McGill-Queen's University Press, 1993) et Katherine Arnup, *Education for Motherhood. Advice for Mothers in Twentieth-Century Canada* (Toronto : University of Toronto Press, 1994). Sur le Québec, François Guérard, «La santé publique», et Denyse Baillargeon, «'Fréquenter les Gouttes de lait.' L'expérience des mères montréalaises, 1910–1965», *Revue d'histoire de l'Amérique française (RHAF)* 50,1 (été 1996) : 29–68.

5 Pour plus de détails sur ces questions, voir, dans ce recueil, l'article de Ann-Emmanuelle Birn qui explore la situation en Amérique Latine et le rôle joué par le Pan-American Sanitary Bureau dans la lutte contre la mortalité infantile dans cette région (Birn, «'No More Surprising Than a Broken Pitcher'? Maternal and Child Health in the Early Years of the Pan-American Sanitary Bureau»).

6 Montréal, *Rapport du Bureau municipal d'hygiène et de statistiques(Rapport)*, 1913, p. xiii.

7 Ainsi, en 1912, New York avait un taux de mortalité infantile de 105 pour mille naissances vivantes, Paris de 103 pour mille et Londres de 91 pour mille, alors qu'à Montréal, ce taux s'établissait à 208 pour mille (Montréal, *Rapport*, 1913, p. xiv, xvi et xvii).

8 Rappelons que ce n'est qu'à partir de la fin de la Première Guerre mondiale que le gouvernement fédéral va mettre en place une procédure uniforme de collecte des données démographiques à travers le Canada. Le Québec ne fera partie de ce «territoire d'enregistrement national» qu'à compter de 1926, mais les données québécoises pour la période 1921–1926 sont généralement incluses dans les tableaux récapitulatifs.

9 «First Report of Vital Statistics in Nine Province», *Canadian Child Welfare News* 3, 3 (août 1927) : 37–38.

10 Selon les tableaux de mortalité infantile par comté publiés dans les rapports annuels du Conseil d'hygiène de la province de Québec (CPHQ), du Service provincial d'hygiène (SPH) et du ministère de la Santé.

11 Le Service provincial d'hygiène remplace le Conseil d'hygiène de la province de Québec en 1922.

12 Québec, *Rapport annuel du SPH*, 1926–27, p. 91.

13 Cet organisme a changé de nom plusieurs fois : nous nous en tenons à cette appellation utilisée à partir de 1918 (Benoît Gaumer et al., «Le service de santé de Montréal, de l'établissement au démantèlement (1865–1975)», *Cahiers du centre de recherches historiques* 12 (avril 1994): 132.

14 Patricia Thornton, Sherry Olson et Quoc Thuy Thach, «Dimensions sociales de la mortalité infantile à Montréal au milieu du XIXe siècle», *Annales de démographie historique* (1988): 299–325; et Patricia A. Thornton et Sherry Olson, «Family Contexts of Fertility and Infant Survival in Nineteenth Century Montreal», *Journal of Family History* 16, 4 (1991) : 401–417.

15 Pour une analyse de la position des médecins ontariens et plus généralement canadiens anglais, voir Comacchio, *Nations Are Built of Babies*.

16 Guérard, «La santé publique», *op. cit.*, p. 245–254. Il reste que certains groupes nationalistes ont aussi lutté contre cette prétention de l'État à assurer la livraison des services de santé à la population. À ce sujet voir Denyse Baillargeon, «Gouttes de lait et soif de pouvoir. Les dessous de la lutte contre la mortalité infantile à Montréal, 1910–1953», *Canadian Bulletin of Medical History/Bulletin canadien d'histoire de la médecine (CBMH/BCHM)* 15 (1998) : 27–56.

17 Pour un exemple d'étude qui insiste sur l'intervention de l'État en matière de santé publique, voir Georges Desrosiers, Benoît Gaumer et Othmar Keel. *La santé publique au Québec. Histoire des unités sanitaires de comtés, 1926–1975*, Montréal, Presses de l'Université de Montréal, 1998.

18 À leur sujet, voir Denyse Baillargeon, «Fréquenter les Gouttes de lait» et «Gouttes de lait et soif de pouvoir».

19 Se penchant sur la contribution de l'hôpital Saint-Paul et du Alexandra Hospital dans la lutte contre la mortalité infantile par maladies contagieuses à Montréal au début du siècle, Marie-Josée Fleury et Guy Grenier soulignent, pour leur part, la modernité de ces structures hospitalières , des techniques utilisées et des traitements en vigueur et le souci des médecins de se spécialiser dans ce domaine en allant se former à l'étranger. Ils constatent par ailleurs que le développement de ces deux hôpitaux a été entravé en raison de leur sous-financement. Voir leur article dans ce recueil.

20 Pour une revue des travaux portant sur la santé publique et de leur apport au débat sur le retard versus la modernité du Québec, voir François Guérard, «L'histoire de la santé au Québec : filiations et spécificités», *CBMH* 17, 1 (2000) : 55–72.

21 De nombreux ouvrages ont traité de ces questions. Voir par exemple Susan Mann Trofimenkoff, *The Dream of Nation. A Social and Intellectual History of Quebec* (Toronto: Macmillan, 1982).

22 Au sujet de ces débats voir entre autres Fernande Roy, *Histoire des Idéologies au Québec aux XIXᵉ et XXᵉ siècle* (Montréal : Boréal, 1993); Yves Saint-Germain, «La société québécoise et la vie économique : quelques échos de la décennie de la «grande ambivalence», 1920–29, dans *Économie québécoise*, dir. Robert Comeau (Montréal : Presses de l'Université du Québec, 1969), p. 439–464; et Jean-Claude Dupuis, «La pensée économique de l'Action française, 1917–1928», *RHAF* 47, 2 (automne 1993) : 193–291.

23 Ibid.

24 Voir par exemple le discours de Joseph Versailles prononcé devant les membres de l'ACJC en 1921, cité dans Saint-Germain, «La société québécoise et la vie économique», p. 456. et les propos d'Esdras Minville cités dans Dupuis, «La pensée économique» p. 214.

25 Mann Trofimenkoff, *The Dream of Nation*, p.113.

26 Esdras Minville, cité dans Jean-Claude Dupuis, «Nationalisme et catholicisme. L'Action française de Montréal, 1917–38», MA (Histoire) Université de Montréal, 1992, p. 69.

27 Sur les préjugés de classe et de genre des médecins, voir en particulier Comacchio, *Nations Are Built of Babies*.

28 Dr. C. N. Valin, «Prophylaxie de la mortalité infantile», *Bulletin sanitaire (BS)* 9, 9–12 (septembre-décembre 1909) : 91. Le Dr Nadeau, directeur-adjoint du SPH, tenait des propos semblables en 1931 dans «Quelques remarques sur l'importance, du point de vue national, de réduire notre mortalité infantile», *Canadian Public Health Journal (CPHJ)* 22, 11 (novembre 1931) : 548.

29 Comacchio, *Nations Are Built of Babies*, p. 85–86; et Mariana Valverde, *The Age of Light, Soap, and Water. Moral Reform in English Canada, 1885–1925* (Toronto : McClelland and Stewart, 1991), p. 104 et ss.

30 Angus McLaren, *Our Own Master Race* (Toronto : University of Toronto Press, 1990).

31 Mentionnons que les théories eugénistes n'ont jamais fait beaucoup d'adeptes parmi les praticiens francophones. Celles-ci allaient trop directement à l'encontre des préceptes de l'Église catholique qui refusait toute forme de limitation des naissances pour quelque raison que ce soit. Réserver le droit de se reproduire aux seuls couples «non tarés» ne cadrait pas de toute façon avec les préoccupations nationalistes de la profession qui accordait la primauté au poids du nombre de la communauté francophone. Au sujet des positions de l'église catholique sur l'eugénisme, voir Hervé Blais, o.f.m. *Les tendances eugénistes au Canada*, Montréal, Institut familial, 1942.

32 Mme Jules Tessier, «The Value of Public Depots», *Public Health Journal* 8, 3 (mars 1917) : 63–64.

33 Valverde, *The Age of Light*, p. 114 et ss.

34 Dr Raoul Masson, «La mortalité infantile dans la province de Québec», *L'Union médicale du Canada (UMC)* 54, 1 (janvier 1925) : 4.

35 R.P. Bernier, omi, *BS* 20, no unique (1920) : 20.

36 Dr Édouard Laberge, «Mortalité infantile et consultations de nourrissons», *La Santé* 1, 4 (octobre 1930) : 20 (Nous soulignons).

37 Le Dr Baudouin exerça plusieurs fonctions au service de santé de la ville de Lachine et au CHPQ. Il fut aussi l'assistant du Dr C.-N. Valin, avant de le remplacer comme titulaire d'hygiène à la Faculté de médecine de l'Université de Montréal. Il a fondé et dirigé l'École d'hygiène sociale appliquée, mise sur pied en 1925, et a été un collaborateur régulier de *L'Action française*. Pour une biographie plus complète, voir Georges Desrosiers, «Joseph-Albert Baudoin (*sic*) (1875–1962) : professeur d'hygiène», *CBMH/BCHM* 10 (1993) : 251–268.

38 Dr Joseph Baudouin, «Nécessité de la lutte contre la mortalité infantile et la tuberculose (suite)», *BS* 23, 1 (janvier-mars 1923) : 32.

39 Ces expressions reviennent sous la plume de diverses personnalités don't plusieurs médecins. Voir par exemple Dr C.-N. Valin, «Prophylaxie de la mortalité infantile», *BS* 9, 9-12 (septembre-décembre 1909) : 91; Dr Séverin Lachapelle, cité dans Joseph Gauvreau, La Goutte de lait, Montréal, École sociale populaire, 1914, p. 7; Madeleine Huguenin, «Entre-nous», *La Bonne parole* 11, 5 (juillet 1911) : 1; Dr René Fortier, «Protection de l'enfance» *BS* 11, 3-8 (mars-août 1911) : 142 et «Considérations pratiques sur l'alimentation artificielle des jeunes enfants», *BS* 18, no unique (1918) : 71; et Dr Joseph Baudouin, «La mortalité infantile», *La Santé* 1, 6 (décembre 1930) : 10.

40 Dr Joseph Gauvreau, *La Goutte de lait* (Montréal : École sociale populaire, 1914), p. 15. Gauvreau a été registraire du Collège des Médecins et Chirurgiens entre 1909 et 1934. Membre du groupe de l'École sociale populaire dans les années 1910, il fut aussi l'un des fondateurs de *L'Action française* et vice-président de la Société Saint-Jean-Baptiste de Montréal (SSJBM). Pour une courte biographie, voir Dr Albert LeSage, «*In Memoriam*. Joseph Gauvreau, 1870–1942», *UMC* 71, 4 (avril 1942) : 329–338.

41 Marie-Gérin Lajoie, «Entre-nous», *La Bonne parole (BP)* 2, 5 (juillet 1914) : 1.

42 L'idée que la mortalité infantile chez les Canadiens français était parfaitement honteuse a souvent été reprise par la suite. Ainsi, en 1921, Victor Morin, alors président de la Société Saint-Jean-Baptiste deMontréal, affirmait que l'aveu de la perte de nombreux enfants «ne devrait se faire qu'à voix basse, au confessionnal, comme un péché honteux contre l'humanité» (Victor Morin, «L'importance de nos groupements nationaux», *BP* 9, 6 [juin 1921] : 5). Au début des années 1940, le Dr Albert LeSage, qui était alors président conjoint de la Ligue de Santé publique du Canada, s'exprimait dans des termes similaires. Constatant que les diarrhées et les entérites faisaient encore des ravages chez les nouveau-nés, il en appelait à l'élimination des causes de cette affection, en particulier le lait non pasteurisé, «sinon, ajoutait-il, nous ne méritons pas d'élever des enfants et nous nous affichons insolemment une [*sic*] race inférieure» (Dr Albert LeSage, «L'hygiène dans la Province de Québec», *UMC* 70, 11 [novembre 1941] : 1208).

43 Marie Gérin-Lajoie, «L'œuvre éducatrice de l'hôpital Sainte-Justine» *BP* 8, 10 (octobre 1920) : 3.

44 Dr E.-M. Savard, «La Sauvegarde de l'enfance», *BP* 9, 9 (septembre 1921) : 4.

45 Dr Arthur Butler Chandler, «The Relation of Child Labour to Child Health», *PHJ* 12, 9 (septembre 1921) : 397. Voir aussi Dr Grant Fleming, «The Present Situation Regarding the Adequacy of Medical Care in Canada», *CPHJ* 30, 9 (septembre 1939) : 422.

46 Québec, *Rapport annuel du sph*, 1934–35, p. 10.

47 Dr Gaston Lapierre, «La mortalité infantile dans la province de Québec», *UMC* 53, 6 (juin 1924) : 266.

48 Masson, «La mortalité infantile», p. 6.

49 Dr Alphonse Lessard, «De l'amélioration des conditions hygiéniques constatées dans les familles», *BS* 18, no unique (1918) : 103.

50 Lapierre, «La mortalité infantile dans la province de Québec», p. 268–269.

51 Dr J.A. Beaudry, «L'hygiène publique dans la province de Québec», *BS* 18, no unique (1918) : 30.

52 Dr. Eugène Gagnon, «La lutte contre la mortalité infantile», *BS* 18, no unique (1918) : 79–80.

53 Dr Jean Grégoire, Adresse présidentielle, *CPHJ* 32, 9 (septembre 1941) : 450.

54 Dr Eugène Gagnon, «Comment diminuer la mortalité infantile», *UMC* 11, 1 (janvier 1911) : 6.

55 Dr Joseph Baudouin, «Nécessité de la lutte contre la mortalité infantile et la tuberculose (suite)», *BS* 23, 1 (janvier-mars 1923) : 30.

56 Dr Émile Nadeau, «A retrospective Study of Public Health Progress in the Province of Quebec during the last Twenty-Five Years», *CPHJ* 20, 11 (novembre 1929) : 537.

57 Père Ernest Savignac, «Vive la santé», *La Santé* 1, 1 (avril 1930) : 3.

58 Masson, «La mortalité infantile », p. 4–5.

59 Le taux de fécondité générale équivaut au nombre annuel des naissances par mille femmes âgées de 15 à 49 ans dans une population donnée. Danielle Gauvreau et Peter Gossage, «Avoir moins d'enfants au tournant du XXe siècle», *RHAF* 54, 1 (été 2000) : 44.

60 Jacques Henripin, *Tendances et facteurs de la fécondité au Canada* (Ottawa : Bureau fédéral de la statistique, 1968), p. 21 et Jacques Henripin et Yves Peron, «La transition démographique de la province de Québec», dans Hubert Charbonneau, *La population du Québec : études et perspective* (Montréal : Boréal Express, 1973), p. 40, cités dans Marie Lavigne, «Réflexions féministes autour de la fertilité des Québécoises», dans Micheline Dumont et Nadia Fahmy-Eid, *Maîtresses de maison, maîtresses d'école; Femmes, famille et éducation dans l'histoire du Québec* (Montréal : Boréal Express, 1983), p. 323.

61 Lavigne, «Réflexions féministes», p. 323. Pour l'ensemble des Québécoises habitant la région métropolitaine de Montréal, Henripin estime que les femmes nées entre 1880 et 1896 donnent naissance à 4,2 enfants; celles nées entre 1901 et 1906 à 3,0 enfants et celles nées entre 1911 et 1916, et qui constituent donc leur famille durant la crise, à 2,6 enfants. Dans la région métropolitaine de Québec, où les francophones sont plus largement majoritaires, les mêmes générations de femmes ont en moyenne 6, 2, 4, 6 et 3, 7 enfants respectivement. Jacques Henripin, *Naître ou ne pas être*, Québec, IQRC, coll. Diagnostic, 1989, p. 50.

62 Lavigne, «Réflexions féministes», p. 325.

63 Les taux de natalité se situaient à 38 pour mille en 1901, à 39 pour mille en 1911, 38 pour mille en 1921 et à 29 pour mille en 1931 (Henripin, *Tendances et facteurs de la fécondité*, p. 21). Il faut souligner que cette mesure ne tient pas compte de la nuptialité, ni de la structure par âge et par sexe de la population (voir Gauvreau et Gossage, «Avoir moins d'enfants», p. 44).

64 Québec, *Rapport annuel du SPH*, 1934–35, p. 6 et 8.

65 Dr Adélar Corsin, «Rapport du comité sur la mortalité infantile», *BS* 16, 2–12 (février-décembre 1916) : 41. Dans la même veine, le Dr Séverin Lachapelle, professeur de pédiatrie et l'un des plus ardents défenseurs de la santé publique et de la lutte contre la mortalité infantile affirmait, en 1904, que si la natalité des Canadiens français «faisait un peu l'orgueil de notre race», sa forte mortalité infantile provoquait «non seulement les lamentations de Rachel, mais le désespoir de ceux qui ont à coeur la force numérique de la nation et les droits qui en résulteraient naturellement.» (Dr Séverin Lachapelle, «Hygiène et médecine infantiles», *BS* 4, 6–7 [juin-juillet 1904] : 5–8).

66 Savignac, «Vive la santé», p. 3.

67 Nadeau, «A retrospective Study», p. 537. Le Dr Lessard affirmait également qu'une haute natalité, «n'appelle pas nécessairement une haute mortalité des enfants de 0 à 1 an» (*Rapport annuel du SPH*, 1930, p. 132).

68 Dr Joseph-Wilfrid Bonnier, «Les statistiques vitales fédérales», *BS*, 26, 5 (septembre-octobre 1926) : 154.

69 Grégoire, «Allocution présidentielle», p. 451.

70 Dr Édouard Laberge, «Mortalité infantile et consultations de nourrissons», *La Santé* 1, 4 (octobre 1930): 20.

71 Dr Joseph Gauvreau, «La mortalité infantile», *Semaines sociales du Canada*, IVe session, *La Famille*, Montréal, Bibliothèque de l'Action française, 1923, p. 166; et Dr Joseph Baudouin, «La Mortalité infantile», *La Santé* 1, 6 (décembre 1930): 10.

72 Grégoire, «Allocution présidentielle», p. 451.

73 Québec, *Rapport annuel du SPH*, 1925–26, p. 4. Le Dr Lessard reprenait cet argument dans «Rural Sanitation in Quebec from the Provincial Standpoint», *CPHJ* 23, 3 (mars 1932) : 104.

74 Savignac, «Vive la santé», p. 4

75 Comacchio, *Nations Are Built of Babies*, p. 45–46.

76 Selon les données publiées dans A.E. Berry, «A Survey of Milk Control in Cities and Towns in Canada», *CPHJ* 29, 6 (juin 1938) : 306–308.

77 La correspondance du CHPQ et du SPH en témoigne : refus de construire, ou de réparer, des canalisations d'eau adéquates, d'installer des usines de filtration, de faire les aménagements nécessaires pour que les égouts ne contaminent pas l'eau potable, etc.

78 Baillargeon, «Gouttes de lait et soif de pouvoir»; Dr Jules Gilbert et C. W. MacMillan, *Rapport sur le service de santé de la Ville de Sherbrooke* (Sherbrooke: Chambre de Commerce, 1949); Dr Fortier de la Broquerie *Au service de l'enfance. L'Association québécoise de la Goutte de lait* (Québec : Éditions Garneau, 1965).

79 Baillargeon, «Gouttes de lait et soif de pouvoir».

80 Comacchio, *Nations Are Built of Babies*.

81 ANQ, Fonds du CHPQ, vol. 90, Mémoire adressé au président et aux membres du Conseil Supérieur d'hygiène de la province, novembre 1920, p. 2.

82 Sur le développement des Unités sanitaires de comtés, voir Desrosiers, Gaumer et Keel, *La santé publique au Québec*.

83 Dr J.-E. Sylvestre, «Les ailes qui s'ouvrent», *UMC* 84, 12 (décembre 1955) : 1413.

Nutrition

❧

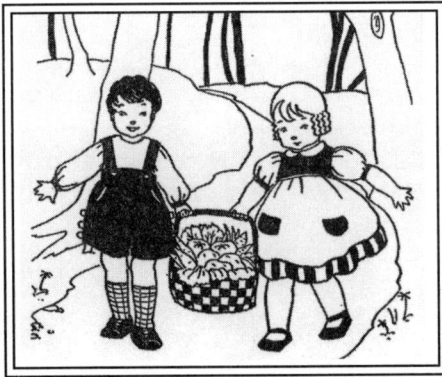

Infant Ideologies

Doctors, Mothers, and the Feeding of Children in Australia, 1880–1910

∝

Lisa Featherstone

The rise of pediatrics as a separate medical discourse is both the symbol and the practical embodiment of a new and fundamental interest in the child. Prior to the 1880s and 1890s, the health and well-being of the child had largely been subsumed into that of the mother: the woman and her child were inextricably linked through the cycles of gestation, childbirth, and lactation. Medically, the child was enmeshed with the mother, and therefore incorporated into the disciplines of obstetrics and gynecology.[1] From the late nineteenth century, however, there was an increasing emphasis on the child as an individual body, as an object of interest in his or her own right. The predominant signifier of such an interest was the rise of a new, specialized discipline to cater to the child: pediatrics. Pediatrics—the study and treatment of the diseases of children—is different from other specialties in that it focuses, not on a single organ, but on the whole body, albeit a different kind of body.[2]

This chapter will first examine the rise of pediatrics, and the emergence of the child as a separate and special body. It will consider the problem of infant mortality, and the increased social, political, and medical concern over the life of the infant in Australia.[3] This medicalization of infant care had important implications for the medical profession and mothers, as well as the way in which children were diagnosed and treated. Second, it will examine the medical discourses of infant feeding. With so few real advances in the care of babies in this period, prevention of disease was crucial, and it was only through the control of infant feeding that doctors had any real impact on infant life. In Australia, breast-feeding was always prioritized, and artificial feeding and wet-nursing were very rarely promoted. Through a consideration of breastfeeding and artificial feeding, we can chart a clear pattern of interest, a movement away from concerns about the mother, to an increasing focus on the child. Infant feeding functions as a key focus for our understanding of medical attitudes towards mothers and babies, and forms a clear signifier of a subtle shift in emphasis from the mother to her child.

The Development of Pediatrics in Australia

In a wide understanding of the term, an interest in children and their diseases can certainly be seen from the late eighteenth century, with a substantial number of important and innovative texts.[4] These texts, however, neither demanded nor constituted a systematic study of the health and diseases of children, and there was little acknowledgment of the need for a discipline to supervise the special or unique body of the child.[5] As a profession, and a discipline separate from obstetrics, pediatrics did not really develop until the early to mid-twentieth century. If an awareness of the need to professionalize and specialize is important, pediatrics began to emerge in the final decades of the nineteenth century.[6] While an interest in the health of the child is very old, the discipline itself did not truly consolidate until much later; in this way, pediatrics is a phenomenon of the late nineteenth and early twentieth centuries.

In one sense, the rise of pediatrics was part of a more general specialization in medicine, and in industry more widely.[7] The professionalization of the medical profession, however, was not enough to guarantee the emergence of a new specialty. A cultural shift was necessary, spanning the separation of child and mother, and the vision of the infant as not only separate, but also special. What was vital was the change from a Romantic concept of the conjoined mother and child, to a more scientific, medicalized concern with the infant alone. The final impetus to the scientific model, encompassing the professionalization of pediatrics, occurred when children were valued, not only for their adorable and precious selves, but also because of their future utility: children would grow to be adults, and be of value to the nation state. Pediatrics as a discipline was justified by the relationship of the child to the future adult, when the child emerged as a potential citizen.[8]

Central to the development of pediatrics was a new and intense anxiety over infant mortality, and the emergence of infant life as a problem of social, political. and medical concern.[9] In Australia, infant mortality was perceived to be worryingly high. In 1885, the death rate was 127.9 per thousand; a decade later it was 101.3.[10] On an international level, Australian infant mortality was not necessarily excessive. Indeed, the infant mortality rate in Australia was significantly lower in this period than that of the United States, England, and most other European nations.[11] In many ways, Australian infants were relatively healthy. In Australia, the mean weight of infants born at full term was eight pounds.[12]

Doctors reported proudly that children were born on average one pound heavier than their English equivalents, and there were commonly extremes in weight not seen in Britain. In the colonies it was not altogether unusual to see an infant born at twelve pounds, while there were cases of children born at eighteen pounds.[13] Children were often taller and sturdier than their European counterparts, the result of better diet, more sunlight, and the absence of the very worst of the British and Continental "slums." Rickets, for example, was not a common problem in Australia, for exposure to sunlight prevented the deficiency of Vitamin D.[14] While there was certainly poverty and overcrowding in Australia, especially in urban areas, in the main the physical environment was preferable to the Old World.

Despite these advantages, anxiety over infant mortality in Australia was pervasive and influential. Such a concern was political, for it was thought that the population was both decreasing and degenerating. In the Antipodes, the crisis was believed to be particularly acute: there were ever-present fears that the populous Asian nations would invade to occupy the vast unsettled lands. Thus the infants described, in both political and medical discourse, were not simply children, but products for the maintenance of the nation. Discussions of infant health were concerned not simply with medical aspects of disease, but were steeped in social, political, and economic beliefs. At a time when the birth rate was declining, it became increasingly important for society to ensure the survival of those babies who were born. Individual babies were rarely the issue, even within medical discourse. The emphasis was instead on the baby as human capital, on the necessity of the child's survival for the nation.[15]

Preventing Infantile Death

Prevention of infantile disease was seen to be the key to forming and maintaining white Australia. More generally, medical progress was aided by advances in antisepsis and anaesthetics, but far less progress was made in the treatment of the diseases of children. The one great advance in pediatric medicine was the introduction of the diphtheria antitoxin in the 1890s. Diphtheria had previously had a mortality rate of over 50 per cent, and careful use of the antitoxin was able to reduce this figure to 23 per cent.[16] Most fatal illnesses, including scarlet fever, diarrhea, and whooping cough were beyond the help of the physician; the most that could be offered was sound nursing and good nutrition. Few drugs had real effect. Only quinine for malaria was truly curative, and opium was of course an effective sedative and pain reliever.[17] Thus while surgical and pharmaceutical science progressed slowly, pediatric medicine was largely preventive: with few effective cures, prevention was the key.

Prevention had long been an important part of the medical regime, in an era when cures were few and far between. Yet preventive medicine had not always been applied to babies, and the emergence of pediatrics as a discipline rested in part in the medicalization of *all* infant life, rather than simply as a response to a specific illness. In Australia, there were significant attempts to regulate the physical environment, particularly in urban areas. Initiatives included slum clearances, an emphasis on clean milk and safe food, and general public works such as sewerage in the cities. Much of this can be read as a middle-class fear of contagion from the lower orders. There was certainly an emphasis on educating the poor in matters of health and hygiene, without ever challenging or changing their material and economic position.[18]

Behind this new emphasis on prevention was a change in attitude towards health and illness. Across time, infants had always been susceptible to illness, disease, and malnutrition, but by the late nineteenth century, such death rates were no longer acceptable to society. Where once high infantile death rates had been greeted with a fatalistic acceptance, late Victorian society believed that this figure could be changed and improved, and that doctors were the vehicle for such change.[19] In fact, it was not necessarily medicine that improved death rates, but the new public health measures. At the same time, however, the image of the medical profession was heightened by the slowly declining death rates.

With prevention the key to infant health, the primary and defining core of the nascent specialty of pediatrics was the control of infant feeding. With contemporary estimates suggesting one half of all infant deaths were caused by stomach disorders, the feeding of babies took on a special significance, and within medical discourses, infant feeding was central to debates over infant mortality.[20]

Doctors, Mothers, and Infant Feeding

Despite the apparent "naturalness" of the act, infant feeding is not simply the provision of nutrition for children, but is represented by a complex set of discourses regarding mother and child. As the anthropologist Vanessa Maher suggests, breastfeeding is not only a matter of food, but is bound by social and economic parameters.[21]

Thus breastfeeding is not as "natural" as it may at first appear. Women make choices, from how often to feed their child, for how long, and indeed whether to feed at all. Breastfeeding is a "cultural action."[22] It is also a biological fact. Mothering in the Victorian period was inextricably tied to feeding, in both ideology, and in real, practical terms. Infant feeding thus acts as an important signifier of the relationship between mother and child. With the intervention of the medical profession, and the emergence of pediatrics, such a relationship is further complicated.

With prevention of disease the key to infant management, breastfeeding was universally encouraged by Australian doctors. In a wider sense, this support can be explained by a broad movement towards breastfeeding and sentimental motherhood, with breastfeeding a key site for the establishment of Romantic maternity.[23] More specifically, medical texts from the eighteenth century onwards encouraged maternal breastfeeding.[24] Even so, the Australian situation is notable for its emphasis on the breast: in the United States, for example, the bottle was increasingly proposed as a more "scientific" approach.[25]

There were good reasons for the calls for maternal breastfeeding. Recent studies of breast milk have revealed that maternal antibodies are passed to the infant through the milk, offering protection from stomach illnesses and respiratory infections. Further, such components may act in the infantile gut itself, making it more capable of resisting infection. Overall, breastfeeding affects infantile health in three ways: there is a decrease in exposure to pathogens, it is nutritionally sound, and it has a positive impact on the immune system.[26] Indeed, historical models suggest that breastfeeding offered the best protection for children, with mortality rates actually increasing when babies were weaned.[27] Certainly, in Australia in the late nineteenth and early twentieth centuries, there were clear and distinct links between infant feeding practices and infantile illness. There was a clear awareness among doctors that infants raised on powdered, condensed, or fresh cow's milk were more susceptible to illness and death.

Much of the debate over infant feeding practices appears to have come out of observations over the pitiful infant mortality in European foundling homes, where death rates could reach over 90 per cent. Similarly, the situation was dire in Australian institutions, where infant feeding and infant mortality were directly related. For example, at the Ashfield Infants Home in Sydney in 1889, of a total of 130 children, eighteen or 13.9 per cent died, all of who were bottle fed. As the medical report for the home suggested, there was a significant "immunity enjoyed by breast-fed children from infectious and contagious diseases."[28] The pattern continued, and in 1891, of eighteen deaths, all were bottle fed. Sixteen of these infants had been artificially fed from birth, while the remaining two had been weaned abruptly in the last six weeks of their short lives.[29] Over a period of twenty years, in only one year does the death rate of breastfed babies rival that of the bottle fed.[30] By the following year, however, the situation was reversed, and bottle feeding continued to be a major causal factor in infant mortality throughout the period.

In the early years of the twentieth century, the link between death rates and feeding was explored by W. G. Armstrong, a Sydney physician who later became involved in infant welfare. Armstrong believed that mortality of infants hand fed either wholly or partially was thirty-seven times that of infants entirely breastfed.[31] He carried out a series of surveys to prove his theory, and he found that in 1903, of the 116 infants who died of diarrhea in the City of Sydney, only five had been purely breastfed, while thirty had never been breastfed. Of the 111 babies reared on breast substitutes, over half were fed solely or mainly on condensed milk.[32] In 1905 of sixty infants who had died of diarrhea before they reached three months of age, only 6.6 per cent had been entirely breastfed. This is compared to a population, he believed, in which 72 per cent of infants were entirely breastfed.[33]

Clearly, breastfeeding was the safest and most effective way of feeding a baby. Nevertheless, doctors were convinced that mothers were abandoning the practice, and while it is difficult to ascertain the number of women who breastfed, this does not appear to have been the case. Some doctors suggested breastfeeding was "fairly general practice."[34] W. A. Verco, president of the South Australian Branch of the British Medical Association, claimed in 1910 that two-thirds of infants were breastfed, but he did not specify to what age.[35] Differences were perhaps class based. The editors of the *Australasian Medical Gazette* claimed in 1907 that a mere quarter of upper-class women breastfed. They also noted that working-class women could rarely breastfeed, as it was necessary for them to earn a living. It was, however, generally believed that the rate of maternal breastfeeding was decreasing.[36]

As doctors believed breastfeeding was declining, and that the result would be an increase in infant mortality, the medical profession attempted to convince women to breastfeed. The advantages of breastfeeding were couched in terms of "naturalness." Breastfeeding was widely seen as "natural," and hence superior. As Nature, personified almost as the loving mother herself, had so cleverly provided breast milk as the "proper" food for infants, it was logical that the "first duty of a mother is to suckle her baby."[37] In a society segregated along the lines of gender, to breastfeed was to be part of the moral order, to obey the laws of both nature and culture. Stemming from this discourse of nature was the idea that it was the mother's obligation to feed her child. As one Sydney doctor wrote in a self-help book aimed at women, "Mother's milk is the inalienable birthright of every child."[38]

The mother was encouraged to feed in a variety of ways. Her milk was portrayed as the ideal: it was perfectly "fresh, sweet and free from germs."[39] Breastfeeding was also idealized in romantic terms. Doctors described the "duty" as a pleasure: "Some intelligent patients have told me that they have never felt so happy as when suckling their baby; and that after each repetition of the pleasing duty, they seemed to have accomplished something worth living for."[40]

Thus doctors reduced women to their biological basis. Just as women were encouraged to reproduce, to breastfeed was also a significant contribution to a gendered society. Women could only gain pleasure, or happiness, through their biological "duty." The breast, and breastfeeding, were thus symbolic of the natural order.[41]

Discourses of naturalness defined and articulated breastfeeding tropes, and the most venomous of terms were used to describe women who did not breastfeed. Such women were seen as "cruel" and "unnatural," as thwarting Nature herself.[42] Women who did not breastfeed stepped outside the "natural" and hence correct gender order; they were described as unwomanly, and "unworthy of the name of mother."[43] In part, to breastfeed was seen as an essential part of married life and the responsibility of a mature woman.[44] More than this, however, such entreaties to breastfeed embraced, and were formed by, wider cultural and biological constructions of womanhood. Women were "governed and defined by their reproductive capacity,"[45] and breastfeeding was a logical and accepted extension of their procreation. Medical discourses on infant feeding thus operated on a number of levels. First, doctors portrayed their interest as a scientific endeavour, using medicine to reduce the infant mortality rate. Science, and science alone, would save the lives of babies. Second, infant feeding was a moral crusade, based at a fundamental level on a gendered view of society. Biological determinism lay at the crux of both the moral order and the scientific regime.

Further, the medical profession was concerned with the individual child in terms of the nation. Using the language of industry, and the rationale of the state, the medical profession attempted to encourage maternal breastfeeding. Breastfeeding, it was believed, would prevent "much wastage of infant life."[46] The medical profession utilized pronatalism, combined at times with overtones of the eugenics movement, and recommended breastfeeding to produce strong and healthy babies for the nation. As one doctor suggested, babies could grow "to fill useful place in society" only if they were properly fed.[47] Correct feeding would both decrease the mortality rate, and produce a better race of stronger, healthier citizens.

Within discussions of infant health, most doctors were highly critical of women, and attacks on mothers could be quite fierce.[48] In general, doctors condemned the ignorance and carelessness of mothers.[49] Stemming from this view was the practical belief that the simplest way to decrease infantile illness and the rate of infant mortality was to educate mothers. Socio-economic realities were rarely mentioned. There were a few exceptions; in an unusual public comment in 1907, the editors of the *Australasian Medical Gazette* claimed that hygienic surroundings would decrease the infant mortality rate and called briefly for better dwellings, with improved ventilation, drainage, backyards, and air spaces.[50] More blatantly, the honorary medical officer at the Children's Hospital in Melbourne claimed in 1908 that treatment was almost useless when the child was to be returned to "the sweltering dusty lanes in the city, to be re-poisoned by dirty milk and city germ-laden air."[51]

More common, however, were critiques of mothers and mothering skills, and an almost universal call for education to overcome these deficiencies. Typical was H. Swift, an Adelaide doctor interested in infantile scurvy, who suggested that mothers should be educated to rear their children on "scientific principles,"[52] while the editors of the *Australasian Medical Gazette* spoke for many when they claimed, "No doubt much can be done in the way of educating mothers."[53] There was an explicit assumption throughout the profession that mothers needed to "be taught how to nourish their infants."[54] Education was so central to an attack on infant mortality that the first two recommendations of the New South Wales Royal Commission on the Decline of the Birth-Rate and on the Mortality of Infants pertained to increasing the education of mothers.[55]

The doctors themselves were to be a crucial part of the educational program: the medical profession clearly believed that mothers could not breastfeed without assistance. Breastfeeding was portrayed as something that women needed to learn, with the help of the medical profession.[56] According to the historian Joan Sherwood, the eighteenth century had seen the new belief that breastfeeding was "a *technology* for producing a new human being."[57] It was the doctor who was in the position to guide and help women to both breastfeed and develop this ideal infant. Doctors therefore promoted breastfeeding as "natural," but at the same time stressed the importance of medical intervention.

Such contradictory discourses continued in medical attitudes towards women's bodies. On one hand, maternal breastfeeding was seen as the ideal form of infant feeding, yet on the other hand, doctors were profoundly critical of those maternal bodies. While breastfeeding was seen as superior in every way, it was still far from perfect, and mothers were told to consult professional help, because the maternal body was often seen as incapable of doing the task correctly. Some women were told they had too little milk, others too much.[58] As J. P. McNeill, who wrote popular self-help books on the raising of infants suggested, there were myriad ways in which the maternal body could cause distress to the child: too much milk, too little, too rich, too thin, too slow, too rapid, or of insufficient quality.[59]

There was, however, very little interest in the emotional advantages of breastfeeding. Doctors judged the issue on medical grounds (breast-feeding was better for the baby's health, and decreased the infant mortality rate), or moral grounds (it was the mother's "duty" to take care of the welfare of the child). A rare exception was Charles Hunter, who in 1878 recommended breastfeeding in part because "babies cannot live by milk alone....A mother's love and petting, and joy in her child go far to carry it safe through the dangers of the first year."[60]

The link between maternal love and infant feeding was then absent from the literature until the royal commission of 1904, where the connection between morbidity and a lack of love and devotion was briefly considered. Dr. Litchfield, an expert on institutionalized children, noted that a child in a foundling hospital, who was merely fed every two hours, but not picked up or played with, would simply "dwindle" away.[61] It is perhaps not surprising that such comments were rare in medical discourse. By claiming maternal devotion was essential to the very survival of the baby, the medical profession would be allowing the mother a significant amount of power in the triad of mother, child, and doctor. The profession preferred to concentrate on such matters that they could more directly control.

Controlling the Breast

Breastfeeding allowed for a number of controls over the freedom of the mother, all for the sake of the child. As such, there was a shift in emphasis from the woman to the infant: the life of the mother was to be constrained for the welfare of her child. It was believed that the "mother's health, temper and habits always affect her suckling child for good or ill."[62] The mother was to control both her physical and psychological well-being, as carelessness on her behalf could lead to danger to the child. In the period from 1880 to around the turn of the century, these controls were of a practical nature. The mother was to eat well, but plainly, renouncing any little delicacies. There was some disagreement among doctors and other "experts" on the use of alcohol during breast-feeding. From the frequency of comments, it is clear that the use of alcohol to stimulate the flow of milk was common, and traditional advice recommended a glass of ale or stout twice a day.[63] Some doctors still prescribed a tumbler of mild ale or porter with dinner and supper,[64] while many of the new experts deplored the taking of any alcohol at all, fearing both mother and child could develop alcoholism.[65] Disagreements over the use of alcohol is an instance of traditional mothering and child-rearing practices being challenged by new, more scientific practices.

The emotional state of the mother was also to be controlled and regulated. It was believed that the infant would thrive only when the mother was "quiet, tranquil, and in a cheerful temper." Normal emotions such as grief, anger, and excitement were seen to pollute the milk, making it "actually poisonous."[66] More than one doctor claimed that a mother who fed her child after a fit of "anger, or excitement, or grief, or worry" could cause a fit of convulsions in the infant, which could even lead to death.[67] A 1905 text was even more explicit: a fretful temper could lead to decreased quantities of very thin milk, which would lead to disturbances of the child's bowels. Anger would lead to irritating milk, which would cause the baby to have diarrhea. Grief or anxiety would diminish the amount of milk, and lead irretrievably to artificial feeding with all its risks.[68] Thus the mother was to moderate her emotional state; there was little recognition of her own needs or desires.

During the entire period, but especially after the turn of the century, the medical profession concentrated on the routines of feeding. Despite its construction of feeding as "natural," doctors proposed a quite rigorous timetable for mothers and babies. If feeding in the late nineteenth and early twentieth century was not yet as "scientific" and controlled as it was to become in the 1920s and 1930s,[69] there was nevertheless a strong emphasis on regularity—an emphasis that does suggest that most women simply fed on demand. This informal method was to be replaced by a schedule of regularized feeds. During the day, the baby should be fed quite frequently: most books recommended every hour or two during the first month or two, then decreasing to every three hours after that.[70] In a list of ten "nevers" for Australian mothers, the first was not to give the infant the breast if she cried. The second was not to give the child the breast in between planned feeds.[71] Feeding was to take precisely twenty minutes.[72] The child was not to be left on the breast overnight, but trained to go without food for a period of some hours. This obviously demanded more of the mother: the child was to sleep in a separate cot, and was not to be fed if it woke. The child should never be fed to relieve soreness in the mother's breasts, nor fed out of schedule if it cried.[73] If the child was not awake when a feed was due, he or she would be wakened, so as not to disrupt the imposed pattern of feeding. To do so was to risk "alimentary derangement" in the child.[74]

Weaning, too, was rigidly controlled. It was strongly recommended that weaning take place between the age of seven months and one year. Few doctors recommended or even discussed the contraceptive value of breastfeeding, probably because of the general belief in pro-natalism, and the reluctance to discuss contraceptive methods more generally. McNeill was an exception: he listed among the advantages of breastfeeding its worth as a birth control.[75] While some, though not all, doctors acknowledged that breastfeeding provided some contraceptive value, it was felt that late weaning was injurious to both mother and child. Albutt strongly condemned those women who fed for up to two years, warning it could lead to pregnancy, miscarriage, general ill health, blindness of the mother, and could also render the suckling child "idiotic." J. E. Usher, a physician and surgeon, claimed prolonged breastfeeding was a sign of the "selfish mother," who was harming her child in order to remain barren. Both mother and child were thus debilitated; the mother from refusing her biological destiny, and the child, for whom breast milk was evidently insufficient. Usher claimed this prolonged feeding was so hazardous that the infant could not really be expected to live.[76] While prolonged breastfeeding without supplementation may be harmful, leading eventually to nutritional deficiencies, it is evident that generally the breast was supplemented from the table. Women might have been better served by prolonged breastfeeding, which can act as a reasonably effective contraceptive, therefore decreasing too frequent childbearing, and its harmful effects on the maternal body. The medical profession, however, stressed the perceived harm to the suckling infant. Rather neatly, such beliefs fitted into a discourse of pro-natalism, and the needs of the nation state.

Throughout medical discourses on infant feeding, doctors' emphasis continued to be on the welfare and well-being of the child. This view was in direct contrast to earlier writings on infant feeding, when maternal breastfeeding was advocated as best for the mother, and the mother–child bond. According to Valerie Fildes in her extensive study of infant feeding from 1500 to 1800, seventeenth- and eighteenth-century doctors believed breastfeeding would offer better health for the mother, both immediately after childbirth and as a preventive, as well as making mothers happier and more content. The mother-infant bond would be stronger, for breastfeeding would encourage love between the two. There were benefits for the child, too, but these were secondary to those of the mother, and were mentioned in only a handful of texts.[77]

In Australia, in the late nineteenth century, however, the situation was reversed. A number of texts did recommend women breastfeed for the sake of their own health; Albutt claimed a woman should feed, as she would be less vulnerable to the "diseases of the womb."[78] In 1878, Charles Hunter claimed cancer arose from a refusal to suckle.[79] Others agreed that the woman who bottle-fed was more prone to peritonitis, abscesses, cancer, and other ailments.[80] Ten years later, McNeill mentioned that suckling could make frail women more robust, and agreed that cancer was less likely in the woman who breastfed.[81] A. W. Gardner, a chemist and author of the popular *The First Few Months of Infancy: Being Hints to Mothers*, claimed the "principle upon which nursing was based was that the infant should derive a positive gain, and the mother no negative loss." (So invisible had the mother become to Gardner that the index to the mother's health was the bowel movements of her child!)[82] Such comments on the mother were always vague and unsubstantiated. Any discussion of benefits to the mother always formed a very marginal argument, a brief comment in a rhetoric of the advantages to the infant, indicating a distinct change over time and space in attitudes to mothers and infants.

Selfish Mothers

Within the medical discourse, the stereotypical target for medical contempt was wealthy women who chose not to feed their own children. The standard mother who abandoned breastfeeding was seen to be the privileged woman: "The frivolous, ballroom, 'society' mother, who objects to nurse her offspring because it would interfere with her social engagements [is] unworthy of the honour of maternity."[83]

The infants were passed to wet nurses, or were hand reared. Given the state of Australian society in this period, however, such women would have been a minority. While there was a distinct gap between the wealthy and the poor, the very wealthy always made up a small proportion of the total.[84] More generally, women were accused of not wanting to face the difficulties of breastfeeding.[85]

There was little recognition of women failing to breastfeed for economic reasons. Attitudes to mothering were firmly constrained by bourgeois notions of family structures. Women had always participated in the Australian economy, and in 1918 the government statistician T. A. Coghlan had noted that around half of all women had been in paid employment, and some 20 per cent remained so over the course of their whole lives.[86] While the ideal of the husband/father as breadwinner and mother/wife as home-maker had infiltrated the dominant Victorian discourses, it was not an ideal achievable by all. Many working-class women and some middle-class women were forced, through economic necessity, to labour outside the home. This reality was not, however, reflected in attitudes to breastfeeding and childrearing.

In an 1886 tract for the Australian Health Society, Dr. Willis does mention that some mothers, most especially single mothers, had to work to support a child, and he recommends partial weaning, with breastfeeding continuing at night.[87] Of all the texts considered, only one discussed the role of the father. Dr. Hunter, also writing for the Australian Health Society, in 1878, blamed the father, who was "too idle, too proud, or too drunken to work," for women's employment, and therefore her perceived failure in her duty as a mother.[88] In general, however, the social and economic causes for the abandonment of maternal breastfeeding were largely ignored. The responsibility for maintenance of child life was strictly gendered, with the father virtually absent from any discussions, not only of feeding, but of infants and infant life.

The poor health of the mother was the main reason given by the medical profession for the abandonment of breastfeeding. Many women were seen as too unhealthy to breastfeed.[89] Underlying this discussion is a cultural assumption of the ill health of women. There is no doubt that many women were exhausted and sickly from too frequent childbearing, poor obstetric care, hard work, and poor diet. Many women may also have suffered with bacterial infections of the breast that prevented feeding.[90] Nevertheless, ideology may have played a part: the "ideal" Victorian woman was frail, sensitive, and wan. With fragility came femininity.[91] While numerous historians have indicated such an ideal was a bourgeois imagining, such a cultural construction of womanhood may have affected attitudes toward women's health generally, and more specifically toward breastfeeding.[92] Recent studies of women in developing nations have indicated that mothers who were undernourished still produced nutritious and plentiful breast milk. It is only the most malnourished of mothers, living in the midst of dire famine, who find it difficult to provide for their infant.[93] Australians during this period were in general well fed, and certainly better so than in the industrial areas of England. As such, it would appear that the idea that large numbers of women could not feed as a result of their health is perhaps misguided, and more of a cultural construction than a reality.

Nevertheless, ill health was the predominant reason given by the medical profession for women not breastfeeding their own children. Women who were seriously ill, with tuberculosis, syphilis, consumption, scrofula, or epilepsy, were exempted from this duty.[94] But there were many other vague admissions of ill health. In his *Illustrated Australian Medical Guide* in 1903, Philip E. Muskett offered two reasons why women could not feed their children: first, her milk might have dried up, and second, her health might be too poor.[95] Other women might have lacked milk; one doctor in 1906 noted, in a case of infantile scurvy, that the child had never been fed, as the mother had never "had a natural flow."[96] There was certainly a belief, among mothers as well as doctors, that, in the words of one Melbourne physician, "very few mothers are able to supply sufficient milk to repair the wear and tear of the growing infant."[97]

Some texts excluded women from breastfeeding on psychological grounds. Breastfeeding was not necessary if the mother had "any marked tendency to nervous diseases,"[98] or suffered with anxiety, hysteria, headaches, or faintness.[99] Tensions are thus evident between the overall insistence on breastfeeding, and the exceptions "allowed" by the medical profession. Indeed, such tensions problematize a simple reading of breastfeeding. On one hand, all women were to breastfeed, and those who did not were seen as both unnatural and unwomanly. On the other hand, exceptions were made for women who were sickly or unwell. While pro-natalism was certainly a dominant discourse in late nineteenth- and early twentieth-century Australia, it was bounded by gender assumptions about femininity, and by the boundaries of the body itself.

Wet Nursing

While maternal breastfeeding was certainly the medical ideal, not all women could or would breastfeed their infant. In contrast to the American model, which highlighted the scientific nature of bottle feeding, in Australia the next best thing to mother's milk was the wet nurse.[100] Wet nursing, for which one woman is paid to suckle the child of another, took two forms in Australia.[101] First, wet nurses were used wherever possible within institutions, such as orphanages and maternity homes. Breastfeeding could help reduce the terrible rates of infant mortality suffered by abandoned babies. Some women would be employed to nurse children other than their own, while destitute women were institutionalized alongside their babies, and could act as a wet nurse for other poor children within the system. Second, wet nurses could be hired, to live in with the parents of the child, much like other types of domestic servants. The live-in wet nurse was available only to reasonably well off families, as a result of the costs involved. This was the preferred form of wet nursing, where both the child and the wet nurse remained in the parental home, under the supervision and care of the biological mother.[102]

Throughout the medical discussion of infant feeding, doctors were concerned with the life of the infant. Their preference for breastfeeding by the mother—or if this was not possible, by her substitute, the wet nurse—are rather indicative of the lowly position of the mother within the discourses of infant feeding. There was little regard for the mother, or even for the bond between mother and child. The mother was central to debates over infant feeding, but it was not for the value placed on her care or devotion. Instead, the concentration on the mother was formed simply because she held the best chance for child survival. It is clear that the woman, whether the mother or the wet nurse, was important only in terms of the baby. In the eighteenth century, there had been a sincere medical interest in the mother, but by the end of the nineteenth century, the child was of profound importance.[103] Such a shift occurs across the West, but was even more pronounced in Australia, where concerns about the population and white babies intensified such beliefs.[104] In Australia, medical discourses on infant feeding serve to almost commodify the mother and nurse: milk became a means to an end, the survival of the child and future citizen.

The Deadly Bottle

The increased interest in infant feeding was not confined to breastfeeding alone. Throughout the last decades of the nineteenth century, there was a rapid increase in interest in the artificial feeding of infants.[105] While breastfeeding was desired and encouraged by the medical profession, concern over the declining birth rate and infant mortality meant articles on artificial feeding substantially increased. Nevertheless, with maternal breastfeeding as the ideal, and the wet nurse a distant second, the medical profession was, in the late nineteenth century, highly critical of attempts to hand feed an infant. Symptomatic of medical views in the late nineteenth century was Dr. Willis. Writing for the Australian Health Society in 1882, he claimed hand feeding was equal to sending the child to an "early grave." If the child did not die outright, Willis felt hand feeding would lead to disaster, "upsetting its digestive system, so deranging its whole economy and maybe laying the foundation of future ills that she will be unable to combat or control."[106]

Bottle feeding had an extremely high mortality rate. In 1878, Hunter claimed that four out of five babies raised by hand died in their first year.[107] In the *Popular Medical Guide*, Dr. Schrader reported that a coroner in Melbourne claimed of every hundred children hand-reared, seventy or eighty would die in the first three months, even when the best of care was taken.[108] The anonymous author of *Healthy Mothers and Sturdy Children*, who claimed to have twenty years experience in general practice, suggested that from every hundred children raised on artificial food, only ten were well developed, twenty-six moderately developed, and the rest badly developed.[109] William S. Byrne of Brisbane claimed in 1904 that nine out of ten babies suffered on an artificial feeding regime. Byrne claimed that of every hundred bottle-fed babies, at least seventy-five died before they reached their first birthday.[110] Certainly, it was believed some 50 per cent of bottle-fed babies died during the Brisbane summer.[111] It is difficult for the historian to verify such claims, given the paucity of information on death certificates; however, it is certain that bottle-fed infants made up the vast majority of the deaths in the first year of life.[112]

The historian Milton Lewis has delineated many of the issues of bottle feeding in Australia, including the fundamental problem of obtaining a clean supply of milk.[113] Once delivered, there was a multiplicity of practical problems within the household. The ice chest did not become reasonably common until 1900, and ice was not available in all areas.[114]

Some families simply could not afford fresh milk even once a day.[115]
Further, fresh milk was not always obtainable,[116] and even when it was,
the use of inferior grade cow's milk was linked to vitamin deficiencies,
such as rickets.[117] Another factor leading to high infant mortality among
bottle-fed babies was cleanliness. Women often did not have the time,
resources, or knowledge to keep equipment adequately sterilized, an
especially difficult task in the heat of the Australian summer.[118]

Despite the rhetoric of "naturalness" surrounding cow's milk, it was
actually quite indigestible for the infant. The medical profession made
frequent and often contradictory comments on the best ways to "human-
ise" milk, and the dilution of cow's milk was a major source of debate
within the medical journals. In the 1880s and early 1890s, such advice
was rough and ready.[119] With the decline in popularity and accessibility
of wet nursing, however, an increased interest in the topic was combined
with a new, more "scientific" approach. Comments on hand feeding
became increasingly complicated as the period progressed. In the early
twentieth century there was an emerging emphasis on calories, and the
chemical makeup of milk.[120] Not all articles were concerned with the
minute details of making milk palatable for infants (some simply stressed
the need for clean supplies),[121] nonetheless there was a clear trend in that
direction. As the life of the infant became increasingly important, investigation into artificial feeding intensified.

While mothers tended to use a simple half-milk, half-water mix,
doctors claimed it was necessary to modify the cow's milk in a more
sophisticated manner.[122] Various combinations were suggested, but most
agreed that sugars must be increased, the proteids diminished, and the
fat levels retained.[123] Some methods relied on percentages, while others
used fat and proteid ratios, all of which depended somewhat on uniformity of cream in the produce.[124] Further, these early infant formulas
were generally developed under laboratory conditions, using test tubes
for ease of measurement, and stable temperatures.[125] They were probably not practical for the mother at home, without excellent facilities and
high level of education. For example, Charles E. Towl, a pharmacist
published in the *Intercolonial Medical Journal*, made the construction of
milk for infants akin to mixing a medicine, using complicated mathe-
matical and chemical procedures.[126]

Because of the limitations of using cow's milk, alternatives were
popular, including goat's milk, tinned milk, condensed milk, and patent
brands of infant formula. Many of them were deficient in fats and vitamins, and were condemned by the medical profession. There was, however, a range of advice provided, with different doctors holding different opinions of the value of these substitutes. Condensed milk is a case
in point. Condensed milk was seen as the cause of rickets and scurvy,[127]

and as the "stock food of the baby farmer."[128] The Melbourne coroner, Dr. Youl, claimed that feeding an infant condensed milk was "equivalent to murdering it."[129] Cheaper brands of condensed milk (and those more likely to be chosen by working-class women) could be low in fat content, which could lead to childhood deficiencies in Vitamins A and D.[130] Some claimed it produced "soft" and "flabby" babies, who looked healthy enough, but had no stamina.[131] There were certainly no guarantees of its purity; in 1910 some twelve thousand tins were confiscated by the Health Department, as unfit for human consumption.[132] There may have been further difficulties with storage; poor homes may not have had a can opener, and so the tin would be opened at the store.[133] Some doctors took a middle line and claimed it was inferior, but usable, especially for poor families who simply could not purchase fresh milk even once a day.[134] Others felt it was "safe and wholesome":[135] it could be preserved for the long term in a "perfectly sweet and fresh condition."[136] Similarly, dried milk could be seen as causing illness such as scurvy, or as a "most valuable and safe food."[137] Mothers were subject to multiple, contradictory advice.

While experts in the 1870s had advocated feeding infants foods such as wheat, oats, and rice,[138] a decade later the medical profession was highly critical of the mother who fed her infant "unsuitable" foods. Feeding a child was not a simple choice between the bottle or the breast.[139] Mothers obviously found it easier to feed babies straight from the family table, and many did not prepare separate meals for their infants.[140] Inexpensive foods such as maize, cornflour (cornstarch), arrowroot, bread and butter, sago, and potato were commonly fed to infants, because of their cost and the ease of preparation.[141] Poor women could often afford no other foods, and the health of the child often quickly suffered.[142] Babies were also given sugar, butter, and gin, and some were given tea, coffee, and "other stimulants" as "common practice."[143] This wide feeding was strongly condemned by doctors, and indeed it is probable that stomach upsets were common. At the same time, mothers were faced with difficult, rather inadequate choices: infant feeding was subject to numerous negotiations between ideals and reality.

Those Less Fortunate

With the increased emphasis on population and children more generally, the late nineteenth and early twentieth centuries saw a wider medical interest in the children of the poor and disadvantaged. New legislation to protect and reform children was instigated, including factory and child protection acts and compulsory schooling.[144] Such measures were designed to more generally control and regulate children, particularly the children of the poor. These children also came under increasing socio-medical surveillance, with medicine keen to explore new ways to improve infant life and health. Doctors and legislators recognized that childhood death rates were substantially higher among illegitimate children, and there was some consideration of the plight of these illegitimate children, particularly those in baby-farms and infant homes. The declining birth rate and high infant mortality made all children, even those without the financial and social support of a father, more important.[145]

This focus is particularly clear in the calls for the increased maternal breastfeeding of illegitimate children. Doctors suggested that mothers keep the babies and suckle them until they reached twelve months, at which time they should be removed.[146] Dr. Wood, of the Children's Hospital in Melbourne, was typical of those interested in the welfare of illegitimate children. He wanted the women to be sheltered from the public gaze before the birth, and suggested confinement within state-run homes for two to three months before childbirth. Such assistance was, however, conditional: all women were to agree to stay on at the institution after the birth for six months, to nurse and feed their children. In this manner, the child was saved, because it was breastfed, and affection and attachment would grow between the mother and her baby. There was little concern for the freedom or life of the mother, only that the child received the breast: "Every infant is entitled to one pair of mother's arms." It was not a solution to the very real problem of single motherhood. While the life of the baby might be saved, there was no explanation of what would become of the mother or baby after the six months of enforced breastfeeding.[147]

In some ways, the new focus on maternal breastfeeding indicates an increase in the importance or worth of the mother. She was someone of value. There had been little examination of the bonds between mother and child, except for in the most cursory assumptions of bourgeois maternal devotion. By 1904, the royal commission briefly though marginally noted that illegitimate children were generally separated from their mothers, and thus lacked the "stimulating influence of the maternal handling and caressing." The report suggested that this need should be considered in future plans for foundling homes and other institutions, proposing that it be compulsory for mothers to be admitted with the child.[148] The key here is "compulsory." While it was understood that women often objected "strongly" to being institutionalized with the child, it was believed that the rights of the mother should be subsumed to the right of the infant to maternal milk.[149] So while the importance of the mother was being "discovered," it was an importance only in relation to the life of the child.

While feeding was central to the rate of infant mortality, such a fact calls into question the role of the mother. While no legislation was enforced, and infant homes continued to take in motherless infants, the calls for the unification of mother and child indicate a distinct disinterest in the mother herself. In many ways, these women were unimportant; by becoming single mothers they had stepped outside the boundaries of social order and polite maternity. They were socially, politically and economically marginal. As such, doctors and the public saw little reason to prioritize their well-being. Emerging ideas about rights were conceived solely in terms of the infant's right to breast-milk, and did not extend to the mother's right to freedom and independence. This seems to be especially so in the case of poor or single mothers, for these were women who transgressed seemingly sacred sexual and social boundaries.

By 1902 the "chief object" of the Ashfield Infants Home, for example, was the "preservation of infant life."[150] This was a change from earlier models, where the emphasis was less explicitly on the child, and more broadly defined in terms of help for destitute women and their babies. The emphasis was altering. When the Sydney Home for Babies was established in February 1910 in Waverley, the "primary reason for our existence" was "To Save the Babies."[151] While the education and training of the mother was important, the most critical issue was "To stem the waste of Child Life."[152] The Benevolent Society agreed; by 1906, "every means" was "adopted in the interests of humanity for the salvation of child life."[153] Indeed, by 1909, the society was to claim that the "Life of the child—as a life—is as precious as the life of the mother, in many cases more so."[154] The voice emphasizing the child intensified.

Conclusion

The emergence of an interest in child health was part of a wider Western awakening to childhood, and the conceptualization of children as both separate and special. The emergence of pediatrics was stimulated in Australia by a concern for high infant mortality and the need to populate a white nation: every baby became increasingly important for the state. Doctors were sufficiently professionalized to be positioned as authorities in infant health, and were able to encourage the status of the child as valuable and needing a specialist's care. The discourses of nascent pediatrics had split the mother and child. They were no longer joined together, physically and ideologically through the practice of obstetrics. Instead, the child was judged as an independent and valuable member of society. The professionalization of the health care of infants and children had important implications for mothers. With the ideological and physical separation of mothers and infants came a change in attitudes towards women and maternity. The professionalization of home life and the care of children led to a devaluation of women's skills and women more generally.[155] Certainly in the case of health care, the increasing emphasis on the knowledge and power of the doctor, and the new importance of the child, led to attacks on women's role as mother. The medical profession frequently attacked mothers, and such attacks were strong, even vitriolic. With child mortality concentrated in the first year of life, and mothers being so closely aligned with the feeding of babies, it is not surprising that these attacks largely centred on infant feeding.

By the late nineteenth century, medical interest in feeding was motivated by a concern for the burgeoning infant life. From practical observations that the breast was best, to a scientific examination of the chemical structures of cow's milk, the infant's well-being (as both an individual and a locus of the state) was the focus. As such, medical views on breast and bottle feeding act as an important signifier of wider attitudes to children and childhood.

Through these discourses on maternal feeding, we can read the changing relationship between mother and child, and among the mother, child, state, and medical profession. For the state, the growing priority was the safety of the child, with only secondary concern for the wishes or needs of the mother. The medical profession was central to such discourses. Despite their assertions that breastfeeding was natural, doctors stressed that medical surveillance and intervention was necessary. Thus the scientific regime was prioritized, and other aspects of infant feeding, such as economics, were rarely noted. The mother herself was marginalized: her role became simply to feed her baby, to maintain the health of her child. The infant was to be the new priority; the idea that children were supremely important, to individual families and to the nation, was an important social, political, and cultural change of the late nineteenth and early twentieth centuries.

Acknowledgement

I would like to thank Dr. Mary Spongberg of Macquarie University for her consideration of an early draft of this chapter.

Notes

1 Fielding H. Garrison, "History of Pediatrics," in *Abt-Garrison History of Pediatrics*, ed. Isaac A. Abt (Philadelphia: W. B. Saunders, 1965), 2; Editorial, "An Hospital for Sick Children," *Australasian Medical Gazette* (January 1861): 36. See also the *Sydney University Calendar 1885*, which clearly indicates the location of infant health within the discipline of Midwifery and the Diseases of Women (Sydney: Gibbs, Shallard, 1885), 241.

2 Abraham Jacobi, "The Relations of Paediatrics to General Medicine," *Transactions of the American Paediatric Society* 1 (1889): 8. Geriatrics is the only other specialty to deal with a special kind of person, rather than a certain part or structure of the body.

3 A brief note on sources. In the late nineteenth century, there were close and continuous relations between British and Australian doctors. In numerous ways, Australian doctors were educated and formed by the British model. To provide a history of Australian medicine, I have focused on Australian texts and journals. The exception, however, is the inclusion of overseas authors whose work was published within Australia. The rationale for choice this was simple: texts published locally were presumably read locally, thus framing and influencing local opinions. Their accessibility is the crucial issue here.

4 Josephine M. Lloyd, "The 'Languid Child' and the Eighteenth-Century Man-Midwife," *Bulletin of the History of Medicine* 75 (2001): 641–79; A. R. Colon with P. A. Colon, *Nurturing Children: A History of Paediatrics* (Westport: Greenwood Press, 1999), 158; and Samuel Kottek, "'Citizens! Do you want children's doctors?' An Early Vindication of 'Paediatric' Specialists," *Medical History* 35 (1991): 105.

5 Colon with Colon, *Nurturing Children*, xiv.

6 A professional body, a sign of the maturation and entrenchment of a discipline, was slow to form. In Australia, the Melbourne Paediatric Society was informally established in 1906, and a paediatric section for the New South Wales Branch of the British Medical Association was formed in 1922. Nevertheless, pediatrics was not officially consolidated until 1950, with the formation of the Australian Paediatric Association. Lorimer Dods, "'As It Was in the Beginning': Some Notes on the Prenatal and Early Postnatal History of the Australian Paediatric Association," *Australian Paediatric Journal* 4 (1968): 204–208. Bryan Gandevia. *Tears Often Shed: Child Health and Welfare in Australia from 1788* (Sydney: Pergamon Press, 1978), 140; and Peter D. Phelan, Don M. Roberton, and Mike South, "Defining Moments in Medicine: Paediatrics," *Medical Journal of Australia* 174 (2001): 16–17.

7 Kathleen W. Jones, "Sentiment and Science: The Late Nineteenth Century Pediatrician as Mother's Advisor," *Journal of Social History* (Fall 1983): 81.

8 Jonathon Gillis, "Bad Habits and Pernicious Results: Thumb Sucking and the Discipline of Late-Nineteenth-Century Paediatrics," *Medical History* 40 (1996): 71.

9 David Armstrong, "The Invention of Infant Mortality," *Sociology of Health and Illness* 11 (1989): 212; and Judith Sealander, "Perpetually Malnourished? Diet, Health, and America's Young in the Twentieth Century," in this volume.

10 Wray Vampleur, ed., *Australian Historical Statistics* (Sydney: Fairfax, Syme and Weldon, 1987), 58.

11 W. McLean, "The Declining Birth Rate in Australia," *Intercolonial Medical Journal*, (March 20, 1904), 109. For an in-depth statistical analysis of infant mortality in Europe, see Carlo A Corsini and Pier Paulo Viazzo, eds., *The Decline of Infant and Child Mortality: The European Experience 1750–1990* (The Hague, The Netherlands: Kluwer Law International, 1997). Statistics from R. I. Woods, P. A. Watterson, and J. H. Woodward, "The Causes of Rapid Infant Mortality Decline in England and Wales 1861–1921: Part 1," *Population Studies* 42 (1988): 349; and Sealander, "Perpetually Malnourished?"

12 Philip E. Muskett, *The Health and Diet of Children in Australia* (Sydney: Edwards, Dunlop, 1890), 96.

13 P. M., "A Review of *A Manual for What Every Mother Should Know*," *Australian Medical Journal* (July 1881): 318.

14 Philip E. Muskett, "Australian Rickets: The Form of Rickets Met with in Australian Children," *Australian Medical Gazette* (July 1891): 285.

15 W. H. Crago, "Presidential Address to the NSW Branch of the BMA," *Australasian Medical Gazette* (April 15, 1895): 149; Gerald E. Cussen, "Infantile Gastro-enteritis," *Australasian Medical Gazette* (May 20, 1899): 189; Editorial, "The Protection of Children," *Australasian Medical Gazette* (June 21, 1909): 321; and W. McLean, "Alleged Artificial Restriction of Families," *Australasian Medical Gazette* (August 20, 1894): 396.

16 P. L. Hipsley, *The Early History of the Royal Alexandra Hospital for Children Sydney, 1880 to 1905* (Sydney: Angus and Robertson, 1952), 67–70.

17 Peter Yule, *The Royal Children's Hospital. A History of Faith, Science and Love* (Sydney: Halstead Press, 1999), 57.

18 See, for example, the Australian Health Society, which from 1875 produced a series of pamphlets aimed at educating the poor. Titles often focused on infant feeding and child mortality. See Australian Health Society Melbourne, "Rules for the General Management of Infants," in *Sanitary Tracts Issued by the Australian Health Society Melbourne*, first series (Melbourne: Australian Health Society, 1882); Board of Public Health, Victoria, on behalf of the Australian Health Society, *Infant Feeding: The Use and Abuse of Artificial Foods* (Melbourne: Board of Public Health, 1896); Charles D. Hunter, *"What Kills Our Babies?"* for the Australian Health Society Melbourne (Melbourne: Mason, Firth and McCutcheon, 1878); James Jamieson, *Diseases Which Should Be Prevented: A Lecture Delivered under the Auspices of the Australian Health Society*, rev. ed. (Melbourne: Australian Health Society, 1892); J. W. Springthorpe, "The Results of Unhealthy Education," in Australian Health Society, *Health Lectures for the People*, first series (Melbourne: George Robertson and Company, 1886), 79–108; and T. R. H. Willis, "The Mortality and Management of Infancy," in Australian Health Society, *Health Lectures for the People*, first series (Melbourne: George Robertson and Company, 1886), 49–78.

19 As Judith Sealander notes in this volume, "it was an 'infant holocaust' that nourished two infant American professions—paediatrics and food science." See page 164.

20 David Hardie, "Presidential Address Medical Society of QLD" *Australasian Medical Gazette* (January 20, 1900): 8; W. F. Litchfield, "Summer Diarrhoea in Infants, from the Public Health Point of View," *Transactions of the Australasian Medical Congress*, 1905, p. 421.

21 Vanessa Maher, "Breast-feeding in Cross Cultural Perspective: Paradoxes and Proposals," in *The Anthropology of Breast-Feeding: Natural Law or Social Construct*, ed. Vanessa Maher (Providence: Berg, 1992), 4.

22 Kirsten Hastrup, "A Question of Reason: Breast-feeding Patterns in Seventeenth and Eighteenth Century Iceland," in *The Anthropology of Breast-Feeding. Natural Law or Social Construct*, ed. Vanessa Maher (Providence: Berg, 1992), 92.

23 Ruth Perry, "Colonising the Breast: Sexuality and Maternity in Eighteenth Century England," *Journal of the History of Sexuality* 2, 2 (1991): 217; and Joan Sherwood, "The Milk Factor: The Ideology of Breast-feeding and Post-partum Illnesses, 1750–1850," *Canadian Bulletin of Medical History* 10 (1993): 30–31.

24 Among the most influential were W. Cadogan, *An Essay upon Nursing and the Management of Children from Their Birth to Three Years of Age* (London: J. Roberts, 1748); Hugh Smith, *Letters to Married Women, on Nursing and the Management of Children*, 6th ed. (London: C. and G. Kearsley, 1792); and Alexander Hamilton,

A Treatise on Midwifery Comprehending the Management of Female Complaints and the Treatment of Children in Early Infancy (London: J. Murray, 1781).

25 Rima D. Apple, *Mothers and Medicine. A Social History of Infant Feeding 1890–1950* (Madison: University of Wisconsin Press, 1987).

26 S. Thapa, R. V. Short, and M. Potts, "Breastfeeding, Birth Spacing and Their Effects on Child Survival," *Nature* 335, 6192 (1988): 679; Gabrielle Palmer, *The Politics of Breastfeeding* (London: Pandora Press, 1988), 46; Barry M. Popkin, Tamar Lasky, Deborah Spicer, and Monica E. Yamamoto, *The Infant-Feeding Triad: Infant, Mother and Household* (New York: Gordon and Breach Science Publishers, 1986), 1, 80; and Thomas W. Hale, *Medications and Mothers' Milk* (Amarillo, TX: Pharmasoft Medical Publishing, 2002), 5.

27 Susan Scott, "Malnutrition, Pregnancy and Infant Mortality: A Biometric Model," *Journal of Interdisciplinary History* 30 (1999): 54–56.

28 Infant's Home, *Fifteenth Report of the Infant's Home Ashfield, for the Year Ending 31st December 1889* (Sydney: J. L. Holmes, 1890), 11.

29 Infant's Home, *Seventeenth Report of the Infant's Home Ashfield, for the Year Ending 31st December 1891* (Sydney: Marcus and Andrew, 1892), 10.

30 Infant's Home, *Seventh Report of the Infant's Home Ashfield for the 18 Months Ending 31st December 1881* (Sydney: Robert Bone, 1882), 8–9.

31 W. G. Armstrong, "Some Lessons from the Statistics of Infantile Mortality in Sydney," *Australasian Medical Gazette* (October 20, 1905): 518.

32 Cited in Milton James Lewis, "'Populate or Perish': Aspects of Infant and Maternal Health in Sydney, 1870–1939," PhD thesis, Australian National University, 1976, 40.

33 Armstrong, "Some Lessons," 518.

34 Walter Summons, "Birth-Rate and Infant Mortality," *Intercolonial Medical Journal* (March 20, 1907): 181.

35 W. A. Verco, "The Influence of the Medical Profession upon the National Life in Australia," *Australasian Medical Gazette* (July 20, 1910): 339.

36 Editorial, "Infant Mortality in Tasmania," *Australasian Medical Gazette* (April 20, 1907): 205.

37 A. W. Gardner, *The First Few Months of Infancy: Being Hints to Mothers* (Melbourne: Kemp and Boyce, 1888), 11.

38 John Service, *On the Natural and Artificial Feeding and Care of Infants* (Sydney: Edwards, Dunlop, 1890), 57.

39 William S. Byrne, "Infant Mortality and Infant Feeding," *Australasian Medical Gazette* (February 20, 1904): 58.

40 George Fullerton, *The Family Medical Guide* (Sydney: William Maddock, 1884), 426. See also the Canadian doctor, P. H. Chavasse, who published in Australia. P. H. Chavasse, *Man's Strength and Women's Beauty: A Treatise on the Physical Life of Both Sexes* (Melbourne: Standard, 1879), 2.

41 As Ludmilla Jordanova suggests, "Links between women, motherhood, the family and natural morality may help to explain the emphasis on the breast." Ludmilla J. Jordanova, "Natural Facts: A Historical Perspective on Science and Sexuality," in *Nature Culture and Gender*, ed. Carol P. MacCormack and Marilyn Strathern (Cambridge: Cambridge University Press, 1980), 49.

42 Chavasse, *Man's Strength*, 295; M. U. O'Sullivan, *The Proclivity of Civilised Woman to Uterine Displacement: The Antidote; Also Other Contributions to Gynaecological Surgery* (Melbourne: Stillwell, 1894), 16.

43 J. P. McNeill, *The Treatment of Children in Health and Sickness* (Sydney: JAS Miller & Co. Machine Printers, 1888), 36; O'Sullivan, *Proclivity of Civilised Woman*, 16; and Gardner, *First Few Months*, 12.

44 Stewart Warren, *The Wife's Guide and Friend*, 5th ed. (Melbourne: Saunders, 1898), 43.

45 Mary Poovey, *Uneven Developments: The Ideological Work of Gender in Mid-Victorian England* (London: Virgo, 1989), 35.

46 Editorial, "Infant Mortality in Tasmania," 205.

47 H. Arthur Albutt, *The Wife's Handbook: How a Woman Should Order Herself during Pregnancy, in the Lying-In room, and after Delivery* (Sydney: Modern Medical Publishing, circa 1890), 27.

48 See, among others, Cusson, "Infantile Gastro-enteritis," 188; J. T. Mitchell, "Summer Diarrhoea of Infants," *Australasian Medical Gazette* (July 15, 1893): 234. William S. Byrne, "Presidential Address to the QLD Branch of the BMA: Medical Matters in Queensland," *Australian Medical Gazette* (December 20, 1904), 608; Chavasse, *Man's Strength*, 295; O'Sullivan, *Proclivity of Civilised Woman*, 16; McNeill, *Treatment of Children*, 6; Willis, "Mortality and Management," 56; Gardner, *First Few Months*, 12; A. Jeffreys Wood, "Preservation of Infant Life," *Intercolonial Medical Journal* (March 20, 1908): 141; Editorial, "Infant Mortality," 205; and Warren, *The Wife's Guide*, 43.

49 Evidently some doctors believed that mothers deliberately harmed their infants. For a counter to this argument, see Philip E. Muskett, *The Feeding and Management of Australian Infants in Health and Disease*, 7th ed. (Sydney: William Brooks, 1906), xxvii. See also evidence from Dr. Worrall, "Report of the Royal Commission on the Decline of the Birth Rate and the Mortality of Infants in New South Wales," *New South Wales Parliamentary Papers*, 1904, 40.

50 Editorial, "Infant Mortality."

51 Wood, "Preservation of Infant Life," 135.

52 H. Swift, "Cases of Infantile Scurvy," *Australasian Medical Gazette* (April 20, 1906): 179.

53 Editorial, "Infantile Mortality," *Australasian Medical Gazette* (September 20, 1906): 461.

54 "Report of the Royal Commission," 40.

55 "Report of the Royal Commission," 43.

56 Gardner, *First Few Months*, 9.

57 Sherwood, "Milk Factor," 27. Italics in original.

58 Service, *Natural and Artificial Feeding*, 8.

59 McNeill, *Treatment of Children*, 21; see also Muskett, *Feeding and Management*, 196.

60 Hunter, *What Kills Our Babies?* 9.

61 "Report of the Royal Commission," 42. Internationally, the links between infantile survival and mother care were noted in the late nineteenth century. It was, for example, reported by the American doctor Joel Foster in the *Medical Record*, of 1873. Foster noted that among institutionalized infants, of those kept with their mother, only 12 per cent died, while of those wet-nursed by another, 72.5 per cent perished. Cited in Janet Golden, *A Social History of Wet Nursing in America: From Breast to Bottle* (Cambridge: Cambridge University Press, 1996), 117.

62 Anonymous, *Healthy Mothers and Sturdy Children: A Book for Every Family* (Melbourne: Peter & Knapton Printers, 1893), 83. In the original, this sentence is in bold type, and enlarged one size for maximum impact.

63 Anonymous, *Healthy Mothers*, 47.

64 Chavasse, *Man's Strength*, 304.

65 Albutt, *Wife's Handbook*, 26; Anonymous, *Healthy Mothers*, 47, 93; and Willis, *Mortality and Management*, 58.

66 Gardner, *First Few Months*, 22. See also Chavasse, *Man's Strength*, 307–308.
67 Anonymous, *Healthy Mothers*, 83. See also McNeill, *Treatment of Children*, 46.
68 F. C. Richards and S. Edin Eulalia, *Ladies Handbook of Home Treatment* (Melbourne: Signs, 1905), 202.
69 Kerreen M. Reiger, *The Disenchantment of the Home: Modernising the Australian Family 1880–1940* (Melbourne: Oxford University Press, 1985), 129.
70 Gardner, *First Few Months*, 12; Philip E. Muskett, *The Illustrated Australian Guide*, 2 vols. (Sydney: William Brooks, 1903), 478; Editorial, "The Diet of Infants Deprived of Breast Milk," *Australasian Medical Gazette* (February 15, 1894): 61.
71 Muskett, *Feeding and Management*, lix.
72 Muskett, *Illustrated Australasian Medical Guide*, 479.
73 Chavasse, *Man's Strength*, 300. Australian Health Society, *11th Annual Report and "Rules for the General Management of Infants as Prepared by the Obstetrical Society of London"* (Melbourne: H. Cordell Printer, 1886), 5; Service, *Natural and Artificial Feeding*, 6; and Anonymous, *Maid, Wife and Mother* (Sydney: n.p., 1883), 57.
74 Willis, *Mortality and Management*, 57.
75 McNeill, *Treatment of Children*, 36.
76 J. E. Usher, *The Perils of a Baby* (Melbourne: Samuel Mullen, 1888), 31. The anonymous author of *Wife, Maid and Mother* claimed menstruation would cause the milk to deteriorate, 8. Chavasse, *Man's Strength*, 329.
77 Valerie Fildes, *Breasts, Bottles and Babies: A History of Infant Feeding* (Edinburgh: Edinburgh University Press, 1986), 112.
78 Albutt, *Wife's Handbook*, 23.
79 Hunter, *What Kills Our Babies?* 10.
80 Willis, *Mortality and Management*, 57; McNeill, *Treatment of Children*, 36.
81 McNeill, *Treatment of Children*, 36.
82 Gardner, *First Few Months*, 22.
83 Service, *Natural and Artificial Feeding*, 4.
84 See, for example, Stuart Macintyre, *Oxford History of Australia* (Melbourne: Oxford University Press, 1986), chapter 1.
85 "Report of the Royal Commission," 40.
86 Beverly Kingston, *My Wife, My Daughter and Poor Mary Ann: Women and Work in Australia* (Melbourne: Thomas Nelson Australia Pty, 1975), 2.
87 Willis, *Mortality and Management*, 14.
88 Hunter, *What Kills Our Babies?* 10.
89 Contemporary estimates suggest some 5 per cent of women are physically (as opposed to emotionally) unable to breastfeed. Golden, *Wet Nursing*, 19–20. Such a figure, however, will not necessarily correlate to women in the past, when health issues were quite different.
90 Fildes, *Breasts, Bottles and Babies*, 111.
91 Barbara Ehrenreich and Deidre English, *For Her Own Good: 150 Years of the Experts' Advice to Women* (London: Pluto, 1979). Ehrenreich and English note, "From the romantic perspective, the sick woman was not that far off the ideal woman anyway. A morbid aesthetic developed, in which sickness was seen as a source of female beauty....The logic which insists that femininity is negative masculinity necessarily romanticises the moribund woman...the romantic spirit holds up as its ideal—the *sick* woman, the invalid who lives at the edge of death" 98–99. Italics in original. See also Elaine Showalter, *The Female Malady: Women, Madness, and English Culture, 1830–1980* (New York: Pantheon, 1985).
92 For a refutation of the idea of the idle Victorian woman, see Patricia Branca, "Image and Reality: The Myth of the Idle Victorian Woman," in *Clio's Conscious-*

ness Raised: New Perspectives on the History of Women, ed. Mary S. Hartmann and Lois Banner (New York: Harper and Row, 1974), 179–91; Nancy Folbre, "The Unproductive Housewife: Her Evolution in Nineteenth Century Economic Thought," *Signs* 16 (1991): 463–84; and Lee Holcombe, *Victorian Ladies at Work: Middle Class Working Women in England and Wales 1850–1914* (London: Newton Abbot, 1973).

93 For example, in one study of well-fed English mothers and less well-nourished Keneba women, their milk output was seen to be the same. See Palmer, *Politics of Breastfeeding*, 44, 88; Vanessa Maher, "Breast-feeding and Maternal Depletion: Natural Law or Cultural Arrangements?" in *The Anthropology of Breast-feeding: Natural Law or Social Construct*, ed. Vanessa Maher (Providence: Berg, 1992), 161. Maher concedes this point, but she questions the load that multiple births and prolonged breastfeeding have on the maternal body, claiming it can be a risk to the mother's own health. Further, as Millard and Bell suggest, the mother's nutritional state during pregnancy readily leads to problems. Lowered levels of nutrition can lead to immaturity of the fetus, and congenital defects. In this sense, the mother's malnutrition may be more likely to affect the infant's health during the neonatal period. See Robert Millard and Frances Bell, "Infant Mortality in Victorian England: The Mother as Medium," *Economic History Review* 54, 4 (2001): 708.

94 Service, *Natural and Artificial Feeding*, 10.

95 Muskett, *Illustrated Australasian Medical Guide*, 479.

96 Swift, "Cases of Infantile Scurvy," 175.

97 Usher, *Perils of a Baby*, 13.

98 Gardner, *First Few Months of Infancy*, 11; Fullerton, *Family Medical Guide*, 471.

99 Chavasse, *Man's Strength*, 329.

100 See, for example, James Jamieson, *How To Feed Infants* (Melbourne: Stillwell and Knight, 1871), 34, 45; Muskett, *Illustrated Australasian Medical Guide*, 480. The only exception to this rule was George Fullerton, a prominent physician in Brisbane. In his 1884 guide to family medicine, Fullerton claimed hand rearing by a loving and careful mother to be preferable to entrusting the care of the infant to another. He cited different cases of neglect by wet nurses who left their charges drugged so they could visit their biological children, spend time with their friends, or visit a lover, while wet nurses kept in the family home could be wilful and disturb the peace. He also claimed that the husband of the wet nurse might be less than thrilled with the arrangement, presumably as it would disrupt his home life and access to his wife's body. Fullerton was, however, a lone voice. Fullerton, *Family Medical Guide*, 474–75.

101 Definition from George D. Sussman, *Selling Mothers Milk: The Wet Nursing Business in France 1715–1914* (Urbana: University of Illinois Press, 1982), 2.

102 For an international perspective, see the definitive work by Valerie Fildes, *Wet Nursing: A History from Antiquity to the Present* (Oxford: Basil Blackwell, 1988.) For a more detailed analysis of the wet nurse, see Lisa Featherstone, "Whose Breast Is Best? The Wet Nurse in Late Nineteenth Century Australia," *Birth Issues Journal* 11 (2002): 41–46.

103 Fildes, *Breasts, Bottles, and Babies*, 112–17.

104 On the international context, see Anna Davin, "Imperialism and Motherhood," *History Workshop Journal* 5 (1978): 9–65; Hilary Marland, "A Pioneer in Infant Welfare: The Huddersfield Scheme 1903–1920," *Social History of Medicine* 6, 1 (1993): 25–50; Jane Lewis, "The Social History of Social Policy: Infant Welfare in Edwardian England," *Journal of Social Policy* 9, 4 (1980): 463–86; Elidh Gar-

rett and Andrew Wear, "Suffer the Little Children: Mortality, Mothers and the State," *Continuity and Change* 9, 2 (1994): 179–84; and Alain Bideau, Bertrand Desjardins, and Hector Perez-Brignoli, eds., *Infant and Child Mortality in the Past* (Oxford: Clarendon Press, 1997). In Australia, see Neville Hicks, *"This Sin and Scandal": Australia's Population Debate 1891–1911* (Canberra: ANU Press, 1978); and Reiger, *Disenchantment of the Home*; Jill Julius Matthews, *Good and Mad Women: The Historical Construction of Femininity in Twentieth Century Australia* (Sydney: George Allen and Unwin, 1984).

105 The term *artificial feeding* is used broadly here, to include all forms of infant nutrition other than human milk. It includes fresh and preserved animal milk, as well as general foodstuffs and a variety of "paps" made from cereals and breads mixed with water.

106 Willis, *Mortality and Management*, 56.

107 Hunter, *What Kills Our Babies?* 10.

108 Christian U. D. Schrader, *Popular Medical Guide* (Sydney: Direct Supply Co., 1887), 78.

109 Anonymous, *Healthy Mothers*, 84.

110 Byrne, "Infant Mortality and Infant Feeding," 56.

111 Muskett, *Feeding and Management*, 229.

112 See death rates within institutions, such as the Ashfield Infant's Home, above. Similar rates were seen in some other Western nations, and in Canada the link between artificial feeding and high infant mortality was well noted. See Aleck Ostry, "The Early Development of Nutrition Policy in Canada," in this volume.

113 On the spread of disease through milk, see Milton Lewis, "Milk, Mothers and Infant Welfare," in *Twentieth Century Sydney: Studies in Urban and Social History*, ed. Jill Roe (Sydney: Hale and Ironmonger, 1980), 193–207. Cow's milk is ideal for the development and growth of micro-organisms, especially diseases. Diseases transmitted through milk include, among others, polio, hepatitis, anthrax, cholera, E-coli, diphtheria, enteritis, listeriosis, dysentery, staphylococcal gastroenteritis, scarlet fever, TB, and typhoid. By the 1880s, it was clear that milk could transmit disease, and several studies in England had linked outbreaks of typhoid and scarlet fever to specific local dairies. P. J. Atkins, "White Poison? The Social Consequences of Milk Consumption, 1850–1930," *Social History of Medicine* 5 (1992): 216–17. On the lack of clean milk available, see Editorial, "Unsound and Adulterated Foods," *Australasian Medical Gazette* (April 1895): 179; Editorial, "Milk Adulteration in New South Wales," *Australasian Medical Gazette* (May 1895): 224; E. Ken Herring, "Infantile Diarrhoea," *Australasian Medical Gazette* (October 1900): 410; Board of Public Health, *Infant Feeding*, 7–8, 13; J. T. Mitchell, "Summer Diarrhoea of Infants"; A. Jefferis Turner, "Infantile Mortality," *Australasian Medical Gazette* (May 20, 1910): 280; A. G. Salter, "The Artificial Feeding of Infants," *Australasian Medical Gazette* (November 20, 1909): 586; Service, *Natural and Artificial Feeding*, 32; Editorial, "The Adulteration of Milk," *Australasian Medical Gazette* (September 20, 1902): 467; Editorial, "Adulterated Milk," *Australasian Medical Gazette* (January 21, 1907): 45; Byrne, "Presidential Address," 608; and D. McFadyen, letter to the editor, *Australasian Medical Gazette* (February 20, 1905): 86. On attempts to clean up the milk supply, see H. S. Cole and Thomas Morris, "Registration of Dairyman," *The Public Health Act 1889* (Melbourne: Charles F. Maxwell London, 1894), 281–83; George Lane Mullins, "Dairies and the Milk Supply in New South Wales," *Australasian Medical Gazette* (October 1896): 417; and "Dairies Supervision Act, Report of the Administration of, for the Year 1894," *Journal of the Legislative Council, New South*

Wales (1894): 1–7. In Canada, there were similar issues, with clean fresh cow's milk available in some regions, while not in others. See Aleck Ostry, "Early Development."

114 Anonymous, "Impure Milk and Infant Mortality," *Intercolonial Medical Journal* (February 20, 1898): 108–109; and Kingston, *My Wife, My Daughte*, 34.

115 Peter Bancroft, "Presidential Address Medical Society of QLD," *Australasian Medical Gazette* (February 1895): 69.

116 Editorial, "Tinned Milk," *Australasian Medical Gazette* (April 1899): 189.

117 Muskett, "Australian Rickets," 285.

118 A sterilizer was out of the reach of most women, costing in 1894 between twenty to thirty shillings. Editorial, "Diet of Infants," 60.

119 See, for example, Board of Public Health, *Infant Feeding*, 6; Wilfrid Nickson, "The Artificial Feeding of Infants," *Australasian Medical Gazette* (October 15, 1893): 329; and Anonymous, *Healthy Mothers*, 90.

120 William MacKenzie, "Caloric Values in Infant Feeding," *Intercolonial Medical Journal* (May 20, 1908): 244–52; A. Jeffreys Wood, "Simple Method for the Quantitative Determination of Proteids in Milk," *Intercolonial Medical Journal* (November 20, 1907): 587–89; and Eleanor E. Bourne, "The Artificial Feeding of Infants," *Australasian Medical Gazette* (December 20, 1909): 638.

121 Wood, "Preservation of Infant Life," 128–41. Dunbar, as late as 1906, stressed the need to avoid bottles with a tube. J. W. Dunbar, "Infantile Mortality," *Commonwealth Parliamentary Papers*, Session 1907–1908, vol. 2. Appendix iv.

122 Salter, "Artificial Feeding of Infants," 586.

123 Byrne, "Infant Mortality and Infant Feeding," 57.

124 Bourne, "Artificial Feeding," 638.

125 Wood, "Simple Method," 587–89.

126 Chas. E. Towl, "Milk Dispensing," *Intercolonial Medical Journal* (October 20, 1900): 482–90.

127 Board of Public Health, *Infant Feeding*, 8; McKay, "Summer Diarrhoea," 257; Bourne, "Artificial Feeding," 639.

128 McKay, "Summer Diarrhoea," 257.

129 Editorial, "Diet of Infants," 61.

130 Lewis, "'Populate or Perish,'" 32.

131 Nickson, "Artificial Feeding," 329.

132 Editorial, "Public Health," *Australasian Medical Gazette* (December 20, 1910): 698.

133 Lewis, "The Social History of Social Policy," 468.

134 Peter Bancroft, "Presidential Address," 69.

135 McNeill, *Treatment of Children*, 23.

136 Service, *Natural and Artificial Feeding*, 27.

137 Salter, "Artificial Feeding of Infants," 588.

138 James Jamieson, *How To Feed Infants*, 34.

139 Vanessa Maher made this observation among contemporary families in the developing world, who also fed even newborns gruels, rice waters, and broths. Maher, "Breast-feeding and Maternal Depletion," 153.

140 Editorial, "Infant Foods," *Australasian Medical Gazette* (June 15, 1894): 205.

141 Anonymous, *Healthy Mothers*, 89; Albutt, *Wife's Handbook*, 31; Sydney Gibbons, *"Notes on Diet: An Outline of the Philosophy and Practice of Nutrition": Lecture for the Australian Health Society* (Melbourne: McCarron, Bird, 1884), 5; and Editorial, "Infant Foods," 33.

142 Benevolent Society of New South Wales, *Annual Report for 1908* (Sydney: W. E. Smith, n.d.), 15.

143 Service, *Natural and Artificial Feeding*, 4; Usher, *Perils of a Baby*, 14.

144 Jan Kociumbas, *Australian Childhood: A History* (Sydney: Allen and Unwin, 1997), 118–27. Chapter 7 offers a comprehensive survey of disadvantaged children.

145 Indicative of the unusual value placed upon illegitimate children in Australia is the Maternity Allowance of 1912. Introduced by Andrew Fisher's Labour Government, the "baby bonus" of five pounds was extended to unmarried women. It was, however, denied to women who were not white, including "Asiatics," Pacific Islanders, and Aboriginal mothers. See Marilyn Lake, *Getting Equal: The History of Australian Feminism* (Sydney: Allen and Unwin, 1999), 75–76.

146 W. F. Litchfield, "The Infants under 'The New South Wales Children's Protection Act' with Some Remarks on Infant's Asylums," *Australasian Medical Gazette* (January 20, 1899), 25.

147 Wood, "Preservation of Infant Life," 135–41.

148 "Report of the Royal Commission," 41.

149 "Report of the Royal Commission," 41.

150 Infant's Home, *Twenty-Eighth Report of the Infants Home Ashfield, for the Year Ending 31st December 1902* (Sydney: G. Watson Printer, 1903), 9.

151 M. C. Luker, *To Save the Babies and To Help the Mothers: The Sydney Home for Babies, Nelson Bay Rd Waverley* (Sydney: D. S. Ford, 1911), 7.

152 Luker, *To Save the Babies*, 11.

153 Benevolent Society of New South Wales, *Annual Report for 1906* (Sydney: Samuel and Lees, n.d.), 12.

154 Benevolent Society of New South Wales, *Annual Report for 1909* (Sydney: W. E. Smith, n.d.), 16.

155 Reiger, *Disenchantment of the Home*; Desley Deacon, "Taylorism in the Home: The Medical Profession, the Infant Welfare Movement and the Deskilling of Women," *Australian and New Zealand Journal of Sexuality* 21 (1985): 161–73.

Perpetually Malnourished?

Diet, Health, and America's Young in the Twentieth Century

ଔ

Judith Sealander

Jacob Riis, New York's most famous police reporter, once again entered the reeking hallway of a familiar Mott Street tenement. Accompanying a "charity doctor" on his rounds, Riis entered a dark room on the top floor. A small girl lay dying of starvation on a makeshift bed of two chairs tied together with rope. Father, mother, and "four other ragged children" sat around her. "Improper nourishment," whispered the doctor. The father, crippled by lead poisoning, could not work. Not a single person in the family had eaten that day. Knowing it could not be fulfilled, the doctor gave an order that the child be given beef broth and left. Instead, by evening's end, she was dead. In *How the Other Half Lives* Riis charged that "hundreds" of other children, also hidden, died from hunger every night in the city's tenements.[1] The book's graphic depictions of want in the midst of great wealth caused a sensation in early-twentieth-century America. Was it true that helpless children wasted away for lack of proper food? Was a rich country neglecting the basic duty of feeding its offspring?

The questions galvanized a generation of reformers and echoed through the twentieth century, as the topic of diet, health, and America's young provoked decades of controversy. The subject of children's nutrition, 1900–2000, is worth reviewing on its own merits, but it also illuminates other themes important to the history of health and children, with lessons relevant to most developed countries, not just the United States. A decline in absolute poverty did not stimulate undisputed improvement in the general nutritional health of the country's young. Instead, a nation with too many stick-thin, underfed children became one with ballooning populations of overfed, fat ones. The century ended with warnings that the United States faced an epidemic of childhood obesity. If the topic shows that prosperity can be a nutritional sword of Damocles, it also illustrates the episodic nature of national attention to hunger in the midst of plenty, and links reform activism to the presence of a thriving, optimistic, middle class. It demonstrates a growing government role as the regulator of food and as an arbiter of what the young should eat. Finally, the subject provides a lens through which to examine the impact of professionalized food study.

The years between 1900 and 2000 spanned the "American century."[2] A big but insular country became a global leader. A nation rich in resources became the richest on earth, and Americans linked faith in progress with worship of expertise. Old occupations such as medicine and law systematized and raised the bars to entrance. New professions—sociology, psychology, and nutrition science—changed culture and government.

Even if rooted in pioneering work done by nineteenth-century European food chemists, the analysis of diet was, as Harvard nutritionist Jean Mayer noted, "the American science."[3] Born in France, Mayer came to the United States to work with leaders of a field increasingly dominated after 1900 by Americans and U.S. universities.[4] However, when called in 1968 to testify before a federal Congressional committee investigating hunger in the American South, Mayer admitted to an ongoing "lover's quarrel" with his adopted country, whose citizens were hopelessly "ignorant" about food. Bad eating habits were the norm, but professional nutritionists often just confused a population already surfeited with conflicting dietary advice.[5]

That was certainly true as several generations of Americans grew to adulthood between the years 1900 and 2000. Consensus about an optimal diet for those under eighteen proved elusive. Some charged that a wealthy country's children were perpetually malnourished, even if by the end of the century that meant that significant numbers of its youngsters ate too much of the wrong foods, not meals that provided too few calories. Decisions about feeding children often nourished professional rivalries, enriched bureaucratic budgets, or fed the demands of food-producer lobbies.[6] Practically everyone saw "money going down the wrong drain."[7]

An overview of the twentieth-century history of professional nutrition science in the United States provides a framework that helps to explain why the task of giving good advice about the feeding of America's young proved so controversial.

The Study of Diet in Twentieth-Century United States: An Overview

The "American science" had German origins. In the 1850s Justus von Liebig separated food into its component parts: proteins, carbohydrates, fats, minerals, water. At least in the West, the act of eating would never be the same. The idea that diets could be judged on the basis on their chemical components was revolutionary. Since ancient times, "well fed" meant a full belly, though clearly all realized that the wealthy had many more choices than did the poor.[8] No, said von Liebig. Good nourishment was not simply a matter of quantity. Expertise was crucial.

American food chemists, especially those employed by the United States Department of Agriculture, eagerly embraced the new view.[9] By the beginning of the twentieth century, a network of government agricultural experiment stations, allied with public land grant colleges, funded and advertised new notions about human nutrition. As rich Americans took up the cause and opened their pockets to create a parallel structure of private institutes and specialized university departments, the "American science" flourished.[10]

Universities, public agencies, philanthropies, and food producers themselves put growing numbers of "household administrators," "home ecologists," "sanitary scientists," "euthenicists," "nutritionists," "dieticians," or "home economists" on their payrolls.[11] The names varied wildly, indicative of the profession's infant status. So too did the advice.

That would prove to be an enduring twentieth-century pattern, as diet experts challenged each other and their predecessors. A first generation of nutritionists, for example, gave short shrift to fresh vegetables, praised protein, and, with an eye to improving working-class diets, elevated turkey backs, beef shinbones, and codfish to a trinity, ideally served in slow-simmered one-dish stews. Successors would damn such a diet as dangerous.[12]

Internecine and intergenerational conflicts characterized twentieth-century professional nutritional advice. So too did nutritionists' anger at an American public perceived to be stubbornly unreceptive. That shaped a century's debate about feeding the country's young, as experts repeatedly scolded parents, politicians, and principals for not choosing correct foods for children. In 1977, the tone of Morgan State University professor of food science Norma Maiden was characteristic: the nation's school boards were the "blind leading the blind."[13] Children could learn good eating habits only if offered some independence, but their choices had to fall within "parameters of good nutrition." That meant public schools must ban chips, cola, and candy, indeed all junk foods. "Whether our nation survives as a free democracy depends upon our educational system being able to teach every child…how to keep a healthy body."[14]

Nutritionists sounded choruses of shrill alarm, but the non-professionals they chastised were often not wilfully feeding themselves and their offspring badly. They were more likely thoroughly confused. The lines between good advice and quackery were never as clearly drawn as each successive generation of nutrition scientists believed. Horace

Fletcher, a wealthy businessman who in retirement recreated himself as a self-taught food expert, was convinced that digestion actually occurred in the mouth. Therefore, all foods had to be masticated until tasteless. Though some disciples thought a hundred chews sufficient, Fletcher himself never attached a number to his technique. Once trained, a practitioner would naturally vomit any food swallowed too soon. If they remembered him at all, later nutritionists thought Fletcher a fraud. But, important to note, a significant number of his contemporaries, including Yale professors of food science, became ardent "fletcherizers." John D. Rockefeller Sr. was only one of a host of American parents who forced children to sit at table silently, stolidly, endlessly chewing their dinner.[15] The fad for fletcherizing died with the man in 1919, though Will Kellogg remained an ardent adherent.

Will Kellogg not only fletcherized. He hired professional home economists, who, not surprisingly, touted his corn flakes as a perfect food for children, epitomizing a final trend in twentieth-century U.S. nutrition science.[16] Governments and academia patronized the new discipline. So did food producers. By the end of the century, hundreds of foundations and institutes supported by food processors competed with associations sponsored by medical professionals and with government agencies to give the public diet advice.[17] The early-twentieth-century milk wars presaged a continuing cacophony, as debates about how best to feed infants began a century in which experts returned repeatedly to child malnourishment as a touchstone.

The Milk Wars: Early-Twentieth-Century Disputes about Infant Feeding

As a new century began, an estimated 16 per cent of babies born in the United States died before reaching a first birthday. In the summer months, the toll rose—to one in three deaths in the first twelve months of life. It was an "infant holocaust" that nourished two infant American professions: pediatrics and food science.[18]

Early-twentieth-century experts blamed many problems for high infant mortality: from the great number of cases of tuberculosis among babies, to alcohol abuse by nursing mothers.[19] Highest on the agenda, however, was improper infant feeding. Some physicians had long suspected that cow's milk spread communicable diseases, but by the late nineteenth century the microscope banished any remaining doubts that unclean milk contained dangerous bacteria.[20] But the search for "pure" milk to give to babies proved controversial.

Indeed, chemists, physicians, and others could not even agree on a common formula for pure milk. Some championed "certified" raw milk produced on approved dairy farms regularly inspected by veterinarians. Others advocated pasteurized milk, which had been heated to 145°F, held twenty minutes, then cooled. Though commonly used in Europe, in the United States, acceptance lagged, even among physicians, who worried that dairymen would employ the process to disguise spoiled product.[21] Some cities banned pasteurization altogether.

If Americans initially regarded pasteurization with suspicion, they quickly embraced another nineteenth-century European innovation, commercial infant formula. By 1900, a significant percentage of middle-class U.S. mothers, the ones who could afford to buy the powdered blends of dried cow's milk, sugar, and malt flour, began to wean their babies earlier. And formula manufacturers advertised products such as Nestlé's Milk Food, meant to be mixed with boiled water, not just as convenient, but as healthful for infants. Breastmilk, they warned, was insufficient.[22]

The stage was set for the entrance of a new group of experts on infant feeding: physicians who specialized in child health, who told parents to trust neither commercial preparations nor the breast. Writing autobiographically in 1954, pediatrician Alton Goldbloom relished the fact that he was no longer a "baby feeder."[23] Yet his use of the phrase reflected the fact that nutritional advice about feeding infants and legitimization of the medical specialty of pediatrics were inextricably linked. As Goldbloom reminisced, "A generation ago, one studied pediatrics with a particular view to infant feeding. It was the key to successful pediatric practice."[24]

Indeed, it was the key to the emergence of pediatrics as a separate medical specialty.[25] As late as 1900, fewer than a dozen American physicians in large East Coast cities devoted themselves exclusively to the care of children. About fifty others called themselves "pediatrists" and saw adult patients as well, usually pregnant women.[26] The split from obstetrics was necessary if pediatrics was to emerge, but how to do it?

Infant feeding provided the way.[27] In the hands of a first generation of American pediatricians, infant formulas became drugs—to be issued only with a doctor's advice. Pediatricians agreed that formulas should be based on diluted cow's milk but warred about the percentages of water, sugar, and fat to add. Some thought "certified" raw milk best. Others started with boiled whole milk or canned condensed milk. All agreed babies should be checked regularly and that formulas might have to be changed from week to week. By the onset of the First World War, however, these internal disputes had largely become moot. During an era when most Americans possessed no health insurance, only the very prosperous could afford to visit any doctor with the great frequency that percentage systems for infant feeding demanded. However, enough parents within this class had begun to consult a doctor about how to feed their babies to create a climate in which pediatricians could reach a truce with their rivals—the nutritionists hired by milk companies to create proprietary infant formula. Food producers began selling their cans of formula only by physician's prescription and removed use instructions from product labels. In turn, pediatricians abandoned their advocacy of home modification of cow's milk.[28]

For the rest of the century, American mothers practised earlier weaning than did their counterparts in other developed countries. By the 1950s, commercial infant formula resumed its old nineteenth-century appearance—sold with directions for mixing with water right on the can. The introduction in 1968 of ready-to-feed canned liquids made an expert's advice about safe preparation completely unnecessary.

By 1918, few American mothers relied on breast milk alone to feed their babies, especially after the infants reached the age of three months. The first nationwide survey of feeding practices in the nation's hospitals, released in 1948, revealed that an estimated 40 per cent of seven-day-old babies leaving U.S. hospitals were already fed by bottle alone. By the end of the century, only about 15 per cent of American infants over the age of two months received breast milk, and that tiny minority also drank supplemental formula, usually at night. By six months, an estimated 95 per cent of American infants were fed formula primarily. Both the American Academy of Pediatrics and the American Dietetic Association advocated breast milk over bottle, whenever possible. Breast milk, they said, was hygienic and nutritious, and it potentially reduced an infant's chance of developing later food allergies. But they also agreed that babies could thrive on commercial infant formula.[29] They seemed to be right.[30] American infant mortality rates dropped steadily throughout the twentieth century, beginning about 1918.[31]

The milk wars had helped establish American pediatrics and nutrition science, but soon ended in truce. Battles about the feeding of older children, however, had just begun, especially since the vaguely defined goal of "child-saving" united many otherwise disparate Progressive Era reform goals. The idea that too many of the country's young were underfed was especially compelling.

"Our Badly Fed" Young: Progressive Reform

While Jacob Riis's exposés were intentionally sensational, his tales of starving and "badly fed" children in fetid slums were not fiction.[32] Early-twentieth-century reformers' focus on child feeding reflected a general awareness that city life worsened chances for bare survival for many of the millions of natives and newcomers who crowded into urbanizing

America. Massive immigration of "non-Nordics" spurred the Progressives' incessant worries about "race suicide." Looking at shorter southern and eastern Europeans through the distorted lens of eugenics, they wrongly saw genetically "weakened stocks."[33] However, reformers' generalized fears about the high health costs of industrialization and urbanization had merit.

Perhaps as many as 40 per cent of city dwellers in turn-of-the-century America faced periodic, but desperate, want. They leased small rooms in crowded tenements that lacked running water or indoor toilets and owned almost nothing, not even cheap furniture or adequate bedding. That too was rented. Poor children rarely wore anything but the made-over hand-me-downs of adults. "Store bought" toys were an unimagined luxury, and everyone in the family was a labourer. Young children helped with infants or a mother's bundle of piecework, ran errands, and peddled in the streets. The absence of sufficient numbers of adolescent breadwinners could throw a family marginally getting by into dire poverty. Even after early-twentieth-century compulsory education laws imposed a new social standard of mandatory schooling for all, most working-class children abandoned books for permanent work by the age of fourteen.

Progressives quite literally turned their eyes—and cameras—to children in crowded cities, but the lives of the rural poor were bleak as well. As the percentage of farms under tenancy increased, especially in the South, rural youngsters worked long hours on somebody else's land and returned home to unheated shacks. Like their urban counterparts, they too often faced hunger or meagre dinners.[34]

America was an emerging colossus, but fear mingled with optimism about the opportunities offered by rapid growth.[35] Could progress be sustained if children grew up malnourished? A dying girl in a New York tenement flat symbolized the ills of rapid social and economic change. Reformers thought her plight threatened America's future health.

Her face and that of many other children entered the nation's consciousness much more easily as technological advances in photography and printing made the mass-marketing of images a new feature of American life. The early twentieth century was visual, in ways no other time had ever been. Mid-nineteenth-century pioneers of photography staggered under the weight of heavy tripods and struggled with boxes of cumbersome and fragile glass plate negatives. Primitive photographic emulsions required subjects to sit rigid for long periods, otherwise their images would blur. By 1900, cameras were far smaller and more sophisticated. Jacob Riis was among the first newsmen to hide a "detective camera" under his coat. Hundreds soon copied him, aided by the new cameras and by dry plates that reduced exposure time and allowed "action" to be captured. Halftone engraving revolutionized the look of books, newspapers, and magazines. No longer did pictures have to be redrawn laboriously and then printed as woodcuts or lithographs. Cheap, dramatic, and "real," the halftone photograph inaugurated a century when Americans judged reality through filmed images.[36] And the middle class, whose numbers increased spectacularly, had only to pick up a newspaper or visit a nickleodeon to see the faces of the "other half."[37]

Prominent among such portraits were those of badly fed children. "Child-savers" agreed: the federal government should actively protect the nation's young. The creation of the United States Children's Bureau in 1912 was a Progressives' victory, and the U.S. Congress explicitly asked the bureau's small staff of under two dozen social workers, physicians, and "household economists" to investigate childhood malnutrition.[38]

Taking this mandate to heart, Children's Bureau agents produced dozens of reports and pamphlets about the subject. Most warned, as did a study published in 1919, that "malnutrition in children is widespread; in some communities it is so common that it is scarcely recognized as an abnormal condition. To combat malnutrition it is first necessary to recognize it."[39] But their own guidelines waffled. A well-nourished child "measures up to the racial and family standards for his age."[40] A poorly fed child was usually quite thin, but he could also be "flabby." His skin might be pale. Then again, it might be "earthy." He might appear to be lazy and listless, or just the opposite: restless and fidgety.

In their attempts to diagnose malnutrition, Children's Bureau dieticians struggled for standards. Frequently they concentrated on relationships between a child's height and weight. Sometimes they also tested eyesight or checked for strength by asking youngsters to lift a brick.[41] During its first decade as a federal agency, the bureau set up temporary examination clinics in public school classrooms around the country to measure and weigh a wide variety of sample groups—from the children of immigrant Italians in New York City to the offspring of Kentucky coal miners. The results of these tests were alarming. Only about 7 per cent of children received "grade one" status and showed signs of "excellent" nutrition. Instead, the bureau reports corroborated those reached independently by other public health officials: from one-quarter to one-third of American children were seriously underweight.[42]

Appearing as tables in dryly written government publications, these figures did not have the shock impact of Jacob Riis's flash-lit photographs. Nonetheless, politicians around the country included them in stump speeches, especially after reform journals such as *Survey* reproduced the results, and state and county health departments used the Children's Bureau reports as evidence that all schools should weigh their students.[43] Like the Children's Bureau, public health departments were new institutions in the early twentieth century, and the issue of malnutrition of the young provided a vehicle that gained both attention and funding.

Children's Bureau definitions of malnutrition depended, as did much of the "American" science's knowledge about diet before 1920, on German research, especially caloric recommendations labelled excessive by late twentieth-century nutritionists. German chemist Carl von Voit, for instance, told adult males to consume at least 3,500 calories daily, and Children's Bureau dieticians used such advice to create their weight charts. Moreover, they, like most Progressives, probably exaggerated connections between shorter immigrant children from southern Europe and underfeeding.[44]

Nonetheless, Progressive concerns were not misplaced.[45] High draft rejection rates in 1917 and 1918 ratified them. The military inducted more than a million and half men but disqualified over one-third of those examined as physically unfit. Great numbers of America's young men weighed under ninety-five pounds, had badly enlarged tonsils, or swollen adenoids, and eyesight so poor it could not be easily corrected. New York State's Commissioner of Health, Dr. Thomas Parran, thought "half-starved" childhoods contributed to the reasons so many of the country's young emerged as military "weaklings." Neglecting the signs of widespread malnutrition in children was, he warned, "expensive stupidity....Malnutrition is our greatest producer of ill health. Like nearly fresh fish, a nearly adequate diet is not enough."[46]

Diet and the Young: Nutrition Advice between the Wars

Victory in 1919 did nothing to quell national unease about high draft rejection rates. If the presence in the population of too many young men who had suffered "half-starved" childhoods played a major role, American politicians were ready to take action; experts were eager to give advice; the public was primed to listen. However, the nutritionists, public health workers, and pediatricians who made children's diets a specialty still could not create a commonly accepted definition of childhood malnutrition.

However, most agreed about its cause—ignorance about proper diet. Why did large numbers of children in the South live on fatback, grits, and molasses? Why, in other parts of the country, did significant percentages subsist on gravy over toast? Everywhere, why did too many drink tea, coffee, even alcohol, regularly?[47] Early-twentieth-century U.S. nutritionists blamed poor parental planning, not poverty, for such inadequate childhood diets.[48]

When, for example, the Children's Bureau mounted a major investigation of children's work, schooling, and home life in the Kentucky coal fields, the agency's field investigators painted a picture of child malnutrition that improved housewifery could solve. Mountain mothers lacked "an understanding of the needs of the growing child." They practised "dangerously unsystematic, promiscuous feeding." They "wasted too much grease in evaporation over great heat." Indeed, Children's Bureau investigators went so far as to rummage through trash cans in several coal camps and reported that "a great deal of it was not legitimate garbage."[49]

The message was clear: Kentucky coal miners' children were gaunt because they lacked sufficiently thrifty mothers, since healthy family meals could be made for pennies.[50] The production of "budget cookbooks" became a cottage industry, providing a living for many practitioners of the new "science of dietary studies," though little evidence emerged that the intended audience embraced the guidance.[51]

Instead, the home economists of the Children's Bureau were members of a larger company who demanded that the poor practise the kind of exquisitely detailed planning that few in any economic situation could manage, much less impoverished mothers unable to control a life governed by unsteady income, the vagaries of charity, or the limited choices of a company store. The idea that impoverished families misused resources was far more comforting than the reality: that a father's injury, a mother's case of tuberculosis, or an older child's loss of a job, could throw even the most carefully drawn working-class family food budget into complete disarray. The same people condemned as wilfully foolish were expected to be preternaturally talented at stretching food dollars. This early-twentieth-century paternalism never really died. When, in 1969, a constituent of Louisiana Congressman Otto Passman demanded that surplus food given to the poor consist of leftover Army C rations placed in garbage dumps, his idea echoed the thinking of the Children's Bureau agents who, decades earlier, pawed through refuse heaps and disapprovingly catalogued cups of potato peels "which could have been used for broth." If the poor were hungry, they must be doing something wrong, and should be set straight, if need be through humiliation.[52]

As the Great Depression replaced the Jazz Age, however, not even nutritionists could argue that childhood hunger was simply a matter of bad menu planning. More experts began to support programs to supply children with extra food in the form of school lunches, reflecting a larger shift in social attitudes about poverty. With more than one-third of its population out of work or underemployed, the country was less inclined to blame the presence of hunger on the hungry themselves.

In 1935, the U.S. Congress passed Public Law 320, allowing surplus commodities to be distributed by the United States Department of

Agriculture to eligible recipients, including public schools that served lunch.[53] When the program ended just after U.S. entrance into the Second World War, over five million schoolchildren ate a federally subsidized lunch daily, though most paid at least five cents to do so.[54]

Between 1942 and 1945 the military disqualified more than one out of three potential soldiers, most because they did not meet the new Army minimum weight requirement of 105 pounds, had lost the majority of their natural teeth, or suffered severely defective vision. The echoes from the Great War were obvious. Once again, the nation worried that badly fed boys grew into adults unable to defend their country. Spurred by the statistics on unfit draftees, as well as by concerns about the physical capabilities of home front workers, President Franklin Roosevelt wondered aloud to Paul McNutt: were Americans eating the right foods? The chair of the War Manpower Commission relayed the question down the line to the United States Department of Agriculture.

There, Secretary of Agriculture Henry Wallace had long been interested in the question. During the Great Depression he had asked his Bureau of Home Economics, which supervised all departmental activities related to human nutrition, to produce tables indicating what kinds and quantities of foods provided maximum benefit. Dietician Hazel Stiebeling of the USDA prepared four: a minimum diet on which a person could survive without starving, a cheap diet, a moderate diet, and a diet for a family with unlimited income. Stiebeling's work immediately got her into trouble, since even her diet for a rich family included relatively small amounts of meat. Outraged farm-belt lobbyists succeeded in attaching a rider to agricultural appropriations, specifying that anyone in the U.S. Department of Agriculture who advocated reduced use of any farm product be summarily fired.[55] Stiebeling kept her job, but only because her bosses retreated, agreeing, in return for removal of the rider, to retire the guidelines.[56]

They stayed on a shelf until the Second World War revived the subject, giving the unlucky Stiebeling another chance to attract rebuke. When she received word that the War Manpower Commission wanted the USDA to create guidelines for an optimal diet, she warily reported that the task would not be easy. In fact, there was vehement disagreement among members of her profession. A chart of "Recommended Daily Allowances" appeared anyway, the product of the National Research Council's Food and Nutrition Committee—which conspicuously did not include Stiebeling.[57]

Prior to the announcement of the RDAs, middle-class parents seeking advice about feeding children often turned to books written by pediatricians, especially Emmett Holt's *The Care and Feeding of Children*. Holt, long-time head of New York City's Babies' Hospital, remained America's most prominent child-rearing guru from the early twentieth century until the 1950s, when a new favourite, Dr. Spock, supplanted him. Holt's lists of forbidden foods were daunting. No child under the age of ten should ever eat any vegetable raw, and even well-cooked celery, radishes, onions, cucumbers, tomatoes, corn, beets, and eggplant could harm young digestive systems. Interestingly, during decades when nutrition-ist-produced recipe booklets urged poor parents to stretch their food budgets with tasty combinations of cabbage, Holt's guide described it as "imperfect for the young."[58] For all foods Holt had one piece of culinary advice: "It is almost impossible to cook (it) too much."[59]

Clearly, in a society increasingly influenced by mass-manufactured imagery and big-budget advertising, a guide written by a pediatrician was not the only source of information about food. Blandishments heard on the radio or seen in magazines spurred food choices, or at least beg-ging from children. But, through the 1940s, most American families ate the majority of their meals at home, and outside of ethnic enclaves, that meant Holt's preferred menu: meat, milk, and potatoes, overcooked and under-seasoned.[60]

The RDAs compiled during the Second World War were also amply laden with fat and protein. Widely distributed as a six-page pamphlet, the Allowances included sample diets, divided into food groups, with chil-dren over the age of two years advised to eat proportionally the same foods as adults. Youngsters should drink at least a pint of milk a day, eat at least one egg, one or more servings of meat, a potato, two servings of vegetables, and two or more servings of fruit. Cereals and bread were optional.[61]

One of the first efforts to see to what degree children were actually consuming recommended foods occurred in 1942. The U.S. Public Health Service and the New York-based philanthropy, the Milbank Memorial Fund, collaborated, using New York City high school students as a sample population. Researchers produced diet histories for over two thousand students and concluded that nearly three-quarters con-sumed far fewer than the number of daily calories the RDA advised.[62]

The report urged schools to supplement inadequate calorie intake at lunchtime, increasing the portion sizes of cheaper dishes. If kids could get inexpensive but big servings of macaroni, spaghetti with tomato sauce, or Spanish rice, they would get more calories, and with the calo-ries, other needed nutrients, while school budgets need not be strained. After all, "a portion of spaghetti can be two or three times the size of a portion of green vegetables and cost no more."[63]

Other studies agreed that, as late as the 1940s, under-feeding of American youngsters was still a significant problem. *Nine Million Weak*, a pamphlet circulated in 1941 by the national Parent-Teachers Association to boost support for subsidized lunch programs, charged that at least that many American children were over 40 per cent underweight.[64] Some nutritionists estimated that four out of every ten American children weighed far less than was ideal.[65]

Government-Sponsored School Lunch

When the U.S. Senate held hearings in 1944 to consider re-establishing a version of federal Depression-era food subsidy programs, the idea that another generation was growing up ill-fed, unfit, and unready for war reappeared, as experts again concluded that poor diets in childhood undermined military preparedness. Thomas Parran, now the nation's surgeon general, reprised his First World War role as prophet of doom: "I am convinced," he intoned, "that probably one half of all men rejected for the draft were rejected because of poor nutrition in childhood."[66] These kinds of warnings rang in politicians' ears and appeared in newspapers.

Senators enthusiastically demanded a return to subsidized lunches for school-aged children, especially since the initiative promised to solve another postwar problem: disposal of record crop surpluses. The National School Lunch Act of 1946 provided federal funding to make widely available a "Type A" hot lunch containing at least two ounces of meat, a tablespoon of butter, two vegetables, and half a pint of whole milk. Such a meal, sponsors promised, would improve nutritional health of the nation's children. It would also increase domestic consumption of agricultural commodities.[67] For the next fifty years, the program promoted these two goals, but the latter always dominated.

In November, 1945, a *New Yorker* editorial gushed, "One of the most pervasive phenomena that ever hit the United States is the hot lunch for school children. It is the warm sun around which American education now seems to revolve. It is clear and plain. It is inescapable; where-ever you go, the hot lunch has got there ahead of you....In the exact center of every school system you find the Mid'Day Bowl, nourishing to young and old alike."[68]

To the general public, school lunch retained that positive image. Few understood the conflicting purposes that had always accompanied the program or examined the ways it actually operated. Officials of the USDA, in charge of a complicated commodities distribution system, required participating school districts to provide detailed reports on food use; in many schools the cafeteria generated over half of all paperwork. Local education officials groused about undue federal interference, but they in turn manipulated loopholes. The program had always required states and localities to match funds, with three dollars from states for every dollar of federal money, but cities and states did not have to raise their share from taxes, and only a handful did. Rather, most sought to make school lunch self-supporting, or even a source of income, something the creators of the program had never envisioned. Most states counted the value of the prices children themselves paid for lunches as part of their contribution. This system almost guaranteed that school administrators would seek to limit the number of free or reduced-price lunches they allowed.

Nonetheless, Congress perennially reauthorized the program. It satisfied the demands of powerful food-products lobbies that the federal government purchase agricultural surpluses, yet could be justified as helping the kids. Few Americans comprehended the complexities of commodities markets, but they could easily support a program that supposedly provided their school-age children with a well-balanced, hot midday meal.

Despite School Lunch, Some Are Still Hungry: Sixties Activism and Its Aftermath

At the end of the Second World War, politicians aware of the potential threats symbolized by the war's high percentages of draft washouts and awash in surplus agricultural commodities embraced school lunch. During the next two decades, record prosperity enabled a great many more Americans to eat the kind of fat- and protein-rich meals the Type A lunch enshrined. Indeed, doing so became easier and easier. The nation that first bought Clarence Birdseye's frozen peas in the 1930s was primed to wolf them down when they appeared in the early 1950s along with buttered, mashed potatoes and meatloaf in gravy—each in its own compartment on an aluminum plate. The new TV dinner eaten in front of the new TV prominently centred in front of the just-installed picture window of a new suburban living room prompted many postwar Americans to congratulate themselves as the best-fed people on the planet.[69] That smugness ignored the perils of a high-fat diet. In a climate of renewed reform activism, it also spurred questions about the hungry left behind.

Several factors combined to reignite national debate about childhood malnutrition in the 1960s. Dramatic economic and social change marked the decade. For the first time in the United States, white- and pink-collar employees outnumbered manual labourers. Married women flooded into workplaces, and an unprecedented majority of all adult women earned wages. A massive internal migration between 1942 and 1960 transformed America's African-American population from the country's most rural to its most urban, as the final mechanization of the South pushed blacks off the farm, and industry beckoned in northern and western cities. The United States dominated world trade.[70]

If photographic images made Progressive Era culture far more visual, the arrival of television accelerated that momentum after the Second World War. Once again, a newly prosperous America examined itself critically with a mixture of dread and faith and turned to government for solutions to social problems. And the country again looked at its "other half."

In 1968 CBS news reporter Charles Kuralt told the country that ten million fellow-citizens, half of them children, were hungry: "Hunger is hard to recognize in America. We know it in other places, like Asia or Africa. But these children, all of them, are Americans. And all of them are hungry."[71] The Citizens' Board of Inquiry into Hunger and Malnutrition in the United States, aided by the Chicago-based Field Foundation, supported Kuralt's charges when it published *Hunger, U.S.A.* in 1968. Too little food caused millions of the country's children to suffer retarded growth, impaired learning rates, and permanent brain damage.[72] For the next two years childhood malnutrition was again a furiously debated subject.

Hunger, U.S.A. identified 256 "hunger counties," primarily in the rural South, where children showed classic signs of malnutrition: anemia, vitamin deficiencies, and eye diseases. The reason was obvious: they lived in families too poor to serve meat more than once a week, too poor to buy milk regularly, too poor to give children eggs.[73]

House Agriculture Committee Chair Bob Poage of Texas mounted a fierce counterattack against *Hunger, U.S.A.* He contacted health officers in all 256 counties and issued a House report based on responses from 212 claiming that the "basic problem is one of ignorance."[74] Adults in poor families who provided their children with diets of clear grease and chitlins, or "dinners of cupcakes and orange soda" were to blame. The only people who missed a meal were just those too lazy to get down to the county seat to pick up their food stamps. The idea that there was a significant problem of hunger in "hunger" counties was the creation of liberals who used the appealing faces of children to hide their efforts to attack states' rights.[75] Called to the Hill to defend low rates of participation in government-subsidized lunch programs in poorer parts of the country, Assistant Secretary of Agriculture Clayton Yeutter indirectly supported Poage's assertions and assured, "Our studies show affluence or lack of affluence is not a factor that leads to low participation or high participation."[76]

Activist Charles Remsberg was just one of many who disagreed. He published a major exposé in 1969 of supplemental feeding programs in Floyd County, Kentucky. There, "lack of affluence" made all the difference. School superintendent Charles Clark insisted that no children went hungry at noon, though some didn't bring or eat lunch. "Look," he told Remsberg, "we can't *force* a child to eat. That would be violating their Constitutional rights." The district, he went on, tried to give parents nutritional advice, but many cared more about "color TVs" than good food for their children.

In a county where more than half of all households earned less than $3,000 annually, and evening meals of flour gravy and mashed potatoes were routine, poor parents charged that Clark and others distributed school lunch tickets as rewards to political supporters who "voted right."[77]

Needy urban children joined their country counterparts. In the nation's cities, kids most at nutritional risk also found a school lunch ticket hard to obtain. The Detroit School District decided, for instance, that all parents seeking a subsidy had to prove that their children could not come home at noon or could not carry a sack lunch to school. A complicated form demanded itemization of the costs of all meals served children at home for a six-month period. Even after principals reviewed these materials and said yes, students could eat free lunches for a maximum period of only one semester, after which the entire application process had to begin again. Detroit school principals regularly received memos from headquarters telling them to exercise a policy of "continuous checking." Without any more specific criteria than that, they were to make sure that no child received an "unnecessary" subsidized lunch.

In 1965 Detroit high schools charged paying students forty-five cents for a school lunch. However, they also created elaborate sliding scales of three-quarters, half, and one-third payment for needy families. All of these were to be constantly updated. In the end, poor children ate few really free lunches, though all of the reduced-price lunches appeared in reports sent to Agriculture in Washington in the "free" column. Detroit had 300,000 pupils in its public schools. Agriculture Department guidelines suggested that over 180,000 qualified for reduced price or free meals. But the Detroit system also faced a seven-million-dollar budget deficit, and a record of failed efforts to win voter support for school levies.[78] In some of the city's poorest neighbourhoods, principals authorized four or fewer lunches per school. Moreover, Detroit used a system common throughout the country. Kids stood in different lines in the lunchroom and received cards to wear around their necks. "Regular" children wore tan cards. Children who paid ten cents instead of forty-five cents received blue cards. The handful who paid nothing got red cards. Obviously the system humiliated those who weren't "tans."[79]

In 1969, as reformers and politicians battled about supplemental food programs for children, the U.S. Congress authorized the federal Centers for Disease Control to conduct the first comprehensive survey of the nutritional status of Americans at all age levels. Researchers collected data from over 40,000 participants, nearly 16,000 of them children, and concluded that the "pot-bellied, spider-limbed malnutrition," so publicized by critics such as Remsberg, was uncommon outside of isolated, poverty pockets.

Poor children, however, were notably smaller, a finding that paralleled early-twentieth-century Children's Bureau's weight–height studies. The survey was meant to be longitudinal, subject to reauthorization after a decade. Instead, after 1971, funds disappeared. A new Republican administration, determined to shrink Lyndon Johnson's Great Society and reorganize federal social spending, prevailed, and Congress cancelled the investigations.[80] Once again, in the aftermath of a war, this time a War on Poverty, horrified Americans discovered underfed children. Then soon their attention drifted to other matters.

Fat and Flabby Kids: The 1970s and After

Between 1942 and 1975, three decades of postwar superpower affluence redefined childhood malnutrition. Ironically, the children of the working classes and the impoverished, in the first half of the century most in danger of weighing too little, were now the most likely to tip the scales as too heavy. To some degree, questions of weight were relative. A first generation of American nutritionists had adopted caloric standards that successors would think over-generous. However, social scientists did not invent the idea that too many early-twentieth-century American youngsters were too thin and too many, at century's end, were too fat. Ordinary people could just use their eyes.[81]

In 1900, working-class Americans spent almost half of their income on food. By 1970, improvements in agricultural productivity dramatically lowered that percentage. But plenty was not making everyone healthier. Instead, it encouraged major increases in clinical obesity at ever-younger ages. By the late twentieth century, the "fat and flabby" child lived in every American community, as malnutrition increasingly emerged as a problem of overweight and over-feeding.

In 1977, *Dietary Goals of the United States*, a benchmark report issued by the U.S. Senate's Select Committee on Nutrition and Human Needs, declared that far too many Americans of all ages weighed too much. The *Goals* urged a diet that reduced fat consumption, sugar and salt intake, while increasing carbohydrates. The report anxiously reported that perhaps one in four school kids was notably over ideal weight.

Not all experts agreed that American children consumed too much sugar, salt, and fats. A minority, in fact, credited high levels of sugar and fats in children's diets as one factor encouraging a steady drop in death rates from infectious illnesses.[82] But beginning in 1968, the National Research Council lowered calorie intake recommendations for the RDAs, a reflection of the fact that most nutritionists thought that American children were, collectively, getting fatter.[83]

School lunch had always been a program guided by agricultural producers' demands for additional uses for surpluses. Whether it ever significantly improved the nutritional health of children most at risk was questionable. Nonetheless, by the 1970s one fact was clear. Fewer kids ate one. School superintendents discovered that vending machines in the hallways stocked with candy, gum, and potato chips made tidy profits for their districts. Aggressively marketing their products, national chains lured administrators with offers to support athletic or music programs in return for control of lunchrooms. By the 1990s Mondays belonged to McDonalds, Tuesdays to Pizza Hut, Wednesdays to Taco Bell.[84]

Increasingly, too, Wednesdays could be Taco Bell day even for those not yet old enough to go to school. At ever younger ages, U.S. kids chose greater percentages of their own meals, and their diets included fat-laden fast food and a wide variety of prepared food products heavily sweetened with corn syrup. At mid-century, an average American child ate three daily meals, with at least two supervised by parents. By the 1990s he or she ate at least five times a day, though for many none of these occasions was a sit-down, adult-controlled event. In the new world of single-parent and two-income-earner families, day care and latch-key children, it began to appear, were feeding themselves as they pleased. By the 1990s, one in three, one study found, was overweight.[85]

Adults and children alike ate fats and sugars on the run, as snacking became an entrenched American habit among all age groups. There was one possible exception—infants and toddlers under age two, the only children left whose foods adults totally selected. A 1995 survey by the Gerber Company found that 20 per cent of parents in a sample of one thousand reported that they had cut the fat in their babies' diets. Experts had not told them to do that, and Recommended Daily Allowances had never included children younger than two. Pediatricians generally thought that infants would fail to thrive if denied sufficient fat, though opinion differed over whether toddlers should drink 2 per cent or full-fat milk. Were large numbers of well-meaning parents just confused?

Studies of the impact of nutritional labelling suggested that the vast majority of consumers did not really comprehend the information they saw, in passing glances, as they shopped.[86] However, the food label was a constant reminder about nutrition, even if Americans were not generally translating it into usable form.[87]

There was one exception to this generalization: parents of children with severe food allergies. Percentages of children whose allergies posed life-threatening risks rose during the last two decades of the century. Some researchers suggested that as many as 8 per cent of children under age three, and 3 per cent of schoolchildren, experienced dangerous reactions to food, especially to nuts and milk-based products. These were the kids whose throats swelled if they so much as touched a piece of cheese, the youngsters who vomited when at a table occupied by a classmate eating a peanut butter and jelly sandwich. As the century ended, many thousands of American children went off to school armed with Epi-pens to use in case they unwittingly came into contact with a forbidden food and went into anaphylactic shock. No one knew exactly why the incidence of such afflictions increased, but one theory suggested that a growing fraction of children raised in a culture that demanded frequent handwashing and daily baths lacked the necessary protections against allergic response that microbes in dirt provided. Others thought that American practices of early weaning, and consequent quick introduction of solids, before children's immune systems had fully developed, were to blame.[88]

Public school principals enacted new policies: no sandwich swapping in the cafeteria, no nut candies in the snack machines. Milk, the very symbol of good nutrition for children, was in the dock as well—not just as a suggested factor in increasing levels of childhood obesity but also as an ingredient some pediatric endocrinologists charged contributed to an earlier onset of puberty in American girls. Had the added hormones given cows to stimulate greater milk production caused an unexpected side effect—encouraging seven- or eight-year-olds to develop breasts and pubic hair?[89]

In the 1990s a few nutritionists even began to challenge the *Dietary Goals* food pyramid, which urged the consumption of carbohydrates. Were children getting too fat because they ate too many servings of potatoes, rice, and bread?[90] Was the most serious problem the couch, not the potato?

Probably both the couch *and* the potato bore blame. Ever since the Second World War, regular exercise declined as a daily activity for U.S. children, who drove or were driven to school, where physical training of any kind was far less likely to be mandatory. Free time increasingly meant television time or Internet time, not time spent playing vigorous physical games.[91]

Peanut Butter: A Coda

Cornflakes made Will Kellogg rich, but peanut butter helped keep his Battle Creek, Michigan, sanatorium open. There, the famous mixed with the ordinary, but all ate a rigorously vegetarian diet heavily reliant on cereal concoctions. In the 1880s, in an attempt to make this bland diet more palatable, Kellogg created peanut butter, an immediate hit.[92] Meant for sick adults, peanut butter became a beloved staple food of generations of American kids. It was cheap, nutritious, and easy to put in lunch boxes. Who could object?

By the 1970s, a food synonymous with twentieth-century U.S. childhood was the subject of furious controversy. A peanut butter, or worse, a peanut butter and jelly sandwich, critics claimed, contained far too much salt, sugar, and hydrolyzed vegetable oils. Moreover, as food allergy concerns increased, peanut butter emerged as a potent threat—and not just to the obese kid who ate too many sandwiches. Some airlines and school systems banned it.

As had been the case since the nutritionist emerged in the early twentieth century as a professional, experts fiercely disagreed. Should children without allergies still be allowed to eat peanut butter regularly? No consensus emerged. If the problem of childhood malnutrition wasn't perpetual, at least it had not yet been solved.

Notes

1 Jacob Riis, *How the Other Half Lives: Studies among the Tenements of New York*, ed. with intro. David Leviatin (Boston: Bedford Books, 1996), 170–71. *How the Other Half Lives* is an American classic. First published in 1890, it was the first book produced anywhere that included large numbers of halftone pictures. Combining sentimentality, hard-bitten reportage, and graphic, candid illustrations, the book was an instant sensation. Riis, once a penniless immigrant from Denmark, toured the country giving hugely successful slide lectures selling *How the Other Half Lives*. The book has been almost continuously in print in several editions since its first publication. David Leviatin, "Introduction," 39–45.

2 The famous phrase is generally attributed to *Life* magazine publisher Henry Luce. For discussion of the impact of Luce's "American Century" essay, see Olivier Zunz, *Why the American Century?* (Chicago: University of Chicago Press, 1998), ix–xiv.

3 "Statement of Dr. Jean Mayer," Problems and Prospects of Nutrition and Human Needs, Hearings before the Select Committee on Nutrition and Human Needs of the United States Senate, Ninetieth Congress, Second Session (Washington, DC: Government Printing Office, 1968), 11 (hereafter cited as Hearings, Prospects).

4 For discussions of the rise of the expert to prominence, see Theodore Porter, *Trust in Numbers: The Pursuit of Objectivity in Science and Public Life* (Princeton: Princeton University Press, 1995); Thomas Haskell, *The Emergence of Professional Social Science: The American Social Science Association and the Nineteeth Century Cri-*

sis of Authority (Urbana: University of Illinois Press, 1977); and Michael Lacey and Mary Furner, eds., *The State and Social Investigation in Britain and the United States* (Washington, DC: Woodrow Wilson Center Press, 1993).

5 Hearings, Prospects, 12.

6 This is a theme echoed by other authors in the volume. See Aleck Ostry, "The Early Development of Nutrition Policy in Canada."

7 John Kramer, a Georgetown University law professor and director of the National Council on Hunger and Malnutrition, lobbying for increased funds for nutrition education for children, made this charge in July 1973, continuing that the "drain" of school budgets was the engine misdirecting the School Lunch Program in America's schools. His claim, however, was one echoed in dozens of different contexts throughout the twentieth century by equally large numbers of advice-givers. "Testimony of John Kramer: A Program of Nutrition Education for Children as a Part of the National School Lunch and Child Nutrition Programs," Hearings before the General Subcommittee on Education of the Committee on Education and Labor, House of Representatives, Ninety-Third Congress, First Session (Washington, DC: Government Printing Office, 1973), 184 (hereafter cited as Hearings, H.R. 4974).

8 Harvey Levenstein, *Revolution at the Table: The Transformation of the American Diet* (New York: Oxford University Press, 1988), 45–47.

9 Again the development crossed borders. A first generation of professional nutritionists found employment in the Canadian federal Department of Agriculture as well. See Ostry, "Early Development."

10 Prior to the early twentieth century, the USDA had studied diet, but the diet of *animals*. John Hillison, "The Origins of Agri-Science: Or Where Did All That Scientific Agriculture Come From?" *Journal of Agricultural Education* 37 (1996): 8–13; and Hamilton Cravens, "Establishing the Science of Nutrition at the USDA: Ellen Swallow Richards and Her Allies," *Agricultural History* 64 (1990): 122–33.

11 Emma Weigley, "It Might Have Been Euthenics: The Lake Placid Conferences and the Home Economics Movement," *American Quarterly* 26 (1974): 79–96.

12 For samples of early twentieth century "ideal" diets proposed by nutritionists, see Adela Beeuwkes, ed., *Essays in the History of Nutrition and Dietetics* (Chicago: American Dietetic Association, 1967), 66–75. Later generations of nutritionists said such advice, which also included injunctions to eat vegetables only after prolonged boiling, encouraged kidney disease and vitamin deficiencies.

13 Testimony of Norma Maiden, "Child Nutrition Act," Hearings before the Subcommittee on Elementary, Secondary, and Vocational Education of the Committee on Education and Labor, Ninety-Fifth Congress, First Session (Washington, DC: Government Printing Office, 1977), 478 (hereafter cited as Hearings, Child Nutrition Act).

14 Hearings, Child Nutrition Act, 480.

15 Fletcher outlined his principles in *Optimism: A Real Remedy* (Chicago: A.C. McClung, 1908). For discussion of the craze for fletcherizing between 1904 and 1918, see Harvey Green, *Fit for America: Health, Fitness, Sport and American Society* (New York: Pantheon, 1986), 294–309.

16 Of course, other nutritionists thought most brands of corn flakes, including Kellogg's sugar frosted, contained far too much sugar. Some even thought sugar was an acquired taste that children would not develop on their own. According to an extreme proponent of this view, William Duffy, sugar was an addictive drug. Parents might just as well let their youngsters smoke cigarettes. William Duffy, *Sugar Blues* (New York: Wang, 1975), 5–12.

17   The explosive growth of industry-supported diet research is discussed in Harvey Levenstein, *Paradox of Plenty: A Social History of Eating in Modern America* (New York: Oxford University Press, 1993), 174–76.

18   J. H. Knox, "Introductory remarks by J. H. Knox," *Prevention of Infant Mortality: Being the Papers and Discussions of a Conference Held at New Haven, Connecticut, November 11–12, 1909* (New York: American Public Health Association [Pamphlet Series], 1909), 7 (hereafter cited as *Prevention of Infant Mortality*).

19   J. H. Knox, "The Relation of Alcohol to Infant Mortality," *Prevention of Infant Mortality*, 6–24; and Clemens von Pirquet, "The Relation of Tuberculosis to Infant Mortality," *Prevention of Infant Mortality*, 25–44.

20   Leonard Wilson, "The Historical Riddle of Milk-Borne Scarlet Fever," *Bulletin of the History of Medicine* 60 (1986): 321–42.

21   For discussion of early twentieth-century pasteurization controversies, see James Giblin, *Milk: The Fight for Purity* (New York: Crowell, 1986).

22   Rima Apple, "Advertised by Our Loving Friends: The Infant Formula Industry and the Creation of New Pharmaceutical Markets, 1870–1910," *Journal of the History of Medicine and Allied Sciences* 41 (1986): 3–24.

23   Alton Goldbloom, "A Twenty-Five-Year Retrospective on Infant Feeding," *Journal of the Maine Medical Association* 45 (1954): 267.

24   Goldbloom, "Twenty-Five-Year Retrospective," 264.

25   As Lisa Featherstone notes, the professionalization of medicine in developed countries was not enough to guarantee the emergence of the new medical specialty of pediatrics. See her "Infant Ideologies: Doctors, Mothers, and the Feeding of Children in Australia, 1880–1910" in this volume.

26   For the emergence of pediatrics, see Sydney Halpern, *American Pediatrics: The Social Dynamics of Professionalism, 1880–1980* (Berkeley: University of California Press, 1988).

27   As Lisa Featherstone remarks, the key was "control" of infant feeding. While a first generation of U.S. pediatricians devised complicated formulas that prosperous women used to modify cow's milk to feed infants, their Australian counterparts advocated breastfeeding as best, whenever possible—a point that the American Academy of Pediatrics come to share. However, Australian specialists felt that without their expert instruction, new mothers were likely to breastfeed improperly. See Featherstone, "Infant Ideologies."

28   Rima Apple, "To Be Used Only under the Direction of a Physician: Commercial Infant Feeding and Medical Practice, 1870–1940," *Bulletin of the History of Medicine* 54 (1980): 402–406.

29   Shirley Walberg Ekvall, "Preventive Nutrition," in *Pediatric Nutrition in Chronic Diseases and Developmental Disorders: Prevention, Assessment, and Treatment*, ed. Shirley Walberg Ekvall (New York: Oxford University Press, 1993), 3–15; and Isadora Stehin, "Infant Formula: Second Best, But Good Enough," *FDA Consumer: The Magazine of the U.S. Food and Drug Administration* 30 (1996): 17.

30   Early weaning, however, which led to quick introduction of solids, remained controversial. Some experts warned that the practice, while it did not kill infants, made youngsters prone to later-in-life food allergies. See Susan Dominus, "The Allergy Prison," *New York Times*, June 10, 2001.

31   Many public health experts credited some of the reduction in infant mortality during the 1920s to pasteurization. As prominent Yale public health public health physician C. E. A. Winslow remarked, "It is an easy matter for a germ to get by a (city milk) inspector, but to escape being cooked at the gates of the city is quite another proposition." "Pasteurization v. Milk Inspection in New York," type-

script, C. E. A. Winslow Papers, Record Group 749, box 33, Yale University Archives, New Haven, CT (hereafter cited as Yale). Long-term declines, some argued, had more to do with better nourishment of pregnant women and improved obstetric care in the U.S., which encouraged safer birthing conditions. For a summary of these arguments, see Levenstein, *Revolution at the Table*, 134–36.

32 The phrase *badly fed* comes from Lydia Roberts, *What Is Malnutrition?* Children's Year Follow-up Series 1, Publication 59 (Washington, DC: United States Children's Bureau, 1919). The cited edition is the 1927 revision, 6.

33 Both politicians and academics raised the issue constantly in the first decade of the twentieth century. President Theodore Roosevelt was only one of its well-known popularizers. After he left the White House, Roosevelt devoted time between 1909 and 1911 to lecture tours where the emphasized the topic. Many of these speeches were later rewritten as essays and published posthumously in collections of the president's writings. In one titled "The Parasite Woman," for instance, Roosevelt said, "We have had six children in this family. We wish we had more. Now the grandchildren are coming along; and I am sure you will agree with me that no other success in life—not being President, or being wealthy, or going to college, or anything else, comes up to success of the men and women who can feel that they have done their duty." Theodore Roosevelt, "The Parasite Woman," *The Foes of Our Own Household* (New York: Charles Scribner's Sons, 1925), 153. A native-born woman, according to Roosevelt, was a "parasite" if she did not try to raise at least four children to adulthood.

34 For discussions of life among the impoverished and working classes in city and countryside in the period 1900–1920, see David Danbom, *Born in the Country: A History of Rural America* (Baltimore: Johns Hopkins University Press, 1995); Michael Katz, ed., *The "Underclass" Debate: View from History* (Princeton: Princeton University Press, 1993); and Ewa Morawska, *For Bread with Butter: Life-Worlds of East Central Europeans in Johnstown, Pennsylvania, 1890–1940* (New York: Cambridge University Press, 1985). Most analysts of early-twentieth-century poverty suggest that an urban family with three children that earned between $500 and $800 annually fit into the extremely broad base of the working poor in America during the first two decades of the twentieth century. Poor people in rural areas operated with far less money, sometimes no money, as members of barter and debt-based household economies.

35 For an overview of economic historians' estimates about general conditions of public health and living standards in the early twentieth century, see John Komlos, ed., *Stature, Living Standards, and Economic Development: Essays in Anthropometric History* (Chicago: University of Chicago Press, 1994); John Komlos and Joo Han Kim, "On Estimating Trends in Historical Heights," *Historical Methods* 23 (1990): 116–20; and Richard Steckel, "Heights, Living Standards, and History: A Review Essay," *Historical Methods* 24 (1991): 183–87.

36 For discussion of the rapidly changing technology of photography, see Leviatin, "Introduction," 23–27; Reese Jenkins, *Images and Enterprise: Technology and the American Photographic Industry* (Baltimore: Johns Hopkins University Press, 1975); and Peter Hales, *Silver Cities: The Photography of American Urbanization* (Philadelphia: Temple University Press, 1984).

37 A number of historians have argued that a focus on poverty has accompanied periods of dramatic increases in the size and status of the American middle class. During periods of rapid economic change, those who have only recently risen, they argue, are more likely to define themselves by looking at those left behind. For a cogent summary of such arguments, see Stuart Blumin, *The Emergence of the Mid-*

dle Class: Social Experience in the American City (Cambridge, MA: Harvard University Press, 1989).

38 In 1912, the U.S. Congress passed a bill authorizing funding for a federal bureau to consider the problems and welfare of American children. The United States Children's Bureau was the first national government agency anywhere exclusively devoted to investigation of childhood and became a widely copied model used by other Western governments. At first a part of the Department of Commerce, in 1913 the bureau became an agency within the just-established Department of Labor. Kriste Lindenmeyer, *A "Right to Childhood": The U.S. Children's Bureau and Child Welfare, 1912–1946* (Urbana: University of Illinois Press, 1997). At the beginning of the century, the field of home economics was another new profession, and several Children's Bureau dieticians and "domestic economists" were among a first generation.

39 Roberts, *What Is Malnutrition?* 1.

40 Roberts, *What Is Malnutrition?* 1.

41 Roberts, *What Is Malnutrition?* 2–3. Anthropometric analysis validates the importance of relationships between stature and weight as an indicator of general health, but by the late twentieth century, experts generally used height as an indication of nutritional deprivation only if used to judge aggregate populations. Few thought height/weight scales of much value in judging the health of individuals. Dora Costa and Richard Steckel, "Long Term Trends in Health, Welfare, and Economic Growth in the United States," *Working Papers Series on Historical Factors in Long Run Growth*, Historical Paper 76 (Cambridge, MA: Harvard University Press, 1995), 12–15.

42 Costa and Steckel, "Long Term Trends," 5–13. For other bureau studies reporting the results of this decade's worth of height and weight testing, see Lydia Roberts, *The Nutrition and Care of Children in a Mountain County of Kentucky*, Publication 110 (Washington, DC: United States Children's Bureau, 1922); Agnes Hanna, *Nutrition Work for Pre-School Children*, Publication 138 (Washington, DC: United States Children's Bureau, 1925); United States Children's Bureau, *What Builds Babies?* Folder 4 (Washington, DC: United States Children's Bureau, 1925).

43 Indeed, speeches that warned of the nation's millions of "dangerously thin" children became common in the 1920s, in part because of public health campaigns that led to regular weighing of significant numbers of the nation's schoolchildren, especially in urban areas with the best organized public health programs. By the end of the decade, scales and height/weight charts were standard school equipment throughout the country. Giving advice that was typical, in 1928, public health officials of Marion County, OR, counselled school principals to establish programs of weighing of all school children. Every six weeks was optimal; three times a year was minimal. W. F. Walker, *Report of Survey of Public Health Activities for Marion County, Oregon, June 19–28, 1928*, folder 3, box 2, series 12, Records of the Commonwealth Fund (hereafter cited as CF), Rockefeller Archive Center, Tarrytown, NY (hereafter cited as RAC).

44 Harvey Levenstein thinks "the great malnutrition scare" was exaggerated. His comments about the unreliability of height/weight ratios, if used to judge individual health, as well as his remarks about the cultural biases inherent in the early-twentieth-century testing regimes, deserve attention. However, he is wrong; the Progessive concern with child malnutrition was not largely a matter of experts' misinformation. Levenstein pays insufficient attention to the reality that only after 1945 did a postwar boom enable the vast majority of married workers and their children to climb above poverty lines. And early-twentieth-century poverty

brought periodic severe deprivation, including food deprivation, to millions of children. For Levenstein's comments about early-twentieth-century malnutrition studies, see Levenstein, *Revolution at the Table*, 114–19. For discussions of how childhood poverty has been "counted," see Althea Huston, ed., *Children in Poverty: Child Development and Public Policy* (Cambridge, UK: Cambridge University Press, 1991).

45 Economists have rightly attacked generalizations made from a "snapshot" approach. Counting height/weight ratios, or any other quantifiable condition, at any given moment, probably underestimates the numbers likely to experience the condition (level of nutrition, poverty, wealth) at some point during a lifetime and simultaneously also overestimates, if the assumption is that the individual caught in the "snapshot" will remain fixed in that condition (malnourished, poor, rich). No universally accepted longitudinal study of childhood underfeeding exists for the years 1900–1920, only "snapshot" anecdotal case studies of groups measured with questionable techniques. However, most analysts think that it was only after 1945 that postwar prosperity enabled the majority of married American workers and their families to rise above poverty levels. See Michael Katz, *Poverty and Policy in American History* (New York: Academic Press, 1983), 17–134.

46 Thomas Parran, quoted in Laurie Schwanenberger, *Introduction to Child Nutrition Programs* (Coolidge, AZ: Central Arizona College Dietetic Education Program, 1993), 3.

47 For examples of these kinds of conclusions, see Mary Frayser, "Children of Pre-school Age in Selected Areas of South Carolina," *South Carolina Agricultural Experimental Station Bulletin* 260 (1929), 29–70; Frank Manny, "A Scale for Marking Malnutrition," *School and Society* 3 (1916): 123–30; Dorothy Mendenhall, *Milk: The Indispensable Food for Children*, Publication 163 (Washington, DC: United States Children's Bureau, 1926); Emma Lundberg, *Unemployment and Child Welfare: A Study Made in a Middle-Western and an Eastern City during the Industrial Depression of 1921 and 1922*, Publication 125 (Washington, DC: United States Children's Bureau, 1923); and Dorothy Bradbury, *Four Decades of Action for Children: A Short History of the Children's Bureau, 1903–46*, Publication 358 (Washington, DC: United States Children's Bureau, 1956). It is interesting that many early-twentieth-century nutritionists who worried about children whose diets were heavily dependent on grits or mush also deplored diets based on beans and rice, meals that by the late twentieth century many experts regarded as more wholesome.

48 Agents for the U.S. Children's Bureau were especially appalled that urban immigrant children frequently made a breakfast of several pickles, bought or swiped from street carts, and that their mothers saw nothing wrong with the practice. Roberts, *What Is Malnutrition?* 9.

49 Quotations and summaries from the Children's Bureau report in Mabel Ellis, "Children of the Kentucky Coal Fields," *American Child* 1 (1920): 385–87.

50 Early-twentieth-century Children's Bureau agents did not consider another possibility. Nor have most historians. But were the parents, especially the fathers, eating before the children? Victorian Americans sentimentalized childhood, as have all successive generations, nourishing a widespread belief that parents sacrifice to give beloved children the best they can afford. In reality, different traditions persisted, even when stereotypes changed. Even in the early twenty-first century, throughout much of the world, children get the leftovers—literally. Adults, beginning with the men in the family, eat first. Anecdotal evidence suggests that such dining practices were still common in the United States through much of the first half of the twentieth century, especially in immigrant families and among the rural poor. For examples of autobiographies that mention children eating last,

see Mary Anderson, *Woman at Work: The Autobiography of Mary Anderson, as Told to Mary Winslow* (Minneapolis: University of Minnesota Press, 1951); Anzia Yezierska, *Red Ribbon on a White Horse* (New York: Scribners, 1950). Significantly, both authors were members of immigrant families. And this sort of message certainly crossed cultures. In this volume, Aleck Ostry and Lisa Featherstone note experts in Australia and Canada were also more likely to criticize mothering skills than call attention to harsh economic realities.

51 For a review of nutritionists' advice about hunger and malnutrition in America in the twenties and thirties, see Levenstein, *Paradox of Plenty*, 1–52.

52 The story about the letter to Passman is told in Nick Kotz, *Let Them Eat Promises: The Politics of Hunger in America* (Englewood Cliffs, NJ: Prentice-Hall, 1969), 229. The constituent was sure that if his recommendation were approved, the poor would be better motivated to seek work, or grow their own vegetable gardens.

53 The federal government was following the example set by private philanthropies. By 1912, dozens of cities had school lunch programs funded by private patrons, who often worked with public officials. For a review of such early-twentieth-century efforts, see "Memorandum: School Lunch Supervisors, August 16, 1943," Records of the General Education Board (hereafter cited as GEB), folder 5741, box 536, sub-series 3, series 1, RAC.

54 "Testimony of Sidney Hall, George Washington University," School Lunch and Milk Programs: Hearings before a Subcommittee of the Committee of Agriculture and Forestry, United States Senate, Seventy-Eighth Congress, Second Session on S. 1820 and S. 1824: Bills To Assist the States To Establish and Maintain School Lunch Programs (Washington, DC: Government Printing Office, 1944), 5–7 (hereafter, Hearings, S. 1820 and S. 1824).

55 In this volume, Aleck Ostry demonstrates a similar influence of food lobbies in Canada, where the dairy industry successfully recruited the country's Department of Agriculture as an ally in its campaign to transform the image of milk from dangerous beverage to perfect food for children.

56 Don Hadwiger, "Nutrition, Food Safety, and Farm Policy," *Proceedings of the Academy of Political Science* 34 (1982): 8–12.

57 Levenstein, *Paradox of Plenty*, 65–66. The Research Council, composed of numerous committees of academic and other experts, had been created immediately after the First World War to be an advisory panel consulted by government agencies.

58 Holt banned pork for children, advice few but the wealthiest families could have followed before the twentieth century. From the seventeenth through nineteenth centuries, Americans were prodigious pork eaters. Only after the Civil War, when a national rail system and centralized stockyards made western cattle-ranching profitable, did the nation begin to turn to beef, and, until after the Second World War, chicken remained a luxury. Richard Pillsbury, *No Foreign Food: The American Diet in Time and Place* (Boulder, CO: Westview Press, 1998), 67–71; and Emmett Holt, *The Care and Feeding of Children*, 136–45.

59 Holt, *Care and Feeding*, 131.

60 A restaurant meal signalled a special occasion, and until after the Second World War, lunch counters and diners were primarily a man's domain, rarely frequented by children at all. See John Jakle and Keith Sculle, *Fast Food: Roadside Restaurants in the Automobile Age* (Baltimore: Johns Hopkins University Press, 1999), 2–23.

61 Food and Nutrition Board, National Research Council, *Recommended Dietary Allowances*, (Washington, DC: Food and Nutrition Board, 1943), 5.

62 It is worth noting that, with no consensus among professional dieticians about ideal daily calorie numbers, the RDAs published during the Second World War

continued the nineteenth-century German research traditions and suggested a very generous caloric intake—2,900 calories for a male adolescent. Nonetheless, the Milbank research indicated that the overwhelming majority of the teenagers in its study consumed not just fewer than that—but *far* fewer than that.

63 Emily Stamm and Dorothy Wiehl, "Medical Evaluation of Nutritional Status, Part 8: The School Lunch as a Method for Improving Diets of High School Students," *Milbank Memorial Quarterly* 20 (1942): 90.

64 "Nine Million Weak," *Consumers' Guide* 3 (1941): 11–14.

65 Dorothy Wiehl, "Medical Evaluation of Nutritional Status, Part 7: Diets of High School Students of Low Income Families in New York City," *Milbank Memorial Quarterly* 20 (1942): 61–82.

66 "Testimony of Thomas Parran," Hearings, S. 1820 and S. 1824, 60.

67 Committee on Agriculture, Nutrition, Forestry, *Child Nutrition Programs: Description, History, Issues, and Options* (Washington, DC: United States Senate, 1983), 13–21; Center on Budget and Policy Priorities, *The Child Nutrition Block Grants* (Washington, DC, 1995), 1–10. For a thirty-year overview of ingredients mandated for a Type A lunches, see Comptroller General of the United States, *The National School Lunch Program: Is It Working?* P.A.D. 77/7 (Washington, DC, 1977).

68 Quoted in Bernard Bard, *The School Lunch Room: Time of Trial* (New York: Wiley, 1968), 17.

69 For discussions of postwar food attitudes and trends, see Jeffry Pilcher, "Food Fads," in *The Cambridge World History of Food*, ed. Kenneth Kiple and Kriemhild Ornelas (Cambridge, UK: Cambridge University Press, 2000), 2:1493. See also John Hess and Karen Hess, *The Taste of America* (New York: Grossman, 1977); for discussion of the social and economic impact of the postwar suburb, see Kenneth Jackson, *Crabgrass Frontier: The Suburbanization of the United States* (New York: Oxford University Press, 1985).

70 By the mid-1960s the country's population owned 1.2 cars and 1.3 televisions per family. Kotz, *Let Them Eat Promises*, 20.

71 Transcript of *CBS Reports*: "Hunger in America," May 21, 1968, in "Hunger and Malnutrition in the United States," Hearings before the Subcommittee on Employment, Manpower, and Poverty of the Committee on Labor and Public Welfare, United States Senate, Ninetieth Congress, Second Session, on S. Res. 281 (Washington, DC: Government Printing Office, 1968), 55–65 (hereafter cited as Hearings, S. Res. 281).

72 Citizens' Board of Inquiry into Hunger and Malnutrition in the United States, *Hunger U.S.A. Revisited* (Washington, DC: Government Printing Office, 1972), 1–4.

73 Hearings, S. Res. 281, Field Foundation report excerpted, 288–95.

74 Congressmen Bob Poague, quoted in Kotz, *Let Them Eat Promises*, 107.

75 For a summary of the Poague report, see "A Nation within a Nation," May 17, 1968 *Time* 91/20: 24–31. Poague even charged, though he offered no plausible proof, that the *Hunger, USA* photographs of children with bloated bellies were not taken in America but came from other countries.

76 "Testimony of Clayton Yeutter," Hearings, H.R. 4974, 97–98.

77 Charles Remsberg, "School without Lunch," *Everyman's Guide to Federal Programs Impact! Reports* 1 (1969): 1–22.

78 "Statement of William Simmons, Deputy Superintendent, Detroit Public Schools," Child Nutrition and School Food Assistance, Hearings before the Subcommittee on Nutrition and Human Needs of the United States Senate, Ninety-First Congress, First Session (Washington, DC: Government Printing Office, 1969), 3454–58 (hereafter cited as Hearings, Child Food Assistance).

188 JUDITH SEALANDER

79 "Joint Testimony of Gloria Atchison and Barbara Quarles," Hearings, Child Food Assistance, 3452–55. Atchison was an attorney who worked for Detroit Legal Aid. Barbara Quarles was a welfare mother who told how her children loathed the separate coloured cards system that declared their poverty.

80 Stanley Garn and Diane Clark, "Nutrition, Growth, Development, and Maturation: Findings from the Ten-State Nutrition Survey of 1968–70," *Pediatrics* 56 (1975): 306–18. For further information about professional attention to the problem of lactose intolerance among black children, see Kenneth Kiple and Virginia Kiple, "Deficiency Diseases in the Caribbean," *Journal of Interdisciplinary History* 11 (1980): 197–215; Kenneth Kiple, "A Survey of Recent Literature on the Biological Past of the Black," *Social Science History* 10 (1986): 343–68.

81 In fact, people had been able easily to judge status for millennia. The rich *were* different: in almost all societies, heavier and taller. In the developed world, late-twentieth-century abundance, combined with historically low prices for food, made relationships among girth, class, and status a fraught topic.

82 For discussions of these controversies, see H. O. Kunkel and P. B. Thompson, "Interests and Values in National Nutrition Policy in the United States," *Journal of Agricultural Ethics* 1 (1988): 241–65; P. L. White, "Nutrition: A Medical, Political, and Public Issue," *Journal of the American Medical Association* 241 (1979): 1407–1408; Food and Nutrition Board, *Research Needs for Establishing Dietary Guidelines for the U.S. Population* (Washington, DC: National Research Council, 1979), 7–16; Louise Russell, *Is Prevention Better Than Cure?* (Washington, DC: Brookings Institution, 1986), 10–28; and Laura Sims, *The Politics of Fat: Food and Nutrition Policy in America* (Armank, NY: M. E. Sharpe, 1998), 213–42.

83 H. O. Kunkel, *Interests and Values in the Recommended Dietary Allowances and Nutritional Guidelines for Americans*, Publications of the Center for Biotechnology Policy and Ethics, CBPE 95-9 (College Station, TX: Center for Biotechnology Policy and Ethics, 1995), 6–11.

84 "Testimony of William Dietz," Delivery of Nutrition by the Domestic Feeding Programs of the U.S. Department of Agriculture, Hearings before the Subcommittee on Departmental Operations and Nutrition of the Committee on Agriculture, House of Representatives, One Hundred and Third Congress, First Session (Washington, DC: Government Printing Office, 1993), 42–43 (hereafter cited as Hearings, Delivery).

85 For discussion of this trend, see Kunkel, *Recommended Dietary Allowances.* Adding to the problem was the fact that in a highly competitive market, food manufacturers by the mid-1990s "supersized" portions, and added ever more fructose-based sweeteners to products, making them richer in calories, even as they advertised, accurately, that these foods were "low fat." See "Snacks Putting on Calories," *New York Times*, April 24, 2001.

86 For further discussion of food labelling in American history, see Alan Marcus, *Cancer from Beef: DES, Federal Food Regulation, and Consumer Confidence* (Baltimore: Johns Hopkins University Press, 1994).

87 Melvin Hinich and Richard Staelin, *Consumer Protection Legislation and the US Food Industry* (New York: Pergamon, 1980), 70–75.

88 For a brief summary of these and other arguments, see Susan Dominus, "The Allergy Prison," *New York Times*, June 10, 2001.

89 For a summary of these charges, see Robert Rosenfield, Laura Bachrach, Steven Chernausek, Joseph Gertner, Michael Gottschalk, Dana Hardin, Ora Pescovitz, Paul Saenger, Marcia Herman-Giddens, Eric Slora, and Richard Wasserman, "Current Age of Onset of Puberty," *Pediatrics* 106 (2000): 622–23; Paul Kaplowitz

and Sharon Oberfield, "Reexamination of the Age Limit for Defining When Puberity Is Precocious in Girls in the United States: Implications for Evaluation and Treatment," *Pediatrics* 104 (1999): 936–41; and Marcia Herman-Giddens, Eric Slora, Richard Wasserman, Carlos Bourdony, Manju Bhapkar, Gary Koch, and Cynthia Hasemeier, "Secondary Sexual Characteristics and Menses in Young Girls Seen in Office Practice: A Study from the Pediatric Research in Office Setting Network Pediatrics," *Pediatrics* 99 (1997): 505–12. The charge, like the causes for the rise of severe food allergies, was controversial. Others challenged the theory that American girls, on average, were entering puberty earlier at the end of the century or argued that they were, but that a trend toward more serious obesity in young girls, not milk, was the culprit.

90 This end-of-the-century research is summarized in Michael Pollan, "When a Crop Becomes King," *New York Times*, July 19, 2002.

91 Public Health Service, U.S. Department of Health and Human Services, *The 1990 Health Objectives: A Midcourse Review* (Washington, DC: Government Printing Office, 1986).

92 Though dated, Gerald Carson's *Cornflake Crusade* (New York: Rinehart, 1957) remains the standard biography.

The Early Development of Nutrition Policy in Canada

Aleck Ostry

Introduction

I n 1921 the Division of Child Welfare in the federal Department of
Health developed Canada's first national dietary guidelines in an
attempt to improve breastfeeding habits and encourage mothers to
feed their babies more cow's milk.[1] These dietary guidelines were developed primarily to reduce infant mortality rates and, not surprisingly,
given the well-known contribution of milk to these persistently high
rates, the guidelines were ambivalent in their advice about the consumption of cow's milk.

The Division of Child Welfare's guidelines were developed during
a transition time in the history of milk as it emerged from its long-held
status as a food easily contaminated and a dangerous carrier of diseases
of infancy and childhood, to its new status as the premier protective
food for children containing life-enhancing vitamins and minerals.[2]
This transition occurred during the 1920s in a Canada covered with a
patchwork system of municipal and provincial sanitary hygiene laws, so
that milk was clean and disease-free in some cities and in some regions,
but not in others.[3] It was also a time of transition for the dairy industry,
which, in the face of declining dairy exports and domestic milk consumption, turned increasingly to public health professionals and nutritionists to increase sales, in particular of fluid milk by changing the status of milk from an unhealthy to a healthy food.

The breastfeeding guidelines developed by the Division of Child
Welfare were widely disseminated to the general public in the interwar
years with the publication of the highly popular Canadian Mothers
Books.[4] Paradoxically, wide dissemination of this advice occurred as
breastfeeding in Canada, and in most of the rest of the developed world,
began a historic and profound fifty-year decline, which was reversed
only in the late 1960s.[5] This occurred as the medical profession in
Canada consolidated control over medical practice and as it increased

191

its oversight of pregnancy and birthing, in part because of growing public concerns over sustained high maternal mortality rates during the
interwar years.[6]

A study of the Division's guidelines and the circumstances of their
introduction and widespread dissemination provides insight into what
was the first nationwide attempt at nutrition policy making in Canada
and elucidates the complex interplay of health beliefs, public health,
economics, and politics in developing Canada's first nationally promulgated dietary guideline.

The general purpose of this paper is to describe Canada's first foray
into the development of national dietary guidelines. Besides this purely
descriptive task the paper seeks to elucidate and explain the interplay
of economics, science, and public health that shaped these early dietary
guidelines and extract lessons that may be relevant to nutrition policy
making today.

Breastfeeding and Doctors in
Canada in the 1920s

There is a long history of artificial feeding from ancient times up to the
nineteenth-century development of modern public health legislation,
which shows that this form of feeding, in unsanitary conditions, generally meant death for an infant.[7] Artificial feeding of infants in cities
undergoing the transformation of an industrial revolution, such as
occurred in Canada towards the end of the nineteenth century and in
the early twentieth century, was a dangerous practice, because it brought
babies into direct contact with contaminated, often germ-ridden water
and cow's milk.[8]

There is some evidence, particularly in North American cities, where
wet nursing was not as popular as in Europe, that the rate of artificial
feeding among poor women increased quickly in the late nineteenth
century.[9] It is likely that poor urban women in the difficult working conditions of the time may had particular difficulty in sustaining breastfeeding. At the same time, these poor women would have faced unsanitary living and difficult working conditions and, if they used artificial
feeding, access mainly to contaminated water and milk for their babies.[10]

Public health reformers were well aware of this situation in the late
nineteenth century. In Britain the scientific links between poverty,
increased artificial feeding, and infant mortality were established by the
turn of the century. In a classic study of infant mortality among the
poor, conducted in London at the turn of the century, Newman (1906)
concluded that "a mother suckling her infant requires nourishment,
and it is lack of nourished mothers among the poor—many of whom are

half-starved—that leads to the inability to provide milk for their off-spring. This, in its turn, leads to early weaning, which involves artificial feeding, which is one of the most difficult undertakings in the tenement homes of the poor. And so it comes about that the early-weaned infant is so often marked for death in infancy."[11]

The links between artificial infant feeding and infant mortality were also well known in Canada.[12] The Industrial Revolution and concomitant social upheavals underway in Canada in the 1880s and 1890s provoked increasing pressure for social reform spearheaded by organizations such as the National Council of Women, the Women's Christian Temperance Union, and the Social Service Council of Canada. These resulted in the establishment of milk depots in some Canadian cities, and Child and Maternal Hygiene Divisions in many municipal public health departments, which educated women to breastfeed their infants.[13]

The social reform movement in Canada achieved much by the First World War, including the development of public health legislation in many provinces and municipalities, and, at the federal level, created the political pressure to establish a national department of health with a Division of Child Welfare. However, by war's end this movement was largely spent as a social force for change.[14] The 1920s was a time of growing public faith and belief in the power of science in general and increased respect for the achievements of medicine in particular, as the medical profession became increasingly better trained, better able to effect cures, and as the profession grew in stature and organizational power.[15]

However, not all medical professionals viewed breastfeeding in a positive light. For example, in the earliest Canadian medical investigation of breastfeeding among 370 children attending the Nutritional Clinic at Toronto's Hospital for Sick Children, investigators claimed that malnutrition cases were to be found in equal proportion among breast-fed and bottle-fed babies.[16] According to the investigator, the cause of malnutrition in approximately half these cases was due to mismanagement and "lack of discipline in the home." In particular, "the first evidence of lack of home control is the fact that the child nurses 15 to 18 months. When the parent fails to control a child of that age, what success need one expect in dealing with this same child at 10 years of age?"[17]

This early medical study of breastfeeding illustrates the distrust the Canadian medical profession displayed towards mothers in general and breastfeeding in particular. The medical profession gained more control over the process of pregnancy and birthing in Canada in the period from 1920 to 1950. For example, by 1939, 41 per cent of women birthed in hospitals, increasing to 67 per cent in 1949.[18] During this time, the advice dispensed by doctors to women increasingly promoted artificial feeding and diminished the importance of breastfeeding.

As Myers has shown, during the 1920s middle-class women moved away from breastfeeding for many reasons. Increasing public faith in science and therefore the science-based feeding increasingly promoted by doctors, and the need for more independence for middle-class women made artificial feeding more appealing.[19] Thus, at the very time when national nutrition guidelines were developed and widely disseminated to promote breastfeeding, new medical, social, and cultural conditions were leading to a profound decline in breastfeeding and increased exposure of very young infants to cow's milk.

The Availability of Disease-Free Cow's Milk in Canada in the 1920s

During the last quarter of the nineteenth century and the first two decades of the twentieth century, rapid industrialization and consequent separation of farm from the urban table stretched the primitive storage and distribution systems of the day, rendering milk an even greater hazard for poor urban children than it had ever been on the farm.[20] Milk had to be transported long distances and stored for relatively long times in the absence of refrigeration, and it was often obtained from tuberculosis-infested cattle living on un-inspected farms and in unsanitary dairy barns.[21]

This began to change in Canada, beginning in Toronto, which passed laws as early as the 1880s to regulate the dairy barns within the city.[22] By 1908 Ottawa passed stringent by-laws requiring the inspection of all cattle supplying milk to the city, in an attempt to extend its dairy inspection regime to its rural milk shed.[23] Toronto passed similar laws at this time, and with growing pressure, in 1911, Ontario passed its Milk Act mandating the inspection of herds and dairy facilities province-wide. In 1914, in a further effort to clean the milk supply, Toronto City Council passed legislation making pasteurization of all milk sold in the city compulsory, so that by the early 1920s milk in Toronto was probably safe.[24]

The first state-level legislation in North America making pasteurization of milk compulsory was passed in Ontario (as an amendment to the Public Health Act) only in 1938. During the 1920s and 1930s, only "fifty municipalities of the eight hundred in the province had passed by-laws requiring the pasteurization of all milk offered for sale."[25] As late as 1922, the head of the National Dairy Council of Canada told a meeting of the Canadian Public Health Association that "milk sold in Ontario for domestic consumption (that is outside of our larger cities), is disgusting, dirty and dangerous."[26] In an article in the *Public Health Journal* he warned that the council required continuing education of farmers, milk processors, and distributors, and greater cooperation between producers and medical officers of health to maintain current standards and further improve the cleanliness of milk.[27]

Even in Canada's most activist public health province through the 1920s and 1930s the milk supply was uneven in its cleanliness. And, outside Ontario, provincial legislation and most municipal by-laws were not as advanced. For example, in Canada's largest city, Montreal, milk was not safe, as evidenced by continuing milk-borne typhoid epidemics through the 1920s.[28]

Thus, in spite of better legislation in some regions, greater awareness within the milk industry, more inspection of cattle and dairy facilities, and greater acceptance and availability of pasteurized milk, much of the Canadian milk supply was unclean and potentially dangerous during the 1920s and 1930s.

Reforming Milk's Image

While most public health professionals had spent the last quarter of the nineteenth century vilifying milk and warning the public of its dangers by the early 1920s, at least in cities where the milk supply had been cleaned up, these same professionals began to extol the virtues of milk. Why this about-face? It came about mainly because of the discovery that besides fats, protein, and carbohydrates, vitamins and trace minerals also were necessary to sustain life. These discoveries came quickly between the turn of the century and the early 1920s.[29] Foods rich in vitamins were dubbed "protective," and milk was quickly identified as the ideal protective food because of its high energy, mineral, and vitamin content.[30]

As well, milk had a special place in early vitamin research. When researchers broke food down into protein, fat, and carbohydrate and fed these constituents in pure form to baby animals, they died. But when fed their mothers' milk, these animals thrived. They used milk as they knew that as nature's food for young animals it contained all the elements necessary for life. And it was, in many cases, from milk that these researchers had isolated the first vitamins.[31]

The publicity around these early vitamin studies was enormous. The role of milk in these experiments was as also well publicized and provided milk with a new image. Following the vitamin discoveries, public health professionals were divided about the impact of pasteurization of cow's milk, as some felt it would denature the vitamins, negating milk's positive impact on health.[32] Once it was discovered that pasteurization only minimally affected vitamin content, public health professionals realized that combined municipal regimes of farm and dairy inspection and pasteurization would make milk safe, and once safe, an ideal protective food.

Thus the early 1920s was a transition time for milk. On the one hand, because of the uneven cleanliness across the milk supply, it was still dangerous, but on the other hand, it was becoming quickly known as the ideal protective food, particularly for children. In order to understand how Canadian health authorities in the 1920s developed guidelines based on feeding cow's milk to babies, children, and pregnant women, it is necessary to consider the position and the needs of the dairy industry at this time, as the 1920s was also a time of transition for this industry as it faced new challenges.

The Relationship between the Federal Government, the Dairy Industry, and Public Health Officials in the 1920s

In the last quarter of the nineteenth and first quarter of the twentieth century, the dairy industry in Canada was overwhelmingly concentrated in the provinces of Ontario and Quebec. The factory system of cheese production, developed in nearby New York State in 1850, had made its way to Canada by the early 1860s, and by the late 1860s there were over 235 cheese factories in the province of Ontario alone.[33] By the 1880s Ontario and Quebec had developed a sophisticated export-oriented cheese and butter factory system, with most exports destined for the British market.

The development of cheese factories and creameries was encouraged by the federal Department of Agriculture through the office of the federal dairy commissioner established in 1890. During the last decade of the nineteenth century, experimental agricultural stations were established across Canada to teach farmers and entrepreneurs the business of factory cheese and butter production. Through these experimental stations the Department of Agriculture subsidized the construction of local factories and the training of personnel. Once these demonstration projects were established, the department would withdraw, allowing local businessmen to finance further operation and expansion.[34] As well, in the 1890s as refrigeration systems developed and became key to the expansion of the export market for dairy products, the Department of Agriculture subsidized the development of refrigeration storage facilities at key export ports.[35]

By the turn of the century, Ontario and Quebec had a sophisticated dairy industry (actively supported by the federal government) based on exporting cheese and butter, mainly to Britain. Exports of cheese and butter peaked in the first decade of the twentieth century and dropped thereafter as local populations expanded and farmers shifted from cheese to fluid milk production to meet this local increase in demand, and as Canadian dairy exports in the British market faced increasingly stiff competition from New Zealand, Australia, and Denmark.[36]

In Canada prior to the First World War, the dairy industry remained remarkably unconcentrated. Fluid milk and butter production was based mainly on single family farms, and while cheese production, with its need for factory facilities, required more capital, it also remained relatively unconcentrated. Concentration in the fluid milk distribution business varied by region and city. For example, in the year preceding the First World War, the cities of Ottawa and Regina were served by one large distributor, whereas Toronto had over fifty distributors.[37]

In 1914, the federal government passed the War Measures Act and created a centralized food control system. In an effort to increase the efficiency of milk production and distribution on the home front, the food controller formed a Milk Committee, which recommend consolidating the dairy industry, particularly its milk distribution component. The committee felt that fewer producers, suppliers, and distributors would increase the economic efficiency of the system, ensuring that farmers obtained better prices and therefore better incentives to produce, and that the reduced number of distributors and producers would make it easier to organize effective systems of public health milk inspection.

While calling for increased consolidation in the milk industry, the federal Department of Agriculture spearheaded an increased drive for agricultural production specifically for export under the slogan "Patriotism, production, and prosperity," resulting in greatly expanded dairy capacity, which peaked just as the war ended and export markets for dairy products dried up.[38] The abrupt shift to dependence on domestic consumption of milk, butter, and cheese, at the end of the war—during a time of growing food price inflation, which restricted the ability of domestic consumers to purchase dairy products—put the dairy industry into crisis.[39] The price of milk increased from 8.8 cents in 1914 to a high of 15 cents a quart in 1920, and for the duration of the decade hovered at 12 cents, approximately 40 per cent higher than it had been at the beginning of the war.[40]

The Food Controller's Milk Committee reported that "any slight increase in the price of milk, unfortunately, has been followed by a largely decreased consumption."[41] Milk consumption was clearly very sensitive to reductions in disposable income. Given the inflationary conditions at that time, the committee recommended that "a campaign of education be undertaken, emphasizing the relatively high food value

Figure 1. Fluid milk prices in Canada, 1914 to 1929

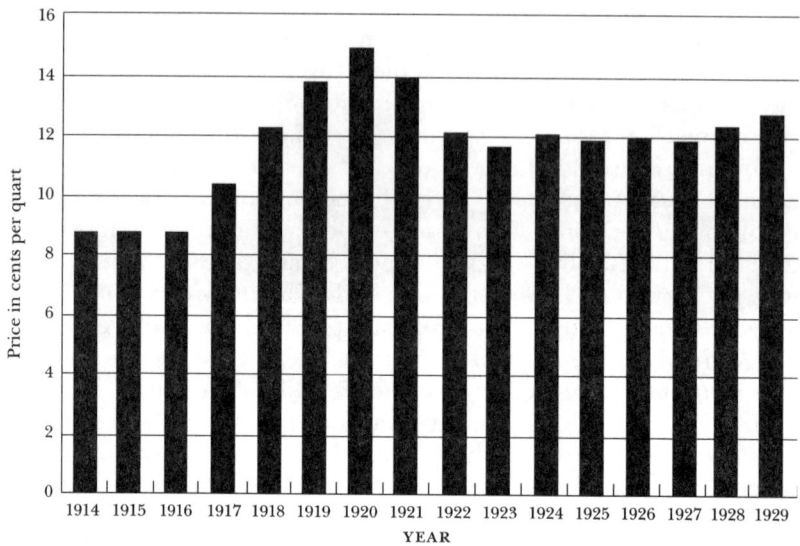

of milk and the many ways of using it. Such a campaign could, perhaps, best be carried out by teachers of Domestic Science and by home economics Associations."[42]

This committee and the dairy industry clearly realized that the price elasticity for milk might be reduced if milk's image could be reformed. The authors of this report understood that enhancing milk's image would take more than a public relations campaign and suggested that the industry work more cooperatively with public health professionals to clean the milk supply.

The process of making milk supplies safe had often involved conflict between dairy farmers, processors, and distributors and municipal public health officers as the last battled to regulate and to convince the industry of the dangers of dirty milk in spreading disease.[43] The process of educating farmers, processors, and distributors, and of cajoling industry into safer practices, involved compromise as well as conflict, both within the industry and between public health and industry officials, so that in many cities by the end of the second decade of the twentieth century, public health professionals and the dairy industry had a long history of working with each other.

For the first time in the history of the urban sanitary reform movement, public health professionals began to recommend clean and inspected milk as the ideal protective food. As early as 1917, as shown by the report to Canada's food controller, the dairy industry also began to campaign harder among its producers, processors, and distributors to improve the cleanliness of the milk supply and harness their relationship with public health officials, nutritionists, and dieticians to promote the protective benefits of milk to children.

An early example of this change occurred in Toronto in 1922 in an extremely well-publicized joint campaign by the Canadian Public Health Association, the Canadian Council on Child Welfare, and the National Dairy Council of Canada. These groups sponsored Milk Week, specifically targeting school children and their mothers to promote increased consumption of milk.[44] The thrust of the campaign was that milk was vitamin and mineral rich with special protective effects for children's health. The message was spread round the city by politicians, public health, and National Dairy Council officials with speeches, carnivals in local parks, and parades, so that it had an extensive reach.

As well, in 1923 officials from the federal Department of Agriculture established strong alliances with the federal Division of Child Welfare and with national child welfare and women's groups, organizing several nutrition-based campaigns to increase the "use of milk for children and mothers."[45] In 1926 the federal Department of Agriculture's Milk Utilization Branch instituted a milk-consumption promotion policy, "cooperating with public health nurses and child welfare workers; assisting in provincial schemes, addressing dairy conventions meetings of school teachers and also public, collegiate and normal school classes. No opportunity is lost for disseminating information as to the dietary value of milk and its products."[46] The Milk Utilization Branch was engaged in "the work of increasing the consumption of dairy products by arousing public interest in their nutritional value."[47] By the late 1920s dieticians were "employed in this work, had booths for demonstration purposes at the leading exhibitions, attended meetings of health and child welfare organizations, women's institutes, dairy conventions and other similar gatherings."[48]

Although the cleanliness of the Canadian milk supply was uneven, particularly in the early 1920s, public health professionals, the dairy industry, and the federal Department of Agriculture increasingly joined forces to promote increased consumption of milk among children. For public health professionals working in cities with clean milk, given the recent discoveries of the vitamin and mineral content of the liquid (and at least thirty years before any hint of a pejorative association between the fat content of milk and ill health), this about-face towards milk made good health sense. For the dairy industry, given decreasing milk consumption following the war, the emerging protective status for milk by the early 1920s was a marketing opportunity. However, as will be shown in the next section, for public health professionals attempting to generate nationwide dietary advice directed primarily at reducing infant mortality, the legacy from milk's past was not so easy to jettison.

The Division of Child Welfare and Canada's First Dietary Guidelines

The Division of Child Welfare was formed in 1919 within the federal Department of Health just one year after it was formed. The mandate of the division was to reduce the persistently high infant mortality rate in Canada.[49] In 1921 the infant mortality rate was 102.1 deaths per 1,000 live births. By 1929 it was 92.9 per 1,000 live births, a reduction of approximately 10 per cent through the 1920s.[50] The federal Department of Health was aware that these were the worst in the industrialized world, noting that in 1921 the infant mortality rate in Canada was more than double that in New Zealand, which had the lowest rate among developed nations.[51]

The gravity of this situation and the well-accepted links among malnutrition, artificial feeding with cow's milk, and infant mortality, as well as the new information on the protective value of milk, figured strongly in the division's first national dietary guidelines directed to expectant and new mothers. These guidelines were first published by the division in 1921 in the *Canadian Mothers Book* (*CMB*), in both English and French and disseminated widely across Canada through the 1920s.[52]

The *CMB* reflected an ambivalence about milk, because it gave general advice to pregnant women to use it as a protective food, but in its specific diets never actually instructed pregnant women to drink milk. And the *CMB* issued dire warnings to mothers against the feeding of cow's milk to babies under nine months of age and strongly advocated breastfeeding for the mother, as "she knows her nursing is the greatest safeguard for the baby's life. She knows that her milk will not only nourish him but protect him from many of the diseases of infancy. She does not want her baby to die. Nursing the baby is the easiest way. No formula with bottles and rubber nipples, and measuring spoons and milk-sugar and sterilizing, and no one knows what else, for the Canadian Mother. These things will get dirty and dirt in milk is death to the baby."[53]

In fact the *CMB* advised mothers to drink cow's milk only after their baby was born. The *CMB* advised women to "keep on the same diet that suited you before the baby came but drink a great deal more—say a pint or more of milk a day and plenty of water three or four times a day. You should have meat at one meal every day. Milk is our greatest protective food. You must have it."[54] Thus, new mothers were specifically advised to drink milk, but pregnant women were not.

After clearly warning Canadian mothers away from feeding milk to babies under nine months of age, the *CMB* described the role of cow's milk in the diet of children once they attained nine months as follows:

Milk is the indispensable food for children. They cannot do without it. The cow has been well called the "the foster mother of the human race." Little children must have milk to enable them to grow properly. No matter what it costs, milk is still the cheapest food for children. Children from nine months to two years should have about two pints of milk every day in addition to other food, and it is really a mistake to give them any less till they are about twelve years of age. Three large cups of milk a day is the very least they should have.[55]

The *CMB* graphically and repeatedly advised that milk for babies over nine months of age should be dirt free, pasteurized, and stored properly, reflecting the extreme unease that professionals in the Division of Child Welfare felt, in the early 1920s, about the safety of the milk supply. In speaking of the situation in the United States around the same time, historian Rima Apple stated that "it is likely that the rising standard of living, greater access to medical care, and improved food and water supplies in the United States in the first half of this century at least in part masked the negative effects of the growing utilization of artificial infant feeding."[56] Infants and children, particularly of poor women, were vulnerable at a time when their mothers were moving away from the practice of breastfeeding under conditions of unavailability or sporadic availability of clean milk and water, and before the era of rapidly rising standards of living and widespread availability of medical care.

The guidelines developed in the *Canadian Mothers Book*, the first guidelines developed in Canada for nationwide dissemination, contained a stark inconsistency, on the one hand promoting cow's milk as *the* protective food, and on the other hand, warning strongly that if used inappropriately it would kill the baby. This message, promulgated given the uneven availability of clean milk in the early 1920s in Canada, may have been more than inconsistent—it was likely quite dangerous.

Throughout the 1920s Canada had the highest rate of infant mortality among industrialized nations.[57] The rate of infant mortality did not begin a steady decline until the early 1930s. It is quite likely that a considerable portion of this mortality during the 1920s was due to continued ingestion of unclean milk during artificial feeding. It is likely that the cow's milk–promotion component of the *CMB*'s dietary guideline was unhelpful in this situation.

The guideline was issued at a time of scientific enthusiasm over the new value of milk in protecting against under-nutrition and promoting optimal health. The public's enthusiasm for the new nutrition science, coupled with local public health promotion campaigns with clean milk, and the unabashed promotion of the protective benefits of milk by industry and Department of Agriculture officials, overwhelmed the ability of the Division of Child Welfare to deliver the best possible dietary guidelines for the times.

Conclusions

This paper demonstrates how, in the absence of a strong nutrition "centre" in the federal government (the Division of Child Welfare was formed only in 1919 and was entirely shut down during the middle of the 1930s), the division's dietary guidelines for infants and children were too easily diluted by the dairy industry and its representative in the federal government, the Department of Agriculture.

The federal Department of Agriculture has figured large in Canada's history, in part because the overarching objective of Canadian national policy in the nineteenth and early twentieth century was to build a strong agricultural sector, particularly in the west, where prior to the building of the transcontinental railway in the 1880s, the Canadian government was concerned with the threat of American expansion into the western provinces. The thrust of agricultural policy after building the railroad was to settle the prairie provinces and create a western Canadian economy on a strong agricultural foundation while strengthening the mixed and dairy farming economy of central Canada.[58]

Expansion of livestock production and the dairy industry was key to this policy, which was threatened by milk surpluses and closing export markets for dairy products in the aftermath of the First World War. In the early 1920s the objectives of the dairy industry and national food policy makers in the Department of Agriculture shifted to active promotion to increase the domestic consumption of fluid milk.

The new science of nutrition with its enthusiastic espousal of milk as the quintessential protective food was harnessed by these interests and new alliances made with public health professionals to garner their support to market milk, particularly to children. Many of the nutrition professionals beginning to emerge from agricultural and home economics programs in the 1920s were employed by the federal Department of Agriculture and the dairy industry to utilize the new science to promote increased milk consumption.[59] The alliance of agricultural interests and their successful harnessing of the new science of nutrition in the 1920s were effective. They were able to market milk to children even in the face of clear evidence of high infant mortality rates, which had been scientifically linked to the ingestion of unclean milk, in the absence of effective provincial public health legislation regulating the milk supply, and even though the price of milk was at historically high levels.

Within the federal government the only resistance to this enthusiastic food policy came from the Division of Child Welfare in the form of the nation's first dietary guidelines warning mothers not to feed cow's milk to babies under nine months of age. This resistance was half-hearted, perhaps because the division itself was also actively involved with the Milk Utilization program within the Department of Agriculture, which specifically and aggressively promoted milk consumption among mothers and school children throughout the 1920s and 1930s.

Acknowledgements

The support of the Canadian Institute for Health Research, New Investigator Fund and the Michael Smith Foundation for Health Research in British Columbia is gratefully acknowledged.

Notes

1 Department of Health, *Canadian Mothers Handbook* (Ottawa: King's Printer, 1923).
2 E. M. Dupuis, *Nature's Perfect Food: How Milk Became America's Drink* (New York: New York University Press, 2002).
3 A. Davidson, *Food and Drug Administration in Canada* (Ottawa: Health and Welfare Canada, 1949); R. E. Curan, *Canada's Food and Drug Laws* (New York and Chicago: Commerce Clearing House, 1954); and H. MacDougall, *Activists and Advocates: Toronto's Health Department, 1883–1983* (Toronto: Dundurn, 1990).
4 Department of Health, *Canadian Mothers Handbook*, 1923.
5 A. W. Myers, "Breast-feeding: A Canadian Perspective on a Global Priority," *Canadian Medical Association Journal* 125 (1981): 1078–1142.
6 J. M. Kerr, *Need Our Mothers Die?* (Ottawa: Division on Maternal and Child Hygiene, Canadian Welfare Council, 1935).
7 N. Baumslag and D. L. Michels, *Milk, Money, and Madness: The Culture and Politics of Breastfeeding* (Westport, CT: Bergin and Garvey, 1993); V. A. Fildes, *Breasts, Bottles, and Babies* (Edinburgh: Edinburgh University Press, 1986); and P. Stuart-Macadam and K. A. Dettwyler, *Breastfeeding: Biocultural Perspectives* (New York: Aldine de Gruyter, 1995).
8 W. P. Ward and P. C. Ward, "Infant Birth Weight and Nutrition in Industrializing Montreal," *American Historical Review* 89, 2 (1984): 324–45.
9 V. Fildes, "Infant Feeding Practices and Infant Mortality in England, 1900–1919," *Continuity and Change* 13, 2 (1998): 251–80.
10 Ward and Ward, "Infant Birth Weight."
11 G. Newman, *Infant Mortality: A Social Problem* (London: Methuen, 1906), 260. Featherstone (2005) also shows that in Australia, in the late nineteenth century, although infant mortality rates were relatively low, the problem of high infant mortality rates also lent urgency to public health reform. She also promotes a view that the Australian medical profession was monolithic in its promotion of breast-feeding. This is in contra-distinction to the situation in Canada (Brown, 1933) and in the United States (Sealander, 2005) where although many in the medical profession advocated breastfeeding, others were actively involved in the promotion of infant formula and methods of supplemental feeding. See A. Brown,

"The Prevention of Neonatal Mortality," *Canadian Medical Association Journal* 29 (1933): 264–68; L. Featherstone, "Infant Ideologies: Doctors, Mothers, and the Feeding of Children in Australia, 1880–1910"; and J. Sealander. "Perpetually Malnourished? Diet, Health, and America's Young in the Twentieth Century," in this volume.

12 H. MacMurchy, *Handbook of Child Welfare Work in Canada* (Ottawa: Department of Health, 1923).

13 R. Allen, *The Social Passion: Religion and Social Reform in Canada 1914–28* (Toronto: University of Toronto Press, 1971); A. Moscovitch and G. Drover, "Social Expenditures and the Welfare State: The Canadian Experience in Historical Perspective," in *The Benevolent State: The Growth of Welfare in Canada*, ed. A. Moscovitch and J. Alberts (Toronto: Garamond, 1987), 13–47; and M. Valverde, *The Age of Light, Soap, and Water: Moral Reform in English Canada, 1885–1925* (Toronto: McClelland and Stewart, 1991).

14 K. McCuaig, "From Social Reform to Social Service: The Changing Role of Volunteers; The Anti-Tuberculosis Campaign, 1900–30," *Canadian Historical Review* 61, 4 (1980): 485.

15 D. Coburn, G. M. Torrance, and J. M. Kaufert, "Medical Dominance in Canada, in Historical Perspective: The Rise and Fall of Medicine?" *International Journal of Health Services Research* 13, 3 (1981): 407–28.

16 C. S. Macdougall, "Malnutrition in Children of School Age," *Public Health Journal* 42, 3 (1922): 28.

17 According to Featherstone, "Infant Ideologies," in Australia at about the same time, the medical profession also often blamed mothers for a lack of mothering skills and general ignorance about breastfeeding and child rearing.

18 A. Y. Burns, "The Child and Maternal Health Division of the Department of National Health and Welfare," *Medical Services Journal of Canada* (April 1967): 688.

19 Myers, "Breast-feeding."

20 R. Cohen and J. Heimlich, *Milk: The Deadly Poison* (New York: Argus, 1998).

21 T. Dormandy, *The White Death: A History of Tuberculosis* (New York: New York University Press, 2000).

22 MacDougall, *Activists and Advocates*.

23 J. B. Hollingsworth, "Milk and Dairy Inspection," *Public Health Journal of Canada* 43 (1922): 223–26.

24 MacDougall, *Activists and Advocates*.

25 E. W. McHenry, "Milk: The Protected, Protective food," *Canadian Public Health Journal* 32, 4 (1941): 227–30.

26 E. H. Stonehouse, "A Safe and Clean Milk Supply," *Public Health Journal of Canada* (1922): 449–54.

27 E. H. Stonehouse, "The Production of Clean Milk," *Public Health Journal of Canada* 21 (1922): 293–302.

28 MacDougall, *Activists and Advocates*.

19 M. Nestle, *Food Politics: How the Food Industry Influences Nutrition and Health* (Los Angeles: University of California Press, 2002).

30 Valverde, *Light, Soap, and Water*.

31 A. Rosen, *The History of Public Health* (Baltimore and London: Johns Hopkins University Press, 1958).

32 Hollingsworth, "Milk and Dairy Inspection."

33 M. G. Cohen, *Women's Work, Markets, and Economic Development in Nineteenth-Century Ontario* (Toronto: University of Toronto Press, 1988); V. C. Fowke, *Canadian Agricultural Policy: The Historical Pattern* (Toronto: University of Toronto Press, 1947).

34 It should be noted that the Canadian experimental agricultural stations had a purely agricultural purpose, unlike the stations established by Atwater in the United States during this same era (Aronson, 1982; Sealander, 2005). In the last decade of the 19th century, Atwater firmly linked the emerging science of nutrition with the problems of efficient labour supply and labour harmony in the rapidly industrializing conditions of America at the time and used agricultural stations established by the USDA to pioneer the new nutrition science (Aronson, 1982). Conditions in Canada were very different at this time. Canada was a small nation, with a small economy and, relative to the United States, an immature industrial infrastructure. In Canada the science of nutrition remained, relative to the United States and Europe, under developed and under appreciated. As an example, in Canada it was only in the late 1930s that the first scientific dietary surveys were conducted whereas the first surveys in the USA were conducted in 1885 (Pett, 1944).

   N. Aronson, "Nutrition as a Social Problem: A Case Study of Entrepreneurial Strategy in Science," *Social Problems* 29, 5 (1982): 474–87; and L. B. Pett, "Malnutrition in Canada," *Canadian Medical Association Journal* 50 (1944): 9–14.

35 G. E. Britnell and V. C. Fowke, *Canadian Agriculture in War and Peace 1935–1950* (Stanford: Food Research Institute, Stanford University Press, 1962); Cohen, *Women's Work*.

36 G. Skogstad, *The Politics of Agricultural Policy-making in Canada* (Toronto: University of Toronto Press, 1987).

37 Food Controller for Canada, *Report of the Milk Committee to the Food Controller for Canada: Including a Plan for the Re-organization of Milk Distribution* (Ottawa: King's Printer, 1917).

38 Britnell and Fowke, *Canadian Agriculture*, 48.

39 Dupuis (*Nature's Perfect Food*, 114) has shown that in the United States the dairy industry faced similar pressures at the end of the First World War.

40 Dominion Bureau of Statistics, Price Division, Retail Prices Section, *Urban Retail Food Prices, 1914–1959* (Ottawa, Queen's Printer, 1960).

41 Food Controller, *Report of the Milk Committee*, 6.

42 Food Controller, *Report of the Milk Committee*, 6.

43 Hollingsworth, Milk and Dairy Inspection.

44 Department of Pensions and National Health, *Health Department Annual Report* (Ottawa: King's Printer, 1923).

45 Pensions and National Health, *Annual Report*, 42.

46 Department of Agriculture, *Agriculture Department Annual Report* (Ottawa: King's Printer, 1926), 34.

47 Department of Agriculture, *Annual Report*, 86.

48 Department of Agriculture, *Agriculture Department Annual Report* (Ottawa: King's Printer, 1927) 40.

49 R. L. Schnell, "A Children's Bureau for Canada: The Origins of the Canadian Council on Child Welfare, 1913–1921," in *The Benevolent State: The Growth of Welfare in Canada*, ed. A. Moscovitch and J. Alberts (Toronto: Garamond Press, 1987), 95–111.

50 Statistics Canada. *Selected Infant Mortality and Related Statistics, Canada, 1921–1990*. Catalogue 82-549 Occasional (Ottawa: Statistics Canada, 1991).

51 Department of Pensions and National Health. *Health Department Annual Report* (Ottawa: King's Printer, 1924).

52 Department of Pensions and National Health. *Health Department Annual Report* (Ottawa: King's Printer, 1923).

53 Department of Health, *Canadian Mothers Handbook*, 72.
54 Department of Health, *Canadian Mothers Handbook*, 82.
55 Department of Health, *Canadian Mothers Handbook*, 107.
56 R. D. Apple, *Mothers and Medicine: A Social History of Infant Feeding, 1890–1950* (Madison: University of Wisconsin Press, 1987), 172.
57 Statistics Canada, *Infant Mortality*.
58 W. J. Anderson, *Canadian Agricultural Policy: A Review*. Occasional Papers on Credit, Livestock, Food Supply (Ottawa: Policy No. 9, Agricultural Economics Research Council of Canada, 1966/67).
59 In *Food Politics*, Nestle has demonstrated the same phenomenon in the United States around this time.

Racial and Ethnic Dimensions

ଓ

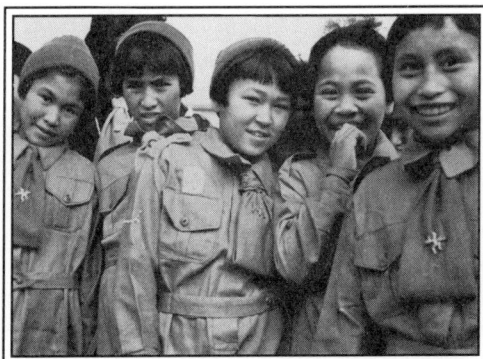

Caring for the Foreign-Born
The Health of Immigrant Children in the United States, 1890–1925

CR

Howard Markel

Introduction

T hat we are, as President John F. Kennedy once wrote, "a nation of immigrants" is indisputable.[1] The founding of the United States of America was a complex process of transforming a vast territory into an established society with its own culture, mores, and institutions dedicated to liberty. This process, of course, relied heavily upon a stream of immigrants who were active participants in the physical, economic, and intellectual development of the nation.

Not surprisingly, historians, journalists, novelists, playwrights, poets, and other observers of the American scene have long paid close attention to the successes and problems engendered by these human migration patterns over the past two centuries. This is particularly true of the era American historians refer to as the "Great Wave of Immigration," 1890–1925, when more than twenty-five million immigrants, chiefly from eastern and southern Europe, arrived at the ports and borders of the United States.[2] But like the confusion that often arises when a patient seeks the opinion of more than one physician, different observers tell this story in markedly divergent ways, reflecting individual views, sources, intellectual contexts, and social beliefs. There are many versions that endorse immigration as a positive contribution to the nation just as there are many others that have decried immigration as an abomination that will inexorably lead to the nation's decline and ruin.[3] Observers of contemporary debates on American immigration policies should take heart in the fact that this is hardly a new debate.

Those of us who study the history of immigration and health in American society have commonly focused on the period of the Great Wave of Immigration, and especially on such issues as the sanitary conditions of steerage travel, the medical inspection process at Ellis Island and similar immigration reception centres, and the occasional health

crises that erupted or appeared to be associated with a specific immigrant group once they settled into the United States.[4] Aside from the
inherent fascinations these topics present, the reason they are so frequently the focus of this field of historical inquiry is that there is such
a huge paper trail left in their wake. Beginning with the Immigration
Act of 1891, the U.S. federal government administered and controlled
immigration on a national basis. During the succeeding years of the Progressive Era (1890–1920), a period marked by the rise of the authority
of the expert and "scientific management," the federal government's
medical inspection of immigrants and similar public health ventures
generated reams of files and reports published by the Government
Printing Office, the home of the largest printing presses in the world
during the time.[5] Local printers who won the lucrative contracts for
publishing the annual reports of state or municipal boards of health also
contributed to a rich documentary archive of the American immigration experience.

One less well-studied aspect of immigrant health in American history, however, is the children of immigrants—both those who may have
immigrated to the United States along with their parents and those who
were born in the United States to immigrant parents. In particular, we
have not yet sufficiently mined the historical record in order to understand the health problems that developed when immigrant children
were examined by physicians of completely different social stations and
culture. Adding to this complex mix were parents of different cultures,
beliefs, and languages. This, obviously, had a significant impact on how
health care for these children was delivered and carried out once they
returned home from a visit to the American physician.

During the Progressive Era, there were three arenas in which children of immigrants were most likely to come in contact with health problems or health professionals: (1) the American city, (2) the medical
inspection of public schools and students, and (3) the urban pediatric dispensaries—milk stations that served impoverished children. These three
arenas will be the focus of this essay. This brief glimpse at children of a
century ago will, I hope, illustrate how barriers of language, culture,
superstition, poverty, education, and numerous other social differences
contributed to negative *and* positive health outcomes. Such backward
glances, however, are not only of interest to the historian of a long-gone
era. They can also provide a social context for emerging problems seen
today as children's health care professionals grapple with providing
health care for increasing numbers of patients from different lands.

The Health of the American City
at the Turn of the Century

Despite the decade's familiar sobriquet, the 1890s were not an entirely carefree period in American history. Economic depressions, massive immigration, and the rise of industry and urbanism all contributed to the deleterious heath conditions of New York City, Boston, Philadelphia, Baltimore, Detroit, Chicago, and beyond. Wealth protected many against the harsher environmental conditions, but for those living in the poorer sections of these cities it was a difficult and dangerous existence. Dirt, filth, noise, overcrowding, and bad odours pervaded almost every aspect and activity of daily life. Foodstuffs ranging from wilting vegetables to rotting fish were sold on open pushcarts in the streets. Transportation was horse-drawn. The noise pollution from the constant clip-clop of horses' hooves on the cobblestones was matched by the massive quantities of horse dung that marked their trails. It was not uncommon for a horse to die suddenly, in harness, and, too often, the carcass was left in the street for days before the municipal authorities arranged removal. Sewage systems, particularly in the poorer districts of the American city, were unreliable and often backed up into already soiled and filthy streets. Toilets in the tenements were often in the form of privies and outdoor outhouses that were inconsistently cleaned by "night soil" removers. Baths were occasional events in many of the lives of urban, poor immigrants, and access to heated water in the proverbial "cold water flat" meant boiling water on the stove and hurrying to a metal basin to bathe.[6]

An excellent contemporary example of these dangers can be found in the pages of the annual reports of the Sanitary Aid Society of the Tenth Ward of the City of New York. Founded in 1884 by a group of prominent New Yorkers that included Theodore Roosevelt and former mayor Abram S. Hewitt, the society's mission was to improve the health and sanitary conditions of the immigrants living on New York's Lower East Side, which at the time was one of the densest urban ghettos on the planet. After a winter-long inspection of every tenement house in the ward, the Sanitary Aid Society reported in 1885, "To get into these pestilential human rookeries you have to penetrate courts and alleys reeking with poisonous and malodorous gases arising from accumulations of sewage and refuse scattered in all directions and flowing beneath your feet....Walls and ceilings are black with the accretions of filth which have gathered upon them through long years of neglect....The rooms were crowded with sick and dirty children."[7]

Mixing the wealthy native-born American's noblesse oblige with a heaping quantity of revulsion, the report, and those that followed in the successive years through the 1890s, only worsen as one continues to read. Inadequately protected against the harsh cold of winter or the stifling heat of summer, children in these urban ghettos often ate poorly, washed sporadically, dodged falling plaster and other environmental hazards, and were exposed to many deadly contagious diseases. Epidemics of diphtheria, smallpox, and whooping cough, to name but a few, were almost annual events during this period. Each summer brought waves of *cholera infantum* or "summer diarrhea," in which thousands of American babies died of dehydration. It was an era when at least two hundred out of every thousand children born in an American city did not live to see their first birthdays; similarly, one out of every five American children did not live to be five years of age.[8] Death was a common visitor, with a frequency and relentlessness that is difficult for most Americans of just a century later to fully comprehend.

The abandonment of babies was another all too common symptom of the dysfunctional American city during the late nineteenth and early twentieth centuries. The social institution we call the orphanage reached its zenith during this period in attempts to grapple with an ever-swelling population of dependent and abandoned children.[9] Not surprisingly, immigrant infants born to those with the fewest social support options were especially vulnerable for this status at the turn of the century. The well-known journalist and photographer Jacob A. Riis, himself a Danish immigrant, achieved national celebrity with his best-selling 1890 account of immigrant life, *How the Other Half Lives: Studies among the Tenements of New York*. It was a book designed to shock and horrify a complacent, native-born American population into doing something about the wretched living conditions of its newest inhabitants. Riis's descriptions of squalor leap off the page. Yet few of Riis's pen portraits of immigrant life are sadder than the following account of the poor "abandon[ing] their children":

Only the poor abandon their children....They come in rags, a newspaper is often the only wrap....[sometimes] a little slip of paper [is] pinned on, perhaps with some such message as..."Take care of Johnny, for God's sake. I cannot." But even that is the rarest of happenings....In midwinter, when the poor shiver in their homes, and in the dog-days of summer when the fierce heat and foul air of the tenements smother their babies by thousands they are found, sometimes three and four in a night, in hallways, in areas and on the doorsteps of the rich....After a night spent in a Police Headquarters, it [the abandoned baby] travels up to the Infants' Hospital on Randall's Island in the morning, fitted out with a number and a bottle, that seldom see much wear before they are laid aside for a fresh recruit. Few outcast babies survive their desertion long. Murder is the true name of the mother's crime in eight cases of ten....The high mortality among the foundlings is not to be marveled at. The wonder is, rather, that any survive.[10]

This was also the era of child labour reform, a wide-sweeping social and legislative response to hundreds of thousands of poor and immigrant children being enlisted into the workforce long before their minds or bodies were ready for such challenges. Prior to this legislation, children as young as six were at work in dirty, overcrowded tenement sweatshops, often operating heavy or dangerous machinery. Many children plied their trades in the city streets, hawking newspapers and delivering messages, some procuring narcotics and prostitutes. Other high-risk activities included petty theft, vandalism, and constant battles with policemen, truant officers, and other symbols of authority.[11]

One major focus of the many efforts to "Americanize" the disparate Irish, Italian, East European, and other immigrant communities was centred on health and hygiene. Following the exciting discoveries of the germ etiologies of specific infectious diseases, public health workers espoused a philosophy whereby teaching immigrants and their children (along with native-born Americans) about proper hygiene and personal cleanliness would make great inroads in improving the nation's public health. As historian Richard Meckel has noted, "Infant mortality was [widely believed to be] a product of maternal ignorance and improper care, and, thus, could be effectively combatted by instruction....the belief that [infant mortality and] many of the social problems besetting urban America could be significantly addressed by acculturating immigrants was one which was central to American progressivism."[12]

Immigrant newspapers and social groups, health departments and civic improvement organizations, home economists, social workers, and government representatives all worked (but not always in concert) to develop culturally sophisticated public health campaigns that explained personal hygiene, disease avoidance, parenting, and personal conduct. Numerous handbooks, pamphlets, newspaper and magazine articles, advertisements for health-related products in the immigrant press, motion pictures, cartoons, lectures, and similar educational materials have, fortunately, been preserved in a number of immigration and governmental archives. The overwhelming majority of these materials reveal a measured understanding for many of the language and cultural differences seen among the immigrant communities, but it was a sensitivity formed in an era when ideas about race, nationality, intelligence, and potential for assimilation were markedly different from our own. But this advice did not always originate from native-born Americans or public health professionals; much of it came through the hard work and cooperation of social institutions founded and maintained by the immigrant communities themselves. Indeed, many of the critical steps in immigrants' assimilation into American practices and hygiene in the past century were undertaken by a predominantly privately funded social network and institutional infrastructure of immigrant peer groups that does not exist in nearly as extensive a manner for today's "newest wave" of immigration.

One small example of this effort can be found in the pages of the major Yiddish-American newspaper of this era, the *New York Daily Forward* (*Forvitz*). For decades, advice on adjusting to a new life in America, politics, family life, social issues, and even personal health were offered up in a daily column called "A Bintel Brief" ("A Bundle of Letters") by the *Forward*'s venerable editor Abraham Cahan. In 1908, for example, a Yiddish-speaking tailor wrote to Cahan about his affliction with "the worker's disease," tuberculosis, and how this condition was affecting his family. The man is a father of a three-year old daughter whom, like any loving parent, he longs to hold and kiss. Yet he realizes that his very kiss might lead to his child's contracting and dying from tuberculosis: "I know I am infecting my innocent child. Every time I kiss the child I feel my wife's eyes on me, as if she wanted to shout, 'Murderer'...What can I do when I cannot control myself?" Along with advice to seek the care of a physician, Cahan patiently prescribed restraint to the tailor in terms of kissing his daughter and some reassurance: "The father could live a long life with his ailment. With good treatment, consumptives can live out their years and he might yet live to have a lot of pleasure from his little daughter."[13]

The Medical Inspection of Public Schools and Students

Coinciding with the rise of the public health movement in the United States, mass public school education was a mid-to-late-nineteenth-century phenomenon. As with any intense phase of institution building, however, the local school districts rarely grew as quickly as the number of students desiring entry.[14] Many urban schools at the turn of the century conducted classes in poorly lit, under-ventilated basements, corridors, and temporary wooden structures called "portables." Inadequate plumbing and sewage systems meant that these "halls of learning" were often filled with the stench of poorly working toilets or overfilled outhouses.[15] Given these conditions, improving the public school facilities and sanitary or health conditions for students became of great concern to the American public. For example, between 1908 and 1909 alone, more than five hundred articles on school hygiene appeared in the medical literature and popular periodicals.[16]

Not surprisingly, these problems were of special interest to children's health professionals and led to the development of the medical inspections of public schools. For example, in 1893, the City of New York appointed the nation's first medical inspector, Moreau Morse. The following year, 1894, the City of Boston appointed Samuel Durgin to organize a team of fifty physicians to oversee the health needs of that city's fifty school districts.[17] A decade later, in 1904, 36 cities and towns had such systems. By 1913, when Luther H. Gulick and Leonard P. Ayers reissued their landmark study, *Medical Inspection of Schools*, there were 443 American cities or towns that conducted medical inspections of schools.[18]

The earliest medical inspection programs in New York (1893), Boston (1894), Chicago (1895), and Philadelphia (1898) were centred on prescribed visits by medical doctors to an assigned district in order to examine the pupils. Most implicit in the motives behind these programs was the surveillance for the many contagious diseases of childhood and, if discovered, their rapid containment in the form of quarantine. In an era framed by the spectre of contagious disease, speed in such endeavours was of the essence. Doctors, nurses, social workers, and, on the front lines, schoolteachers worked assiduously to facilitate these methods of disease control.

During the first two decades of the twentieth century, medical inspection of the schools became more formalized and broader in reach. Many individual schools were staffed with full-time nurses. There were organized plans for the isolation of children suspected of a contagious disease. Vaccinations for smallpox were offered routinely. Vision, hearing, and dental examinations were instituted. Developmental and physical abnormalities began to be addressed by pediatricians of this period as well. Some of the most common concerns were the predicted effects of enlarged tonsils and adenoids on a child's health and development; pediatricians ascribed almost everything from mouth-breathing and apnea to a propensity toward tuberculosis, hyperactivity, enuresis, and feeble-mindedness to the hypertrophied lymphoid tissues.[19] The inspection of school buildings by sanitary engineers and public health workers also became routine during this period. But perhaps the widest-reaching activities of this endeavour revolved around the education of children and their parents about personal hygiene and disease prevention. Indeed, these topics were standard elements of most public school curricula well into the 1950s. Public schools became the homes of "Health Leagues," "100% Hygiene Classes," and "Little Mother's Clubs," all to promote the gospel of public health for the children and, by extension, to their parents and families.

Applying the tools of Americanization and public health education to the diverse immigrant communities during the first three decades of the twentieth century was, indeed, a challenge. Yet one does not have to look far in the annals of history to find dedicated, zealous Americans who lived in and worked with these communities for such a cause. Lillian Wald, a New York City nurse who founded the Henry Street Settlement and the Visiting Nurse Service;[20] Jane Addams, a Chicago social worker and children's advocate who founded Hull House;[21] and Michael M. Davis, the director of the Boston Dispensary who wrote one of the first textbooks on immigrant health care,[22] are but a few of the many dedicated professionals whose work we now take as a matter of course when delivering health care for immigrants and their children and maintaining a healthy environment in the classroom.

There were, of course, many tensions that resulted in a milieu where members of a dominant culture provided health care and education for immigrants within (and without) the public school setting. Historians Charles Rosenberg and Judith Walzer Leavitt have described the ambivalent progressive stance taken by many urban professionals of this era assigned to work among immigrant communities. To be sure, many shared traditional (and decidedly negative) American-born, Protestant, middle-class views about the immigrants flooding into the cities in the years before the First World War; at the same time, their zeal for reform compelled them to try to improve the lot of the immigrant, albeit from a world view of elitist assumptions.[23]

One example of this ambivalence can be found in the memoirs of S. Josephine Baker. Baker was a tireless, compassionate public health physician and advocate for impoverished urban children. She spent much of her career with the New York City Health Department, where she organized the Bureau of Child Hygiene. She was also the author of the major textbook *Child Hygiene* and ultimately went on to head the U.S. Children's Bureau.[24] Yet even her descriptions of work among the children of Irish, Italian, Jewish, and Russian immigrants in the New York City public schools were often framed with occasional condescension and some disapproval:

The children's parents were painfully astonished at finding that Giuseppe and Isador and Sonya were being kept out of school because of inconspicuous troubles to which no one had ever paid attention in the old country...the famous melting-pot of Manhattan Island had long since become a huge germ culture....It was a thoroughly insane situation. Not the least ridiculous detail of it appeared when the truant-officers, finding the schools emptied of pupils, began going around and ordering these children back into school. Here was one city department prohibiting the children from attending school and another city department commanding the parents to send them to school. At this point, I suppose, the children's parents concluded that without exception, all government officials in this new country were crazy.[25]

The Pediatric Dispensary and Milk Station

Much of the social activism of the Progressive Era centred on a concern over the health of the nation and its citizens. During this period, some older American institutions of caring, such as orphan asylums and dispensaries, had to adapt to new demands, missions, and patient populations; many other new social agencies, such as immigrant aid societies and hospitals that boasted the technological advances of the early twentieth century, were created in response to the rapidly changing face of the nation.

Perhaps more than any other means of health care delivery, the dispensary was "the primary means for providing the urban poor with medical care and a vital link in the prevailing system of medical education" during the nineteenth century. Consequently, it was inevitable that immigrants and their children had an intimate acquaintance with dispensaries. In these freestanding, neighbourhood outpatient clinics, medical examinations and minor operations were performed and medicines were dispensed. Originally developed in Great Britain during the late eighteenth century, dispensaries soon appeared in American cities: the Philadelphia Dispensary was established in 1786; New York in 1791; Boston in 1796; and Baltimore in 1800. These dispensaries were established by socially conscious Americans with a sincere interest in improving the conditions of the poor. Although many of these dispensaries were operated on a minuscule budget, they grew dramatically both in size and number of patients treated during the nineteenth century; in 1860, for example, all of New York City's dispensaries treated 134,069 patients; in 1900, the number was 876,000.[26] By this point, the great majority of patients being treated in urban dispensaries were foreign-born.

What constituted the urban poor and immigrant community during the late nineteenth and early twentieth centuries shifted markedly with each decade. The Irish, Germans, Italians, East European Jews, Chinese, and Japanese, to name a few of the major groups arriving during these years, were all in their turn derided by native-born Americans as an impoverished, disease-ridden lot. Mixed into these assessments were judgments on the immigrants' morality and religious or cultural beliefs. Yet it was in this social milieu that American-born physicians provided medical care for immigrants and their children. As in other social settings in which immigrants and native-born Americans had close dealings, the social and cultural disparity between these two groups was palpable. To many of the physicians and nurses who staffed the dispensaries, the immigrants were distinctly alien, troublesome, and often defiantly resistant to even the most basic forms of medical advice. To the immigrants, however, the medical attendants may have seemed rude or, because of language differences, unintelligible.[27]

The dispensaries served more than the health needs of the urban poor and immigrant communities; they were also the training centres for a large group of elite American physicians who often went on to become leading members of the medical profession. It was here that ambitious men (and a few women) gained clinical experience and reputations in the competitive urban medical marketplace. In that dispensaries were often organized along specialty lines (e.g., pediatrics, obstetrics, gynecology, medicine, ophthalmology, etc.), young physicians seized the opportunity to embark upon careers as specialists. Indeed, this de facto system of postgraduate medical education remained an important part of the elite American physician's curriculum vitae well into the early years of the twentieth century. As medicine became increasingly more centred in the hospital, more reliant on medical technology, and hospitals and medical schools instituted their own outpatient clinics, the dispensaries lost their cachet for many ambitious young physicians. By the end of the 1920s, these institutions were all but moribund; poorly staffed, they were gradually replaced by other types of outpatient clinics such as the neighbourhood health centre.[28]

That post-mortem aside, the rise of the medical specialization during the late nineteenth and twentieth centuries and the active clinical work of the dispensaries proved to be powerful forces in developing the field of pediatrics and children's health care in the United States. For example, when reviewing the careers of the forty-three founding members of the American Pediatric Society, which was established in 1888, one should not be surprised to discover that all forty-three were male. Less well known to the modern-day children's health professional is that 85 per cent of these men spent significant time learning their specialty as an attending pediatrician in a public or charitable dispensary or orphan asylum–based clinic.[29] Indeed, those few founding members of the American Pediatric Society (APS) who did *not* spend time training in a pediatric dispensary or similar institution were not actually pediatricians at all, although they occasionally saw children in their busy practices. Instead, these few men were prominent medical statesmen—such as internist William Osler of Johns Hopkins, Victor C. Vaughan, dean of the Michigan Medical School, and Simon Baruch, a New York City physician and proponent of public baths for the poor—who were invited to help found the APS because of their international stature as prominent physicians.[30] These few exceptions aside, one can safely posit that it was in the dispensaries where some of the most successful academic pediatricians of the early twentieth century in the United States learned the clinical nuances of the diseases of infancy and childhood.[31]

One of the greatest medical concerns these pediatricians had was the alarmingly high numbers of infant deaths, particularly among the urban poor and immigrant communities, ascribed to diarrhea and dehydration. A common culprit for these waves of infantile diarrhea was contaminated milk. In the days before the advent of widespread pasteurization and refrigeration, milk typically was collected at the dairy farms in the rural areas close to a particular city. While some dairy farmers were scrupulous in the proper handling of milk products, many others were not. Milk then travelled by horse-drawn cart in milk pails that may or may not have been set upon melting cakes of ice. Finally, it was sold in tiny grocery stores and from pushcarts in the urban slums. Many an immigrant mother living in the tenements simply hung the milk pail out on the fire escape in an attempt to keep it cool.[32] Such a method worked far better in the colder months of fall and winter than during the summer. As journalist H. L. Mencken glibly overstated in 1910, "When a cow is milked, the milk takes up floating germs from the air which it passes in its descent to the can, just as raindrops of a summer shower take upon 'the gay motes that dance along a sunbeam.' These germs, finding milk a fertile soil, begin to multiply at once with enormous rapidity."[33]

In response to these glaring health challenges, a large number of pediatricians, chemists, public health workers, and other professionals directed their scholarly attentions to discerning the biochemical composition of human and bovine milk, the development of safe, nutritious, artificial infant formulas (i.e., modified cow's milk products fed using a bottle), and the development of milk laboratories for the proper handling, bacteriological analysis, and distribution of infant formula. Indeed, it would not be an overstatement to note that the study of milk and infant nutrition were the cutting-edge topics of study for many of the most celebrated American pediatricians at the turn of the century.[34]

Not coincidentally, then, pediatricians working at the urban dispensaries began to develop programs that combined medical examinations and health education with the distribution of clean, inexpensive milk for babies. Such prominent pediatricians as Abraham Jacobi, the "father of American pediatrics," Henry Koplik, best remembered for describing the pathognomic sign of measles, Henry Coit, who worked to have milk certified by local boards of health, and Thomas Morgan Rotch, the first professor of pediatrics at Harvard, were instrumental in the spread of pediatric milk stations across the United States. So, too, was the philanthropic support of Nathan Straus, scion of the New York City merchant family that owned R. H. Macy and Company.[35]

With the passage of time, however, we should not conclude that the dispensaries were the ideal means of providing health care for immigrant children. For example, in 1921, public health researcher Michael M.

Davis documented a wide disparity of immigrant satisfaction with the dispensaries and similar urban health care clinics. Ukrainians in Davis's study reported feeling "very strange and lost" in these institutions, while the Jewish immigrants "flocked" to the dispensaries, knowing that "they will receive the care of a specialist, a professor, and they are only too glad to avail themselves of the opportunity." Similarly, a citywide study of the dispensaries of New York, conducted by the New York Academy of Medicine in 1919, revealed a wide disparity of satisfaction with the care provided for immigrants and the urban poor.[36] Imperfect institutions though they were, the dispensaries were the "birthplace" of the well baby examination, the training ground for two or more generations of American pediatricians, an integral part in the movement to provide clean, fresh, and cheap milk for poor infants, and the primary site of medical care for the majority of first-generation immigrant children in American cities during the Progressive Era.[37]

Conclusion

Americans as a society are particularly prone to relegating valuable lessons from the past to the overflowing dustbin of history. This is an unfortunate national trait as consideration is begun for the needs of immigrant children living in the United States, today. Indeed, there is much to be gleaned from the social activism and sense of community responsibility that spawned the health efforts described in this essay. And while there were conflicts and cultural disparities that played themselves out daily between foreign-born patients (and parents) and American health professionals, from the viewpoint of a century later, these health care efforts were remarkably successful. Infant mortality rates dramatically decreased during the course of the twentieth century; the catechism of scientific motherhood was preached to native-born American mothers and their immigrant counterparts across a huge spectrum of socio-economic classes; the health of students and the health conditions in American public schools were significantly improved by medical inspections; health care and nutrition were delivered regularly to millions of impoverished and immigrant children in the form of dispensaries, neighbourhood health centres, and school clinics; and a legion of health care professionals, ranging from pediatricians and nurses to social workers and bacteriologists, obtained impeccable training within these community settings.

In the current era of anti-immigrant sentiment, social and economic scapegoating has returned, as well as a distressing potential for punitive laws directed at immigrants wanting access to health care. There also exists a morass of confusion and misguided finger-pointing by many Americans over the distinction between legal and illegal immigrants.

In a social milieu where federal, state, and municipal welfare support systems are being markedly altered or scrapped altogether, it obliges those who are concerned with the needs of this diverse patient population to reconsider the vital partnerships that once existed among philanthropic social agencies, public health and medical professionals, schoolteachers, social workers, the immigrant communities, *and* the government. All of these historical actors and social institutions played integral roles in improving the physical, mental, and social welfare of the newcomer. Yet these efforts did not fulfil a utopian version of "how things ought to be." Volunteer community efforts, then as today, often combine diverse groups with markedly different goals and agendas. Such efforts are as fragile as a powerful engine whose parts are held together with chewing gum. There are "engineers" who can pull off such a feat, but only with back-breaking work and constant attention.

Many of today's immigrant health care issues, including the barriers of language, education, and culture, would be very familiar to the health worker of a century ago. As a result of abrupt and chaotic human migration patterns, however, a number of new paradigms have emerged. For example, the new immigrant groups of the 1980s and 1990s have had difficulty creating social support networks de novo when compared to their predecessors of a century ago. Further, many immigrants from Africa, Eastern Europe, the Middle East, and other politically unstable areas are currently fleeing from their native lands to seek political asylum; a large percentage of these immigrants have experienced some form of physical torture or abuse. Another challenging group are the illegal immigrants who smuggle themselves across our borders and, thanks to an international trade in counterfeit passport and identification dossiers, through our major airports. Undocumented by definition, these immigrants have little, if any, access to health care. The potential for significant health problems, including epidemic disease, that can result from such an underserved segment of our population is alarming, to say the least.[38]

Pediatricians and children's health professionals have a major stake in the success of meeting these challenges with creative and culturally sensitive solutions. These include the refinement and development of community and school-based clinics in immigrant neighbourhoods; linkage of such efforts with educational training programs for today's health professionals in training; and active research that investigates the social, cultural, and health needs of these diverse communities. Surmounting overwhelming obstacles seems to accompany almost every valuable human endeavour. Often these obstacles seem so great they inspire frustration, avoidance, and indifference. But history teaches us, time and again, to seek better solutions than the tried-and-true response of social paralysis, and, more specifically, the history of American child care over the past century suggests we are soundly up for this challenge.

Acknowledgements

This research was generously supported by a Robert Wood Johnson Generalist Faculty Scholars Award, the James A. Shannon Director's Award of the National Institutes of Health, and the Burroughs-Wellcome 40th Anniversary History of Medicine Award. A version of this paper was previously published in *Archives of Pediatrics and Adolescent Medicine* 152 (1998): 1020–27.

Notes

1 John F. Kennedy, *A Nation of Immigrants*, rev. and enlarged ed. (New York: Harper Perennial Library, 1986).

2 John Higham, *Strangers in the Land: Patterns of American Nativism, 1860–1925* (New York: Atheneum, 1963).

3 P. F. Hall, *Immigration and Its Effects on the United States* (New York: Henry Holt, 1908); Mary Antin, *They Who Knock at Our Gates: A Gospel of Immigration* (Boston: Houghton Mifflin, 1914); E. A. Ross, *The Old World in the New: The Significance of Past and Present Immigration to the American People* (New York: Century, 1914); Oscar Handlin, *The Uprooted: The Epic Story of the Great Migrations That Made the American People* (Boston: Atlantic Monthly, 1973); and J. Bodnar, *The Transplanted: A History of Immigrants in Urban America* (Bloomington: University of Indiana Press, 1985).

4 A. M. Kraut, *Silent Travelers: Germs, Genes and the Immigrant Menace* (New York: Basic Books, 1994); Elizabeth Yew, "Medical Inspection of Immigrants at Ellis Island, 1891–1924," *Bulletin of the New York Academy of Medicine* 56 (1980): 488–510; Rosebud T. Solis-Cohen, "The Exclusion of Aliens from the United States for Physical Defects," *Bulletin of the History of Medicine* 21 (1947): 33–50; A. E. Birn, "Six Seconds per Eyelid: The Medical Inspection of Immigrants at Ellis Island, 1892–1914," *Dynamis. Acta. Hosp. Med. Sci. Hist. Illus.* 17 (1997): 281–316; and Howard Markel, *Quarantine! East European Jewish Immigrants and the New York City Epidemics of 1892* (Baltimore: Johns Hopkins University Press, 1997).

5 Thomas L. Haskell, ed., *The Authority of Experts: Studies in History and Theory* (Bloomington: University of Indiana Press, 1984); Robert H. Wiebe, *The Search for Order, 1877–1920* (New York: Hill and Wang, 1967); Robert Kanigel, *The One Best Way: Frederick Winslow Taylor and the Enigma of Efficiency* (New York: Viking, 1997); and Richard H. Hofstadter, *The Age of Reform: From Bryan to F.D.R.* (New York: Alfred A. Knopf, 1956).

6 David Nasaw, *Children of the City: At Work and at Play* (New York: Oxford University Press, 1985); Deborah Dwork, "Health Conditions of Immigrant Jews on the Lower East Side of New York: 1880–1914," *Medical History* 24 (1981): 1–40; Maureen Ogle, *All the Modern Conveniences: American Household Plumbing, 1840–1890* (Baltimore: Johns Hopkins University Press, 1997).

7 Sanitary Aid Society of the Tenth Ward of the City of New York. *Annual Report for 1884–1885* (New York: Sanitation Aid Society, 1985).

8   Richard Meckel, *Save the Babies: American Public Health Reform and the Prevention of Infant Mortality, 1850–1929* (Baltimore: Johns Hopkins University Press, 1990); and S. H. Preston and M. R. Haines, *Fatal Years: Child Mortality in Late Nineteenth Century America* (Princeton: Princeton University Press, 1991).

9   Nurith Zmora, *Orphanages Reconsidered: Child Care Institutions in Progressive Era Baltimore* (Philadelphia: Temple University Press, 1994); Reena S. Friedman, *These Are Our Children: Jewish Orphanages in the United States, 1880–1925* (Hanover, NH: Brandeis University Press/University Press of New England, 1994).

10 Jacob A. Riis, *How the Other Half Lives: Studies among the Tenements of New York* (New York: Charles Scribner's Sons, 1890).

11 Jeremy P. Felt, *Hostages of Fortune: Child Labor Reform in New York State* (Syracuse, NY: Syracuse University Press, 1965), vii; and Harpo Marx and Rowland Barber, *Harpo Speaks!* (New York: Freeway, 1974), 36.

12 Richard Meckel, *Save the Babies*, 131; see also George Rosen, *Preventive Medicine in the United States, 1900–1975: Trends and Interpretations* (New York: Prodist/Science History Publications, 1975), 47; Elizabeth Ewen, *Immigrant Women in the Land of Dollars: Life and Culture on the Lower East Side, 1890–1925* (New York: Monthly Review, 1985); and Andrew R. Heinze, *Adapting to Abundance: Jewish Immigrants, Mass Consumption, and the Search for American Identity* (New York: Columbia University Press, 1990).

13 Isaac Metzker, ed., *A Bintel Brief: Sixty Years of Letters from the Lower East Side to the Daily Forward* (Garden City, NY: Doubleday, 1971), 87–89; and The interactions of health, Americanization, and the immigrants during the Progressive Era have been deftly discussed in Nancy Tomes, *The Gospel of Germs: Men, Women and the Microbe in American Life* (Cambridge, MA: Harvard University Press, 1998). For an elegant analysis of the teaching of personal hygiene, nutrition, and other health issues in American schools during the 1920s, see Naomi Rogers, "Vegetables on Parade: American Medicine and the Child Health Movement in the Jazz Age," in this volume.

14 John Duffy, "School Vaccination: The Precursor to School Medical Inspection," *Journal of the History of Medicine and Allied Sciences* 33 (1978): 344–55.

15 John Duffy, "School Buildings and the Health of American School Children in the Nineteenth Century," in *Healing and History: Essays for George Rosen*, ed. C. E. Rosenberg (New York: Science History Publications, 1979), 161–78.

16 Howard Markel and Frank A. Oski, *The H. L. Mencken Baby Book: Comprising the Contents of H. L. Mencken's What You Ought To Know about Your Baby with Commentaries* (Philadelphia: Hanley and Belfus, 1990).

17 J. T. Sullivan, T. J. Murphy, and M. J. Cronin, "Medical Inspection of the Schools from the Standpoint of the Medical Inspector," *Boston Medical and Surgical Journal* 160 (1909): 746–48; and W. P. Coues, "The Medical Inspection of Schools in Boston: The Present Limitations and Future Possibilities," *Boston Medical and Surgical Journal* 160 (1909): 746–48.

18 Luther H. Gulick and Leonard P. Ayers, *Medical Inspection of Schools* (New York: Russell Sage Foundation/Survey Associates, 1913), 15–16; Lewis M. Terman, *The Hygiene of the School Child* (Boston: Houghton Mifflin, 1914); and L. H. Gulick and L. P. Ayers, "Medical Examination of Schools and Scholars in the United States of America, in *Medical Examination of Schools and Scholars*, ed. T. N. Kelynack (London: P. S. King and Son, 1910), 341–58.

19 Josephine E. Young, "Hygiene of the School Age," in *Pediatrics*, ed. I. A. Abt, vol. 1 (Philadelphia: W. B. Saunders, 1923), 866–1131. Although much has been written by historians about medical inspection of the schools in the United States, lit-

tle has been done to analyze this movement in other parts of North America. Fortunately, this oversight has been corrected in a superb study by Mona Gleason, "Race, Class, and Health: School Medical Inspection and 'Healthy' Children in British Columbia, 1890 to 1930," in this volume; L. E. Holt, *Diseases of Infancy and Children*, 3rd ed. (New York: D. Appleton, 1907), 299–307.

20   Lillian Wald, *The House on Henry Street* (New York: Holt, Rinehart and Winston, 1915); and Wald, *Windows on Henry Street* (Boston: Little, Brown, 1934).

21   Jane Addams, *Twenty Years at Hull House, with Autobiographical Notes* (1910; repr., Chicago: University of Illinois Press, 1990).

22   Michael M. Davis, *Immigrant Health and the Community* (New York: Harper and Bros., 1921).

23   C. E. Rosenberg, "Social Class and Medical Care in 19th Century America: The Rise and Fall of the Dispensary," in *Sickness and Health in America*, ed. J. W. Leavitt and R. L. Numbers, 157–71 (Madison: University of Wisconsin Press, 1997); and Judith Walzer Leavitt, *Typhoid Mary: Captive to the Public's Health* (Boston: Beacon Press, 1996).

24   S. Josephine Baker, *Child Hygiene* (New York: Harper and Bros., 1925).

25   S. Josephine Baker, *Fighting for Life* (New York: Macmillan, 1939), 79–80.

26   Rosenberg, "Social Class," 157.

27   Helen Campbell, *Darkness and Daylight, or Lights and Shadows of New York Life* (Hartford, CT: Hartford, 1898), 318–34; and Rosenberg, "Social Class," 163–65.

28   Howard Markel and Henry Koplik, "The Good Samaritan Dispensary of New York City and the Description of Koplik's Spots," *Archives of Pediatrics and Adolescent Medicine* 150 (1996): 535–39; and George Rosen, "The First Neighborhood Health Center Movement: Its Rise and Fall," in *Sickness and Health in America*, ed. J. W. Leavitt and R. L. Numbers (Madison: University of Wisconsin Press, 1997), 185–99.

29   American Pediatric Society, *Semi-Centennial Volume of the American Pediatric Society, 1888–1938* (Menasha, WI: George Banta, 1938), 1–76.

30   Howard Pearson, with the assistance of A. K. Brown, *The Centennial History of the American Pediatric Society, 1888–1988* (New Haven: Yale University Printing Service, 1988), 2–12.

31   H. K. Faber and R. McIntosh, *History of the American Pediatric Society, 1887–1965* (New York: McGraw-Hill, 1965); see also George Rosen, *The Specialization of Medicine with Particular Reference to Ophthalmology* (New York: Arno, 1972); and Sydney A. Halpern, *American Pediatrics: The Social Dynamics of Professionalism* (Berkeley: University of California Press, 1988).

32   M. J. Wasserman, "Henry Coit and the Certified Milk Movement in the Development of Modern Pediatrics," *Bulletin of the History of Medicine* 46 (1972): 359–90.

33   Markel and Oski, *H. L. Mencken Baby Book*, 86.

34   Rima D. Apple, *Mothers and Medicine: A Social History of Infant Feeding* (Madison, WI: University of Wisconsin Press, 1987).

35   Meckel, *Save the Babies*, 78–79; Howard Markel, "Academic Pediatrics: The View from New York City a Century Ago," *Academic Medicine* 71 (1996): 36–41; and George Rosen, *A History of Public Health* (New York: MD Publications, 1958), 330–31.

36   Davis, *Immigrant Health*, 328–34; M. M. Davis and A. R. Warner, *Dispensaries: Their Management and Development* (New York: Macmillan, 1918); Public Health Committee of the New York Academy of Medicine, *Report on the Study of New York Dispensaries, 1919* (New York: Public Health Committee, 1919).

37 S. S. Goldwater, "Dispensaries: A Growing Factor in Curative and Preventive Medicine," *Boston Medical and Surgical Journal* 172 (1915): 613–17.

38 T. A. Ziv and Bernard Lo, "Denial of Care to Illegal Immigrants: Proposition 187 in California," *New England Journal of Medicine* 332 (1995): 1095–98; S. Asch, B. Leake, and L. Gelberg, "Does Fear of Immigration Authorities Deter Tuberculosis Patients from Seeking Care?" *Western Journal of Medicine* 161 (1994): 373–76; Selma Canto Berrol, *Growing Up American: Immigrant Children in America Then and Now* (New York: Twayne, 1995); E. Harney and D. J. Henandez, eds. *From Generation to Generation: The Health and Well-being of Children in Immigrant Families* (Washington, DC: National Academy Press / National Research Council / Institute of Medicine, 1998); A. Hulbert, *Raising America: Experts, Parents and a Century of Advice about Children* (New York: Alfred A. Knopf, 2003); and H. Markel, *When Germs Travel: Six Major Epidemics That Have Invaded America since 1900 and the Fears They Have Unleashed* (New York: Pantheon/Random House, 2004).

La médicalisation de la mère et de son enfant

L'exemple du Vietnam sous domination française, 1860–1939

ᚻ

Laurence Monnais

Introduction

L'histoire de la médicalisation de la mère et de son enfant est relativement bien connue pour l'Occident. Elle l'est beaucoup moins
pour ce qui est des contrées tropicales et des anciennes colonies
européennes, en particulier asiatiques, qui se sont affranchies au cours
du XXᵉ siècle[1]. Remédier en partie à cet oubli s'avère utile, ne serait-ce
que pour mieux souligner la mondialisation d'un processus et en marquer de nouvelles phases et de nouveaux aspects, parallèles ou décalés
dans le temps, à l'exemple de ce que proposent d'autres articles de cet
ouvrage et en particulier celui d'A.-E. Birn. Mais il s'agit surtout de
marquer, au travers d'un exemple à la fois expressif et original, celui
du Vietnam sous domination française, que l'histoire de la santé maternelle et celle de la santé infantile ne font qu'un; qu'elles s'inscrivent
dans le champ de la santé publique née avec la deuxième moitié du
XIXᵉ siècle et en révèlent ensemble des orientations majeures[2].

Cette étude viendra par ailleurs appuyer certaines convictions quant
à la signification profonde d'une *médicalisation coloniale*, aux moyens mis
en place pour en obtenir une efficacité maximale, au rôle précis joué par
la prise en charge de la mère et de son enfant dans cette dynamique générale. On évoquera alors aussi bien le personnel utilisé pour cette double gestion que l'évolution des structures mises à sa disposition ou encore
le pourquoi et le contenu des principales mesures préventives et cura-
tives prises à l'endroit de ces populations[3].

Finalement, alors que l'hégémonie de la gynéco-obstétrique et l'interventionnisme sanitaire dans le domaine de la surveillance maternelle et infantile n'ont pas partout la même histoire, ne sont pas partout
au même stade de maturation et ne suivent pas les mêmes modalités
d'application, la présente analyse veut apporter une pièce supplémen-
taire au puzzle éclairant l'imbrication du politique, du médical et du
social. Le cadre géographique vietnamien – pour contourner l'anachro-

nisme qui consiste pour l'époque à employer le terme de «Vietnam»[4] – est un territoire aux traditions et comportements socioculturels souvent éloignés de repères occidentaux. Mais, de par sa condition de «colonisé», il se trouve en effet dès les années 1860, en position de recevoir un programme de santé et de médicalisation aux objectifs précis. En outre, son entrée en dépendance coïncide avec un temps médical et scientifique idéal pour l'épanouissement de ce volet incontournable de la colonisation.

Colonisation du Vietnam et Organisation d'une Politique de Santé Locale : L'enfant Devient Logiquement un Bénéficiaire Prioritaire

En France, la conjoncture démographique alarmante des années 1860–70 encourage la promulgation des premières lois d'assistance à l'enfance (initiée en 1874 par la loi Roussel de protection à l'enfance du premier âge) qui s'insèrent dans un mouvement plus large de développement d'une couverture sociale[5]. C'est à cette même époque que les troupes métropolitaines achèvent de pacifier la Cochinchine et le Cambodge (1858–67). L'Annam, le Tonkin puis le Laos suivront (1873–97). A partir de 1887 néanmoins, le territoire formé par ces cinq pays constitue déjà une entité politique, administrative et dominée par un gouvernement colonial : l'Union indochinoise ou Indochine française.

Au lendemain d'un conflit particulièrement meurtrier (1914–18), la Troisième République conjugue sa préoccupation anti-malthusienne avec une prise de conscience du droit de l'enfant à bénéficier d'un cadre de vie sain, une sorte d'assurance-vie. On retrouvera le même genre d'attention en Indochine et surtout cette idée alors commune à tous les pays occidentaux qu'il faut par tous les moyens arrêter le «massacre des innocents». A la hantise, double, de la chute démographique et du risque de dégénérescence, amplifiée et justifiée par la Grande Guerre, se surajoutaient des objectifs impérialistes anciens. Mais la réalité ne ressemble pas toujours à la théorie, surtout en matière de politique de santé et quand cette politique fait l'objet d'une application outre-mer à des fins précises. Faisons justement un bref retour sur les principales directions en matière de santé proposées par la France à sa dépendance extrême-orientale pour évaluer ce hiatus initial.

Brève Histoire de la Colonisation en Indochine et de Son Volet Santé

Dès son installation définitive en Cochinchine, la France fait de la santé un des fers de lance de sa politique générale. Il faut dire que la foi dans la science et le «progrès» de ses dirigeants s'exprime pleinement dans ce domaine. L'avènement de médecins auprès des instances gouverne-mentales, *médecins-hygiénistes* au secours de la santé collective, est en voie d'être assuré. Réclamant, entre autres, le développement de la pué-riculture et une réglementation de la prostitution, cette investiture médi-cale et la politisation du champ de ce que l'on nomme désormais *santé publique* concordent. Les conditions sont réunies pour une utilisation du praticien outre-mer : insufflateur de la bonne santé nécessaire à l'ex-ploitation[6], ce dernier s'imposera également en superviseur de la crois-sance démographique des «races» indigènes[7].

Or, les premiers médecins, militaires, envoyés en mission en Indo-chine se trouvent rapidement démunis. Leur méconnaissance de la pathologie tropicale, l'étendue des ravages épidémiques et endémiques (variole, choléra, paludisme, maladies vénériennes, parasitismes intes-tinaux, dysenteries, béribéri) s'associent pour les empêcher de dépas-ser la mise en place d'un cordon sanitaire capable de protéger de la contamination humaine les «Blancs» et les colonnes en mission de paci-fication. Par le biais de campagnes de vaccination antivariolique de masse et la construction des premiers hôpitaux civils dès les années 1860, on commence pourtant à envisager un plan sanitaire à destina-tion directe des colonisés. Quelques mesures urbaines de santé publique (décrets de police sanitaire et d'assainissement, création de comités d'hygiène entre 1895 et 1899), la surveillance de populations «à risque» et en particulier des prostituées et des élèves des premières écoles franco-indigènes viennent confirmer qu'une véritable programmation sanitaire est imminente.

L'année 1897 marque à notre avis la véritable intronisation d'un système de santé à destination des Indochinois et en priorité des Viet-namiens. Dix ans après la création de l'Union indochinoise en effet, le Gouverneur général P. Doumer officialise une première «assistance médicale» civile : il nomme un directeur de la santé dans chacun des cinq pays et fait appliquer en Cochinchine la loi métropolitaine de 1892 sur l'obligation du doctorat en médecine pour exercer. Puis, c'est au tour du Gouverneur P. Beau de proposer des textes qui entérinent la mise en place d'une Assistance Médicale Indigène (AMI, 1905), vaste plan à la fois préventif et curatif. Il détermine deux ans plus tard des principes généraux *d'hygiène et de protection de la santé publique*». Les directives contenues dans ces documents resteront les piliers d'un plan de médi-calisation qui ne cessera alors de se développer, entre autres, autour de la mère et de l'enfant.

Au cœur de cette action sanitaire définitivement formulée au début du XXe siècle, le combat farouche mené contre la variole, considérée comme la principale cause de mortalité épidémique et surtout infantile, se poursuit. L'obligation pour tout enfant cochinchinois d'être vacciné était intervenue dès 1871[8]; elle sera étendue à l'ensemble de l'Union en 1908. Dans cette même optique d'immunisation à grande échelle et collective, les femmes vénériennes font l'objet d'une surveillance drastique en milieu urbain (entreprise à Saigon, capitale de la Cochinchine, dès les années 1860–70). Les premiers signes d'attention à l'individu, son éducation hygiénique et son bien-être sanitaire ont également paru, en milieu scolaire et hospitalier (1880–90). L'enfant s'avère au centre de ce processus de sensibilisation alors que les résultats des premières années de l'AMI, obtenus au moyen de statistiques hospitalières, nécessitent des réorientations majeures. Il faut dire que les médecins ont largement participé à dénoncer certaines inadéquations et carences.

Dès son arrivée en 1911, le Gouverneur général A. Sarraut propose en conséquence de nouvelles réformes avec l'aide de l'inspecteur des services de santé, A. Clarac. Un premier programme d'envergure sur plusieurs annuités et avec prévision de ressources financières adaptées est alors enfanté[9]. Ses orientations sont ambitieuses. Il prône l'exécution continue des mesures d'hygiène et de prophylaxie des maladies endémiques, épidémiques et transmissibles. Il insiste sur l'isolement des contagieux, la mobilité d'un personnel médical plus nombreux, la prophylaxie des maladies vénériennes, l'adduction d'eau potable et l'importance de conférences d'hygiène. Si l'hospitalisation et la consultation continuent de diriger l'assistance médicale proprement dite, d'autres méthodes sont proposées, comme l'organisation de l'assistance aux lépreux, aux aliénés, aux femmes enceintes mais aussi et surtout l'extension des bienfaits sanitaires coloniaux aux populations rurales et isolées.

L'entre-deux-guerres va poursuivre dans les directions proposées par Sarraut, en essayant bien sûr toujours de s'acclimater davantage aux contextes locaux, qu'ils soient d'ordre géographique, pathologique, socioculturel ou économique. En France, c'est avec le XXᵉ siècle que le champ de la santé publique s'était vu augmenté d'un secteur «d'hygiène sociale». En Indochine, c'est après la Première Guerre mondiale, que le qualificatif «social» fait son apparition dans les textes de l'Inspection générale des services de santé. Premier objectif, prioritaire : la lutte contre les «maladies sociales» justement, pulmonaires, oculaires, vénériennes et les cancers. En parallèle, un réseau essentiellement rural de dispensaires, d'infirmeries, de maternités, de lieux de consultation médicale, se densifie assez rapidement. En fait, c'est le discours tout entier en arrière plan de cette réorientation infrastructurelle qui s'est modifié. Il insiste désormais sur une plus grande présence physique du médecin, français et indochinois, qui doit impérativement «aller vers le malade».

Plusieurs enquêtes sanitaires et épidémiologiques permettent d'affiner le contenu de ces nouvelles directives dans les années 1920 et surtout 1930. En 1925, une section de démographie et de préservation sociale est officialisée auprès de l'Inspection générale de la santé; un programme d'Assistance Rurale est confirmé pour 1927. Enfin, un service indépendant d'Assistance sociale voit le jour en 1929. En 1937, le dernier programme sanitaire à destination de la péninsule indochinoise résumera ces nouvelles préoccupations et les premiers bénéfices qu'elles ont entraînés, évoquant même pour la première fois officiellement un recours organisé à la médecine traditionnelle[10].

En 1937, la mère et l'enfant sont assurément toujours en bonne position dans l'échelle des inquiétudes administratives. Ils le sont aussi dans les résultats positifs avancés. Il faut dire que leur médicalisation remonte relativement loin et qu'il s'était assez rapidement agi de réduire deux processus (de médicalisation) en un pour optimiser les chances de réussite du plan.

La Place des Activités Confessionnelles et Privées et les Pratiques Locales Entourant la Femme Enceinte, L'accouchement et le Nourrisson

Le peu d'informations dont on dispose sur les actions médicales concernant l'enfant vietnamien dans la deuxième moitié du XIXe siècle, en dehors des campagnes d'immunisation contre la «petite vérole», pourraient laisser croire que la lutte contre la mortalité infantile n'était alors pas favorisée. Pourtant, en métropole, plusieurs lois sur l'assistance à l'enfance avaient déjà révolutionné la conception de la naissance, on l'a dit, et sonné l'heure d'un embryon d'assistance sociale les concernant. On vient de le voir également, les médecins étaient à même et en position de tirer la sonnette d'alarme et de proposer des mesures concrètes pour non seulement arrêter une hémorragie dangereuse mais fortifier le potentiel humain qui leur était confié. Il doit donc y avoir une autre explication à ce silence, peut-être même deux. D'abord, l'administration coloniale se contentait alors de laisser cette question aux institutions religieuses et privées, installées avant la colonisation et dotées de prérogatives et d'une influence qu'il n'y avait pas lieu de remettre en cause. S'ajoutant à cela, la médecine militaire, en mission d'occupation dans les années 1860–90, n'eut longtemps pas pour mandat officiel de s'en préoccuper en priorité.

Les religieuses, et en particulier l'Oeuvre des Sœurs de la Providence de Portieux et celle de Saint Paul de Chartres, dominent incontestablement le champ de la protection infantile en Cochinchine et au Cambodge dans le dernier quart du XIXe siècle. A la fin des années 1870, elles avaient tissé un premier réseau d'assistance charitable, plusieurs de leurs orphelinats devenant bientôt le prolongement logique et nécessaire à quelques crèches où les nourrissons affluaient. Pour autant, il ne s'agissait pas pour elles de prendre en mains une assistance plus strictement maternelle, en dehors de quelques petites institutions hospitalières sans médecin ni équipement adéquat. Leur prise en charge des prostituées, limitée le plus souvent à un simple internement proche de l'incarcération pénale, est une preuve saillante tant de leur peu de moyens que de leurs connaissances médicales réduites[11].

L'administration coloniale commence dès 1905 à leur disputer cette activité médico-sociale, défendant sa laïcité avec vigueur et réclamant l'exclusivité pour son programme d'AMI et son personnel médical. Elle ne remettra cependant jamais clairement en cause leur rôle caritatif dans la protection de l'enfance : en 1935, 1 039 enfants sont encore accueillis à la crèche cambodgienne des Sœurs de la Providence de Culao Gien ouverte en 1878; au premier juillet, 997 autres sont élevés dans les six orphelinats de la Mission. Entre-temps l'initiative privée s'est par ailleurs étoffée, forte de la participation financière de notables indigènes, essentiellement dans les grands centres urbanisés. Ainsi, l'Association Maternelle de Cholon, dirigée par le médecin maire de la ville, le Dr Drouhet, devient-elle en 1901 l'emblème applaudi d'un partenariat efficace avec l'élite chinoise locale[12]. Mettant en marche un asile municipal pour enfants malades et abandonnés (1902), l'Association s'introduit surtout à la maternité de Cholon et supervise sous peu son bon fonctionnement, soulageant des services publics ayant fort à faire pour penser une intervention plus globale. On retrouvera ce genre d'initiative dans tous les protectorats de l'Indochine, en priorité au Cambodge et dans les principaux centres urbanisés.

Il n'est pas ici question de s'étendre davantage sur l'activisme social des collectivités religieuses et privées. Avant 1929, il se propage effectivement en marge du système sanitaire officiel, se contentant de combler les lacunes du plan républicain. Si les deux systèmes parallèles convergent parfois pour obtenir de meilleurs résultats, il faudra attendre les années 1930 pour voir s'affirmer une orientation commune structurée. En attendant, ce sont plusieurs médecins coloniaux qui, de leur propre chef, avaient entrepris une guerre féroce contre la mortalité infantile et certaines pratiques traditionnelles jugées hérétiques.

Il ne faut effectivement jamais oublier que l'accouchement est autant acte biologique que construction culturelle et sociale; qu'il révèle par ailleurs un ensemble de techniques, de rites et de croyances qui conditionnent largement et profondément la vie et la santé des futures mères et de leur progéniture. La grossesse, la femme enceinte, l'accouchement, le nourrisson sont autant de situations, d'actes et d'acteurs dirigés (pour ne pas dire normalisés), en terre vietnamienne comme ailleurs. Pour autant, il est très difficile d'introduire à leur encontre et pour le XIXe siècle le qualificatif de «médicalisés». Il a donc fallu que la France frappe doublement fort dans le domaine. Et il est clair que de nombreuses incompréhensions entre les deux systèmes de valeurs et leurs représentants allaient rendre difficile l'application de certaines décisions sanitaires. Mais, on empiète là sur des développements ultérieurs. Revenons pour l'instant sur quelques clés de compréhension d'un univers conceptuel complexe.

La fécondité et une natalité forte sont partie intégrante de la vie familiale et communautaire vietnamiennes parce qu'elles sont fragiles, mais en premier lieu parce qu'elles répondent à des principes primordiaux : le culte des ancêtres transmis au fils aîné; le fait que l'enfant est la première et la plus importante richesse d'une famille vietnamienne. Dans un autre domaine, la variété des règles entourant la grossesse et de comportements symboliques déterminent non seulement la place de la femme et de la mère dans cette société du Sud-est asiatique et confucéenne mais aussi préparent la naissance et la place de l'enfant à naître. Tout aussi cardinale, la protection ancestrale de l'enfance transite par l'affection de la mère, l'éducation et bien sûr par un ensemble de précautions ritualisées et magiques devant l'assurer d'une croissance sans heurt. Il est évident que ces dernières préoccupations marquent davantage une sollicitude culturelle traditionnelle qu'une efficacité dans les objectifs de défense préventifs et curatifs poursuivis.

Une multitude de convictions, règles, mais aussi beaucoup de mystère gravitent autour de la grossesse vietnamienne. Pour un médecin occidental de l'époque, la connaissance locale de l'anatomie s'avère particulièrement lacunaire. Par exemple, on reconnaît le rôle du sperme dans la fécondation mais on ignore la participation des ovaires, la mère offrant abri et substance à l'embryon conçu par le père dans le cadre de la théorie vietnamisée du *yin* et du *yang* chinois. En parallèle, la femme enceinte concentre sur elle toutes les superstitions collectives liées aux notions d'impureté (développée entre autres par la rétention de sang souillé liée à son état). Si le temps de gestation voit se rapprocher «impur» de «néfaste», il n'en demeure pas moins entouré d'interdits et de recommandations devant mener à un terme le plus heureux possible : enfant unique, en bonne santé, de sexe masculin bien sûr. Une kyrielle de conseils, d'attitudes corporelles, d'interdits de gestes ou de tâches à signification symbolique[13] et de précautions alimentaires complètent cette surveillance rapprochée.

L'épreuve de l'enfantement appelle quant à elle des gestes et un «savoir-faire» séculaire particulièrement éloignés des balises occidentales modernes. Ainsi peut-on citer l'isolement de la parturiente dans un lieu exigu et fermé en lien avec cette impureté funeste que son état stigmatise; le recours très fréquent à une matrone formée sur le tas qui se contente la plupart du temps d'assister l'opération et en fait surtout d'intercéder auprès des puissances sacrées. Pour résumer, l'accouchement est une affaire privée au Vietnam dans la deuxième moitié du XIXe siècle, presque cachée, et c'est l'affaire exclusive des femmes. Suivent un ensemble de coutumes concernant la délivrance (l'expulsion et l'usage du placenta, la coupure du cordon ombilical) qui, là aussi, contreviennent aux règles les plus élémentaires de l'hygiène moderne[14].

De même, la toilette du nourrisson est une attention plus métaphorique (à des fins de purification toujours) qu'hygiénique. Quant à sa nourriture, elle continue de lui être exclusivement transmise par sa mère. La pratique du «prémâchage du riz» surtout est chargée par la tradition vietnamienne de participer à véhiculer l'énergie nécessaire au nourrisson[15]. Enfin, l'accouchée doit également suivre certains préceptes tout au long d'une période de relevailles extrêmement réglementée : position particulière, alimentation strictement codifiée, réchauffement externe du corps avec un brasero pendant un mois.

C'est sans peine que l'on peut établir là une liste conséquente de risques d'infections susceptibles d'attaquer l'enfant et la mère. Et même l'existence avérée d'un champ vietnamien de pratique pédiatrique ne peut être considérée comme une protection réelle, mis à part peut-être au travers du contenu d'un arsenal thérapeutique relativement complexe. Néanmoins, ne nous méprenons pas sur ces comportements «dangereux». Premièrement, ils perdurent pour la plupart d'entre eux, sous une forme similaire ou différente, en Occident, en particulier en milieu rural. En second lieu, ils ne sont pas considérés comme imprudents par les populations locales et relèvent au contraire tous d'une volonté de protection et de soins optimaux à l'égard de l'enfant, de sa conception à son âge adulte. Paradoxalement, il s'agit donc là d'un indice qu'il pouvait y avoir une ouverture, une certaine bienveillance face aux propositions médicales de la France.

Vers une Prise en Charge Acclimatée des Enfants Vietnamiens

On a déjà démontré la constance de la priorité, quels qu'en soient les termes, donnée à la santé des enfants, de leur naissance à leur adolescence. Cette réalité ne fait pas que confirmer un contexte métropolitain particulièrement propice à ce favoritisme, mêlé à des ambitions coloniales limpides, économiques, politiques et humanitaires. Les agressions dont étaient victimes les jeunes Vietnamiens y furent aussi pour beaucoup. Il suffit à ce sujet de prendre quelques statistiques, d'évoquer le poids ancestral de la variole et du tétanos ombilical pour le comprendre.

Désignation d'un meurtrier: le tétanos ombilical

Les premiers médecins militaires, extrêmement choqués par la mauvaise santé indochinoise, l'avaient été en grande partie du fait de forts taux de morbidité et mortalité infantiles[16]. S'il subit, plus inhumainement à leur avis, les grands fléaux épidémiques qui touchent ses parents, l'enfant indigène est surtout la victime désarmée, dès les premiers jours de sa vie, du tétanos[17]. Remarquant en outre des signes très fréquents de variole, de «syphilis héréditaire», une alimentation défectueuse, certains se sentirent sans aucun doute investis d'une mission envers ces jeunes êtres et, par extension, d'une mission de surveillance rapprochée de l'accouchement et de la femme enceinte. Compulser la littérature médicale coloniale de la fin du XIXe siècle et des premières années du XXe siècle convainc de la véridicité de ce cheminement[18].

Les préoccupations du médecin français trouvent bientôt leur écho auprès de supérieurs ayant tiré quelques effrayantes conclusions des premières recensions de population et de statistiques hospitalières passées entre leurs mains, surtout du premier âge (0 à un an). Ensemble, ils décident de remédier au plus vite à une situation jugée affolante pour éloigner le spectre d'une dépopulation qui pourrait contrecarrer les plans de la République. Les premières enquêtes des médecins coloniaux le démontrent alors chiffres à l'appui, le tétanos ombilical joue un rôle de premier plan dans les hécatombes infantiles vietnamiennes. Elles montrent du doigt ces coutumes, largement répandues dans toute la péninsule, qui veulent que l'accouchement se fasse en dehors de toute présence masculine et médicale; que seule cette fameuse matrone (*Ba mu* en vietnamien), aguerrie aux techniques les plus courantes, assiste l'accouchée et s'occupe de sectionner le cordon. De l'avis, justifié, de leurs auteurs, c'est là que le mal fait son entrée, l'opération se réglant rapidement à l'aide d'un instrument qui n'a d'approprié que sa faculté à couper. Utilisant un simple tesson de bouteille ou ramassant à terre n'importe quel objet pourvu de cette propriété, la sage-femme sectionne sans précaution. Elle ne procède à aucune désinfection, n'appose jamais de pansement protecteur.

Le Dr M.L.R. Montel, médecin municipal à Saigon, est le premier à articuler un véritable programme de surveillance de la natalité et de prophylaxie du tétanos ombilical pour sa ville en 1904–05[19]. Jusqu'en 1902, les statistiques de la maternité de Cholon estimaient à 40 % les décès de nouveau-nés dus au tétanos; sa propre enquête sur Saigon était parvenue à des résultats analogues. Il n'y avait donc pas à tergiverser. Selon lui, il fallait rapidement trouver des moyens d'encourager les femmes à venir accoucher à la maternité et, à défaut d'y parvenir, d'entreprendre l'éducation des accoucheuses indigènes. Montel met par conséquent l'accent sur le rôle de la consultation municipale gratuite qu'il vient de fonder :

Dans le local de cette consultation gratuite une consultation spéciale vient d'être instituée pour les femmes enceintes et cela dans le but précis de lutter contre la mortalité infantile de la première année, due très souvent à la faiblesse congénitale, à l'hérédité morbide. Procréés par des parents débiles, impaludés, par des syphilitiques jamais traités, par des fumeurs d'opium, ces enfants viennent au monde petits, malingres, mal constitués (...) Donner de la quinine aux paludéennes, des toniques aux anémiées, du mercure aux syphilitiques, soigner les mères en un mot, n'était-ce pas augmenter pour l'enfant les chances de santé et de vie? Cette sorte de thérapeutique du fœtus in utero, de prophylaxie avant la lettre, a déjà fait ses preuves en Europe (...). En ce qui concerne les soins à donner aux nourrissons, la meilleure prophylaxie consiste à éduquer les futures mères.[20]

En employant les expressions de «prévention in utero», «éducation de la mère», en confirmant que soigner la famille équivaut à optimiser les chances de voir grandir un enfant en bonne santé, le médecin municipal entrevoyait précocement de construire une sorte d'environnement sain et salutaire pour le développement des générations futures. Ces générations de colonisés à venir deviendraient en outre des défenseurs idéaux de la médecine occidentale, convaincus de la nécessité de se plier aux exigences d'une santé publique et d'état[21].

La municipalité de Saigon s'engage donc sur la voie tracée par le Dr Montel, bientôt suivie par Hanoi, admirative des résultats obtenus et bien entendu victime de problèmes similaires[22]. Mais, en dehors de ces enclaves peuplées, on n'obtient aucune information à ce sujet, signe encore une fois – indépendamment du fait que les rapports sanitaires restent rarissimes avant la législation de 1905 – que la grande majorité des médecins s'attardaient sur d'autres problèmes de santé publique dans les années 1910. Par ailleurs, on sait que l'application des principes du fonctionnaire municipal s'arrêta le plus souvent à une surveillance des accouchements volontaires en milieu institutionnalisé. Enfin, il faut savoir que, pour beaucoup de médecins, les manifestations pathologiques de la mortalité infantile indochinoise ressemblaient à celles de la métropole, tétanos et paludisme en sus. Si cette assertion permet de justifier une attention exclusivement portée sur les premiers jours du nouveau-né, elle dénote un parti pris et une action qui risquait d'atteindre rapidement ses limites.

Dans une étude consacrée à la mortalité infantile, de la ville de Hanoi cette fois, en 1928, le Dr A. Le Roy Des Barres se dit justement peu convaincu des choix qui ont jusque là prévalu en matière de protection de l'enfant. S'appuyant sur les statistiques de l'état civil et surtout sur les renseignements du bureau d'hygiène et de démographie municipale qui vient d'ouvrir ses portes, il démontre que pour la période

1902–28, 50 % des décès ont été des décès d'enfants, que 35 % de ces enfants n'avaient pas atteint 13 ans, dont un quart pas même un mois[23]. Rapport éloquent mais qui ne pouvait avoir tenu compte de réorientations par trop récentes en matière de protection infantile. Quant à l'antitoxine tétanique destinée à protéger les nourrissons, elle n'était apparue dans les statistiques des sérums thérapeutiques envoyés par l'Institut Pasteur de Paris qu'en 1925.

Au-delà du tétanos ombilical : le tournant des années 1920

En Indochine, les années 1920 sont des années de recherche et de prospection qui tentent de rattraper le temps perdu. Désormais, l'observation de médecins plus à l'aise dans leur pratique tropicale précède souvent la mesure législative. En outre, cette dernière n'est plus une simple reproduction de textes métropolitains mais s'adapte aux réalités vietnamiennes[24]. Observations soutenues par un arsenal juridique renouvelé donc qui génèrent alors une pléthore de statistiques et d'enquêtes sur des groupes d'enfants ciblés avant de prendre des mesures plus adéquates.

En 1922, un rapport synthèse sur la «mortinatalité et la mortalité infantile dans les colonies françaises» marque autant cette adaptation que la teneur des préoccupations coloniales de lendemain de guerre. Les Drs Nogué et Adam, responsables du projet, y tirent leurs conclusions des réponses à un questionnaire envoyé aux directeurs locaux de la santé du Tonkin et du Cambodge et au médecin chef de la maternité de Hué (Annam). Le questionnaire, précis, concerne la fécondité, la stérilité et l'état général de «l'oeuvre française». Les réponses obtenues montrent que les efforts portent déjà sur la lutte antivénérienne, les vaccinations, la multiplication des maternités; on parle même déjà de «la condition sociale de la femme, les travaux pénibles qui lui sont imposés» (provoquant apparemment nombre d'avortements). Les superviseurs jugent néanmoins que beaucoup de problèmes restent entiers[25].

Les premiers symptômes d'adaptation aux besoins des populations vietnamiennes apparaissent naturellement dans les villes, dans la continuité des expériences du Dr Montel. En quelques années toutefois, on repère à l'échelle de l'Union tout entière une réorganisation de la lutte contre les maladies qui affaiblissent les parents (paludisme et affections vénériennes principalement). Le développement d'un plan de vaccination rationalisé (antivariolique, désormais obligatoire à trois reprises au cours de l'enfance et de l'adolescence, mais aussi antituberculeuse dans les écoles cholonaises à partir de 1924[26]) est complété par un programme d'éducation. Pour essayer de régler certains problèmes comme l'avortement ou inculquer des notions d'hygiène de la grossesse, la maternité jouera un rôle d'éducateur. Quant aux enfants, cette mission revient à un autre centre de protection ad hoc : l'école. Le développement de l'hygiène sociale coïncide pour sa part avec la multiplication de centres de puériculture – crèches, pouponnières cherchant à contrôler l'hygiène de la femme qui allaite puis nourrit, autant que celle du nouveau-né[27].

L'évolution de l'obstétrique, l'évolution en matière de nutrition, celle de la lutte contre les maladies infectieuses et l'amélioration des structures hospitalières participent conjointement à ériger l'enfant en bénéficiaire prioritaire. Ce dernier reçoit des soins adaptés à sa condition dans des hôpitaux pour enfants, des maternités dotées de consultations externes et spécialisées. Alors qu'avec le XXe siècle les politiques familiales et natalistes s'épanouissent, l'activité «sur le terrain» se déploie autour de visites à domicile et de Gouttes de lait. La fonction de médecin inspecteur (précisée en 1915) dans les établissements scolaires et l'éducation des femmes s'imposent en valeurs sûres de la politique de santé. Enfin, la collaboration entre institutions religieuses, privées et publiques de protection de l'enfance relève désormais d'un enjeu capital qui ne peut plus se permettre d'être altéré par des conflits de principe ou d'intérêts[28].

En novembre 1934, une circulaire du Ministère des Colonies se contente finalement de condenser dans un texte officiel ce que les médecins en poste en pays vietnamien, relayés par l'Inspection des services sanitaires et le Gouvernement général, ont entrepris depuis plusieurs années déjà. La même année d'ailleurs, le Congrès de l'Enfance organisé à Saigon entérine de nouvelles convictions quant à l'importance de l'état psychologique de l'enfant, de sa scolarisation ou encore de ses droits juridiques[29].

D'une lutte contre le tétanos ombilical qui donnait lieu à une éducation post-partum sommaire et d'un encouragement à l'accouchement au sein des premières maternités de l'AMI à un programme complet de défense du bien-être de l'enfant et de l'adolescent, la progression de la double médicalisation était nette bien que quelque peu déséquilibrée. Et les activités des maternités et des sages-femmes y étaient incontestablement pour beaucoup.

Deux Outils de Médicalisation Indispensables

Pour revenir à l'exemplarité de l'expérience du Dr Montel, on voit se développer avec lui diverses méthodes d'encouragement à l'accouchement en maternité mais, surtout, pour obtenir des résultats plus immédiats, un système d'enseignement à destination des sages-femmes locales. Maternité et sage-femme, voici en effet les maîtres mots d'une politique bicéphale, renvoyant à des outils de propagande et de propagation incontournables.

Maternités urbaines, maternités rurales

Après un demi siècle environ d'un dynamique mouvement de construction hospitalière (1860–1905), l'Union indochinoise est divisée en circonscriptions médicales pourvues d'une organisation théoriquement identique: au chef-lieu une formation principale dirigée par un médecin chef, formation à laquelle est annexée une maternité provinciale tenue par une sage-femme et sous le contrôle de ce praticien superviseur. Dans l'intérieur même de ce périmètre sanitaire se sont installés au fil des années des infirmeries, d'autres maternités, des dispensaires – maternités et des dispensaires ruraux. Le paysage infrastructurel de chaque capitale provinciale domine cette distribution verticale. Hôpitaux et structures spécialisées de l'AMI, établissements privés y prolifèrent côte à côte. Hors de ces centres, le tissu hospitalier reste d'importance variable, résultat d'une attention plus ou moins soutenue des autorités coloniales et des possibilités locales[30].

Cet organigramme apparaît bien rodé. En 1931, l'Inspecteur général des services de santé le Dr L. Gaide apporte pourtant lui-même un bémol, ajoutant qu'il est encore loin d'être étendu à l'ensemble du territoire et que toutes les formations sanitaires ne suivent pas ce découpage. On peut avancer une explication: la politique de construction a été orchestrée par vagues successives, selon les régions, selon les moyens à disposition. Dans ce contexte, le fossé entre l'hôpital citadin, moderne, offrant des services diversifiés et spécialisés, et le poste médical provincial se comprend aisément. Pour autant ne serait-il pas honnête d'affirmer que la politique sanitaire en milieu urbain reçut toutes les attentions. La question, beaucoup plus complexe, fait entrer en jeu une multitude de paramètres.

La courbe de croissance globale du nombre d'établissements de santé rend incontestablement compte aussi de plusieurs innovations dont la dispersion «dans les campagnes» de petites structures théoriquement faciles à construire, à entretenir et à gérer. Ce qui frappe d'ailleurs dans la physionomie hospitalière de 1930, c'est le nombre d'infirmeries rurales, établissements qui ont connu depuis cinq ans environ une formidable croissance (432 sur 594 établissements hospitaliers de tous ordres à la charge de l'AMI). On tente en fait d'installer davantage de relais ruraux, surtout des maternités et des dispensaires, qui seront desservis, soit par des médecins, soit par des sages-femmes ou encore par des infirmiers indochinois. Cette impulsion répond évidemment à plusieurs textes du Gouvernement général, mais aussi à des initiatives plus régionalisées, en provenance des Résidents supérieurs et des directeurs locaux de la santé conjuguant parfois leurs compétences avec talent[31].

Dans les villes comme dans les campagnes, la maternité sert la politique infantile, ce à plusieurs titres. Lieu d'accouchement, elle devient aussi celui de consultations prénatales, de stérilité, postnatales et, par là même, d'éducation des mères[32]. En milieu rural et dans les régions les plus isolées, seul centre de soins à des kilomètres à la ronde, elle est même souvent l'unique manifestation concrète des «bienfaits» de l'AMI, seul contact entre populations indigènes et médecine occidentale[33]. La plus grande question reste cependant de savoir si les femmes s'y rendaient réellement et dans quelle proportion. On aura l'occasion de revenir sur les mythes et réalités entourant ce point nébuleux.

La décision de 1908 d'autoriser l'ouverture de «maternités libres» aurait davantage répondu à un besoin (entre autre financier) qu'à une volonté confiante de la part des autorités coloniales et sanitaires. Elle permet néanmoins et rapidement de voir s'installer plusieurs sages-femmes dans l'agglomération saigonnaise capables de concurrencer leurs consœurs acquises à des méthodes plus traditionnelles. En 1925, il existe déjà huit maternités libres dans la seule capitale méridionale, dont sept sont dirigées par des diplômées d'une école professionnelle et une seulement par une *Ba mu*. C'est sans compter sur dix autres diplômées pratiquent à leur compte des accouchements à domicile. Ce pari hasardeux constituait la première phase, urbaine, d'une politique de récupération du champ d'activité des accoucheuses.

Le système diffère au-delà des zones urbanisées. Les maternités commencent certes à être dispersées dans l'ensemble de l'Union, mais les sages-femmes ne sont pas en assez grand nombre pour faire fonctionner les plus isolées. De plus, lorsqu'elles doivent s'occuper seules de quelques dizaines de lits au chef-lieu d'une province, il leur est matériellement impossible de se déplacer au domicile des femmes enceintes et des parturientes. On en est conscient au siège de chaque direction locale de la santé: les statistiques, encourageantes, d'accouchements et de consultations pré- et postnatales ne donnent aucune information sur les femmes – on les sait néanmoins nombreuses – qui font appel à l'accoucheuse de leur village, une femme disponible, une femme en laquelle elles ont confiance ou tout au moins dont la réputation a encouragé leur entourage à requérir sa présence.

En conclusion de sa thèse de médecine soutenue en 1934, le Dr Marie-Laure Blot, consciente de l'importance de cet auxiliaire féminin, n'a qu'un vœu, révélateur, à former : que soit développée cette «corporation» féminine pour «apprivoiser» la femme indochinoise[34]. Or, pour forcer les résistances ou transformer des habitudes, il faut pouvoir compter sur un personnel abondant et mobile; pour que la maternité fonctionne, il faut des sages-femmes acquises aux valeurs de la médecine – science.

La sage-femme vietnamienne en contexte d'indigénisation du personnel médical

Dès 1902, Montel avait aussi demandé aux autorités municipales de lui offrir leur appui en signifiant aux sages-femmes installées dans la ville l'obligation d'appliquer le fameux pansement cicatrisant. Il proposait aussi que, chaque fois que l'une d'entre elles viendrait annoncer une naissance au préposé administratif, ce dernier se rende sur place, regarde le pansement et fasse son rapport au médecin responsable qui se déplacerait ensuite auprès du nouveau-né, treize jours après la délivrance. En cas de plaie fermée, la sage-femme recevrait une prime d'encouragement. Montel obtenait gain de cause en 1904[35].

Une fois de plus, cette expérience se retrouve au cœur d'un processus en marche plus large, à savoir la formation d'un personnel indigène, médical et surtout subalterne[36]. Dans le contexte indochinois, il semble en tous cas particulièrement indispensable de remplacer «l'accoucheuse empirique» par une sage-femme éduquée ou, à défaut, éduquer la première pour optimiser les chances d'introduction de la médecine moderne dans le don de vie. Aux côtés de Montel, ou dans d'autres centres urbanisés, les Drs Drouhet (à Cholon), Déjean de la Bâtie (à Saigon) et Angier (à Phnom Penh) font les premiers pas dans cette direction. C'est d'ailleurs à ces médecins que l'on allait demander conseil à l'heure de la création d'écoles professionnelles locales[37].

L'Ecole de médecine de Hanoi, lieu de formation des médecins auxiliaires indochinois à partir de 1902, s'érige en école professionnelle, centre d'apprentissage à l'occidentale du métier de sage-femme dès 1904. Des cours similaires sont alors déjà offerts depuis quelques mois à Cholon dans l'enceinte de sa maternité modèle. En clair, alors que le recrutement européen en la matière s'avérait de plus en plus ardu (en temps de séparation de l'Eglise et de l'Etat et surtout rapporté aux besoins croissants d'une politique de santé s'étendant au monde rural), l'appel aux vocations indigènes devait se systématiser rapidement. Pour les autorités coloniales, cette *indigénisation* ne pouvait de toute façon pas être aussi lourde de conséquences politiques que la formation d'une élite de médecins. Elles s'engagèrent donc sur cette voie en relative quiétude.

Prenons l'exemple de l'école de Choquan pour mieux comprendre en quoi consistait cette formation institutionnalisée. En avril 1903, le Gouverneur de la Cochinchine Rodier décide de constituer une commission en vue d'organiser une *Ecole pratique de médecine indigène*, destinée aux Cochinchinois pour la santé de la Cochinchine. Il se sait soutenu par les populaires initiatives de certains de ses fonctionnaires médicaux[38]. La commission, réunie en mai, se penche sur la délicate question de la section des sages-femmes que l'on veut localiser à Cholon, près de la principale maternité de la ville chinoise. Il faut en effet essayer de prendre en considération certains principes directeurs: il s'agit de les former à la pratique et non à une théorie inutile; elles devront être mobiles et leur exercice fera l'objet d'une surveillance serrée et régulière. Enfin, l'interventionnisme qui vaut pour l'infirmier ne vaut pas forcément pour cette accoucheuse: «Il ne faut pas chercher à faire des sages-femmes mais des assistantes, des infirmières. L'indigène accouche très facilement, ce qu'il faut surtout, c'est inculquer à la *Ba Mu* indigène, cette idée que le mieux est de ne pas intervenir, de laisser la nature agir»[39].

Persuader la *Ba mu* de son incapacité et de la nécessité d'appeler le médecin français en cas de complication, voilà les directions à suivre. Lui enseigner l'hygiène sera la deuxième grande règle à observer. On précise qu'il existe des sages-femmes en pays vietnamien faisant partie intégrante de l'univers médical traditionnel local et qu'il faut tenter dans ce cas non pas de les combattre – on n'est pas certain de vaincre et le prix d'une victoire serait de toute façon trop élevé – mais de les rééduquer. En effet, à cet obstacle que peut constituer la forte présence d'accoucheuses traditionnelles s'ajoute le fait que cette profession féminine semble paradoxalement jouir de peu de crédit auprès des populations. La tâche de Choquan était donc double, surtout que l'on voulait doter chaque chef-lieu de province et chaque village important d'au moins une *Ba mu*.

L'Ecole de médecine pratique ouvre ses portes au lendemain de l'adoption unanime de ces préceptes en janvier 1904. En raison des obstacles évoqués précédemment, aucune condition d'âge ni d'instruction n'est requise[40]. Les premières années de recrutement sont malgré tout difficiles : 14 élèves seulement forment la première promotion. En 1908, l'école tente de profiter de la disgrâce dans laquelle se trouve sa rivale tonkinoise pour renforcer son statut[41]. Les résultats ne s'améliorent pas pour autant, au contraire. En 1916, la section cholonaise se retrouve véritablement sur la sellette[42]. Selon une commission de réorganisation de l'école formée cette année-là, il faut surtout et au moins «relever aux yeux des indigènes la profession de sage-femme»[43]. Ainsi doit-on être plus exigeant sur les modalités de recrutement, imposer un examen à la fin de chaque année. Vœu pieu que les effectifs des années suivantes accusent: en 1918 toujours, 4 sages-femmes seulement sont reçues, une promotion qui ne pouvait assurément pas faire face à la demande provinciale ni détrôner des concurrentes bien installées.

En dehors des périmètres de Saigon et de Hanoi, où les problèmes de recrutement – formation – emploi sont globalement identiques, d'autres méthodes sont à la même époque employées pour essayer d'utiliser au moins, et au mieux, les vocations locales avérées. A l'échelle de certaines provinces, on décidait en conséquence de se focaliser sur la *réédu-*

cation des *Ba mu* pour servir au mieux les objectifs de pénétration en milieu rural sans trop grever les budgets coloniaux. Formule dont on attendait un (double) franc succès et qui recevait bien évidemment l'aval des médecins comme des autorités. Dès 1907, la Direction locale de la santé du Tonkin avait d'ailleurs donné l'avantage à ce personnel féminin «rééduqué» sur le cadre infirmier en le dotant de trousses de chirurgie, indice de confiance en ses capacités et moyen simple de lui faire prodiguer des soins au-delà du cadre strict d'assistance médicalisée à l'accouchement[44].

Avec les réorientations de la politique sanitaire dans les années 1910–20, les deux pôles urbains de formation ne suffisent de toute façon plus du tout à la demande et aux compétences réclamées qui doivent désormais dépasser le «pansement du cordon» et une surveillance passive de l'accouchement. Hanoi et Cholon se contentent en réalité de proposer pour les hôpitaux principaux des chefs-lieux de province une frange aristocratique, diplômée et en grande majorité d'origine vietnamienne. De plus, la sage-femme de Hanoi et de Cholon, détentrice d'un diplôme reconnu, coûte cher et s'octroie parfois des privilèges qui ne cadrent pas avec la volonté de l'heure «d'aller vers le patient» et de l'assister dans ses besoins les plus courants. Plusieurs rapports dénoncent certaines attitudes condescendantes et des aspirations mercantiles[45]. L'équation «sage-femme + diplôme = succès rural» était complètement fausse dans un cadre comme celui de l'Indochine.

Au lendemain de la Première Guerre mondiale, la stratégie de l'Inspection des services sanitaires est la suivante: à l'échelle de chaque province, une (ou plusieurs) diplômées de Hanoi ou Cholon aura pour mission de former, à la maternité, quelques consœurs adeptes de pratiques jugées surannées. Cette préparation contrecarrera les habitudes hygiéniques de ces dernières. Guidées par «cette amie» avertie, ces matrons seront par la suite habilitées à s'occuper des accouchements à domicile, devenant de véritables sages-femmes mobiles[46]. Recrutées dans les villages, il n'y aura plus à s'interroger sur le degré de confiance des femmes à leur intention. Formées pour se déplacer, il ne sera plus non plus question de rivaliser de persuasion pour obliger la future mère à accoucher à la maternité. A la même époque, une poignée de sages-femmes décide de prendre en mains quelques lits dans des petites maternités rurales complètement isolées. Certaines autres, c'est le cas en Cochinchine, se conforment à la demande locale en servant comme accoucheuses à l'hôpital du chef-lieu en même temps que comme infirmières dans les postes moins bien équipés. Devant ce genre d'initiatives aussi, le gouvernement colonial acquiesce.

En second lieu, les autorités coloniales prennent acte de l'erreur majeure et toute occidentale qui consistait à employer des femmes viet-

namiennes au Cambodge, au Laos et auprès des minorités ethniques[47].
Elles ont eu le temps de remarquer que beaucoup de futures mères de
ces pays et de ces ethnies préféraient la sage-femme française à son
alter ego vietnamien, aspiration que les maigres effectifs français, surtout féminins, ne pouvaient satisfaire. La grande innovation se trouve toutefois ailleurs, même si elle inclut cette correction. La création d'un
cadre de *Ba mu* au Tonkin en 1927 fait en fait figure de décision tant
audacieuse que vitale. Progressivement, chaque province se dote d'un service personnalisé faisant appel aux bonnes volontés locales, surtout
financières, pour l'organiser. Dans la province de Hai Duong, par exemple, un rapport sanitaire du médecin chef rapporte que les populations
villageoises ont offert 4 000 piastres[48] pour concourir aux dépenses
occasionnées par la mise en place de ce cadre, répondant ainsi aux
espoirs du Résident R. Robin. Exclusivité du pays tonkinois dans ces
termes, le principe se propage néanmoins hors des frontières du protectorat pour tout au moins essayer de suppléer à une disette en personnel de plus en plus préoccupante[49]. Ainsi en Annam, à partir de 1935,
les accoucheuses vietnamiennes doivent accomplir à tour de rôle un
stage de deux à trois mois à l'hôpital provincial. Si ce roulement permet
à l'hôpital d'avoir un personnel auxiliaire à moindres frais, cela donne
aussi à ces dernières l'occasion de se refamiliariser régulièrement avec
les pratiques occidentales[50].

Formelles ou informelles, toutes les bonnes idées reçoivent l'assen-
timent de Hanoi. Quelle que soit la proportion d'accoucheuses qui vou-
dra bien se recycler, les sages-femmes diplômées continueront de contrer les activités des plus irréductibles d'entre elles avant de pouvoir
toutes les remplacer. A la fin des années 1930, et bien que certaines
régions soient encore à la traîne (un service de *Ba mu* fonctionne au
Cambodge à partir de 1936 alors qu'au Laos il n'existe encore que sur
le papier), la grande majorité des sages-femmes en activité sert en tant
qu'accoucheuse rurale.

A cette époque, les effectifs de *Ba mu* ont déjà largement dépassé
ceux des sages-femmes diplômées, malgré la jeunesse de leur cadre
(graphique 1). Par ailleurs, non seulement les effectifs confondus des différents profils de sages-femmes (privées, fonctionnaires, indochinoises
et *Ba mu*) ont augmenté de près de 50% entre 1930 et 1939 mais ils ont
permis, en outre, de mieux quadriller de structures sanitaires (184 maternités en 1936) le Vietnam rural et surtout de faire augmenter de façon
extraordinaire le nombre d'accouchements assistés par un professionnel
de santé. Pour ce qui est de ceux assistés en milieu hospitalier (tableau 1),
on sait ainsi qu'ils représentaient en 1936 près de 25 % des entrées dans
les hôpitaux vietnamiens (le total des entrées y est estimé à 309 000
pour l'année).

Graphique 1. Composition du milieu des auxiliaires médicaux indigènes en 1930 et 1939[51]

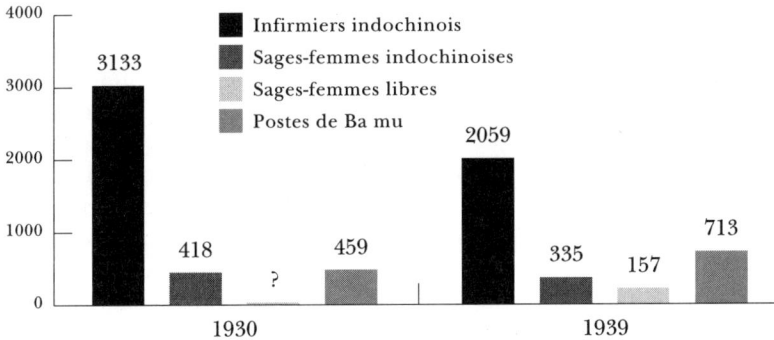

Tableau 1. Sages-femmes et *Ba mu*: Le poids de leur mission de protection des enfants vietnamiens (1936)[52]

	Tonkin	Annam	Cochinchine	Total
Sages-femmes diplômées	62	35	199	296
Ba mu	726	102	—	828
Maternités isolées	18	15	36	69
Maternités rurales	115	—	—	115
Accouchements en milieu hospitalier	19 528	11 328	44 179	75 035
Accouchements/ par des accoucheuses	86 633	2 104	—	88 737

On aimerait achever cette étude du personnel médical féminin au service de la protection maternelle et infantile en évoquant la place des femmes médecins. Malheureusement, les données à cet égard manquent cruellement, illustrant dans une certaine mesure la mise à l'écart systématique ou presque dont elles étaient l'objet. Citons néanmoins les noms de M.-L. Blot, dont on a déjà parlé; du Dr J. Eliche, auteur d'une thèse datant de 1924 sur le paludisme du nourrisson, médecin-chef de la maternité de Cholon et professeur à son école de sages-femmes dans les années 1930; du Dr Fabre, employée comme médecin contractuel à l'AMI, spécialisée en puériculture et épidémiologie (à l'hôpital de Cholon en 1920–23); et du Dr Larochas, auteur d'une étude sur le sevrage en 1935[53]. Parmi les diplômées vietnamiennes, on retiendra pour la même époque – il est en effet intéressant de remarquer que françaises ou vietnamiennes les femmes médecins font leur entrée simul-

tanément dans le système de santé local – , les noms d'Henriette Bui
Quang Chiêu, médecin sous les ordres du Dr Eliche avant de prendre
sa place, ou encore celui de Le Thi Hoang, directrice du service de santé
de la province annamite de Bana à partir de 1938[54].

L'étude du personnel médical subalterne et féminin a mis en lumière,
dans nos travaux antérieurs, le rôle primordial de la sage-femme indigène, de la *Ba mu* rééduquée à la jeune femme instruite à l'hôpital du
chef-lieu ou encore dans les écoles de Hanoi et Cholon. Par ce biais, il
nous a été donné d'observer la naissance d'une profession, bientôt pilier
de la médicalisation rurale dans les années 1920–30 travaillant auprès
de catégories des populations à convertir d'urgence. La sage-femme
indochinoise, quelle que soit son origine, sa formation et sa fonction,
obtenait en fait un rôle *social* autant que médical. Et, à l'inverse de ce qui
se passe dans le monde occidental à l'époque, elle semblait prendre une
place primordiale, peut-être même la plus importante, dans la gestion
de la parturition et de la parturiente, que ce soit en milieu rural ou
urbanisé. Mais que doit-on pour autant penser et dire de l'efficacité de
leur embauche et de leurs actes? Quels sont finalement les résultats,
pour ceux qui sont repérables, de ces efforts de médicalisation? Et qu'en
était-il de la santé des mères et plus largement des femmes vietnamiennes à l'heure des bilans?

Les Adaptations de la Politique Sanitaire Française en Pays Vietnamien : La Femme et L'enfant Sont-Ils de Bons Révélateurs?

Ce dernièr developpement n'a pas pour objectif de proposer des résultats chiffrés précis. L'impossibilité de comparer et de valider des données
statistiques coloniales et lacunaires nous en empêche. Pour autant, nous
estimons que quelques pistes méritent d'être suivies et plusieurs enquêtes sanitaires et démographiques examinées à la lumière de la politique
qui vient d'être évoquée. Ainsi, plusieurs études statistiques s'accordent
a posteriori pour dire que la fécondité des femmes indochinoises, très
élevée, est longtemps restée «compensée» par une mortalité infantile
importante (en moyenne proche de 50 %). Le statisticien H. Brénier
affirme en 1914 qu'il n'est possible de compter qu'une moyenne de 3
enfants par famille pour aboutir à des résultats proches de la réalité[55].
En 1932, 42 % des décès totaux seraient encore des décès de jeunes
Indochinois, dont 58 % de moins de 5 ans et 62 % de moins de 15 ans.
Cette constance veut-elle pour autant dire que l'action menée contre la
mortalité infantile avait obtenu des résultats négligeables?

Une Nouvelle Génération D'enquêtes Sur La Mortalité Infantile : Quelques Repères Sur Une Chute Controversée

Alors que les deux premières décennies du XXe siècle ont vu se multiplier des études en rapport direct avec les principales préoccupations sanitaires de l'époque – lutte contre la mortalité infantile en première ligne – , les années 1930 font intervenir un médecin plus indépendant, aux ambitions élargies. Il cherche de plus en plus à évaser l'horizon de ses investigations pour tenter de parer à la méconnaissance des comportements démographiques indochinois[56]. Peut-être s'efforce-t-il, par la même occasion, de mieux comprendre son patient. Quoiqu'il en soit, c'est en dehors des villes et des chefs-lieux qu'il veut porter son regard et trouver des solutions pour épargner les populations rurales[57]. Avant d'avancer quelques hypothèses quant à l'évolution du taux de mortalité infantile[58], donnons quelques repères sur le contenu des enquêtes parmi les plus remarquées dans les années 1930.

Les interventions des Drs Chesneau et Darbes au Congrès international de la population en 1937 montrent, parmi les premières, une utilisation renouvelée de l'enquête de terrain : une enquête correctrice, à des fins sanitaires et sociales élargies. Chesneau avait déjà pu déterminer un taux de natalité mais aussi de fécondité, de stérilité et même d'avortements pour l'Annam en suivant ce schéma[59]. Il avait, de surcroît, établi un taux moyen de mortalité infantile ainsi qu'un âge moyen des décès d'enfants et leurs principales causes (et donc l'impact des différents moyens de lutte mis en œuvre depuis plusieurs années). Les chiffres que le médecin avance dans ses publications de l'époque sont signes d'une extrême rigueur et d'une grande acuité. Selon lui, la fécondité dans le Nord Annam des années 1930 était de 577 enfants pour 1 000 femmes, de 568 pour 1 000 dans le sud du pays. La stérilité atteignait entre 2,2 et 3 % des Annamites. Quant à la mortalité infantile, elle frappait environ 42 % des enfants, en Annam comme au Tonkin. A partir de comparaisons entre pays, il déclarait avec aplomb que la natalité était assurément plus élevée dans les régions à forte densité de population[60].

Le Dr Chesneau propose des taux de mortalité encore alarmants pour l'ensemble de l'Union indochinoise au milieu des années 1930. Il semble, en outre, croire à une mortalité plus élevée en Cochinchine et au Tonkin qu'en Annam ou au Laos, avec 424 enfants morts pour 1 000 vivants dans les deux pays les plus densément peuplés et les plus urbanisés, 422 pour l'Annam et 375 seulement pour le Laos. Sa moyenne des décès d'enfants représenterait environ 25 % de la totalité des décès déclarés[61]. Quant aux déclarations officielles de la ville de Hanoi, considérées comme relativement fiables, elles donnent 1 710 décès de moins d'un an pour 3 978 au total, soit effectivement un taux de 430 pour 1 000, taux qui atteindrait les 458 pour 1 000 en 1930 (1 900 sur 4 150).

Echelle différentielle à propos de laquelle s'inscrit en faux, par exemple, une modeste enquête d'observation des comportements démographiques de 24 familles lao entreprise par le médecin de la province de Xieng Hou en 1924. Cette enquête aboutissait en effet aux conclusions suivantes: ces familles ont en moyenne cinq enfants, la mortalité touche deux tiers des naissances; la mortalité maximale se situe entre l'âge de 1 et 10 ans et, enfin, les enfants forment encore deux tiers de la mortalité totale[62]. Fait régionalisé? La mortalité infantile restait-elle finalement plus élevée en région densément peuplée ou urbaine qu'en milieu rural où les mesures sanitaires auraient mieux réussi à maîtriser l'impact morbide (une morbidité rurale peut-être même plus inoffensive)? Quelques chiffres précis concernant la mortalité des enfants de moins d'un an au Tonkin apportent d'autres éléments de réponse, sans pour autant pouvoir encore prétendre répondre franchement aux interrogations du Dr Chesneau.

Graphique 2. Evolution de la mortalité des enfants tonkinois de moins de un an rapportée à la mortalité totale du protectorat dans les années 1930[63]

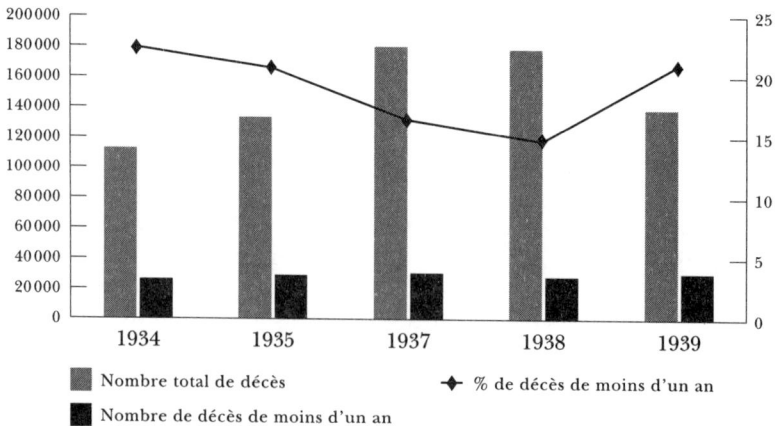

Assurément, la mortalité infantile continuait de peser lourd dans la balance démographique du Tonkin, en particulier entre la naissance et la première année de vie. Et si donc on tient pour acquis qu'elle était encore un facteur particulièrement aggravant dans l'histoire coloniale de la mortalité indochinoise, il est en conséquence normal de croire que la chute de la mortalité générale a pu, de ce fait, être ralentie.

En 1943, une enquête du Dr Jouin portant sur les populations minoritaires de la province annamite du Darlac décimées par le paludisme, révèle que la mortalité infantile y atteint entre 60 et 70 % des enfants de 0 à 1 an et entre 10 à 15 % de ceux âgés de 1 à 5 ans (ce qui signifierait un total de 700 à 850 décès pour 1 000 naissances). Cette enquête met aussi à jour le fait que les femmes, sur lesquelles repose l'économie de ces communautés, surmenées et malades, avortent et meurent en plus grand nombre qu'ailleurs, contrariant encore une natalité à l'avenir aléatoire[64]. L'enquête menée en 1950 par une équipe de spécialistes envoyés par le Haut Commissariat de France dans plusieurs régions encore mal connues et isolées du Sud Annam rapporte des résultats moins alarmants mais qui remettent tout autant en cause l'idée communément acceptée que la mortalité infantile a chuté partout et de façon marquée en Indochine[65].

Quoique l'on puisse penser de ce genre de séries statistiques, on envisage bien des disparités dans l'exposition de l'enfant à la mort, disparités qui recoupent à la fois une opposition urbain – rural et une entre les pays vietnamiens et le reste de l'Union indochinoise. Pour autant, il semble que, influencée par de trop fortes concentrations humaines (théorie du Dr Chesneau), par certaines insalubrités régionales ou encore «pas suffisamment influencée» par la médecine occidentale, surtout préventive (accès demeuré restreint aux structures hospitalières, au personnel sanitaire ou encore aux campagnes de vaccination régulières), la mortalité infantile a régressé lentement, maintenant finalement, par son incidence considérable sur la mortalité globale, des taux de mortalité élevés[66]. Mais cette régression a incontestablement eu lieu, même si les résultats sont apparus plus tard que prévu et dans des proportions que l'on connaît mal, faute, une fois de plus, de repères sur la gravité des mouvements démographiques vietnamiens au XIXe siècle. Sinon, comment expliquer, seule certitude que nous ayons, cet accroissement démographique qui, pour l'Indochine entière (taux d'accroissement annuel estimé à 2 % en 1939 contre 0,5 % en 1907) ou relatif à chaque pays (près de 2 % en 1937 en pays vietnamien; aux alentours de 1,3 % en pays khmer et lao[67]) a augmenté régulièrement à partir des premières décennies du XXe siècle pour ne plus jamais fléchir?

Une Nouvelle Donne Significative

D'autres chiffres, peut-être moins aléatoires, sont eux aussi significatifs d'une nouvelle donne, sans compter qu'ils mettent directement en avant cette fois le rôle de la médicalisation engagée par la France et en particulier le poids des structures hospitalières (hôpitaux et maternités) et du personnel qui tend à prendre de plus en plus en charge les femmes en même temps que leurs enfants.

Tout d'abord, nombreuses sont les données hospitalières qui montrent que les mères ont peu à peu pris l'habitude d'accoucher à l'hôpital mais que les parents ont également pris celle de conduire leur progéniture malade dans les formations de l'Assistance. Par exemple, on comptabilise 13 361 enfants recensés dans les structures annamites en 1937 sur un total de 71 813 hospitalisations comptabilisées cette année-là. Cela revient à dire qu'un hospitalisé annamite sur 5 avait alors moins de 5 ans[68]. Le total d'hospitalisés âgés entre 2 et 5 ans, plus élevé de 50 % que celui des hospitalisés âgés de 0 à 2 ans, renforce la réalité de nouveaux réflexes parmi la population vietnamienne. Certes, ces petits malades souffrent comme les adultes de paludisme, d'affections pulmonaires ou encore de maladies cutanées. Mais la mortalité consécutive à ces pathologies plus ou moins graves (plus proche de 0 que de 1 %) reste très nettement en deçà de taux de mortalité hospitalière des adultes[69], appuyant la confirmation que le mythe de l'hôpital mouroir est à bannir à la veille de la Seconde Guerre mondiale en pays vietnamien.

Sans avoir les moyens informatifs et statistiques suffisants pour contredire des taux de mortalité infantile qui avoisineraient encore à l'époque les 40 %, ni d'être, à l'inverse, en mesure d'en éprouver l'éventuelle véridicité, il faut aussi incontestablement surligner l'intérêt grandissant des femmes pour une offre de plus en plus adaptée, intérêt renforçant cette idée que partout «plus la fonction de survie s'est rapprochée de la courbe idéale, plus a grandi l'exigence de l'atteindre»[70]. Ne serait-ce que les progrès de l'obstétrique, de la chirurgie occidentale apparaissent par ailleurs comme des outils efficaces de conversion des femmes vietnamiennes à la médecine et au médecin occidentaux, comblant de plus en plus des exigences grandissantes[71].

Il est impossible de chiffrer de façon exacte l'évolution du recours à la sage-femme, particulièrement en milieu rural. Il est par contre relativement facile de comptabiliser celle du recours à la maternité qui confirme une acceptation d'un acte d'accouchement médicalisé. Un rapport sanitaire (tableau 2) consigne ces données pour l'ensemble de la péninsule:

Tableau 2. Protection de la maternité et de l'enfance indigène en Indochine en 1935[72]

Nature de la consultation	Nombre de consultants	Nombre de consultations
prénatales	13 558	31 026
postnatales	10 202	25 004
Enfants 0–2 ans	27 974	43 786
Enfants 2–5 ans	86 030	207 702

Il faudrait bien sûr rapporter ces chiffres au nombre total de femmes enceintes, de naissances cette année-là, au nombre d'enfants de 0 à 5 ans, au taux de mortalité infantile ou encore les comparer avec les mêmes données d'autres colonies pour évaluer la portée de l'effort et des résultats locaux. Il faudrait aussi pouvoir opérer une répartition par pays et calculer un taux régional de recours à la maternité. Quoiqu'il en soit, ces données ponctuelles donnent une indication précieuse sur l'utilisation qui est faite de la maternité, en dehors de l'épisode d'accouchement. Ainsi, pour 1935, le total des naissances est évalué à partir de rapports sanitaires à 618 221. Ceci permet d'estimer la fréquentation des consultations postnatales à 1,65 % des naissances, un chiffre certes peu élevé mais qui renvoie à une nouvelle réalité. Quant au nombre d'accouchements justement – assistés par un personnel médical employé du gouvernement colonial, *intra* et *extra* maternités – , il serait passé de 2 604 en 1904 à 12 501 en 1920, puis 84 384 en 1929, multiplié en 25 ans par plus de 32[73].

Les répercussions de la circulaire du Ministère des Colonies de 1934 sur les réorientations à donner à la protection maternelle et infantile outre-mer avaient été immédiates en Indochine parce que les initiatives locales l'avaient devancée. Entre autres, la réponse du Résident supérieur d'Annam à propos des suites qu'il désirait personnellement donner aux propositions ministérielles ne s'était, pas fait attendre. Ce dernier faisait en effet parvenir à son supérieur des indications plus que pertinentes au travers d'un compte-rendu minutieux sur l'organisation régionale de la protection de la maternité et de l'enfance en mars 1935[74]. En 1936, le Dr Brindaux, revenant justement d'Indochine, abondait dans son sens, rapportant à la métropole des statistiques engageantes sur l'année qui venait de s'écouler et ce pour l'ensemble de l'Union (Tonkin et Annam en tête des succès) (tableau 1).

Quoiqu'il en soit, à l'aube de la défaite métropolitaine de 1940 et considérant l'étendue de la tâche, bon nombre de médecins avouent sans détour qu'il reste encore beaucoup à accomplir : «D'après le dépouillement méthodique des déclarations d'état civil effectuées à Hanoi depuis 1925, à Saigon-Cholon depuis 1936, le taux de natalité est environ de 40 pour mille dans les deux agglomérations -taux stable-, le taux de mortalité environ de 30 pour mille. La moitié des décédés sont des enfants de moins de 15 ans. La mortalité de la première année est en général de 25 à 35 % du nombre des naissances»[75]. L'enquête effectuée par le Dr Chesneau sur la mortalité infantile du Tonkin dans les années 1930 corrobore ces dires et la vision alarmiste du rapport.

Phénomène citadin à propos duquel il faut accuser l'insalubrité et les dangers pathologiques d'une trop forte densité humaine? Faut-il plutôt admettre que l'insuffisance des données démographiques en matière de natalité[76] et de mortalité pourrait expliquer l'optimisme de quelques médecins qui ne voyaient, depuis plusieurs décennies, que les résultats ponctuels et relatifs obtenus dans leur service hospitalier ou à leur poste? Ou alors, les données antérieures étaient-elles tellement fantaisistes et en deçà de la réalité que l'on a encore du mal à voir que les efforts ont porté un minimum leurs fruits? Certes, les enfants continuaient de payer un lourd tribut à un environnement morbide particulièrement néfaste. Il ne faudrait pas pour autant remettre en question les efforts coloniaux et médicaux qui les visaient, efforts qui participaient à une politique médico-sociale d'envergure.

Dans cette mise en perspective, il ne faut pas non plus oublier l'importance d'un contexte de protection de la femme enceinte et surtout de l'enfance dans la société vietnamienne traditionnelle susceptible d'avoir largement aidé à développer la médicalisation de ces populations constamment menacées. Si les chiffres sont globalement indicateurs d'une amélioration de la santé, ils sont aussi la démonstration, plus indirecte, de l'acceptation par la population locale du programme d'action médicale français[77]. Bien sûr, la réponse française à cette demande sociale de santé ne fut pas partout la même, quand elle existait : une disparité qui oppose en premier lieu les milieux urbanisés aux régions les plus rurales et les moins peoples, une disparité qui s'avère encore plus flagrante entre le Vietnam et les deux autres pays de l'Indochine que sont le Cambodge et le Laos actuels.

D'où ce seul élément de réponse assuré à propos de la situation de l'époque en matière d'évolution de la mortalité et de la morbidité des parturientes et de leurs enfants : une situation en lente mais ascendante évolution, dépendant davantage de moyens défectueux que de réticences locales. L'ensemble des rites entourant traditionnellement la naissance étaient finalement davantage dépendants d'une appréhension de la mort, quelle soit celle de la mère, de l'enfant ou des deux, que de convictions proprement médicales. Et parmi les défauts de fabrication du système de santé colonial, il y avait aussi la lenteur de l'organisation d'une politique de protection de toutes les femmes. Pour ne prendre qu'un exemple symptomatique, il faut savoir que le Dr Joyeux parlait en 1933 de 96 % de femmes infectées par une maladie vénérienne à sa consultation municipale de Hanoi[78].

Conclusion

Au vu de ces développements, il apparaît difficile de ne pas remarquer la place de la protection maternelle et surtout infantile dans le processus global de médicalisation proposé par la France à l'Indochine. Ayant connu une évolution continue et une adaptation globalement linéaire, ce fer de lance de la politique sanitaire aide à concevoir une acceptation progressive de la politique sanitaire française par les populations indigènes, révélant une hausse dans le recours (statistiques hospitalières à l'appui) à ses propositions, surtout hospitalières. Ajoutons, à cet égard, que le cadre général de la médicalisation indochinoise et les objectifs impérialistes s'étaient conjugués pour faire de l'éducation médicale de ces populations un des murs porteurs d'un plan d'acculturation.

Dans ce contexte, et on l'a également noté, la médicalisation de la femme, de ses grossesses et de ses accouchements a servi en priorité la protection d'une population infantile agressée de toutes parts et décimée. En fait, le contrôle maternel, plus qu'une attention périnatale structurée, conduisait au développement de nouvelles générations plus saines acquises aux idées et principes occidentaux, futures générations de colonisés «idéaux» dans la lignée des objectifs coloniaux. Il faut par ailleurs souligner que cette politique a d'abord obtenu des résultats en milieu urbain, et donc en sol vietnamien (le plus «urbanisé»), pour diverses raisons qui se sont combinées : structures, personnel plus nombreux, populations mieux sensibilisées, mieux éduquées mais aussi mieux surveillées en matière de santé publique.

Reste que, relativement à ce sujet délicat et encore controversé, il ne faut pas oublier non plus que, à la même époque en Occident, le regard médical sur la grossesse était encore en période d'essai. Il essayait de s'affirmer auprès des femmes, réussite qui dépendait entre autres de progressions dans la prévention, les soins offerts, les techniques et les outils de persuasion. L'approche, résolument moderne, s'était finalement retrouvée proposée presque simultanément aux femmes vietnamiennes dans les années 1930. En rappelant les objectifs coloniaux de sensibilisation sanitaire, d'attention à l'histoire pathologique et sociale des femmes enceintes, les enquêtes sur la fécondité, la stérilité, les maladies vénériennes, la mobilisation médicale face à l'environnement social de l'enfant, le développement de consultations prénatales, on doit alors et surtout apprécier la précocité et les conditions d'existence et la valeur de l'effort.

Enfin, l'héritage de la période coloniale dans le domaine de la protection de la mère et de l'enfant peut corroborer certaines de nos hypothèses, en particulier en ce qui a trait à l'emploi d'un personnel féminin compétent et à des mesures de prévention ciblées (surveillance de la grossesse, attention à l'alimentation de la mère et du nourrisson, vaccinations obligatoires, développement de consultations spécialisées et de centres de planning familial en milieu urbain et rural). Le gouvernement vietnamien actuel s'en défend. La dénonciation de la colonisation française dans son ensemble participe en effet, et logiquement, à asseoir l'indépendance depuis 1945 et à valoriser les activités socialistes de la République démocratique du Vietnam. Il semble quoiqu'il en soit évident qu'un retour sur ce passé médical colonial apporte sa pierre à l'édification solide d'une histoire nuancée de la médicalisation maternelle et infantile moderne.

Annexe : La Médicalisation Maternelle et Infantile en Indochine Française : Quelques Repères Chronologiques

Années	La santé des femmes et des enfants en métropole	Repères sur la colonisation et la politique sanitaire en Indochine	La prise en charge des mères et des enfants indochinois
1858		Conquête de la Cochinchine (1858–67)	
1860		Le premier hôpital est installé à Saigon (Cochinchine)	
		Les dispensaires des Missions reçoivent des subventions du gouverne-ment français	
1863		Lalhuyeaux d'Ormay organise le premier réseau d'assistance médicale (1863–74)	
1864		Ouverture de l'hôpital indigène de Choquan (Cochinchine)	
1866		Premières mesures d'hygiène publiques à Saigon; Construction de l'hôpital de Cholon; Création d'un comité de vaccine à Saigon	
1870	Avènement de la IIIe République		
1871		Arrêté qui rend obligatoire la vaccination antivariolique en Cochinchine	
1873		Début de la première phase de conquête de l'Annam et du Tonkin	
1874	Loi Roussel sur la protection des enfants en nourrice; Loi sur le travail des enfants		
1882	Obligation de cours d'hygiène dans les écoles primaires	Reprise de la conquête de l'Annam et du Tonkin (1882–97)	
1883		Organisation d'un Etat civil en Cochinchine	
1886	Création de la fonction de médecin inspecteur des écoles primaires		
1887		Création de l'Union indochinoise; Début de la période du Gouvernement général (1887–1945)	Installation de la première creche missionnaire à CulaoGien (Cambodge)
1889	Création de la Ligue antituberculeuse; Loi sur les enfants abandonnés		

Annexe (cont'd)

Années	La santé des femmes et des enfants en métropole	Repères sur la colonisation et la politique sanitaire en Indochine	La prise en charge des mères et des enfants indochinois
1891		L'Institut Pasteur de Saigon produit ses premiers vaccins antivarioliques	
1892	Instauration de consultations gratuites de nourrissons et de gouttes de lait à Paris (1892–94) Loi sur l'obligation de posséder un doctorat pour exercer la médecine		
1893	Loi sur l'Assistance Médicale Gratuite (AMG)	Institution du protectorat du Laos	
1894		Inauguration de l'hôpital indigène de Hanoi	
1897		Une direction de la santé est créée dans chaque pays de l'Union La loi de 1892 sur l'exercice médical est appliquée à la Cochinchine	
1898	Loi sur les enfants maltraités		
1900			
1901		Le Dr Angier ouvre la première clinique privée de Saigon	Le Dr Drouhet fonde l'Association Maternelle de Cholon Premier enseignement donné à de futures sages-femmes vietnamiennes
1902	Loi sur la santé publique, première du genre en France	Fondation de l'Ecole de médecine de Hanoi Les services de santé de l'Indochine sont mis sous l'autorité d'un directeur	L'Association Maternelle de Cholon fonde un asile municipal pour enfants malades et abandonné
1903			Le Dr Déjean ouvre la première consultation gratuite à l'intention des indigènes dans sa clinique privée à Saigon
1904	Loi sur les enfants assistés	Institution d'une direction générale de la santé auprès du Gouvernement général	Ouverture d'une section de sages-femmes à l'Ecole de médecine de Hanoi Ouverture de l'Ecole de médecine pratique de Choquan

Annexe (cont'd)

Années	La santé des femmes et des enfants en métropole	Repères sur la colonisation et la politique sanitaire en Indochine	La prise en charge des mères et des enfants indochinois
1905	Séparation de l'Eglise et de l'Etat	Organisation de l'AMI (Assistance Médicale Indigène)	Obligation de cours d'hygiène dans les écoles franco-indigènes
1906			Organisation de la Société de Protection de la natalité au Cambodge
1907		Instructions relatives à la protection de la santé et de l'hygiène publique	
1908			Apparition des premières maternités libres L'Ecole de Choquan devient «Ecole des infirmiers-vaccinateurs et des sages-femmes indigènes de Cochinchine» La vaccination antivariolique est rendue obligatoire en Indochine pour la 1ère, 11ème et 21ème année
1911		L'Inspection générale des services sanitaires et médicaux remplace la direction général de la santé Début du Gouvernement général d'A. Sarraut (1911–14) Proposition d'un premier programme sanitaire quinquennal	Ouverture d'une école d'infirmières-sages-femmes indigènes à l'hôpital central de Hué (Annam)
1912			Première enquête sur la tuberculose à Hué
1914		Réorganisation des services d'AMI et du personnel concerné Programme sanitaire pour l'agglomération de Saigon-Cholon Second mandat de Sarraut (1917–19)	
1917			
1922	Rapport sur «la mortinatalité et la mortalité infantile dans les colonies françaises» Mise au point du BCG (1922–23)		
1923			Organisation d'un comité d'études de la tuberculose à Cholon

Annexe (cont'd)

Années	La santé des femmes et des enfants en métropole	Repères sur la colonisation et la politique sanitaire en Indochine	La prise en charge des mères et des enfants indochinois
1924	Mise au point par le pastorien Ramon de l'antitoxine tétanique		Les médecins et les sages-femmes diplômés de Hanoi obtiennent le droit d'exercer une médecine libérale Enquêtes sur la tuberculose dans les écoles franco-indigènes de Cochinchine (1924–25) Le vaccin BCG est utilisé pour la première fois en Cochinchine et au Cambodge
1925	Rapport de l'Académie des sciences coloniales sur l'insuffisance alimentaire des populations des colonies françaises	Création à l'Inspection des services sanitaires d'une section de démographie et de préservation sociale	
1927		Officialisation d'un programme d'assistance rurale	Premières vaccinations BCG au Tonkin Mise en place d'un cadre de *Ba mu* au Tonkin Ouverture de l'Institut de puériculture de Cholon
1928			Premières vaccinations BCG en Annam à Hué Création d'un dispensaire antituberculeux à Hué
1929		Organisation d'un service d'Assistance sociale indépendant	
1930			Création de la Ligue antituberculeuse du Tonkin Congrès de l'Enfance à Saigon
1934	Circulaire du Ministère des colonies sur la protection de la maternité et de l'enfance		
1937	Mise en place de la Commission Guernut par le Front Populaire pour évaluer l'état social des colonies	Mission Godart du Front Populaire en Indochine Programme sanitaire du Dr Hermant	
1938			Enquête sanitaire sur l'enfant indochinois

Notes

1   Il faut noter un intérêt, encore discret mais réel, des historiens pour l'évolution démographique de la région du sud-est asiatique : Peter Boomgaard, *Children of the Colonial State. Population Growth and Economic Development in Java, 1795–1880*, (Amsterdam : Center for Asian Studies, 1990), p. 256; Norman G. Owen, *Death and Disease in South East Asia : Explorations in Social, Medical and Demographic History*, (Singapour : Oxford University Press, 1987), p. 288). On n'oubliera pas pour autant quelques études ethnologiques autour de pratiques traditionnelles dont l'ouvrage de Do Lam Chi Lan : *La mère et l'enfant dans le Viet-Nam d'autrefois*, (Paris : L'Harmattan, coll. «Recherches Asiatiques», 1998). Enfin notre propre ouvrage a tenu à combler certaines lacunes en proposant plusieurs chapitres sur ces questions (Laurence Monnais-Rousselot, *Médecine et colonisation. L'aventure indochinoise, 1860–1939*, (Paris : CNRS Editions, 1999), p. 456).

2   Il faut en effet préciser que généralement l'histoire de la médicalisation infantile est dissociée de celle de la médicalisation maternelle. La plupart des auteurs arrêtent leur analyse à la fin de l'allaitement, à la séparation effective de la mère et de son nouveau-né, après avoir traité des questions entourant la grossesse, l'accouchement, le post-partum (et, connexes, l'avortement, la sexualité ou la contraception) les techniques (gynéco-obstétrique) et professionnels (médecins, sages-femmes) intervenant sur ces aspects. Un cloisonnement dans les thèmes abordés qui tend à exclure les liens, pourtant forts, entre intervention médicale sur les populations féminines et celle sur les populations infantiles. Dans le cas vietnamien, il y a de toute façon obligation d'opérer ce rapprochement dans un contexte de développement d'une santé publique qui a d'emblée englobé dans une même vision le vaste domaine du «maternal and child care» (voir «Maternal and Child Health in Primary Health Care» dans *Maternal and Child Care in Developing Countries*, dir. Elton Kessel, Asghari K. Awan. Proceedings of the 3rd International Congress for Maternal and Neonatal Health, Lahore, 1987, (Lausanne : Ott Publishers Thun, 1989), p. 19–25; et *La protection de la mère et de l'enfant au Vietnam* (Hanoi : Editions en Langues Etrangères, 1979).

3   Cette étude reprend effectivement certaines des réflexions en maturation qui ont parsemé une thèse de doctorat (Laurence Monnais-Rousselot, «Médecine coloniale, pratiques de santé et sociétés en Indochine française [1860–1939]», thèse de doctorat en histoire «nouveau régime», Université Paris VII–Denis Diderot, 1997), p. 1079.

4   L'Indochine française englobe à partir de 1887 cinq territoires administratifs sous la houlette d'un Gouverneur général, dont trois à population majoritairement vietnamienne : la colonie de Cochinchine et les protectorats d'Annam et du Tonkin, en plus donc des protectorats lao et khmer. S'il existe alors une identité vietnamienne, liant les habitants des territoires de Cochinchine, Annam et Tonkin (grossièrement l'actuelle République Démocratique du Vietnam), il reste impossible de parler de «Vietnam» en tant qu'entité administrative et politique. Précisons à ce sujet que nous avons décidé de nous attacher à parler ici en priorité des régions vietnamiennes pour deux raisons principales : le manque flagrant de sources concernant les deux protectorats restant; le fait, avéré par nos recherches antérieures, que le territoire vietnamien est celui qui a le plus uniformément reçu le plan sanitaire métropolitain. On pourrait même ajouter que le poids numérique à joué dans le sens où la population vietnamienne représente environ les 4/5èmes de la population indochinoise en 1906 comme en 1936. Pour de plus amples informations sur la période de colonisation de la péninsule indochi-

noise, voir : Pierre Brocheux, Daniel Hémery, *Indochine. La colonisation ambiguë, 1858–1954*, (Paris : La Découverte, 2002, 2ᵉ éd.), p. 427; et plus généralement, sur l'histoire de la colonisation française : Charles-Robert Ageron, Catherine Coquery-Vidrovitch, Gilbert Meynier, Jacques Thobie, *Histoire de la France coloniale*, (Paris : Armand Colin, 1991), p. 654.

5 La loi votée sous l'impulsion de Théophile Roussel prévoit que «*tout enfant placé, âgé de moins de deux ans, devient l'objet d'une surveillance de l'autorité publique ayant pour but de protéger sa vie et sa santé*». Le texte repose surtout sur la présence d'inspecteurs des enfants assistés auxquels sont adjoints des médecins inspecteurs chargés de visiter les enfants en nourrice. Cette loi s'intègre à une activité de protection de l'enfance qui dépasse là le champ médical avec des réglementations subséquentes sur la protection des enfants abandonnés (1889) et sur les enfants maltraités (1898) (voir la chronologie proposée en annexe).

6 Sans disserter outre mesure sur un concept de colonie «d'exploitation», discutable, précisons que la colonisation de l'Indochine eut initialement un triple objectif : politique (étendre la présence et l'influence française dans le monde et en Extrême-Orient en particulier), économique et humanitaire (la colonisation étant considérée comme pouvant aider les «sociétés primitives» à évoluer). Porteurs d'un savoir médical scientifique, au cœur d'un mouvement eugéniste et hygiénique, les médecins français pouvaient alors, en tant que *médecins coloniaux* intervenir sur la réalisation de ces trois objectifs.

7 Tout comme les termes de «indochinois», «annamite» (synonyme à l'époque de vietnamien), ceux de «race» et d'«indigène» sont ici utilisés sans aucune connotation péjorative, pour coller à une réalité coloniale et ainsi contourner toute espèce d'anachronisme.

8 A noter que la vaccination antivariolique ne sera obligatoire en France qu'avec la grande loi de santé publique de 1902, c'est-à-dire plus de trente ans plus tard.

9 Archives Nationales du Vietnam (ANVN), centre n°1 (Hanoi), Fonds de la Résidence Supérieure du Tonkin (RST), dossier 10 999.

10 Centre des Archives d'Outre-Mer, Aix-en-Provence (CAOM), Fonds de la Commission Guernut, carton 22, dossier Bb.

11 Voir à ce sujet : Laurence Monnais-Rousselot, «Colonisation et problèmes sociaux : une intervention médicale. L'expérience de l'Indochine française, 1860–1954», dans *Nouvelles configurations des problèmes sociaux et l'intervention*, dir. Henri Dorvil et Robert Mayeur (Sainte Foy : Presses de l'Université du Québec à Montréal, 2001) p. 511–540.

12 ANVN, centre n°2 (Ho Chi Minh Ville), Fonds du Gouvernement de la Cochinchine (Goucoch), dossier IA.7/286 (1).

13 Ces interdits ne sont par exemple pas en rapport avec la dureté physique de certaines tâches. On croit, au contraire, chez les Vietnamiens que la femme doit continuer à travailler dur pour avoir un enfant robuste et courageux.

14 Le terme de «moderne» est ici à utiliser avec circonspection. Comme l'expose très bien Francine Saillant, par exemple, il est important de rappeler que perdurent en Occident à la même époque des pratiques, des rites, des croyances du même genre que celles qu'on peut évoquer pour le Vietnam (voir à ce sujet : Jacques Barbaut, *Histoires de la naissance*, (Paris : Editions Plume, 1990), p. 178–184; et Edward Shorter, «Un accouchement traditionnel : une affaire de femmes» dans *Le corps des femmes*, (Paris : Le Seuil, 1984), p. 57–73), une perdurance qui oblige à la nuance, à une distinction complexe entre univers professionnel et profane et qui appuie aussi la nécessité de ne pas simplement faire une histoire «moderne» positiviste de la grossesse et de l'accouchement depuis deux siècles (Francine

Saillant, *Accoucher autrement. Repères historiques, sociaux et culturels de la grossesse et de l'accouchement au Québec* (Montréal : Editions St Martin, 1987). Le principal décalage finalement se trouve dans le fait que les populations vietnamiennes n'étaient pas préparées à recevoir d'un seul coup ces nouvelles visions non seulement coloniales (donc dans une certaine mesure imposées et dirigistes) mais occidentales. Le prosélytisme de la médecine dite moderne dans ce contexte ne pouvait alors qu'entraîner des réticences, surtout lorsqu'il contrevenait à des règles socioculturelles bien établies.

15 Voir sur ce point : Do Lam, «La prémastication du riz», dans *La mère et l'enfant*, p. 155–156.

16 Les premiers taux moyens de mortalité infantile calculés par ces médecins ne pouvaient effectivement qu'attirer l'attention et révéler l'urgence de mesures spécifiques. Ces taux, d'environ 400 décès pour 1 000 naissances, étaient loin devant ceux de la métropole où, en moyenne de 150 pour 1 000, ils continuaient pourtant de mobiliser les esprits médicaux et hygiénistes. Si, à Paris, ville de mortalité infantile par excellence, il pouvait encore varier en 1860 entre 20 % et 80 %, il restait plus proche des 20 % au tournant du XXe siècle (Rollet-Echallier, *La politique de la Troisième République*, Paris : Presses Universitaires de France/INED, 1990).

17 Le tétanos ombilical, ou néonatal, est consécutif à une coupure du cordon ombilical dans des conditions d'antisepsie et/ ou d'asepsie inadaptées ou inexistantes permettant l'introduction du bacille de Nicolaïer. L'affection a de quoi intriguer et mobiliser les médecins coloniaux. En premier lieu, parce qu'elle n'existe pas dans les statistiques de morbidité infantile métropolitaine; deuxièmement parce que, à l'inverse d'autres affections infantiles, le tétanos est, avec un minimum d'hygiène, facilement évitable. Il reste intéressant de préciser que cette affection néo-natale n'a pas disparu pour autant (ou a-t-elle réapparu?), restant dans de nombreux pays en développement un problème important de santé publique, entre autres en Asie du Sud-est. Le Vietnam reste d'ailleurs parmi les pays touchés par cette affection (A. Galazka, F. Gasse, R. Henderson, «Neonatal Tetanus and the Global Expanded Programme of Immunization», dans *Maternal and Child Care*, p. 109–123).

18 Ce travail permet aussi de mesurer le fossé que certains auteurs dénoncent entre les traditions locales et la médicalisation dont ils sont les agents, faisant des réticences des femmes et de leur entourage le symptôme révélateur de cette incompréhension mutuelle. Voir à titre d'illustration : Dr Bonifacy, «Certaines croyances relatives à la grossesse chez les divers groupes ethniques du Tonkin», *Bulletin de l'Ecole Française d'Extrême-Orient (BEFEO)* 7 (1907); et Dr Duvigneau, «La grossesse, l'accouchement et le nouveau-né chez les Annamites à Hué», *Annales d'Hygiène et de Médecine coloniale (AHMC)* 10 (1907).

19 Cette entreprise lui tiendra d'ailleurs longtemps à cœur comme le montrent ses nombreuses interventions et publications dans le domaine tout au long de sa carrière outre-mer. Citons : «La surveillance de la natalité indigène, de la prophylaxie du tétanos ombilical à Saigon, 1905–07», *AHMC* 11 (1908) : 72–85; «La prophylaxie du tétanos ombilical à Saigon», dans Comptes-rendus du 2e congrès de la Far Eastern Association for Tropical Medicine, Hong Kong, 1913, p. 251–262; et René Montel et Tran Van An, «Sur la mortalité infantile en Cochinchine. Notes statistiques sur la mortalité infantile de la ville de Saigon», *Bulletin de la Société Médico-chirurgicale de l'Indochine (BSMI)* 11 (novembre 1926) : 572–576.

20 Dr. Montel, «Notes d'hygiène et de démographie : pourquoi doit-on faire de l'assistance medicale en Indochine» *BSMI* 60 (1911) : 15.

21 «C'est en apprenant aux enfants ce qu'est une maladie infectieuse et comment on s'en préserve, c'est en enseignant aux fillettes leurs devoirs de futures mères et tout ce que l'on a appelé du nom pompeux de puériculture, c'est en insistant surtout sur les soins à donner aux nourrissons, que l'on formera des générations saines et robustes, esprits sains dans des corps sains, aptes à se défendre intelligemment contre les causes des maladies. Cette bonne semence qui germe difficilement dans le cerveau de l'adulte trouvera chez l'enfant terre vierge merveilleusement fertile et la mission féconde se fera plus tard...naturellement...» (Montel, «Notes d'hygiène», p. 17).

22 ANVN, Centre n°1, Fonds de la direction locale de la santé du Tonkin, dossier 442.

23 Dr Le Roy des Barres, «La mortalité infantile au Tonkin», *BSMI* (juin 1928) : 245–260. Si la fiabilité des sources dont se sert ce praticien dépend largement des déclarations de l'état civil, le fait qu'il dirigeait lui-même le bureau d'hygiène de la ville et qu'il connaissait parfaitement bien les données chiffrées des établissements hospitaliers donne (et donnera) toujours un crédit particulier à son travail.

24 Un grand nombre d'articles publiés dans le *Bulletin de la Société Médico-chirurgicale de l'Indochine*, revue médicale publiée à Hanoi par les médecins de l'Indochine et pour information sur la situation médicale indochinoise, rend compte de cette attention.

25 ANVN, Centre n°1, Fonds de la direction locale du Tonkin, dossier 447.

26 Sur ces nouvelles campagnes de prévention infantile et leur incidence, le lecteur pourra se reporter à deux articles parus dans les *Archives des Instituts Pasteur d'Indochine* en octobre 1925: Drs Guérin, Lalung-Bonnaire, Advier, «Premiers résultats de l'enquête sociale sur la tuberculose dans les écoles de Cholon», (1) : 189–208; Jean Bablet, «La prémunition antituberculeuse des nouveaux-nés par ingestion de BCG en Cochinchine», (1) : 208–213.

27 Avec les années 1920, on ne se focalisait plus seulement sur la pratique de «prémâchage du riz» mais bien plus généralement sur la question de l'alimentation quotidienne du nouveau-né (surveillance de l'allaitement en priorité) en faisant toutefois attention de ne pas contrevenir aux règles élémentaires dans le domaine relevant de conceptions sociales et traditionnelles liant la mère à son nouveau-né (voir Blot, *Natalité et obstétrique*, p. 103).

28 Pour l'historien engagé qu'est Nguyên Khac Vien, la réutilisation massive de l'œuvre religieuse dans les années 1930 ne répond en effet pas seulement à des problèmes d'ordre financier et à des carences en personnel. Selon lui, l'administration coloniale était allée jusqu'à favoriser son activité (rarement remise en question par les populations qui en bénéficiaient) pour reprendre en main des régions troublées (Nguyên Khac Vien, *Vietnam, une longue histoire* (Hanoi : The Gioi, 1993), p. 228).

29 Circulaire du Ministère des Colonies (n°29–4/ S), 7.11.1934; Congrès de l'Enfance, Saigon, 1934, *Rapports du congrès* (Saigon, 1934). Pour une autre perspective sur la complexité et l'ambiguïté de la position sociale de l'enfant dans un contexte coloniale et de «hiérarchisation» ethnique, voir l'article de M. Tennant («Complicating Childhood: Gender, Ethnicity and "Disadvantage" within the New Zealand Children's Health Camps Movement») dans le présent ouvrage.

30 Partout, la majorité des formations relève du budget local de chaque pays, les plus citadines dépendant des budgets municipaux.

31 Le Tonkin, par exemple, sous la houlette de son Résident René Robin, instaure un programme d'Assistance Rurale, fondé avec efficacité sur la dissémination de

dispensaires et de postes de *Ba mu*, sages-femmes rurales, élevés aux frais des villages qui en font la demande, on aura l'occasion d'y revenir (ANVN, Centre n°1, Fonds de la Direction locale de la santé du Tonkin).

32 Ces consultations, organisées en effet autour de la transmission de quelques principes d'hygiène et d'attention à soi, permettent en outre de repérer d'éventuels signes de syphilis chez la mère. Pour ce faire, la Cochinchine bénéficie d'ailleurs à partir de 1927 du concours de l'Institut prophylactique antivénérien de Saigon. Pour autant, il faut bien considérer que là comme ailleurs la médecine périnatale est encore très immature.

33 ANVN, Centre n°1, RST, dossier 48 024.

34 Blot., «Natalité et obstétrique».

35 Montel, «Notes d'hygiène» p. 10.

36 Voir Laurence Monnais-Rousselot, «La professionnalisation du «médecin indochinois» au XXᵉ siècle: Des paradoxes d'une médicalisation coloniale», *Actes de la Recherche en Sciences Sociales* 143 (2002) : 36–43.

37 ANVN, Centre n°2, Goucoch, dossier IA.7/286 (1)/ dossier IA.8/042 (2).

38 ANVN, Centre n°2, Goucoch, dossier IA.7/286 (1).

39 ANVN, Centre n°2, Goucoch, dossier IA.8/042 (2).

40 ANVN, Centre n°2, Goucoch, dossier IA.8/042 (3).

41 CAOM), Fonds du Gouvernement général (Gougal), dossier 6 733.

42 ANVN, Centre n°2, Goucoch, dossier IA.8/031 (4).

43 ANVN, Centre n°2, Goucoch, dossier IA.8/031 (5).

44 ANVN, Centre n°1, RST, dossier 6 576. On retrouve le même genre de pratique auprès des sages-femmes françaises dès la deuxième moitié du XVIIIᵉ siècle (Jacques Gélis, *L'arbre et le fruit. La naissance dans l'Occident moderne, XVIᵉ-XIXᵉ siècles* [Paris : Fayard, 1984] p. 189).

45 Dong Bao, «Sage-femme moderne», *L'Ami du Peuple*, 3.02.1934.

46 L'Inspection sous-entend par là que les diplômées, cette nouvelle élite, resteront au service sédentaire des maternités les plus importantes.

47 Il faut en effet savoir que le territoire indochinois et d'abord vietnamien est peuplé d'une multitude d'ethnies : au-delà de l'ethnie majoritaire «Viet», on retrouve bien sûr des Khmers, des Lao, des Chinois et des Sino-vietnamiens mais également de nombreuses minorités ethniques (Mnongs, Méo, Thaï entre autres) alors nommés «Moïs» par les autorités coloniales et les populations d'origine Viet (le terme signifiant «sauvages» en vietnamien).

48 A la même époque, un ouvrier vietnamien gagne aux environs de 70 piastres par an; un médecin vietnamien, selon son statut, entre 300 et 1 200.

49 ANVN, Centre n°1, RST, dossiers 32 119/ 37 301–50/ 37 355.

50 ANVN, Centre n°2, Goucoch, dossier IA.8/031 (5).

51 D'après les données lacunaires des *Annuaires statistiques de l'Indochine* publiés par le Gouvernement général de l'Indochine (Hanoi : Imprimerie d'Extrême-Orient, 1923) 42.

52 Dr Brindeaux, «A propos d'un voyage en Indochine, 1937», *Paris Médical* 2 (juillet–1er octobre–3 décembre 1937).

53 Les informations, minces, glanées sur ces quelques femmes médecins proviennent de plusieurs dossiers personnels éparpillés dans les archives aixoises et vietnamiennes (ANVN, Centre n°1, RST, dossier 49 258; CAOM, Gougal, dossier 31 419; ANVN, centre n°2, Goucoch, dossier 4 216).

54 ANVN, Centre n°2, Goucoch, dossier 1353; ANVN, Centre n°2, RSA, dossier 3 878.

55 Henri Bernier, *Atlas statistique de l'Indochine* (Hanoi : Imprimerie d'Extrême-Orient, 1914).

56 Voir entre autres à ce sujet : Dr Borel, «Contribution à l'étude de la mortalité infantile en Cochinchine,» *BSMI* 10 (novembre 1926) : 577–81; Pierre Chesneau, «Natalité et mortalité infantile au Nord Annam», *Archives de Médecine et de Pharmacie Coloniale (AMPC)* 35 (juillet–septembre 1937); Jeanne Eliche, «Notes statistiques sur la mortalité infantile indigène à Cholon» 10 (novembre 1926) : 570–571; Dr Lavau, «Notes sur la mortalité infantile en Cochinchine», *BSMI* 8 (septembre 1926) : 472–473; «Deuxième enquête sur la mortalité infantile en Cochinchine particulièrement dans ses rapports avec la syphilis», *BSMI* 6 (juillet-août 1928) : 355–359; Montel, «Sur la mortalité infantile en Cochinchine», *BSMI* 10 (novembre 1926) : 572–574; Georges Muraz, «La mortalité infantile et la tache mongoloïde dans la région de Saigon-Cholon», *Anthropos* 45 (1935) : 254–255; Nguyên Van Luyen, *Etude médico-sociale de la mortalité des enfants du premier âge*, thèse de médecine, Faculté de médecine de Paris, 1928; et Tran Van An, «Notes statistiques sur la mortalité infantile dans la ville de Saigon», *BSMI* 10 (novembre 1926) : 575–576.

57 Voir : Dr Jouin, «Enquête démographique au Darlac», *Bulletin de la Société des Etudes Indochinoises (BSEI)* 25 (1950); Dr Pietrantoni, «La population du Laos en 1943 dans son milieu géographique», *BSEI* 32 (1957) : 238–241; Haut Commissariat de France en Indochine, Services du conseiller à la Santé Publique et aux affaires économiques, Drs Farinaud, Choumara, Royer, *Infestation palustre et démographie dans les populations montagnardes du Sud indochinois*, 1950; et Nguyen Thieu Lau, «La mortalité dans le Quang Binh», *BEFEO* 16 (1951) : 131–143.

58 L'absence de données quantitatives et qualitatives concernant la mortalité féminine et en particulier des femmes en couches ne nous permettent en effet pas de prendre cette population comme un révélateur.

59 Pierre Chesneau, «Natalité et mortalité infantile au Sud Annam», dans Congrès international de la population Paris, 1937, t. 6, «Démographie de la France d'outre-mer» (Paris : Hermann & Cie, 1938); et «Natalité et mortalité infantile au Nord Annam», *AMPC* 35 (juillet–septembre 1937).

60 Philippe Ariès en arrive à la déduction inverse lorsqu'il étudie les comportements démographiques de la Touraine aux XVIIIᵉ et XIXᵉ. Selon lui, on assistait à une régulation qu'il qualifie de naturelle des naissances, dépendant des caprices de la nature (épidémies, famines). Donc, quand la quantité humaine serrait de trop près les ressources, ce qui est le cas des provinces vietnamiennes très densément peuplées, il y avait chute consécutive et inéluctable de la natalité (Philippe Ariès, *Histoire des populations françaises* (Paris : Le Seuil, 1971), p. 40–41).

61 Pierre Chesneau, «Natalité et mortalité infantile au Cammon (Laos), au Sud Annam et au Nord Annam», dans Congrès International de la population; Pierre Chesneau cité par Henri Ulmer dans *Les statistiques dans les pays coloniaux* (Paris : Berger Levrault, 1938), p. 10.

62 CAOM, Fonds de la Résidence Supérieure du Laos, D9.

63 Ces taux proviennent de sources statistiques médicales (ANVN, Centre n°1, RST, dossiers 3679–99). Ils n'ont bien sûr qu'une valeur d'approximation et sont ici utilisés pour donner une tendance générale. Pour autant, précisions qu'ils ont fait l'objet de comparaison avec d'autres statistiques, en particulier administratives (rapports coloniaux, recensements), pour éprouver leur degré de réalisme et de fiabilité (voir Monnais-Rousselot, «Médecine coloniale, pratiques de santé», p. 675–785).

64 Jouin, «Enquête démographique», p. 3. A l'heure de son enquête, le Dr Jouin travaillait depuis plusieurs années déjà à protéger la santé de ces régions annamites. Il n'hésite d'ailleurs pas, devant l'ampleur des hécatombes qui s'offraient à

ses yeux, à parler de peuples en voie de disparition tant la situation sanitaire, et plus généralement sociale (due aux menaces de famine, entre autres, résultat d'un environnement géographique peu cultivable) et donc démographique lui apparaissait critique.

65 Farinaud, Choumara, Royer, *Infestation palustre*. Selon Albert-Marie Maurice, régulièrement victimes de la variole (responsable du dépeuplement de certains cantons) et du paludisme, les Mnongs des hauts plateaux annamites voyaient leurs enfants mourir en masse: sur une moyenne de 5 à 6 enfants par famille, la moitié n'arrivait pas à l'âge adulte et le paludisme aurait été responsable des 4/5 de ces décès (Albert-Marie Maurice, *Les Mnongs des Hauts Plateaux* (Paris : L'Harmattan, 1993).

66 Cette remise en question d'une importante chute de la mortalité infantile constitue pour Philippe Ariès le meilleur indice d'une médecine mal implantée, encore peu acceptée par les populations. Il part en effet du fait que, pour que la médecine-science du XIXe ait réussi en France métropolitaine, il avait fallu au préalable que les mœurs y changent, que les populations se préparent à la recevoir, en modifiant entre autres leur conception de l'enfant ou de la durée de leur vie : «*Le goût de la vie chez le vieillard a précédé les progrès de la médecine*», aime-t-il écrire (Ariès, *Histoire des populations*, p. 373–398). On l'a vu, l'univers mental indochinois traditionnel savait mettre en échec le médecin français et sa médecine occidentale. De là à dire que la permanence d'une forte mortalité infantile pouvait devenir un des exemples les plus concrets de ces réticences populaires, il y a un grand pas à franchir.

67 Ces chiffres, calculées à partir de nos différentes sources statistiques (archives, rapports médicaux, données administratives du Gouvernement Général de l'Indochine) concordent dans une certaine mesure avec ceux avancés par des projections rétrospectives de démographes dont : Nguyen Shui Meng, *The Population of Indochina*, (Singapour : Institute for the South East Asian Studies, 1974), p. 126; et Jacques Migozzi, *Les facteurs du développement démographique au Cambodge*, Paris : CNRS, 1971, p. 303.

68 ANVN, Centre n°2, RSA, d. 3727.

69 La mortalité hospitalière des adultes est encore estimée (en moyenne) aux alentours de 4 %. Dans les tableaux conservés par les hôpitaux annamites, on remarque parmi les taux les plus frappants : 0,09 % de mortalité paludique (la deuxième cause de morbidité) pour les enfants de 0 à 2 ans; aussi peu que 0,02 pour ceux de 2 à 5 ans; du côté maladies cutanées (la première cause de morbidité hospitalière); côté affections pulmonaires (principale cause d'entrée avec les maladies cutanées) respectivement 1,09 et 0,15 %.

70 Edward Shorter évoque ce même passage pour l'Occident pour une période s'étendant selon les régions de la fin du XVIIIe au début du XIXe siècle («L'émergence de l'accouchement vécu», dans *Le corps des femmes*, p. 133–167). Ce qu'explique finalement aussi Do Lam en disant que voyant les «succès» de la médecine occidentale en termes de vies infantiles sauvées les Vietnamiennes ne pouvaient qu'adhérer à ses principes (Do Lam, *La mère et l'enfant*, conclusion).

71 Le contenu de la principale revue médicale publiée à Hanoi à partir de 1910, le *Bulletin de la Société Médico-chirurgicale de l'Indochine*, est à ce sujet parlant. On y remarque nettement, au fil des années, un développement de la considération et de l'expertise face aux grossesses à risque, à la gestion des malformations, des naissances gémellaires; on note encore des études probablement en rapport avec un contrôle prénatal sur le bassin des femmes vietnamiennes, certaines caractéristiques de l'anatomie féminine vietnamienne, la croissance des jeunes

filles....En 1934, la bibliographie de la thèse de médecine de M-L. Blot contient pour sa part plus de 130 articles traitant de l'une ou l'autre de ces questions. En outre, elle met en évidence, l'ancienneté du regard (certes très critique jusque dans les années 1920) d'une minorité de médecins posé sur les pratiques traditionnelles entourant l'accouchement, les rapports mère–enfant, les rites de *post partum*.

72   R. Beaudiment, «Protection de la maternité indigène dans les colonies françaises en 1935», *Archives de Médecine Navale et coloniale* 35, 2 (1937) : 504–564.

73   Laurent Gaide, *L'Assistance Médicale et la protection de la santé publique en Indochine* (Hanoi : Imprimerie d'Extrême-Orient, 1931). Sans pouvoir avancer des taux de recours à la maternité, il faut bien considérer que, à la même époque, la structure hospitalière est loin de convaincre toutes les femmes occidentales : en 1924, seules 9 % des femmes allemandes y auraient eu recours; en 1935, 27 % contre 37 % aux Etats-Unis (chiffres tirés de Shorter, *Le corps des femmes*, p. 150) et il s'agirait d'une majorité de femmes des «classes moyennes» et non plus seulement des femmes indigentes ou filles mères comme c'était le cas jusqu'à la fin du XIXe siècle.

74   ANVN, Centre n°2, RSA, d. 3363. La réponse tonkinoise interviendrait l'année suivante (ANVN, Centre n°1, RST, d. 74025).

75   *Rapports au grand Conseil des intérêts économiques et financiers et au Conseil du gouvernement* (Hanoi : Taupin, 1938).

76   En matière d'évolution de la natalité, qui pourrait, elle aussi, être un indicateur précieux non seulement de «succès» médicaux mais aussi de changements dans les comportements vietnamiens face à la grossesse et la naissance, les chiffres font encore trop largement défaut pour avancer plus que des hypothèses timides. Toutes les études statistiques dignes de ce nom, rapports du bureau d'hygiène de Hanoi invariablement en tête, donnent à observer un accroissement important du taux global de natalité indochinois. Très probablement parce que les fonctionnaires avaient appris à recenser plus exactement les naissances que la population dans son intégralité, largement épaulés dans cet objectif par le corps médical et l'aura grandissante des maternités. Prenons un dernier exemple avec les séries statistiques de Le Roy pour Hanoi: on constate une progression linéaire et non négligeable du nombre de naissances pour le seul périmètre urbain, passant de 29,3 pour mille en 1923 à 37,6 en 1928, pour finalement atteindre un taux record, voire étonnant, de plus de 49 pour mille en 1936. Taux que certains médecins remettaient d'ailleurs en question en dénonçant les sous-estimations dont avait été victime le recensement de 1936.

77   Même s'il reste à comprendre les prémisses et les logiques de cette acceptation, probablement fluctuantes dans le temps et surtout dans l'espace, dans sa linéarité globale : qu'est-ce qui a décidé les premières citadines à accoucher à l'hôpital? Y avait-il demande de la part des femmes enceintes ou davantage coercition coloniale? Quel rôle ont pu jouer les premiers résultats dans le domaine, l'éducation en milieu scolaire et des jeunes mères?

78   Dr Joyeux, «Organisation de l'hygiène et de la protection de la maternité et de l'enfance à Hanoi», *BSMI* (mai 1934) : 503–522.

Complicating Childhood

Gender, Ethnicity, and "Disadvantage" within the New Zealand Children's Health Camps Movement

œ

Margaret Tennant

Over the first part of the twentieth century, health camps, residential open-air schools, and tuberculosis "preventoria" were presented in many Western societies as models of healthy lifestyles for children, incorporating into their programs wholesome and plentiful food, exposure to sunshine and fresh air, and regular rest and sleep. As sites that captured populations of children for varying periods of time and exposed them to ideal regimes, they also provided a stage on which wider social concerns were acted out. In New Zealand, a children's health camp movement has been in existence for over eighty years, bringing together state medicine and voluntary endeavour in its evolution and administration. Its longevity and high profile within a relatively small nation state with a strong and increasingly vocal indigenous population make it an ideal base from which to study challenges to the undifferentiated category of "the child." Gender and ethnicity were key components of such challenges in New Zealand and are highlighted in this article, but "disadvantage," variously constructed, was also a consideration. Over the twentieth century socio-economic status, race, and gender were respectively suppressed, ignored, and selectively highlighted in the children's health camps movement.

New Zealand's health camps were part of broader international initiatives highlighting personal over environmental health during the early twentieth century: a preventive medicine based upon health education, personal hygiene, and nutrition. School children became a focus of concern and school medical inspection an important adjunct to these health campaigns, as Mona Gleason shows for British Columbia in chapter 10. The New Zealand experience was not unique, and even its health camps were inspired by the example of open-air schools elsewhere. Individual doctors in New Zealand's School Medical Service were aware of the work of Auguste Rollier in treating tuberculosis in the Alpine sun at Leysin, Switzerland, and of an open-air school established at Charlotten-

berg near Berlin in 1904. However, their most direct knowledge was of
the open-air school movement in the United Kingdom, where a number of day and residential open-air schools were in operation by the
end of the First World War. Some such operations functioned initially as
camp schools held under canvas, but all were based upon the idea of
exposing children, especially pre-tuberculous children, to fresh air, sunlight, and a healthy regimen based on personal hygiene and regular
habits. By 1937 there were ninety-six open-air day schools and fifty-
three open-air residential schools in Britain.[1] Similar schools had
emerged in the United States from 1908, along with "preventoria" and
camps aimed at "building children up," redressing existing defects, and
very often inculcating moral values. In many countries, charitable holiday camps for underprivileged city[2] children provided an additional
model, while camping, outdoor activities, and contact with nature had
long been part of the repertoire of youth groups, especially for boys.[3]

All these strands of influence fed into the children's health camp
movement in New Zealand, but in this instance they acquired a distinctive, nationally organized institutional form. Harnessing both state and
voluntary sector resources, children's health camps reached their fullest
expression in the mid-twentieth century, when the open-air school movement had waned in Britain. Health camps developed from 1919 as
short-term summer holiday camps held in the country, at the seaside, or
in some other temporary venue. Supported partly from voluntary donations, they drew on growing government financial and personnel support, and by 1945 had evolved into year-round operations, located in permanent buildings with attached schools. They remain in existence in
six venues, funded overwhelmingly from government contracts.[4] The
heyday of the health camp movement was from the 1940s to the 1960s,
during which time the camps gained iconic status within New Zealand.
A major contributor was the annual health stamp campaign, which saw
the issue of a special postal stamp with a "health" surcharge dedicated
to the camps. This campaign drew upon the resources of youth groups,
service clubs, and schools, as well as New Zealand's Health and Post and
Telegraph Departments and was a predecessor of the now commonplace annual marketing campaigns employed by most national charities.
The stamps, associated films, and other publicity linked the camps with
ideal childhood in New Zealand. Their images were of active, happy, and
until recent times, white-skinned boys and girls playing sport, frolicking
in the sea, and generally enjoying a vigorous outdoor existence. For two
months each year, children's health was promoted as a national issue, and
a campaign, unrivalled until the 1960s by any equivalent peacetime voluntary cause, foregrounded these images in schools, post offices, cine-
mas, and other public spaces. In mid-century "homogenising narratives

of nationhood,"[5] the health camps movement became a fulcrum of concern for childhood. The image of childhood promoted was cosily optimistic and determinedly uncomplicated.

Internationally, a good deal has been written about the transformation and idealization of childhood over the later nineteenth and early twentieth centuries. The boundaries between childhood and adulthood were seen as becoming increasingly firm across social categories, while childhood itself became a distinctive, protected, and sometimes romanticized stage of human development.[6] Over the first half of the twentieth century, "the child" was firmly identified as the key to social betterment. As Roger Cooter has pointed out, this process largely de-sexed children, casting them into a "gender-free zone of attributed innocence,"[7] though notions of childhood were early intersected by class in the British context. In New Zealand, too, variations in socio-economic status were sometimes acknowledged, but as the twentieth century progressed and the welfare state expanded its outreach, such differences were increasingly downplayed. In this former British colony with a Maori population increasing in numbers and in political assertiveness, race was to become a sharper point of intersection after the 1950s—though earlier silences about Maori children were significant in themselves. However, there were moments when gender also posed a challenge to unitary concepts of childhood and where the respective needs of boys and girls were explicitly or implicitly asserted over each other.

As Naomi Rogers points out elsewhere in this volume, the First World War politicized the problem of human resources on a national and international stage. In New Zealand, as elsewhere, there was shock about the rejection rate among army recruits, and a consciousness about the need for a healthy generation to replace those fallen in the war. New Zealand was an Anglo-settler dominion, and "race" effectively meant whiteness of Anglo-Saxon origin, which needed to be defined against racial "others." These others varied according to circumstance.[8] In New Zealand, as in Australia, Anglo-Saxon purity was seen to be threatened by Asian peoples to the north, who were supposedly casting covetous eyes on the Antipodean outreaches of British empire. Internally, there was some paranoia about Asian migrants, but as the majority of New Zealand immigrants were still British, a more insidious threat was identified *within* "the race." As a 1924–25 Committee of Inquiry into Mental Defectives and Sexual Offenders concluded,

New Zealand is a young country already exhibiting some of the weaknesses of much older nations, but it is now at a stage where, if its people are wise, they may escape the worst evils of the Old World. It has been rightly decided that this should be not only a "white man's country," but as completely British as possible. We ought to make every effort to keep the stock sturdy and strong, as well as racially pure....The Great War revealed that from [the] loins [of the pioneers] have sprung some of the finest men the world has ever seen, not only in physical strength, but in character and spirit. It also revealed that an inferior strain had crept in and that New Zealand was already getting its share of weaklings....In these beautiful and richly dowered islands we have a noble heritage—to be in keeping and to ensure the full development of their resources and enjoyment of their blessings the inhabitants should be of the highest type obtainable by human effort.[9]

The eugenicist orientation of the committee is clear in its report, but in New Zealand eugenics always had a strong environmental orientation, with some of its most vocal advocates acknowledging that heredity might be modified by early intervention in a child's rearing.[10] Significantly, half the members of this committee were officials from the School Hygiene, Education and Child Welfare sections of the public service and one, school doctor Ada Paterson, was to be a leading light in the health camps movement.

A number of international studies compare the experiences of indigenous peoples in the face of European settlement, some of them focusing on British settler colonies.[11] Inasmuch as they were included in racial discourses, Maori were perceived as closer to whites than most brown-skinned indigenes, and therefore potential candidates for assimilation with the majority of settler descent. They figured more ambivalently in health treatises than the First Nations people discussed by Gleason in chapter 10 of this volume, for example, since Maori were sometimes commended for their physical stature and racial vigour at the same time as their villages were denounced for lack of hygiene and ability to spread disease. While Maori had lost the best of their lands and had largely been reduced to the position of a rural proletariat by the early twentieth century, Maori values remained strong, as did traditional leadership, despite the emergence of new forms of political expression and new Maori leaders who were conversant with both Maori and Pakeha worlds.[12] To this extent they were in a stronger position than many indigenous peoples after the First World War. Nonetheless, "similarity" and relative proximity to whites on the racial scales of the time was a double-edged sword. Social policy was predicated on the assumption that Maori assimilation into the majority population would occur quite readily. Although at a local level there were attempts at Maori autonomy and self-determination in health service delivery, official policies were increasingly geared to the integration of Maori services.[13] There was a separate Maori Division of the Department of Health in existence under Maori doctor and former parliamentarian Peter Buck (Te Rangi Hiroa) during the 1920s, but it was later disbanded, and from 1930 Maori health was added to the general work of medical officers of health and district nurses. Such "mainstreaming" (as it would now be termed) did little to underline differentials in health status between Maori and Pakeha, though one significant study published in 1935 showed a Maori death rate from tuberculosis ten times that of Pakeha.[14] It also meant that Maori perceptions of health were subordinated to Western medicine, though many of the district nurses did learn to take account of local custom in delivering services.[15]

Ironically, while the first children's health camps were promoted as a major force in the campaign against tuberculosis, Maori children were not targeted as recruits. Where race fused with gender in the consciousness of early organizers, it reflected the concerns about white superiority, numerical and physical. Other writers have commented on women's role in maintaining the racial boundaries of nationhood, both as biological reproducers of racial and ethnic groups and as transmitters of group and cultural ideologies.[16] In New Zealand, as elsewhere, debates about racial efficiency took their most prescriptive form in relation to the mature, fecund female body, but this was one time when they also encompassed the health of pre-pubescent Pakeha girls. Boys needed to grow up fit and strong to defend the British Empire—of which New Zealand was a fiercely loyal component—but girls were its future breeders and, even before puberty, they were never free of their adult destiny. Infant welfare authority Frederic Truby King founded the Plunket Society in 1907 and went on to become one of New Zealand's most vocal child health advocates and director of the Child Welfare Division of the Department of Health in the 1920s.[17] He was just one of those asserting the need for young girls to be kept in the "best possible physical condition"[18] but, as some school doctors were also pointing out at this time, school medical inspections suggested that girls' incidence of "defect" in nearly every category of examination exceeded that of boys. One school doctor, Ada Paterson, pointed out,

In modern civilization the girl is brought up under less favourable circumstances than the boy....In the poorer homes [the girl] has a considerable amount of indoor work, which curtails the time spent out-of-doors. In the better-class homes she is often a victim of parental ambition and is made to spend profitless hours at practising [music] or producing useless fancy-work. Her clothing does not give her the same opportunities for healthy development as does that of the boy.[19]

Health camps were seen as exposing housebound girls, in particular, to outdoor exercise and fresh air, and releasing them from the constraints of domestic tasks and responsibilities. And at a time when the camps were supposed to turn recruits into "health missionaries," who would take new ideals of personal hygiene and good habits back into the

family setting, girls were considered the more effective promulgators
of such doctrines, both as children and as future mothers.

It is worth noting that while Paterson peripherally acknowledged
socio-economic differences in this report, she and other school doctors
increasingly underplayed their importance to child health in the New
Zealand context. Some of the first, informal health camps of the 1920s
and 1930s were certainly run by committees of local worthies who saw
themselves as providing holidays for the poor. However, parental consent was needed for a health camp stay, and any charitable connotations
were soon suppressed as discouraging parents' cooperation. Official discourses increasingly presented "needy children" as coming from all sections of the community and, as the prime agents of health camp selec-
tion, school doctors and nurses made a point of sending children from
a range of social backgrounds.[20] Paterson was later to insist, "Extremes
of poverty and riches found in older lands and incidental to industrial-
ism are absent [in New Zealand], the necessities for healthy growth being
available for almost all,"[21] and even in the Depression she publicly attributed poor nutrition to maternal mismanagement.[22] Disadvantage was represented by Paterson and her successors in the movement as a matter of
rearing rather than resources. No child was exempt from inadequate
mothering, and here the lifestyle education of girls was critical.

The first children's health camps of the 1920s seem to have taken
in boys and girls in roughly equal numbers, both sexes participating in
vigorous outdoor activities inspired by military routine and precedents.
(This replicated the usual pattern in New Zealand primary schools of the
time, which were overwhelmingly coeducational.) But it is significant
that the few single-sex camps were for girls, and were run in the 1930s
by the Christchurch-based Sunlight League. Inspired by the British association of the same name, the Sunlight League wrote admiringly of Nazi
attempts to restrict the procreation of the unfit, but generally placed a
stronger emphasis upon positive eugenics and exposure to sunlight and
fresh air.[23]

The local leader of the Sunlight League, Cora Wilding, went in for
small-scale health camps that catered for girls aged nine to twelve.
Accused of discriminating against boys, Wilding defended all-girl camps
on the basis that girls would in future have the main work of teaching
laws of health and physical fitness to succeeding generations. As she
pointed out, they had less opportunity than their brothers to enjoy
camping and outdoor life in the normal course of events.[24] In later years
the sheer physicality of the health camp routine was criticized for failing to meet the needs of children of a more contemplative bent, and girls
in particular. In the interwar period it was seen as releasing girls from
the gendered constraints of their normal existence.

← M/female difs

Nonetheless, the protests at all-girl camps anticipated a shift in the discourse about child health over the next decade. Despite advocating all-girl health camps in the 1930s, Cora Wilding participated in a more general shift in emphasis that came with the Second World War and with the advent of permanent, year-round health camps. Acknowledging that the first camps had been for girls as "mothers of the future," she explained in the mid-1940s that changed conditions had made *boys'* camps the more important. Boys at an impressionable age missed the influence of fathers on service overseas, she explained, and boys' camps, run by the right kind of man, would provide excellent training grounds in the democratic principles believed necessary in the postwar era. While school doctors some twenty years earlier had highlighted the inferior health of school girls, by 1940 their annual reports were supplying statistical evidence that boys' nutritional status was the poorer.[25] One newspaper commented in 1944 that the overwhelming predominance of boys on health camp waiting lists confirmed a popular belief that little boys were "harder to rear" than girls.[26] The First World War and racial discourses of the interwar period had seemed to foreground the importance of the female body—including the pre-pubescent female body—as the bearer of future generations, but the Second World War coincided with closer attention to the health and well-being of boys. Boys' future participation in public life made them the more effective vehicles for the optimistic, democratic values of the postwar era. There may also have been another factor operating here: the mid-century has been seen as a period of increasing anxieties about the male role in New Zealand. As society became more urbanized and distanced from the "pioneering" period, as distinctive male enclaves were restricted and controlled, and more and more New Zealand men saw themselves locked into the breadwinner role, definitions of masculinity became more complicated. Boys were variously future leaders and family men or, more problematically, delinquents or possible homosexuals.[27]

This development was tied up with broader definitions of health, which became firmly established over the mid-century. Admissions to health camp were justified less exclusively on physical grounds and began to take on behavioural dimensions of well-being.[28] Associated with this change was a decline in the reported incidence of physical disorders such as tuberculosis and other infectious diseases and, with antibiotics, alternative ways of treating them. Nationwide height–weight surveys of primary school children also suggested improved standards of nutrition.[29] Broader conceptions of health reflected international trends for a wider range of professional "experts" to have access to school-aged children, most particularly through child guidance and psychological clinics. Such clinics were first established in the United States in the late

1900s and in Britain over the 1920s, with New Zealand facilities opening from the late 1930s. A special committee was convened by the
national board of the children's health camps movement in 1957 to consider the implications of an apparently changing clientele, and it recommended that better quality staff be sought to handle intakes that included
"emotionally disturbed" children. In his evidence to the committee,
New Zealand's director-general of Health estimated that health camps
had a mixed clientele, which was approximately 50 per cent physically
debilitated and 50 per cent emotionally disturbed.[30] The conceptualization of the healthy child now included a sturdy mind as well as a sturdy
body—the potential health camp recruit was as likely to display a problematic psyche as a physical ailment, and to be identified as coming
from a home in some way disordered.

Boys appear to have dominated waiting lists for a health camp placement from the 1940s to the present day.[31] However, most of the permanent health camps were built with equal numbers of beds for boys and
girls (the exception was the last to be opened, in 1983, which had two
boys' units and only one for girls). Before the 1980s there was surprisingly little analysis of this disproportion. Statistics on admissions were
seldom broken down by gender, and complex cases were usually translated into health terms, the vague classification of "debility" providing
a useful catch-all for statistical purposes. But case materials from the
mid-century suggest a growing preoccupation with the inappropriate
home and classroom behaviour of boy recruits to health camp, in particular. In the 1940s and 1950s this frequently encompassed concern
about insufficiently masculine behaviours, characterized by "nervous-
ness" and excessive tears, clinging to adults, and generally "sissy" or
effeminate behaviour, some of which was blamed upon mothers' own
nervous tension and possessive behaviour. It reflected insecurities about
the male role mentioned earlier.

Health camps files provide examples: "Martin" was an eleven-year-
old boy selected by a local public health nurse in 1955 to go to a South
Island health camp. Martin was recommended for health camp because
he was highly emotional, found school life a severe strain, and was frequently reduced to tears. His father was described only as a dairy farmer,
and his mother—by implication the cause of Martin's problems—as a
"tense, energetic woman of spare frame and severe mien—whose life
was a continuous frantic cycle from cow-shed to farm-yard to house and
children and back again." The report noted that "her standards for her
children appeared always a little beyond their capabilities or rather
impressed the boys with a sense of inadequacy." She provided good
nourishing food but "anxious urging destroyed appetites and the possibility of failing to meet the standard at school gave restless nights." Mar-

tin was listless and uncooperative at school and burst into tears on the slightest provocation.

As a result of a health camp stay, the public health nurse reported that Martin was much less easily upset than previously, had realized his abilities and the benefits of helping the teacher and being an example to younger boys. He was still among the academic plodders in class but was no longer crushed by this state. The opportunity of community life in health camp, and of seeing others less fortunate than himself was said to have given him a "broader and steadier" approach to his problems. But significantly, the mother had also seen the light and, the report said, was less openly critical of her "nervy children" instead extolling their prowess at athletics. The case says as much about the pressure on a rural mother to be a virtually full-time farm worker while meeting new standards of motherhood, as it does about the child. Here, as in so many of the cases of the time, the mother was said to have learnt about the management of her own child, who had returned from health camp no longer "nervous and emotional" but a "real boy."[32]

By the 1960s and 1970s concern focused more on the *excessive* masculinity of boy recruits to health camps, manifest in aggression and destructiveness. There was a marked increase in reports of breakages, "hooliganism," and absconding from health camps over the period.[33] Health camp managers complained about unbalanced intakes of children, with too many instances of behaviour problems among them, as both parents and teachers sought a period of relief from difficult children. The gender dimension of the situation was barely touched upon in the health camps' published reports, though matrons' notes and registers were often more specific: "The boys were a very difficult group, many breakages of furniture"; "It has been a pleasure to have this group of girls, no problems at all with them. Most of the boys have been a very trying group, with many behaviour problems."[34] It was not until a ministerial inquiry into the health camp movement was initiated in 1983 that gender was officially problematized as an issue the movement would have to deal with. This, the so-called "Hancock Inquiry," was headed by a former child welfare officer, university lecturer, and private counsellor who was also heavily involved in the Men against Violence movement and was influenced by feminist analyses of gender inequities. It took place in an environment where discrimination against women was being recognized within official agencies and at a stage when sexual abuse was being identified as a child welfare issue. In terms of an ongoing subtext within the movement, it is worth noting that the inquiry also took place against a background of declining real incomes for low-income families, and that this was highlighted as a matter of concern in the report. However, the suggestion of possible socio-economic differentials in health camp intakes was politically unpopular and continued to be down-played in broader publicity.[35] Dependent as it was on government fund-ing, the health camps movement could not afford to be the centre of debate on government policies inimical to the interests of children.

By the 1980s more complete statistics were being kept on health camp intakes. The 1984 Hancock report noted a significant difference between the sexes in reasons for health camp referral, with boys being referred for behavioural problems and girls for such family reasons as parental illness and stress or family tension. In other words, girls were being admitted for reasons outside themselves, while boys were more likely to be seen as the cause of their own admission, and to be exposed to specialist programs to deal with their problem. Where camps had a 50:50 admission quota, public health nurses frequently had trouble fill-ing beds for girls and were sending them on less well-substantiated grounds. But the inquiry also suggested that the demand for services for boys was so strong that it may have been masking girls' real needs, that the pattern of upbringing in New Zealand households made their behav-iour at home and in schools less demanding. In this situation, the inquiry suggested, the needs of depressed or unhappy girls may have been over-looked. The inquiry suggested the need for differential responses to boys' and girls' health requirements and occasional separate camps for boys and girls where demand existed.[36] It is worth noting that where the latter recommendation was implemented, it usually involved health camps held solely for boys in an attempt to reduce waiting lists, and that experiences of all-boy camps in the 1990s were considered so dif-ficult for staff that camp managers often declined further such experi-ments. Health camps, like other agencies, came to share in the flourish-ing "anger management" industry, and girls continued to be regarded as a moderating influence on male behaviour.

The 1984 inquiry pointed to another dimension that the health camps had often ignored in their publicity as well as practice: the chang-ing ethnicity of health camp recruits. This development, even more than gender, had come to undermine the cosily inclusive categoriza-tion of childhood promulgated in health camp publicity. As noted ear-lier, the movement's origins were firmly embedded in a particular con-ception of race that, if it did not specifically exclude Maori, certainly did not embrace Maori childhood. An episode at one of the first children's health camps, at a North Island beachfront site in 1929, encapsulates their Pakeha orientation. As the girls paddled or washed their hair in a nearby stream, and the boys "played red indians" and mounted raiding parties in the hills, "Good-natured Maoris came from the neighbourhood to conduct a haangi [Maori oven]." The Maori cooked a meal for the chil-dren and "gave folk songs and a war cry," their leader, Mr. Ngakihi

Tamihana, expressing pleasure at being able to help European children. His party donated fruit, vegetables, and eggs to the camp, and endowed it with a Maori name after an ancestor of their people.[37] Interestingly, this exchange undercuts some of the usual paternalist assumptions about interactions between Maori and Pakeha: here it is Maori acting as donor to European children perceived in need of help; it is Maori giving permission, in effect, for the use of the area, and stamping their authority by conceding a Maori name for the camp. But the perception by Maori and Pakeha alike is of the camp as a Pakeha enterprise.

Nonetheless, as Maori urbanization accelerated over subsequent decades and Maori came under school medical inspection, even in rural areas, more Maori children were selected by district nurses for a stay in health camp.[38] Their "Maoriness" was seldom acknowledged, only Maori names in case notes indicating that certain children might somehow be different from the main body of recruits. Where the admission of Maori children drew comment at the national Health Camps Board level, it was simply to endorse broader policy goals of integrating Maori into the Pakeha mainstream. As early as 1937 the board had rejected holding separate camps for Maori children, and administrators agreed in subsequent years that it was mutually advantageous for Maori and Pakeha children to be admitted to camps together.[39] The camps' already strong socialization function took on an assimilationist thrust, and where reports did acknowledge Maori entrants to health camps, it was to commend their adoption of approved habits. Occasionally case reports noted with satisfaction how Maori-speaking children left camp chattering away in English.[40] For public consumption, however, the inclusion of Maori children was deliberately underplayed: as one medical officer of health privately warned the Health Camps Board in 1957, there was a need to tread warily lest a stigma be attached to the camps, either from their charitable associations, from the reflection they were seen to cast on mothers of children selected, or from a "race consciousness, as in some quarters there is the perception that camps are primarily for undernourished Maoris of the worst type."[41] A national consensus about the importance of child health and welfare depended upon the erasing of difference and simplistic responses to problems when they became apparent.

Health camps consequently played their part in perpetuating mid-century ideals of New Zealand as a classless and raceless society where Maori and Pakeha were equal, largely by rendering invisible the Maori needs, culture, and differentials in well-being. This went along with a muting of earlier Pakeha claims to Anglo-Saxon identity. By the mid-century,

No one thought of New Zealand identity in "racial" terms as White. New Zealand society and Pākeha culture were valued for their own sake as normal and necessary, without requiring any justification along racial or ethic grounds....It would take a more concerted effort to pry open the realisation that New Zealand identity was inextricably linked with European culture, infused with colonialist assumptions, overwhelmingly White in orientation, and larded with self-serving myths.[42]

The concept of "whiteness" was soon to be reasserted, but in a critical mode that overturned earlier, celebratory usage of the term.

In the 1980s the children's health camp movement was just one of a number of longstanding institutions caught up in what has been termed the "sovereignty bombshell."[43] Ever since the nineteenth century, Maori tribes had protested loss of land and autonomy, though armed conflict had largely subsided by the 1870s. In the later twentieth century a stronger Maori (as opposed to tribal) identity emerged from participation in the war effort during the 1940s, and from the subsequent migration of more than 75 per cent of the Maori population from rural tribal areas to towns and cities.[44] Led mostly by young urban radicals, some of them well-educated and with experience in the union movement, modern Maori activism was expressed in a number of ways: a nationwide petition to have the Maori language taught in primary and secondary schools, land occupations, and a major land march in 1975.[45] The initial focus on land grievances took an even sharper turn in the following decade with claims that ranged from an end to Pakeha monoculturalism, to absolute Maori ownership of New Zealand. This was part of a broader, international assertion of indigenous rights challenging white settler governance in the most fundamental ways. Although Maori protests reflected global trends, they also included elements that were embedded in New Zealand's past, most particularly a grounding in New Zealand's "foundation document," the Treaty of Waitangi.[46] The treaty, signed in 1840 by Maori chiefs and representatives of the British Crown, accorded British citizenship and gave other significant guarantees to Maori in exchange for Crown authority. While treaties were signed with indigenous peoples elsewhere, as Ken Coates has pointed out they did not generally involve "negotiated rights, established between two sovereign powers and designed to forge lasting relationships," as did the Treaty of Waitangi—in theory at least.[47] In the years following 1840, the treaty was often ignored, but in the 1980s it was strongly reasserted as the basis of New Zealand's ethno-politics. One consequence of its authority was the privileging of biculturalism as official policy at a time when Australia and Canada, countries with more diverse immigrant populations, were moving towards multiculturalism.[48] Although challenged from some quarters, biculturalism in New Zealand acknowledged contemporary Maori and Pakeha as descendants of the treaty signatories. Indigenous rights were defined as Maori rights, though at various times and on various issues, the notion of a Maori collectivity was contested by tribal ethnicity and identification. The situation reflected "a clearly identifiable cultural homogeneity, expressed in a commonality of language and customary practice" among Maori, compared with First Nations peoples elsewhere.[49] Although losing much of their land, Maori had not been placed in reservations, had political representation, and represented a higher proportion of the total population than indigenous populations in Australia and Canada, for example—all factors affecting attempts to improve Maori health status.[50]

This summarizes in very simple form developments and debates that have generated an enormous literature, judicial and political processes, and a good deal of institutional and personal angst in recent years. What did they mean for an established organization dealing with children's health and well-being, a body that was already accused of being stuck in the 1950s? The Maori language version of the Treaty of Waitangi, which, translated, is broader than the English, saw Maori accepting Crown authority in return for a guarantee of *te tino rangatiratanga*, or chieftainship, and *taonga katoa*, loosely translated as "treasures" or "all things precious."[51] *Te tino rangatiratanga* came to be equated with Maori autonomy and control over issues concerning Maori, including social policy concerns, while the term *taonga* was taken to include cultural as well as material properties,[52] and was extended to children, language, and health. The "ownership" of Maori children was especially contested in the child welfare field, but their removal from *whanau* (extended family) even for a temporary stay in a health camp was also questioned. Following the 1988 report of a Royal Commission on Social Policy, three key principles were seen as linking the Treaty of Waitangi and government social policy: the principles of partnership, participation, and protection. All of this had implications for children's health camps, which, like other bodies in receipt of government funding, were vulnerable to accusations of "institutional racism," and were required to assume a commitment to treaty principles over the 1980s and 1990s.

While the 1984 Hancock inquiry into children's health camps had not directly referred to the treaty, it had certainly identified a lack of Maori input to the movement: a lack of partnership in consultation over policy, negligible Maori participation in camp management, and little that was deliberately targeted towards the protection of either Maori children's health or their culture.[53] The report had also foregrounded the changing ethnicity of health camp intakes, showing that whereas 12.5 per cent of the population in the five-to-twelve-year age group was Maori, 33 per cent of those entering health camps in early 1983 were Maori (and 6 per cent, mostly those attending the Auckland health camp, were from Pacific Island backgrounds).[54] Maori and Pacific Island children differed from European children entering health camps on a number of counts. They were more likely to be living with a family member other than a biological parent, came from larger families on average, and from homes characterized by referral agencies as having poor hygiene, nutrition, or home management, or as being overcrowded.[55] The supporting study on which these conclusions were based noted that health camp recording systems were largely silent on the subject of ethnicity, only one camp specifically including the information on its admission form. When approached to supply information, some districts were reluctant to do so, fearing to be labelled "racist" merely by recording such details. "Unfortunately," it noted, "a frequent corollary of this perspective is the notion that all children, whether Pakeha or Polynesian, should be treated the same. Inevitably, the ethnocentric view of the dominant culture determines the manner in which children will be treated."[56]

From the mid-1980s, then, the ethnicity of children admitted to health camp, and of Maori children in particular, became an issue. The all-inclusiveness of the category of "child" was officially fractured and the cultural homogeneity of the health camp experience publicly challenged. Maori—and to a lesser extent, Pacific Island—children became visible, literally and figuratively: for the first time, health stamps showed children of markedly darker hue, and posters and other publicity included children of obvious Polynesian descent. The response at health camp level varied according to the ethnicity of local intakes. At the Gisborne camp, on the east coast of the North Island, as many as 60 per cent of children were Maori, and attempts to make the camp a comfortable environment for Maori children preceded the Hancock report.[57] The camp was adopted by a local Maori community, representatives from the local Department of Maori Affairs were included in case discussions over the 1980s, and by 1990 a *kohanga reo* or Maori language pre-school was based at the health camp. Other camps gained funding for a *kaumatua* or elder, or a Maori field worker to liaise with Maori parents and local *marae*, and there were attempts to employ Maori staff in positions other than domestic.[58]

At national Health Camps Board level, the response was slow, but it was hastened by a government shift away from deficit funding through the Health Department to more competitive funding models in the early 1990s. As has happened among First Nations peoples in Canada,[59] tribally based Maori authorities successfully claimed government funding for their own, autonomous ventures. Other organizations wanting a share in government health revenues had to demonstrate a commitment to treaty principles. Contracts signed between the Children's Health Camps and government health funding authorities in the 1990s required the camps to "apply the principles of partnership, participation and active protection of Maori interest in their management, employment and service delivery policies and practise."[60] Reference to the treaty was made in the service requirements and was expected in the inevitable mission statements issued from the late 1980s. The Children's Health Camps Board began to speak of "holistic" conceptions of health, which were seen to be in keeping with a Maori integration of the spiritual and physical, to emphasize the movement's "long, close and positive" relationship with Maori, and its delivery of programs in a "culturally appropriate manner."[61] Within the camps the visibility of Maori children was now an asset to the movement, an avenue to continued funding, and an indicator of the camps' relevance to contemporary New Zealand. Ethnicity overshadowed gender as an issue of concern, and although a majority of male Maori children was sometimes implied, ethnicity and gender were not correlated. A 1999 evaluation of children's health camps for the government's Health Funding Authority gave no gender breakdown of intakes, instead constructing "equity" as a rural–urban access issue or as one relating to Maori health.[62] The report mentioned only in passing that 29 per cent of health camp children lived with two parents and that the principal source of income for 56 per cent of attendees' households was a social welfare benefit.[63]

As an organization existing for more than eighty years, one that is still "a national icon well loved by politicians and supported by local voluntary action groups"[64]—as even its critics reluctantly concede—the children's health camps movement illustrates many broader themes in New Zealand society writ small. Not least, it shows changing conceptions of health over time, as reasons for referral shifted from risk of tuberculosis and nutritional deficiency to behavioural problems and mental and emotional health. But from the perspective of this article, the movement shows how a blanket categorization of "childhood" was challenged at certain moments in the movement's development, by gender, and later, and more substantially, by an appreciation of the ethnicity of health camp recruits. "Disadvantage" was a constant subtext, but its link with socio-economic status was muddied by reference to inadequate parenting, "overenthusiastic" or anxious mothers, the continued referral of children from relatively comfortable homes, and the suppression of poverty in official health camp discourses. Disadvantage could take various forms, and gender was highlighted first in the 1920s and 1930s, when girls' health needs were informed by (white) racial anxieties. Thereafter the physical and mental health needs of boys underwrote health camp recruitment procedures and programs, even if it was not always formally acknowledged. It was not until the 1980s that an official inquiry influenced by feminist concerns recommended differential responses to boys' and girls' health needs, in the same way that the special health needs of women had been recognized. But gender was quickly subordinated to the growing focus on Treaty of Waitangi issues and relationships of Maori to social services. Official policies of biculturalism and the need for accountability with regard to treaty principles saw Maori children become visible in New Zealand's health camps as never before.

In the long run, this more recent fracturing of childhood has created problems for health camps as a national organization receiving over $NZ7.2 million annually from government. The success of the movement and its high public profile over the mid-twentieth century were based on a highly unitary conception of childhood and an uncomplicated view of child health. This meshed well with the tranquil discourses of mid-century New Zealand as a homogeneous society where children were supposedly better off than anywhere else in the world—and if they were not, matters could readily be put in order through mass health camp intakes and exposure to a simple routine of sleep, good food, and fresh air. The acknowledgement of children's varying health needs and ethnic and socio-economic status, and the suggestion that boys' and girls' requirements may be different raised the prospect of specialist programs better provided by competing agencies. More generally, it has led to decreased optimism about children's health and undermined consensus about appropriate solutions. The complicating of childhood has led to a multiplicity of responses to health needs and ongoing debates about the appropriate targeting of funds on the basis of ethnicity or "need."[65]

Notes

1 Linda Bryder, *Below the Magic Mountain: A Social History of Tubercolosis in Twentieth-Century Britain* (Oxford: Oxford University Press, 1988), 148. See also Linda Bryder, "'Wonderlands of Buttercup, Clover and Daisies': Tuberculosis and the Open-Air School Movement in Britain, 1907–39," in *In the Name of the Child: Health and Welfare, 1880–1940*, ed. Roger Cooter (London: Routledge, 1992), 72–95.

2 Barbara Bates, *Bargaining for Life: A Social History of Tuberculosis, 1876–1938* (Philadelphia: University of Pennsylvania Press, 1992), 273–78.

3 Colin Ward and Dennis Hardy, *Goodnight Campers! The History of the British Holiday Camp* (London: Mansell, 1986), 1–8.

4 For a survey of the movement's early years, see Margaret Tennant, "Children's Health Camps in New Zealand: The Making of a Movement, 1919–1940," *Social History of Medicine* 1 (1996): 69–87.

5 Radhika Mohanram, "(In)visible Bodies? Immigrant Bodies and Constructions of Nationhood in Aoteroa, New Zealand," in *Feminist Thought in Aotearoa/New Zealand*, ed. Rosemary du Plessis and Lynne Alice (Auckland: Oxford University Press, 1998), 24.

6 For a review of this in the Canadian context, see Robert McIntosh, "Constructing the Child: New Approaches to the History of Childhood in Canada," *Acadiensis* 28, 2 (Spring 1999): 126–40. An early but key work discussing this process in New Zealand is Dugald McDonald, "Children and Young Persons in New Zealand Society," in *Families in New Zealand Society*, ed. Peggy G. Koopman-Boy-

den (Wellington: Methuen, 1978), 44–56. A more recent history of child welfare also touches on the construction of New Zealand childhood: Bronwyn Dalley, *Family Matters: Child Welfare in Twentieth-Century New Zealand* (Auckland: Auckland University Press, 1998).

7 Roger Cooter, *In the Name of the Child: Health and Welfare 1880–1940* (London: Routledge, 1992), 9.

8 For a useful discussion of this in the Canadian context, see Mariana Valverde, *The Age of Light, Soap and Water: Moral Reform in English Canada 1885–1925* (Toronto: McClelland and Stewart, 1991), chap. 5; and Angus McLaren, *Our Own Master Race: Eugenics in Canada, 1885–1945* (Toronto: McClelland and Stewart, 1990), chap. 3

9 New Zealand Committee of Inquiry into Mental Defectives and Sexual Offenders, "Report of Committee of Inquiry into Mental Defectives and Sexual Offenders," *Appendices to the Journals, House of Representatives* (1925), H-31A, 28.

10 Philip Fleming, "Eugenics in New Zealand 1900–1940" (MA thesis, Massey University, 1981).

11 For earlier comparisons between Maori and First Nations peoples in Australia and Canada, see, for example, Robin Fisher, "The Impact of European Settlement on the Indigenous Peoples of Australia, New Zealand and British Columbia: Some Comparative Dimensions," *Canadian Ethnic Studies* 12, 1 (1980): 1–14; for a comparison with Australia, K. R. Howe, *Race Relations: Australia and New Zealand* (Wellington/Sydney: Methuen, 1977); for more recent works published within New Zealand, see Ken S. Coates, "International Perspectives on Relations with Indigenous Peoples," in *Living Relationships/Kōriki Ngātahi: The Treaty of Waitangi in the New Millennium*, ed. Ken S. Coates and P. G. McHugh, 19–103 (Wellington: Victoria University Press, 1998); Paul Havemann, *Indigenous Peoples' Rights in Australia, Canada and New Zealand* (Auckland: Oxford University Press, 1999).

12 The term *Pakeha* is commonly used in New Zealand to refer to non-Maori persons of European descent.

13 Mason Durie, *Whaiora: Maori Health Development* (Auckland: Oxford University Press, 1994), 43, 47.

14 Derek Dow, *Safeguarding the Public Health: A History of the New Zealand Department of Health* (Wellington: Victoria University Press, 1995), 119. See also Derek Dow, *Maori Health and Government Policy 1840–1940* (Wellington: Victoria University Press, 1999). Earlier comparative work by the author of the tuberculosis study, H. B. Turbott, suggested Maori superiority over European children in physique and dental hygiene, but a higher Maori incidence of conditions linked with indigence, poor diet, and poor housing, most especially infectious skin, eye, and ear disease, along with respiratory disease. "Maori and Pakeha: A Preliminary Study in Comparative Health," *Appendices to the Journals, House of Representatives* (1929), H-31, 73–74.

15 For a discussion of changing interests in Maori health, see Derek Dow, "Driving Their Own Health Canoe: Maori and Health Research," in *Past Judgement: Social Policy in New Zealand History*, ed. Bronwyn Dalley and Margaret Tennant (Dunedin: Otago University Press, 2004), 91–107 .

16 Mohanram, "(In)visible bodies?" 23; see also Nira Yuval-Davis and Floya Anthias, *Woman-Nation-State* (London: Macmillan, 1989).

17 Linda Bryder, *A Voice for Mothers: The Plunket Society and Infant Welfare 1907–2000* (Auckland: Auckland University Press, 2003), 8–17.

18 F. Truby King, "Education and Eugenics," *Australasian Medical Congress: Transactions of the Tenth Session* (1914), 84–85.

19 Department of Education, "Annual Report," *Appendices to the Journals, House of Representatives* (1916), E-2, Appendix F, iv.
20 This is reinforced by oral evidence and written recollections gathered in the course of my research, where informants who regarded themselves as from comfortable homes reported being sent to health camp for reasons that mystified them and seemed to have been taken personally by their mothers.
21 Department of Health, "Physical Growth and Mental Attainment: New Zealand School-Children," Appendix to Annual Report, *Appendices to the Journals, House of Representatives* (1927), H-31, 61.
22 "Address by A. Paterson to School Committees Association, September 21, 1932," H1 35/70 (B.11), Archives New Zealand, Wellington [hereafter ANZ].
23 S. K. Wilson, "The Aims and Ideology of Cora Wilding and the Sunlight League 1930–36" (master's extended essay, Canterbury University, 1980).
24 Draft of letter [1936?], Cora Wilding Papers, 1.7, University of Canterbury Library.
25 Department of Health, "Annual Report," *Appendices to the Journals, House of Representatives* (1939), H-31, part 3, 42.
26 Unidentified press cutting [1944], Press Cuttings Book, Roxburgh Health Camp Records, Roxburgh.
27 On this, see a key work in the history of masculinity in New Zealand: Jock Phillips, *A Man's Country? The Image of the Pakeha Male: A History* (Auckland: Penguin Books, 1997).
28 This conclusion is based upon comments in health camp annual reports, intermittent series of registers from the Roxburgh, Pakuranga, and Gisborne camps, unpublished reports undertaken by medical students and other professionals, Health Department memos, and a 1957 Committee on Children's Health Camps, which was established especially to consider the question of a changing clientele and how best to respond to this more varied intake. See "Committee on Children's Health Camps," 1957, H1 261/3 (26743), ANZ.
29 For example, a 1954 survey suggested that a fifteen-year-old boy was, on average, 100 mm taller than his counterpart in 1934. See H1 35/37 (33808), ANZ.
30 H. B. Turbott to Committee on Children's Health Camps, 1957, H1 261/3 (26743), ANZ.
31 Health Camp annual reports occasionally refer to "catch up," all-boy camps held in an attempt to reduce the number of boys on the waiting lists, and references to more applications for boys than girls are numerous. See, for example, *Eleventh Annual Report of Wellington Children's Health Camp Association* (1945), 4, Alexander Turnbull Library, Wellington; "Matron's Report to Maunu Health Camp Committee, March 12, 1947," Maunu Children's Health Camp, Whangarei; "Report on Pakuranga Health Camp by Dr S. Godfrey, June 6, 1973"; and "Report on Otaki Health Camp," *Annual Report, Children's Health Camp Board* (1980), 7, Te Puna Whaiora, Children's Health Camps, Wellington; Committee to Review the Children's Health Camps Movement, *Children's Health, Tomorrow's Wealth* (Wellington: Department of Health, 1984), 53.
32 "Glenelg Follow Up by Nurse Inspector," 1955, H1 261/16 (31850), ANZ.
33 See, for example, "Medical Officer's Report on Otaki Health Camp," April 12, 1965, J. Murphy to medical officer of health, March 3, 1965, H1 263/2 (32851), ANZ.
34 Quotes from Gisborne Children's Health Camp Register, 1941–1976, matron's comments on intake, June 18, 1970 and November 4, 1975.
35 M. Hancock, interviewed by M. Tennant, June 5, 1991.

36 *Children's Health, Tomorrow's Wealth* (Wellington: Department of Health, 1984), 53.
37 *Auckland Star*, January 7, 1929, reprinted 1944. Education Department files, Waikato Museum.
38 Although more heavily concentrated in some parts of New Zealand than others, Maori had never been shifted into reservations. In 1951, 19 per cent of Maori lived in boroughs and cities; by the 1970s this figure had increased to 75 per cent. See Ranginui J. Walker, "Māori People since 1950," in *The Oxford History of New Zealand*, ed. Geoffrey W. Rice (Auckland: Oxford University Press, 1992), 500–503.
39 Secretary, Auckland Central Council, to Dominion Advisory Board, Children's Health Camps, November 12, 1937, H1 262 (16969), ANZ.
40 See case materials, H1 261/18, ANZ.
41 J. D. Murray to director-general of health, August 22, 1957, H1 261/22 (50520), ANZ.
42 Augie Fleras and Paul Spoonley, *Recalling Aotearoa: Indigenous Politics and Ethnic Relations in New Zealand* (Auckland: Oxford University Press, 1999), 43.
43 Fleras and Spoonley, *Recalling Aotearoa*, 45.
44 Walker, "Maori People," 519.
45 Walker, "Maori People," 511–13.
46 Coates, "International Perspectives," 19–21.
47 Coates, "International Perspectives," 30.
48 Fleras and Spoonley, *Recalling Aotearoa*, 232–36.
49 Fleras and Spoonley, *Recalling Aotearoa*, 31.
50 On this, see Susan J. Elliott and Leslie T. Foster, "Mind-Body-Place: A Geography of Aboriginal Health in British Columbia," in *A Persistent Spirit: Towards Understanding Aboriginal Health in British Columbia*, ed. Peter H. Stephenson, Susan J. Elliott, Leslie T. Foster, and Jill Harris (Victoria: University of Victoria Western Geographical Press, 1995), 95–127.
51 Durie, *Whaiora*, 48; and Mark Barrett and Kim Connolly-Stone, "The Treaty of Waitangi and Social Policy," *Social Policy Journal of New Zealand* 11 (December 1998): 31.
52 Durie, *Whaiora*, 84.
53 *Children's Health*, 51.
54 *Children's Health*, 22.
55 *Children's Health*, 26–27.
56 Mary Routledge and Craig Johnston, *Going to Health Camp: An Investigation of the Referral and Follow-up Process* (Wellington: Department of Health, 1984), 38.
57 See [Wellington: Children's Health Camps Board] *Annual Report, Children's Health Camps Board* (1983), 11.
58 Information taken from [Wellington: Children's Health Camps Board] *Annual Report, Children's Health Camps Board*, 1984–1998.
59 James B. Waldram, D. Ann Herring, and T. Kue Young, *Aboriginal Health in Canada: Historical, Cultural, and Epidemiological Perspectives* (Toronto: University of Toronto Press, 1995), chap. 10; and Mary-Ellen Kelm, *Colonizing Bodies: Aboriginal Health and Healing British Columbia 1900–50* (Vancouver: UBC Press, 1998), 178.
60 Felicity Dumble, *An Evaluation of New Zealand's Children's Health Camps against the HFA's [Health Funding Authority's] Prioritisation Principles* (Hamilton: Health Funding Authority, 1999), 11.
61 See, for example, pamphlet entitled *Health Camps: "The Modern Perspective,"* Wellington: Children's Health Camps Board, 1999.
62 Dumble, *An Evaluation*, 10–11.

63 Dumble, *An Evaluation*, 5.
64 Dumble, *An Evaluation*, 5.
65 In 2000 new health legislation proposed by New Zealand's Labour government included a controversial Treaty of Waitangi clause, which was denounced by opponents as guaranteeing indigenous people superior levels of health care on the basis of indigeneity rather than need, and giving Maori a basis for litigation against the government if Maori health indicators continue to lag behind those of the rest of the population. Backlash against the proposal from the predominantly Pakeha population caused the government to back away from the scheme and to quickly drop its title of "Closing the Gaps" from policy papers and statements. Ian Templeton, "Balancing act to close the gaps," *Sunday Star-Times*, September 10, 2000, C2.

Race, Class, and Health
School Medical Inspection and "Healthy" Children in British Columbia, 1890–1930

CR

Mona Gleason

Introduction

P ublic health reform in British Columbian schools at the turn of the twentieth century reflected the values and priorities of white middle-class professionals. First Nations children on the Inkameep Reserve in the early 1930s, for example, learned that "good health" meant conforming to the expectations of the dominant society. As the school nurse at Inkameep remarked, "Health lessons are necessarily very elemental when one remembers that most of the children have previously never seen a tooth-brush, a bath-tub was unheard of, and a balanced diet beyond the limits of imagination....Surely our chief aim in this special branch of our work is to help develop the Indian into a healthy, respectable, self-supporting citizen."[1] Such connections between health and social acceptance worked to legitimize dominant–subordinate relations in the province in the early decades of the twentieth century.[2]

This study explores how and which standards of health identified by medical and educational professionals were applied to children. Like Myra Rutherdale's focus on northern missionaries' health initiatives and Margaret Tennant's work on health camps for New Zealand children in this volume, I focus on school medical inspection as a window on the social process of "constructing" healthy children. Within the context of the history of public health reform in British Columbia, I investigate what the crusade to encourage clean, disease-free school children reveals about the social construction of health. In particular, I am interested in how race and class mattered in this construction. Second, I evaluate the gaps and contradictions in what public health reformers claimed for children, their families, and their health, and what their work in British Columbian schools actually meant for students, parents, and teachers. As my analysis will show, school medical inspection attempted to "discipline" children by pathologizing those whose race, class, and location put them beyond the boundaries of white middle-class urban British Columbia.[3] In response, and often constrained by racism, classism, and sexism, children and their families found ways to variously accommodate, resist, and ignore the health demands placed upon them.

Prevention, Surveillance, and Race: The Origins of Public Health Reform

The Public Health Act of British Columbia, passed in 1893, was not proclaimed until 1895.[4] The government nominated five male doctors as the Provincial Board of Health. The Public Health Act provided for sanitary surveillance and intervention by local boards of health mandated for each municipality.[5] White, middle-class professional men, intimately connected with the formal structure of governance, guided these boards. At this time, public health was frequently construed as a problem rightly managed in the first instance to preserve civic order rather than promote the social welfare of the less-well-to-do.[6]

To justify their crusade against unsanitary conditions in the province, public health officials pitted modern science against superstition and quackery, knowledge against ignorance, right against wrong, life against death. "People commonly speak of death from diphtheria, typhoid fever, consumption, cholera, etc., as a visitation from God," John Chapman Davie, first secretary of the Board of Health, complained in 1893. "Modern scientists," he continued, "know they are nothing of the kind...death from such causes arises from ignorance and the non-observance of the laws of hygiene."[7]

Race was an integral part of the discourse on public health from its earliest days. For those at whom such rhetoric was aimed, particularly non-whites, the stakes could be very high: hefty fines, court appearances, evictions under city health by-laws, and routinely penalized contravention of specific notions of "filth" and "sickness."[8] Protecting the "public" health revolved around a paradox: it meant excluding and demonizing a particular portion of that public. Asian immigrants were condemned as simply incapable of obeying sanitation laws. After a visit to Japan and China in 1894 to "acquaint myself, as far as possible, with the health condition of the people from which at present British Columbia draws the bulk of her immigration," George Duncan, medical officer of health for Victoria, concluded simply that "Chinese immigration is, from the point of view of health, the most dangerous element against which we have to contend."[9] Cholera, smallpox, bubonic plague, typhoid fever—Chinese immigrants personified all of these deadly killers. And public health officials drew repeated and unmistakable connections between Asian newcomers and filth and disease.[10] Citing the example of the bubonic plague then raging in India, Davie typically noted that its inhabitants were dying in larger numbers than whites because "the natives live in unsanitary conditions...in defiance in every way of the laws of hygiene...the White population, comparatively speaking, obey sanitation laws."[11]

Health officials subscribed to the notion that different communities had differing immunities to diseases and that some had an inherited distaste for modern (and in their minds, superior) methods of disease control and prevention.[12] Reporting in 1903, C. J. Fagan, secretary of the Provincial Board of Health, remarked that "the Indians, like the Chinese, have a hereditary dislike for modern methods of treating and stamping out disease, and are apt not only not to co-operate with the authorities, but to attempt to hide themselves away among their own people, and thus indefinitely and indiscriminately spread disease."[13] He did not consider that Natives and Asians, who often sought refuge in their communities, might legitimately have been fearful or distrustful of treatment at the hand of white health officials.[14]

The assumed inferiority of First Nations peoples was, ironically enough, also used to justify neglect and inaction. In 1909, much to the chagrin of local health officials, smallpox ran rampant on the Nanaimo Indian Reservation. Rather than focusing on treatment, health officials censured the Indian Department in Victoria for its failure to supply "guards" on reserves to prevent "a general epidemic over the whole Province." Commenting on the situation, Walter Bapty, the local medical officer, complained that "notices were placed on the houses, but no guards were placed to strictly carry out isolation...many of the milder cases have occurred in the large lodge-houses, or 'rancheros,' and contacts have been into town, and to all the neighbouring reservations."[15] This neglect of First Nations peoples in terms of contagious diseases extended even into the 1920s and beyond. While officials claimed "reports of infectious diseases have shown a marked decrease," rates of death from tuberculosis among Native peoples were five times that of whites in 1929.[16]

Several enduring features of public health reform as a disciplining force in British Columbia were thus established early. White middle-class male professionals were dominant. It was organized along defensive lines, dependent on surveillance of the public, driven by the (supposedly) superior laws of European science, and thoroughly developed along racial lines.[17]

Sanitation, Scabies, and Schools

While all residents fell within their mandate, public health reformers identified youngsters as particularly appropriate targets of their work. The origins and orientation of public health reform in British Columbia, particularly after 1890, had an enduring impact on attitudes towards healthy children. The fact that many schools housed large numbers of children, and that children were believed to be particularly vulnerable to such ailments as tuberculosis, smallpox, diphtheria, and typhoid fever, made them natural targets for sanitary surveillance.[18] Outbreaks of these diseases around the province in the 1890s haunted public health officials and helped spur on their attention to school children.[19] Reformers legislated their connection to schools and students and concentrated on building mechanisms of surveillance to root out "defective" children. They saw medical inspection as part of a scientific approach to the detection of diseases.

Detecting contagion in schools was not left to voluntary compliance. The 1893 health act legislated cooperation among teachers, parents, and inspectors. Initiating a web of scrutiny and examination, the act made parents the first line of defence. Within eighteen hours of discovering an infectious or contagious disease (including smallpox, cholera, scarletina, diphtheria, whooping cough, measles, and mumps), they were expected to notify their children's school and the local board of health. No member of a suspected household could attend without a certificate indicating that the disease was no longer present, and "that the sick person, their house, clothing, and other effects had been disinfected to the satisfaction of the Medical Health Officer."[20] Members of local boards of health were expected to act similarly decisively if they found evidence of contagion. For their part, teachers were instructed to notify the medical officer of health (or the local board, if no medical officer existed) about suspicious children. Official forms had to be sent to the local authorities. Until the claims of the teacher were investigated, students under any suspicions whatsoever were forbidden to attend.[21] Reporting a child with a contagious disease was considered both a moral and a legal responsibility. In 1908, C. J. Fagan made the connection especially dramatically: "For every death resulting from typhoid fever someone ought to be hanged....This bring(s) home to the minds of thinking persons the criminality of carelessness."[22]

In terms of the amount of work and responsibility required of individual parents and teachers, and by virtue of the assumption that everyone had the capacity to be both urban and middle-class, the health act was fraught with problems. It is unclear how many British Columbian parents and teachers would have been capable of identifying diseases, espe-

cially in the early period of incubation when they were most dangerous. Even medical doctors often had difficulty correctly diagnosing contagion such as diphtheria. Its initial symptoms, sore throat and mem-
brane formation, were considered very similar to those of scarletina.[23]
In 1906, the Vancouver School Board appointed its first full-time medical inspector of schools, Georgina Urquhart, because neither parents nor
teachers were found to be reliable and/or knowledgeable about the detection of disease among school children.[24]

Urquhart had graduated from Trinity Medical College the preceding year with a Doctor of Medicine and a Master of Surgery degree.
Before taking up her post, she had worked in private practice in Vancouver. The school trustees appreciated her work, but she gave up the post
in 1909.[25] Given that she was required to examine children in the fourteen city schools twice during the year without assistance, it is reasonable
to speculate that she might well have sought less onerous work elsewhere.[26]

Enforced quarantine and the costs of confining breadwinners would
have made the willing identification of disease problematic, particularly
for working-class families. Details of police enforcement of health by-laws
in Vancouver confirm that citizens, including the occasional public health
nurse, were regularly fined either for breaking quarantine or for failing
to report infectious diseases. Despite the rhetoric regarding the inability of Chinese immigrants to obey health laws, white British Columbians
appear to have been as likely as any other citizens to contravene the by-
laws.[27] In any case, loss of income and social stigma appeared to be of
little concern to public health officials.

An integral strand in the web of health surveillance, teachers were
expected, as part of their professional commitment, to be vigilant about
dirt and disease. As early as 1872, the official "rules and regulations" governing provincial public schools stated that part of the "duty of every
Teacher of a Public School" was to "promote, both by precept and example, CLEANLINESS, NEATNESS, AND DECENCY...to personally
inspect the children every morning to see that they have their hands and
faces washed, their hair combed, and clothes clean. The school apartment, too, should be swept and dusted every morning."[28] In the name
of cleanliness, children were to be taught to wash hands and faces, to keep
fingers out of mouths, to blow their noses, and to sneeze and cough
without infecting others. Sharing food, eating utensils, cups, and "bean
blowers" was discouraged, and the dust and dirt that came with life in
growing urban centres and rural backwaters alike were targeted. Classrooms and halls were to be swept every day, windows opened, and the
schoolhouse scrubbed with soap and water as often as possible. In order
to kill germs, teachers were to "wash walls, floors, desks, etc., and to wet

them over with a mixture of carbolic acid and water" during their Christ-mas holidays.[29]

Given the often extremely difficult conditions under which many British Columbian teachers worked, especially those in the more remote areas of the province, the necessities of school hygiene made their jobs harder.[30] In 1912, school medical inspectors in Kaslo, Harrop, and Salmo in the Kootenays complained about inadequate school buildings that were draughty, poorly lit and ventilated, without running water, and overcrowded.[31] Into the 1920s and 1930s, a significant gap contin-ued between the demanding rhetoric of health reform and the realities of those in British Columbian classrooms. Abigail Nicholson, a teacher in Port Alberni on Vancouver Island in the 1920s, complained that because the school building doubled as the community centre, "men smoke and throw matches, partly used cigarettes and cigars on the floor, desks, and blackboard ledges."[32] Norval Brown recalled teaching in a one-room schoolhouse in Narcosli Creek in 1933. Carried over a distance of three-quarters of a mile for drinking and washing, the water often froze before it got to the school.[33]

Even in more populated urban areas, significant structural prob-lems existed. R. Eden Walker, medical health officer for the municipal-ity of Coquitlam reported in 1896, for example, that the New Westmin-ster schoolhouse was clean, "but not well ventilated." He also cautioned that "the well was closed up and the pump did not work," both of which had to be remedied, since "children are liable to drink foul water out of the ditch or any other convenient place." In the same year, despite the fact that no serious infectious diseases were reported, J. Kerr Wilson, med-ical health officer for Delta, complained about the deplorable condi-tions in the village of Ladner. He was outraged by the prevalence and "taken-for-grantedness" of scabies in the local schools. Capturing some-thing of the inflated rhetoric that framed much of the discourse of early public health reform, Wilson ended his report by declaring, "We must not forget that in matters of sanitation, eternal vigilance is the price of liberty and freedom from disease."[34]

"Protecting the Students": The Evolution of School Medical Inspection

The terms of the Schools Health Inspection Act for British Columbia reveal the disciplinary goals of the framers and their conception of "healthy" children.[35] Also clearly reflected are the limitations and prob-lems that plagued its operation. Provisions of the act set out a list of priorities in terms of disease and disease prevention. At the top of the list was the longstanding concern about contagion. Pupils absent from school for prolonged periods were referred to the medical officer. Inspectors were also expected to pay closer attention to the condition of individual children, specifically to note conditions that "prevent his receiving the full benefit of his school work, or as to whether he requires a modification of the school work in order to secure the best educational results." If a student was found to have a "defect," the medical officer was to recommend appropriate treatment to his or her parents by postcard. Health records for each student, containing information gathered during inspections, were to be kept on file.[36] In endeavouring to organize, inspect, diagnose, categorize, and segregate "diseased" children, medical inspection disciplined the student body, reassured observers, and legitimized medical expertise.[37]

In practice, the provisions contained in the act were applied unevenly and with mixed results. Total school enrolment figures and the number of children inspected by school doctors and nurses rarely corresponded. Almost one-quarter of the students registered in the province's schools in 1914 did not receive a school medical examination.[38] Clearly, as Mary Ellen Kelm has shown, residential schools for First Nations children in the province were rife with contagious diseases over the entire twentieth century. The death rate of Aboriginal children in residential schools from contagious disease, particularly tuberculosis, demonstrated that even this most basic line of defence was inadequately enforced.[39]

Since school medical inspectors did not have to be doctors, teachers were often burdened with a task for which they were not trained. This duty often fell on women, the majority of BC teachers. Their reports reveal that most did their best to protect their young students. In Columbia Gardens, J. Pipkin, the schoolteacher, endeavoured to keep "a careful watch over the pupils." In Edgewood, teacher Margaret Timeaus reported that the eleven children in her school, "as far as (she) could judge," were remarkably healthy. Yet even when intentions were the best, thorough inspection did not always occur. If some teachers, like the one for Alice Landing, were able to give a detailed accounting of children's "defects," others such as Coquitlam's inspector complained, "I have been so overworked that it has been impossible for me this past two months to keep up with daily events and get sufficient rest, so that I postponed making this report until I could get time undisturbed for it."[40]

School medical practitioners themselves acknowledged the shortfall between the promise of the inspection system and the reality of its efficacy. Early defenders of the system suggested that initiatives were still in their infancy and that improvements would come.[41] Evidence from doctors suggests that examinations of some children remained less comprehensive than intended, for many years. Although the Schools Health Inspection Act called for full examination, including stripping children to the waist, F. W. Brydone-Jack, Vancouver's school medical officer between 1910 and 1919, confessed, "I don't know any place, in British Columbia at least, where that examination is carried on in that way."[42] Since one might suspect parental objection, particularly from parents of girls, it is not surprising that such potentially compromising and embarrassing directives were not followed.

The equal application of the Schools Health Inspection Act across the province was difficult, if not impossible. The depth of reportage and the variety of problems identified in British Columbian schools were highly dependent on the thoroughness, commitment, qualification, and personality of individual inspectors. In 1912, the inspector for Alice Siding in the south-eastern part of the province noted that of the "sixteen pupils examined...only two are poorly nourished; three have enlarged turbinates; four have enlarged tonsils; one adenoids; one presents a pigeon-breast; one has ichthyosis; one a goitre; six have been vaccinated; six had measles last year; one is neurasthenic."[43] In sharp contrast, his counterpart for Cache Creek School remarked that he "made one trip there last fall, and found the children all in good health...I will call in at the school the next time I go up the road." At the Lower Bella Coola School, teacher and inspector were one and the same. "As you possibly are aware," he noted, "I am teaching in the above-mentioned school, and can say that no sickness of any kind, except a slight cold once in a while, has been in the school...I have never examined any of the pupils minutely, chiefly because I am no medical man and therefore not qualified to do so."[44]

School district reports beyond the Lower Mainland averaged about three paragraphs in total. These contrast sharply with those of F. W. Brydone-Jack in Vancouver, which typically ran to three to four pages. Even taking into account the fact that Brydone-Jack had many more children and schools to inspect, his reports nevertheless offer much more depth and detail regarding his efforts to secure sanitary schools and healthful children.[45] While Brydone-Jack, along with his staff of three, including two nurses, was by 1917 advocating "not school medical inspection but school medical service," rural respondents such as the school board trustees from Hope regretted that they continued to have no medical practitioner, let alone a report on the conditions of the schools.[46]

Complaints about overcrowding, poor ventilation, grimy appearance, inadequate and damaged supplies, and poor sanitary provisions came largely from rural schools. Urban school inspections could muse about expanding health services, but most rural schools could barely keep up with the minimum of inspection. Over the course of the early twentieth century, medical inspectors in other rural communities continued to complain: "I found Readers in a filthy condition—soiled and torn"; "I found desks all loose, the floor rather dirty from wax"; "recommended that seat of closet be regularly cleaned when school-room is being done"; "the draught along the floor of the school-room is, at least during winter, liable to give rise to cold feet"; "the building is simply the most miserable I have ever seen used as a school building."[47] Outdoor water closets plagued schools beyond city limits. The inspector for the Erie district reported, "The boys' and girls' closets should be separated from each other, more for moral than sanitary reasons."[48] In Box Lake, the inspector noted that the situation was "primitive; one earth-closet for each sex....I think there should be a closet with two seats for each sex at least, and either a partition separating the closets outside, or, what would be more satisfactory, two separate buildings." At Foster's Bay School, the inspector noted, "closets clean and in good condition, but those for boys and girls are side by side with no screens."[49] Concerns about public health often elided with notions of gendered propriety. Regardless of the circumstances and in keeping with the disciplinary thrust of surveillance, inspectors were anxious to replicate middle-class standards of privacy.

Like the work of southern missionaries in the North and attitudes among health camp officials in New Zealand, school medical inspection in British Columbia involved changing habits most often associated with the working-class and non-European peoples. Urban schools, as easily as rural ones, could be problematic in these terms. Cleanliness, for example, was repeatedly held up to British Columbian school children as the epitome of acceptability. In the early decades of the twentieth century, however, abundant hot water in Vancouver was associated only with the middle classes.[50] Jennie Schooley, a teacher at Strathcona School in Vancouver's downtown eastside, remembered that "they had a bathtub down in the Senior Building, and children who were really unclean were sent down there to wash...but what could you expect—many of the kiddies lived in these apartment buildings in just a cold-water flat....Some of them didn't even have cold water, they had a sink and a toilet down at the end of the hall on each floor."[51]

Children could readily experience the "cleanliness imperative" as violent, repressive, and shaming. Strathcona teacher Gertrude Doyle recalled her principal physically assaulting a student who refused to comply with socially constructed standards of cleanliness.

After lots of warning, [the principal] said, "Now if you come back again in this mess, I'm going to take you down to the basement, and I'm going to bath you."...But the boy came back dirty again, and he took him down and he turned the hose on him, with cold water, and everybody in the building could hear his kid screeching at the top of his voice, "You're killing me, you're *killing* me." And he never came back dirty.[52]

The link among notions of cleanliness (defined and enforced by those in positions of power), moral righteousness, and middle-class membership was clear. Youthful transgressors, particularly those perceived to be worthy of such "education," risked not only chastisement but also enforced compliance.

While reports cannot be relied upon to reflect accurately the state of children's health, they do suggest a great deal about whose interests were served by school medical inspection. First, between 1910 and the late 1930s, inspectors exposed the sharp contrast between the ability of rural and urban schools to carry out government health demands. Second, the reports also reveal that teachers in a number of communities were carrying out the tasks of medical officers and that the focus of inspection, whether on individual "defects," general conditions, or something in between, was somewhat arbitrary, depending on the inclination, expertise, and energy of individual inspectors. Third, parents were regularly characterized as helpful or a hindrance in the work of school medical inspection, with the distinction highly influenced by supposed racial traits.

Health officials routinely lamented that, given parents' critical importance to the successful surveillance of their offspring, ignorance, indifference, or hostility in the home undermined their important work. In 1909, for example, the medical officer for Vancouver schools, Lazelle Anderson, suggested that while most dealt promptly with conditions such as scabies, ringworm, and pediculosis, conditions "left to the discretion of parents" often went untreated. He noted that less serious conditions were often treated with "indifference." In some cases, parents pleaded financial hardship as an obstacle.[53] In 1913, Anderson's successor, F. W. Brydone-Jack, noted that "parental apathy and ignorance" accounted for 65 per cent of Vancouver students' receiving insufficient attention. Brydone-Jack reasoned that only "education" would improve the situation.[54]

In 1914, the provincial medical officer categorized parents as belonging to one of three "types": the "appreciative," the "indifferent," or the "rebellious."[55] Given the deeply racialized undercurrent shaping public health discourse, transgressing parents, or those in need of paternalistic guidance by medical officials, were likely to be working class, Asian, Native, or members of other minority cultures. Elizabeth Breeze, head nurse for Vancouver Schools, wrote in 1911 that "among the foreigners, Italians, Greeks, and Russians, many cases of overcrowding are suspected, and in one case we found a family of seven, not including three boarders, living on a small scow in two rooms."[56] Commenting on her experiences in 1916, another Vancouver school nurse hoped to amuse readers by reporting that she was very rarely asked in to her client's homes for afternoon tea, "although I have had Christmas cake and tea at 10 a.m. and been offered beer at an Italian's house in the afternoon."[57] Appreciative parents held a "profound sense of duty towards their children" and moved quickly to follow the advice of doctors. Conversely, indifferent parents lacked the "finer maternal or parental instincts that should arouse them to a sense of duty regarding the health of their children." Rebellious parents could, with "a little tact and diplomacy," be persuaded to follow the doctor's recommendations and "benefit their children's health and education."[58] Given that women were expected to look after young children, such typology also carries a gendered subtext. "Proper" maternal behaviour demanded self-effacement, obedience, and deference to the disciplining activity of (male) experts.[59]

Medical inspection officials were guided by telling assumptions, as their attitudes towards parents suggest. They appear to have accepted their diagnoses as unproblematic and always worthy of compliance. When it came to treating children, however, doctors were not always right. In 1907, for example, an irate father complained to the Vancouver School Board that the medical superintendent had sent his daughter home with a diagnosis of head lice. When he duly had the child examined by the family doctor, she was declared perfectly healthy and pest free. When he complained to the superintendent, the father reported that "the only satisfaction I received from the official was a threat that if I didn't send the child to school I would be sent to Police Court." The school board promised a quick and speedy investigation.[60]

While school medical inspectors assumed that parental compliance was in the best interest of children's health, this too was not necessarily so. The contentious issue of vaccination justified some parental opposition. Controversy around vaccination was not unique to British Columbia. Across the country, concerned citizens debated and actively resisted public health officials' attempts to vaccinate all children.[61] The effectiveness of such measures was not clear. Some doctors themselves openly questioned the benefits of vaccination. In 1914, Dr. Dyer, a Vancouver doctor, suggested that while vaccination and antitoxin injection for the prevention of smallpox were favoured by the provincial Board of Health, they were often more troublesome than the disease. "A typical 'good' arm is looked on as 'blood-poisoning' by the parents," he pointed out, "a diagnosis often confirmed by the nurse."[62] From the point of view of children, vaccination promised immediate pain and stress. They might well plead with sympathetic parents to escape this invasive procedure. Growing up in Fernie, BC, for example, Sydney Hutcheson recalled that vaccination time was to be avoided if at all possible.

All of the pupils in the Public School in Fernie were sent in groups to the old Fernie Hospital (under guard so we didn't run away) to be vaccinated against smallpox. We stood in line in the hallway of the hospital and stepped up to a long table one at a time with our arms bared. A huge man by the name of Dr. Corson scraped your arm with a small knife and put some serum in the cuts. A light bandage was then put on the arm and you were sent back to school.[63]

This memory testifies to the fact that vaccination was, at times, not only physically painful but also psychologically difficult, reminding children of their often-debilitating powerlessness in the midst of medical "expertise."

Medical school inspectors did not actually treat the children they diagnosed. It was up to parents to seek out treatment. The rhetoric of public health officials positioned parents as real obstacles to children's good health.[64] In order to improve parental compliance, school nurses were charged with the task of visiting the homes of children in need of treatment.[65] In the late 1920s, school medical inspectors typically placed the lion's share of work publicizing the health message on their shoulders: "By home visiting, nurses discover the reasons for lack of treatment and so are able to deal with the cases...home visits afford the nurses many opportunities for teaching health and hygiene...in many ways our nurses are the social workers for the schools."[66] Nurses themselves characterized such outreach as challenging. Foremost was the recurring need to provide assistance for low-income and poor households to make them approximate middle-class standards of health care. This could well require charity. As a school nurse in Vancouver in 1916 reported, "Although a great deal of parents are unable to afford even the simplest of treatments, we are able to a certain extent to overcome this difficulty through the kindness of the different specialists in the city."[67] The irony inherent in admonishing mothers and fathers to provide treatment that they could not afford went unnoticed. Grinding poverty and/or lack of choices were never tackled as a root of parental reluctance.

For Mary Jong, one of many Chinese Canadians whose families settled in Armstrong, BC, over the course of the nineteenth century, the inculcation of "Canadian" standards of health and cleanliness was both racist and exclusionary. She remembered her teacher's disciplining techniques with heartbreaking clarity. Students' hands, hair, and clothes would be routinely checked and passes and failures firmly separated. "Clean" students would receive stars. "My row always came in last," Mary recalled, "because of me...everyone blamed me and didn't want me in their group...how could they know that I had to work in the vegetable garden every morning before school and didn't have time to clean up?"[68] Unacknowledged here, except as cause for punishment, was the fact that work, both paid and unpaid, was a routine part of childhood for many youngsters. Most particularly, labour on the part of poor immigrant youngsters was critical to the well-being of many families.[69]

Conclusion

The interest of public health reformers in shaping attitudes towards healthy children was inextricably bound up in concerns about racial and class "contagion." School medical inspection, and the considerable social surveillance and disciplining it made possible, enabled white middle-class professionals, primarily but not exclusively male, to infuse notions of "health" with the values and priorities of white middle-class and urban British Columbia.

In both form and content, school medical inspections in British Columbia over the turn of the century conveyed powerful messages about "healthy" and "unhealthy" children. In the memories of some children, encounters with health professionals and with health imperatives were coloured by fear and/or racial and class discrimination. For other children, the provision of health services in schools was woefully inadequate or completely absent. The reports of school medical inspectors around the province make clear that their services varied widely in frequency, thoroughness, and, indeed, aims. Some school medical inspectors set out to improve the health of children in their jurisdiction; others merely sought out contagion as the end goal; others sought to use standards of health to discipline subordinate groups. For most, a mixture of motives held sway. Far from simply signalling the triumph of sanitary science, school medical inspection was a powerful means of legitimizing existing relations of power and confirming social boundaries. In 1930, Rita Mahon, Inkameep Indian Reserve public health nurse, made clear the function that learning "modern hygiene methods" had for Native school children: "The Indian will be an ever-present factor in our affairs for years to come…thanks to his adaptive and imitative faculties, he himself is making a valiant effort to adapt himself to our modern parade."[70] Provincial school inspection often implied, however, that Native peoples and their children, like others who had difficulty meeting the health standards of the day, would never direct a pageant scripted and managed by settler society.

Acknowledgement

I wish to thank the members of the Department of Educational Studies History Group at the University of British Columbia for their insightful comments on an earlier version of this paper.

Notes

1   Rita M. Mahon, "Inkameep Indian Reserve, Oliver District," *Public Health Nurses Bulletin* 2, 2 (April 1935): 11–14.

2   Taking her lead from anthropologist Mary Douglas, historian Anne McClintock has more recently underscored the notion that "filth" is a socially constructed and determined label. "Nothing is inherently dirty," she argues. "Dirt expresses a relation to social value and social disorder…it is that which transgresses social boundary." Anne McClintock, *Imperial Leather: Race, Gender, and Sexuality in Colonial Conquest* (New York: Routledge, 1995).

3   My use of the term *discipline* evokes Michel Foucault's work on the nature of normalizing power. In Foucaultian terms, *discipline* is a dynamic phenomenon that describes the flow of power between those in varying positions of power. In the case of school medical inspection, I focus on how surveillance techniques employed by doctors and nurses, including examination, categorization, diagnosis, and segregation of patients, worked not simply to produce "healthy" children, but to solidify traditional relations of power. On Foucault's conception of normalizing power, see *Discipline and Punish: The Birth of the Prison* (New York: Vintage, 1979). For the application of Foucault's normalizing power in the Canadian context, see Mona Gleason, *Normalizing the Ideal: Psychology, Schooling and the Family in Postwar Canada* (Toronto: University of Toronto Press, 1999).

4   Margaret W. Andrews explores Vancouver's relatively early provision of public health services as a sign of municipal progress. Any analysis of the role that race played in this development is absent. See "The Best Advertisement a City Can Have: Public Health Services in Vancouver, 1886–1888," *Urban History Review/ Revue d'histoire urbaine* 12, 3 (February 1984): 3–27. Studies that do acknowledge this link between the development of public health and racism in British Columbia at the turn of century include Kay Anderson, *Vancouver's Chinatown: Racial Discourse in Canada, 1875–1980* (Montreal and Kingston: McGill-Queen's University Press, 1991), 53, 81–88; John Atkins, *Strathcona: Vancouver's First Neighbourhood* (Vancouver: Whitecap Books, 1994), 47–52; Robert A. J. MacDonald, *Making Vancouver, 1863–1913* (Vancouver: University of British Columbia Press, 1996), 87–88; Paul Yee, "Chinese Business in Vancouver, 1886–1914" (MA thesis, University of British Columbia, 1978); and Paul Yee, *Saltwater City: An Illustrated History of the Chinese in Vancouver* (Vancouver/Toronto: Douglas and McIntyre, 1988), 8–30.

5   In city municipalities, local boards of health consisted of the mayor (ex-officio chairman), the police magistrate, the clerk of the municipal council, the city engineer, and the medical health officer (appointed by municipal councils). In township municipalities, the reeve (ex-officio chairman), the clerk of the municipal council, the medical health officer, and the justice of the peace made up the board.

6   Alan Sears, "Before the Welfare State: Public Health and Social Policy," *Canadian Review of Sociology and Anthropology* 32, 2 (1995): 169–88.

7   Province of British Columbia. "Introductory Report by the Chairman," *Second Report of the Provincial Board of Health* (Victoria: Queen's Printer, 1897), 687.

8   For the city of Vancouver, for example, a surviving record book listing offences against health by-laws between 1900 and 1902 suggests that offenders (overwhelmingly Chinese or Japanese) were fined amounts ranging from two dollars to twenty dollars, primarily for overcrowding, running unlicensed boarding houses, or "blowing or causing to be blown, water from the mouth" in the oper-

ation of laundry and ironing services. The city addresses of offenders suggest that police did frequent sweeps of Chinatown in East Vancouver. As noted in the record book, officers had discretionary power to suspend charges and to give offenders a chance to comply with the regulations, if they chose to do so. This occurred almost exclusively only in the case of offenders with Anglo-Celtic surnames rather than those of Asian descent. See *Health By-laws Record Book,* 1900–1902, 37-C-7, series no. 188, Vancouver (BC) Police Court, City of Vancouver Archives (hereafter cited as VA).

9 Province of British Columbia, *First Report of the Provincial Board of Health* (Victoria: Queen's Printer, 1895), 541–42.

10 British Columbia, *First Report.* As Duncan concluded, "Canton, from which the greatest part of Chinese immigration flows to these shores, is regarded as the most filthy city in the world, and is known to be continually impregnated with cholera" 545.

11 B.C., "Introductory Report," 690.

12 Michael Worboys, "Tuberculosis and Race in Britain and Its Empire, 1900–1950," in *Race, Science and Medicine, 1700–1960,* ed. Ernest Waltraud and Bernard Harris, 144–66 (London and New York: Routledge, 1999).

13 "Report of the Provincial Board of Health, 1902," in *Sessional Papers,* Fourth Session, Ninth Parliament of the Province of British Columbia (Victoria: King's Printer, 1903), J34.

14 Mary Ellen Kelm, "Medical Pluralism in Aboriginal Communities," in her *Colonizing Bodies: Aboriginal Health and Healing in British Columbia, 1900–1950* (Vancouver: UBC Press, 1998), 146–62. On medical involvement in First Nations lives as part of larger colonial praxis, for example, see chapter 6, "Acts of Humanity: Indian Health Services."

15 Province of British Columbia, *Sessional Papers* (Victoria: King's Printer, 1911), F12–F13.

16 See Province of British Columbia, *Thirty-Fourth Report of the Provincial Board of Health* (Victoria: King's Printer, 1930), R18–R19. In 1929, 31 per cent of all deaths in the Native community were due to tuberculosis, compared to 6.7 per cent in the white community. On the devastation to Native communities caused by tuberculosis, see Kelm, *Colonizing Bodies.*

17 On the development of public health during this period as a response to fears of racial contamination and decline, see Patricia Jasen, "Race, Culture, and the Colonization of Childbirth in Northern Canada," *Social History of Medicine* 10, 3 (1997): 383–400; and Mariana Valverde, *The Age of Light, Soap, and Water: Moral Reform in English Canada, 1885–1925* (Toronto: McClelland and Stewart, 1991).

18 The fact that schools were often quite unhealthy places for children to be was not simply a Canadian phenomenon. Conditions in schools in the United States and New Zealand, for example, were also often judged by public health officials to be deplorable. See, for example, William A. Link, "Privies, Progressivism, and Public Schools: Health Reform and Education in the Rural South, 1909–1920," *Journal of Southern History* 54, 4 (November 1988): 623–42; and Pamela J. Woods, "Hazardous to Children's Health? New Zealand Primary Schools, 1890 to 1914," *Historical News* 66, 4 (May 1993): 4–8.

19 Union, Rossland, and Kamloops were singled out in the Board's report of 1896 as suffering previous unchecked epidemics. *Second Report,* 688. See also Neil Sutherland, *Children in English-Canadian Society: Framing the Twentieth-Century Consensus* (Waterloo: Wilfrid Laurier University Press, 2000), especially 39–55.

20 *Second Report,* 688.

21 *Second Report*, 688.

22 Board of Health, *Annual Report of the Provincial Board of Health* (Victoria: King's Printer, 1907), G5.

23 Catherine Braithwaite, Peter Keating, and Sandi Viger, "The Problem of Diphtheria in the Province of Quebec, 1896–1909," *Histoire Sociale/ Social History* 2, 57 (May 1996) 74–75.

24 *Vancouver Daily Province*, February 8, 1907, 6, as quoted in Ruth Wells, "'Making Health Contagious': Medical Inspection of the Schools in British Columbia, 1910–1920" (unpublished extended research paper, University of Victoria, 1981), 21–22.

25 See, for example, the words of praise for Urquhart from R. P. McLennan, chairman of the Vancouver School Board Management Committee, in the 1908 *Vancouver School Board Annual Report*, 20.

26 Urquhart is no longer listed in the Vancouver city directory by 1911 and most likely left the province, given her withdrawal from the College of Physicians and Surgeons of British Columbia. Neither the reports of the Department of Public Health nor the reports of the Public Schools of British Columbia make clear why she decided to leave. Her successors, however, did not stick with the post for lengthy periods either. Her replacement, E. Lazelle Anderson, occupied the post only until 1912, to be replaced by F. W. Brydone-Jack, who held the post between 1910 and 1919. Brydone-Jack's father was a prominent member of the Vancouver School Board during the first few years of his position as school medical inspector. Drs. Wightman and Hogg succeeded the junior Brydone-Jack. In 1925, H. White acted as medical inspector of Vancouver's public schools.

27 *Health By-laws Record Book*. Over these years, for example, seventeen people were found to have either broken quarantine (ten) or failed to report the presence of contagious diseases in their homes (seven). Of those who broke quarantine, two were public health nurses. Of this total of seventeen, only four had Chinese surnames.

28 *First Annual Report of the Public Schools in the Province of British Columbia* (Victoria, Queen's Printer, 1872), 18–19. Emphasis in original.

29 [n.a.] "Public School Sanitation," *Thirty-Eighth Annual Report of the Public Schools of the Province of British Columbia, 1908–1909* (Victoria: King's Printer, 1909), A64–A65.

30 As the annual public school reports make clear, rural and assisted schools in the province were severely underfunded and understaffed. On the conditions of rural schools in British Columbia, see J. Donald Wilson and Paul J. Stortz, "'May the Lord Have Mercy on You': The Rural School Problem in British Columbia in the 1920s," in *Children, Teachers, and Schools in the History of British Columbia*, ed. Jean Barman, Neil Sutherland, and J. Donald Wilson (Calgary: Detselig Press, 1995), 209–34.

31 *First Annual Report of the Medical Inspection of Public Schools of the Province of British Columbia* (Victoria: King's Printer, 1912), M32, M38, M64.

32 As quoted in Wilson and Stortz, "'May the Lord Have Mercy,'" 214.

33 Norval Brown, "Johnny of the Spot," in [n.a.] *Kindling the Spark: The Era of One-Room Schools* (Vancouver: British Columbia Rural Teachers Association, 1996), 3.

34 [n.a.] "Supplementary Report of the Provincial Board of Health Being the Annual Reports of Medical Health Officers and Local Boards of Health for Year 1896," in *Second Report of the Provincial Board of Health of British Columbia* (Victoria: Queen's Printer, 1897), 970–71.

35 Province of British Columbia, "An Act to Provide for the Medical Inspection of Schools," *Statutes of the Province of British Columbia* (Victoria: King's Printer, 1910), 379–82.

36 Province of British Columbia, "Act to Provide for Medical Inspection," 379–80.

27 On Michel Foucault's conception of normalizing power in these terms, see Mona Gleason, "Disciplining the Student Body: Schooling and the Construction of Canadian Children's Bodies, 1930–1960," *History of Education Quarterly* 41, 2 (Summer 2001): 189–215.

38 Province of British Columbia, *Sessional Papers* (Victoria: King's Printer, 1915), A7–A11; Province of British Columbia, *Nineteenth Annual Report of the Provincial Board of Health* (Victoria: King's Printer, 1915), I 31. Students enrolled in the province's schools totalled just fewer than 62,000 in 1914. The total number of children inspected was just under 47,000.

39 Kelm, *Colonizing Bodies*, 57–80.

40 Kelm, *Colonizing Bodies*, M12.

41 Blanche Swan, "Report of School Nurse," *Nineteenth Annual Report of the Provincial Board of Health* (Victoria: King's Printer, 1915), I 31.

42 Province of British Columbia, *Seventeenth Annual Report of the Provincial Board of Health* (1914), U72. This gulf between what was expected of inspection, and its practice for children, echoes the tragic death from appendicitis of an eleven-year-old Kwakiutl girl, Renee Smith, of Alert Bay, BC, in 1979. Dara Culhane Speck argues that racist attitudes towards Native people continue to shape European-influenced medical practice and were a significant factor in the unnecessary death of Renee. Dara Culhane Speck, *An Error in Judgement: The Politics of Medical Care in an Indian/White Community* (Vancouver: Talon Books, 1987).

43 Province of British Columbia, *Seventeenth Annual Report of the Provincial Board of Health*, M6. *Turbinates* refer to spongy, scroll-shaped bones in the nasal passages, *ichthyosis* is associated with eczema, and *neurasthenic* signifies a person suffering from nervous breakdown.

44 Province of British Columbia, *Seventeenth Annual Report of the Provincial Board of Health*, M7, M10, M13.

45 In the report for 1911, for example, Brydone-Jack explains in detail how examinations of children are carried out, the role of both doctors and nurses in the schools, the details of reporting diseases and illnesses, special classes and activities related to sanitary science, and details of the physical plant of the school. His report also often included three or four photographs of the work in progress. See a reprint of his report in "Medical Inspection," *Vancouver School Board Annual Report, 1911*, 50–61.

46 Trenna G. Hunter and C. H. Gundry, "School Health Practices: Ritualistic or Purposeful?" *Canadian Journal of Public Health* 46, 1 (January 1955): 9–14.

47 *First Annual Report on the Medical Inspection of Public Schools of the Province of British Columbia* (Victoria: King's Printer, 1913): M5–M91.

48 *First Annual Report on the Medical Inspection*, M25.

49 *First Annual Report on the Medical Inspection*, M22, M25, M27.

50 Public sanitary conveniences grew in the city between 1886 and 1926 as a response to increasingly socially unacceptable "frontier toilet behaviour." See Margaret W. Andrews, "Sanitary Conveniences and the Retreat of the Frontier: Vancouver, 1886–1926," *BC Studies* 87 (Autumn 1990): 3–22.

51 Daphne Marlatt and Carole Itter, eds., *Opening Doors: Vancouver's East End* (Vancouver: Sound Heritage, n.d.), 8:94. Strathcona School is one of the earliest schools in Vancouver. The first building on the grounds was completed in 1891 and was known as the East School until 1900.

52 Marlatt and Itter, eds., *Opening Doors*, 94. Emphasis in original.

53 *Vancouver School Board Annual Report* (1908), 40–41.

54 [n.a.] "Medical Inspection," *Vancouver School Board Report* (Victoria: King's Printer, 1913), 34.

55 [n.a.] "Medical Inspection from the Standpoint of the Parent, the Teacher, and the Physician," *Seventeenth Annual Report of the Provincial Board of Health and Proceedings of the Meeting of Medical Health Officers of British Columbia Held in Vancouver, B.C., June 17th and 18th, 1914* (Vancouver: King's Printer, 1914), U66–U68.

56 "Medical Inspection (Nurse Report)," *Vancouver School Board Annual Report (1911)*, 63.

57 M. Ewart, "Home Visiting in Connection with School Nursing," *Canadian Nurse* 12, 6 (June 1916): 308.

58 Provincial Board of Health, *Proceedings of the Meeting of Medical Health Officers of British Columbia Held in Vancouver, B.C., June 17th and 18th, 1914* (Victoria: King's Printer, 1914), U66–U67.

59 Katherine Arnup, *Education for Motherhood: Advice for Mothers in Twentieth-Century Canada* (Toronto: University of Toronto Press, 1994); and Cynthia Comacchio, *"Nations Are Built of Babies": Saving Ontario's Mothers and Children, 1900–1940* (Montreal and Kingston: McGill-Queen's University Press, 1993).

60 *Vancouver Daily Province*, November 9, 1907, 4.

61 Anti-vaccination riots occurred in North American cities like Montreal and New York in the early part of the century, largely because deaths from tetanus had resulted. In Saint John in 1901, for example, a six-year-old girl died as a result of tetanus after being vaccinated. Such episodes caused understandable fear and concern among parents. Michael J. Smith, "Dampness, Darkness, Dirt, Disease: Physicians and the Promotion of Sanitary Science in Public Schools," in *Profiles of Science and Society in the Maritimes Prior to 1914*, ed. Paul A. Bogaard (Halifax: Acadiensis, 1990), 200–203. Debates about the efficacy of vaccines for both adults and children continue today. See Martin Mittelstaedt, "Taking shots at vaccine," *Globe and Mail*, April 11, 2000, R6–R7.

62 Provincial Board of Health, *Proceedings of the Meeting of Medical Health Officers*, U57.

63 Sydney Hutcheson, *Depression Stories* (Vancouver: New Star, 1976), 85–86.

64 See the thorough discussion of parents' role in school medical inspections in Wells, "'Making Health Contagious,'" 16–27.

65 I surveyed a number of professional journals in order to get a clearer idea of the perspective of school nurses, including *Reports of the B.C. Medical Inspection of Public Schools, Public Health Journal, Public Health Nurses Bulletin, Canadian Public Health Journal, Canadian Journal of Public Health, Canadian Medical Association Journal*, and *Canadian Nurse*.

66 Hunter and Gundry, "School Health Practices," 10.

67 Ewart, "Home Visiting," 307–308.

68 Peter Critchley, "The Chinese in Armstrong," *Okanagan History* 63 (1999): 1–12. I am indebted to Jean Barman for this reference.

69 Neil Sutherland, *Growing Up: Childhood in English Canada from the Great War to the Age of Television* (Toronto: University of Toronto Press, 1997). See particularly chapters 6 and 7.

70 Mahon, "Inkameep," 12.

Ordering the Bath

Children, Health, and Hygiene in Northern Canadian Communities, 1900–1970

CR

Myra Rutherdale

istorians have recently started to pay close attention to the increased surveillance of Aboriginal children in residential schools.[1] Teachers, missionaries, doctors, and nurses routinely inspected Aboriginal bodies in their desire to reform or "colonize bodies." Informed by Michel Foucault's analysis of power and surveillance, and influenced by post-colonial critiques, we now understand how, as Mary-Ellen Kelm argues, "the drama of colonization" was acted out on Aboriginal bodies.[2] Those involved in colonizing Aboriginal bodies believed that to "capture" the minds of Aboriginals, they had to "capture" their "bodies first."[3] Aboriginal autobiographies, biographies, and oral histories on residential schools inevitably turn to a discussion of bodily matters, from cleanliness and clothing, to hair and health.[4]

While our attention has so far been drawn to residential schools, this chapter shows that whether in or out of school, children experienced greater and greater surveillance and control. The central focus here is on methods used by newcomers, especially missionaries and nurses, in northern Canadian and Arctic communities to actively introduce children to Western hygienic and medical practices.[5] Newcomers' perceptions and prescriptions about how Aboriginal bodies, especially children's, should be shaped were numerous. Children's bodies were particularly appealing because they were believed easier either to shape or reform than were adults'. From infancy, to young childhood, to adolescence, youngsters were routinely watched over and commented upon. Their bodies were the sites of numerous efforts at reform. Western sleeping habits, hygiene, clothing, and medical care were solutions offered in a broad campaign to reconstruct northern bodies. Visitors from the south generally shared a profound belief that traditional cultural practices could and should be displaced, if not eradicated.[6]

As this chapter makes clear, church workers, just as much as nurses and doctors, were insistent on reshaping Aboriginal children. The missionaries being discussed here worked under the auspices of the Church of England, one of the main Christian institutions in northern Canada, which arrived on the mission scene as early as the 1860s.[7] Missionaries attempted to convert to Christianity as many Aboriginals as possible. Many of their early efforts centred on separating local people from their customary practices, including their medicine-makers or shaman. For many decades Anglican missionaries, often with very little medical training, attempted to offer cures and reconfigure public and personal hygiene. By the early 1930s they began to raise funds to build and staff hospitals with missionary nurses. The result was that by 1943 there were eleven hospitals in northern Canada, nine of which were operated by either Catholic or Anglican missions.

While missionaries were often the first newcomers to live in Aboriginal communities, they paved the way for secular workers, who were increasingly present in northern Canada after World War Two and included not just traders and RCMP officers, but also doctors and nurses. These secular authorities turned their attention—as had their religious predecessors—to children's bodies.

The provision of medical services was, however, all too often perceived as burdensome, particularly by the federal government. As Sharon Richardson points out in her essay in this volume, rural and northern communities in Alberta were served by "ad hoc endeavour, largely dependent on political whim and travelling conditions."[8] This can be said about Canada's Arctic too, but, as a result of the federal government's initiative to create permanent northern settlements, Inuit, Inuvialuit, and northern Indian children, from birth onward, were regularly exposed to newcomers and their foreign bodily practices.[9]

Birthing

Newcomers' scrutiny of Aboriginal bodily practices started at birth. Throughout the twentieth century, birthing became a contested site between Aboriginals and newcomers.[10] Patricia Jasen traces the evolution of childbirth practice throughout twentieth-century northern Canada and concludes that Aboriginal women lost their sense of empowerment through the erosion of their control over childbirth. In her view, responsibility lay with "a process of colonization that introduced new health risks," and a "civilizing mission that undermined old knowledge."[11] Consistent with Jasen's argument, the impact of colonization upon childbirth in the north intensified during the 1960s, especially once Aboriginal women began to be evacuated from their communities to give birth to their children in the northern regional centres or in the south. Yet even after reformist newcomers arrived, Aboriginal women still retained some degree of autonomy over pregnancy's outcome, although this was not always the desired outcome. Newcomers frequently commented on the birthing rituals of Aboriginal women, usually in a comparative context to assure themselves and their readers that white ways of birthing were much more civilized and safe.

Donald Marsh and his wife Winifred were stationed as Anglican missionaries at Eskimo Point, Northwest Territories, from 1926 until 1944. In his memoir Rev. Marsh recalled how Winifred employed her skills as a trained midwife to help the Padlimiut women deliver children in a new way. He described the "dangers" of delivery in traditional communities: "At the first signs of labour, usually before the end of full term, a rope was placed around the pregnant woman just below the breasts and knotted tightly. Then, with her kneeling with legs apart, her upstretched arms held by two women (often female angakoks), the rope was forced downwards until the child was expelled."[12]

Children delivered using long-standing methods, according to Marsh, were at risk of being born prematurely, with low weight and broken ribs. Marsh portrayed the moment of transformation for Padlimiut women occurring when Caroline Gibbons, a Christian Aivilingmiut who apparently rejected older methods in the delivery of her baby, sent for Winifred Marsh to help her. In the Anglican minister's retelling of the story, Winifred's first job upon arrival at Caroline's tent was to establish herself as the one in charge:

Inside were Caroline and her mother-in-law (also a Christian Aivilingmiut), all the camp midwives and angakoks. Win stopped, looked around, and asked Caroline, "Do you want to have your baby this way?" The answer was a quick "No!" Win politely asked the angakoks and midwives to leave and then rolled down the tent flaps, restoring privacy. Quickly and smoothly (and without ropes) the newborn baby appeared, a beautiful boy of 7½ pounds. Caroline's mother-in-law carried out the entire procedure.[13]

After Winifred determined that she was in control, she asked "the angakoks and midwives" to leave. Only Caroline's mother-in-law, a Christian, was allowed to stay, presumably because she could be trusted to follow directions. The implication here was that, as a (presumably modern and up-to-date) Christian, she would listen to Marsh. In his narrative of this "turning point" for women at Eskimo Point, Donald Marsh emphasized the desire of local women to mimic Caroline's birthing experience. They were, he suggested, rejecting "the cruel ways of the past."[14] Although the comfort of delivering a child "naturally," could offer considerable advantage, this point was ignored. "Natural" childbirth as Marsh referred to it, required the absence of ropes and a supine posture. Far greater emphasis was placed on the new and modern methods, possible only when the angakoks and midwives were removed from the scene. Marsh's narrative suggests that the transition from a traditional to a modern birthing ritual was rapid, but other birthing stories suggest that this was not the case across northern Canada.

For example, when Amy Wilson worked in the Yukon in the late 1940s, she was occasionally called in to attend births deemed by Aboriginal community members to be risky. The federal Department of Health and Welfare hired Wilson as the official Alaska Highway nurse in 1949. Her territory covered northern British Columbia to points beyond Whitehorse, in the Yukon Territory. She was field nurse to the approximately three thousand Aboriginals who lived in communities along the Alaska Highway. Increased contact from American military personnel as well as highway construction workers threatened Native well-being.

Wilson's duties varied from day to day, but she came into contact with hundreds of children, sometimes commencing from their birth. In one instance recounted by Wilson, she was alerted by the Signals Station in Whitehorse to an emergency maternity case 160 miles north near Minto, Yukon. With maternity kit, sleeping bag, and medical bag in hand, she flew north. The patient's delivery turned out to be straightforward, but the retelling of this story prompted Wilson to remember what she viewed as a traditional Aboriginal woman's delivery. At the time of birth a favourite midwife, usually a mother or mother-in-law, would be invited to assist, unless an abnormal delivery was anticipated, when all of the women in the community would be asked to help. The mother would stand or squat over a pole in the tent. Her abdomen would be "pummeled and squeezed." Pressure was applied: "Often a blanket is tied around her as tightly as two women can pull it. They think this will force the baby's birth. Nothing particularly clean is used, yet it is surprising how few die."[15]

While Wilson's description sounds similar in some respects to Marsh's, she did not appear to want Aboriginal women to give up the entirety of their traditional practices. She participated in the delivery, adding modern practices as they seemed appropriate. She applied silver nitrate to the infant's eyes, and tied the umbilical cord. She stayed to bathe the newborn, and remembered how all the women stood near to watch: "They were delighted when I took a small spring scale out of my kit and weighed the little fellow. He was tied in the towel the way the stork brought him, and weighted 9 lbs. and 4 ozs."[16] In the process she observed that although there were few diapers, muskeg moss had been gathered to use instead. This she saw as a fine alternative: "One seldom sees a baby with sore buttocks if muskeg moss has been used as a diaper."[17]

Wilson differed from the Anglican minister in her sensitivity to the value of some practices. She did not appear to advocate change. Rather, she was more circumspect in her advocacy, as the last quotation demonstrates. Her medical bag was jammed with previously foreign objects like spring scales and silver nitrate. New technological apparatus and medicinal supplies introduced the possibility of early intervention in the lives of northern Aboriginal infants. Wilson also was subtle. She tied the umbilical cord, which may well have seemed unusual for the women who watched. As the nurse herself acknowledged, mothers often would trim the cord off with their teeth if there was too much left after the first snip. Wilson also claimed that sometimes the cord was carried in a buckskin bag around the neck of the infant: "It is a common belief among the native people that if the cord is carried by the child throughout his or her childhood it will insure health, intelligence and good nature."[18] It may well have appeared strange to the Native women in this region to see the nurse tying the umbilical cord, with all its long-standing spiritual meaning and set of rituals.

In the 1950s Dorothy Knight, hired to work as a nurse in Lake Harbour on the southern coast of Baffin Island, also remembered her first experience of a midwife-supervised delivery and the treatment of the afterbirth. Knight's new home of Lake Harbour had been occupied by newcomers since the early twentieth century, and like other Arctic communities, it was home to a coterie of southern officials—traders, RCMP officers, and missionaries. Except for the few who were locally employed, the Inuit were not settled permanently in the community. They moved seasonally and were, for the most part, engaged in the fur trade.

Since it seemed unlikely that she would be spontaneously invited to attend a delivery, Knight asked her hospital interpreter and helper, a man named Ishawakta, if he could arrange it for her. Tagalik, an expectant mother, and two midwives, Oola and Pitsulala, agreed to have her in attendance. During the birth she watched Tagalik squat on a sealskin, with two wooden crates supporting her elbows. Each time she had a contraction, the midwives on either side of her massaged her abdomen, or as Knight's biographer put it, "the midwives kneaded and pushed at the woman's swollen belly."[19] The Inuit woman took occasional sips of tea and became increasingly "shiny with sweat," and weary, until finally the baby boy was born. The midwives cut the umbilical cord, wrapped the afterbirth in sealskin and arranged to have it taken outside. The mother sipped tea and relaxed with her son, Nootoosha, named after a well-respected hunter from the community. In this instance Knight served more as an observer than Wilson or Marsh. While somewhat judgmental, she did not interfere. She did not attend the birth as a participant or necessarily with reform as her goal. Her narrative demonstrates that Inuit women in Lake Harbour maintained traditional birthing practices and rituals, like the placement outside of the afterbirth, as late as 1957.

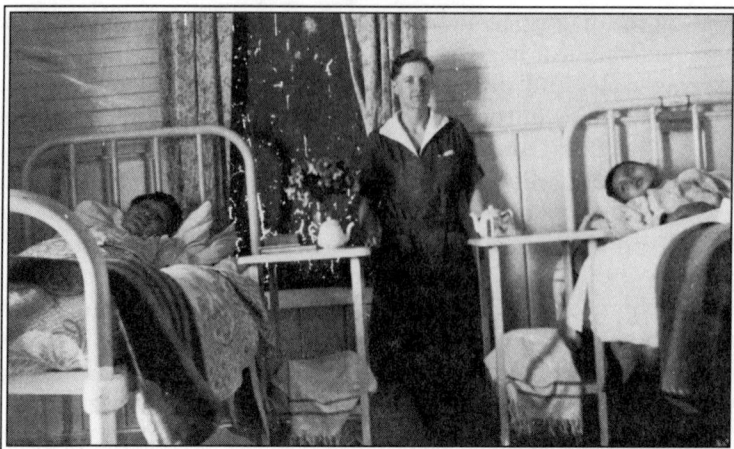

Captain Nurse Mildred Rundle and two young patients, All Saints Hospital, Aklavik, late 1930s (Fleming/NWT Archives n-1979-050-0053)

Lake Harbour residents, unlike some other Aboriginal mothers in northern Canada, had not been exposed to the most dramatic intervention in childbirth practices, that of evacuation.

Birthing traditions were, however, changing. In the early 1950s, Lilian Lucey worked as an Anglican nurse/missionary at Old Crow in the Yukon and later at Fort McPherson, along the Mackenzie River. In her memoir she recalled being awakened from her sleep at 3:30 a.m. to the sight of an expectant woman and prospective grandmother. Since this patient previously had both a Cesarean section and a difficult birth, the itinerant doctor had recommended she fly north to Aklavik for her confinement. He was concerned that the third delivery would also be hazardous. The woman refused to leave her home and instead she landed on Lucey's doorstep just at the onset of labour. The southern nurse recalled: "I inwardly gulped—admitted my mother, prepped her, no getting HER to Aklavik." The baby arrived very soon after. The next day Lucey learned that her early morning visitors had deliberately avoided going to Aklavik: "I was told afterwards the mother and daughter put their heads together after the doctor's visit and told it around the village. 'Mrs. Lucey was as good as any doctor!'"[20] This report gave the nurse the shivers, since she was well aware of the risks, but she was forced to accept her patient's determination to maintain some control over natural processes.[21]

Evacuation from northern communities represented intervention at its most dramatic. Apphia Aglakti Awa, who was flown from Pond Inlet to Iqaluit in 1966 for a hospital delivery, reflected on the meaning of her experience. She was born in 1931 and had eleven children. Interviewed by anthropologist Nancy Wachowich in 1993, she recalled how her first children were born on the land: "We used to deliver in camp without nursing stations or nurses to help us. We delivered in sod houses, and we delivered in tents, and we were fine."[22] When her last child arrived, it took her four days of hospital labour. In comparison to her typical birthing experiences, she found her hospital confinement traumatic.[23] In her own lifetime, Apphia Aglakti Awa found out what it meant to shift between old and new routines of childbirth and judged the latter as less than satisfactory.

Missionaries and nurses believed they were providing invaluable services, and in some cases they were. However, they seemed rarely to appreciate the meanings attached to umbilical cords, or the taboos associated with the afterbirth. Nor could they relate to standing deliveries, or the prospect of an involved audience of women. First-person accounts suggest that missionaries and nurses remained for the most part wedded to the belief that life had to change for Inuit mothers.

Nonetheless, the delivery of children served as a significant meeting ground between Natives and newcomers. Deliveries represented the first moment of intervention in Aboriginal lives. Infants were exposed to regimes that were foreign to their own culture. Perched between the traditions of their mothers and midwives, and the new nurses with their technologies rooted in Western medicine, newborns from the moment they entered the world were caught between the old and new. In fact, babies provided a major justification for intervention into Aboriginal lives. Missionaries and nurses felt that *because of the children*, they had a mission. The infants were born to Aboriginal women, but were born under the close scrutiny and measurement of newcomers.

White scrutiny was justified by the federal government's periodic and fleeting attention to infant health in the north. In the mid-1950s concern mounted when statistical data pointed to high infant mortality rates, particularly among the Inuit. However, there was very little discussion about the relationship between these deaths and the new economic conditions. The mortality rates, which by 1958 were significant, were in most cases not related to birthing practices, so intervention at birth may not have made much difference.[24]

Dressing

While the birth of children attracted attention and activity, newcomers remained attentive to youngsters as they grew. In particular, their gaze focused on clothing, or lack of such, as a key signifier of the move from "barbarism" to "civilization." From the early twentieth century right through until the end of the 1950s, infant clothing prompted constant

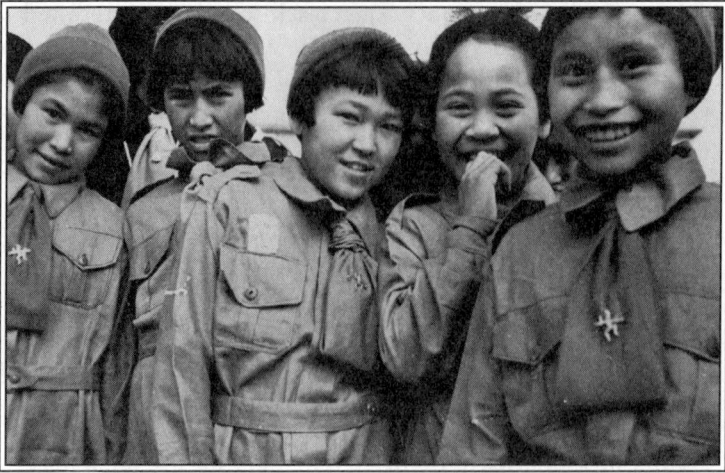

Aklavik Loucheux Brownies, 1943 (Fleming/NWT Archives n-1979-050-0098)

criticism from missionaries and nurses. Southerners wrote endlessly about their perception that Inuit women did not dress their infants in warm clothing in the face of excessively cold winters. They wondered if the high rates of pneumonia and respiratory illnesses might be attributed to apparently insufficient covering. Again, as in the case of delivery, children's bodies provided the testing ground for exchanges between adult Aboriginals and newcomers.

Southern clothes represented civilization, health, and progress to outsiders. Newcomers came to expect that northerners would, to some extent, mimic their clothing style. In 1928 Minnie Hackett, an Anglican missionary/nurse stationed at Aklavik, was inspired to compare Dene and Inuvialuit infant fashion:

When the babies are born I visit the mothers, and see that they are getting the right care, and show the mother how to dress the baby—advice which is neglected as they prefer their own way. The Indians put a flannelette shirt or dress (I don't know what they call it) on the baby, and wrap several squares of the same material around it, in a moss bag, which is laced in front with moose-hide strings. It is a good method in this country as the baby keeps warm, but I want to teach them to use the barracoats, and by persevering I hope to succeed—after several years. The Eskimos do not use a moss bag; the baby has just one flannelette shirt and is placed inside the mother's dress on her back and a belt around the waist saves the baby from falling through.[25]

Less frustrated with Dene than Inuvialuit mothers, Hackett nonetheless wanted to introduce the babies to "barracoats." Her preferences were shared by Donalda McKillop Copeland, a nurse at Southampton Island in the early 1950s. The latter revealed her dismay about the condition of Inuit infant attire. Her housekeeper, Kitty, was late for work one day, and when she finally showed up, Copeland noticed that she was especially joyful: "In a moment she revealed the reason for her joy. She lifted the hood of her loose kooletah to show me. Snuggled down within the warm enclosure was Okalik and Eyakak's new-born daughter, deep in slumber. And [the child was] stark naked. I stifled an exclamation of shock and dismay."[26]

Kitty announced that she and her husband had just adopted the baby. Instead of ruining Kitty's surprise, Copeland congratulated her, and then proceeded to "hunt out warm clothing for the babe—shirt, diaper, sweater, bonnet and blanket."[27] These were the proper garb for a newborn, not naked shelter in her mother's hood. Even though the baby girl was in a "warm enclosure" in the *kooletah*, Copeland still expressed her sense of "shock" when she saw her naked.

From their delivery, to their attire, Aboriginal youngsters attracted the attention and reform efforts of missionaries and nurses. Delivery and clothing shifted slowly under the critical eyes of newcomers, who saw both as threatening children's well-being. Across the north, newcomers increasingly did not hesitate to make suggestions about clothing, or as Minnie Hackett put it, she wanted to show mothers "how to dress" their babies. From the point of view of most newcomers, health and hygiene were at stake, and the emphasis was to be placed on Western medical practices over more traditional methods. Properly delivered babies, clad in Western costumes, symbolized the start of new regimes that required the setting aside of old practices. In response, Inuit women usually resisted the appeal of southern infant wear and generally remained unenthusiastic throughout most of the twentieth century.

Bathing

Efforts at intervention continued as children grew. Attention to hygiene and cleanliness were overwhelmingly visible in both the mission record and in northern nursing narratives. Aboriginal children in northern communities, and in mission schools, were bound at one time or another in their early years to encounter a newcomer determined to convert their bodily practices. Hygiene was an utter obsession for newcomers, as they came in to contact with children in communities and schools. Beyond the gaze of parents, missionaries or nurses would make little effort to disguise their disdain for the past and their determination to impose a new order.

In 1909, at the beginning of what would be a long missionary career in the north, Archibald Fleming was sent by London's Church Missionary Society to Lake Harbour in the eastern Arctic. This was the same com-

munity that Dorothy Knight would be sent to nearly fifty years later.
The Rev. Fleming, along with his housemate, J. W. Bilby, were the first
missionaries to live in that small community. Fleming remembered being
enthusiastically greeted by the Inuit who were camped in the area. Cheerful women with babies in their hoods helped unload the ship and welcomed the newcomers. The local Inuit were no strangers to contact,
having previously engaged in trade with Euro-American whalers.

As Reverends Bilby and Fleming settled into their newly constructed
house, Fleming quickly realized that Bilby hated having any of the Inuit
touch his food. However, because of the demands of mission work,
including their efforts to translate the Bible, as well as keep up with
their own domestic tasks, Fleming convinced the reluctant Bilby that it
would be wise to hire a young Inuk boy to help out. Fleming set to work
to find the right candidate. He watched the community children at play,
and, as he claimed, "It seemed to me that one, named Yarley, was particularly bright. He was a dirty little barbarian, good natured, ragged,
rotund, and ridiculously amusing."[28] Yarley was just the boy Fleming
was looking for. He approached the youngster, offering him work and
undertaking to train him in cooking and cleaning. The next hurdle
came with Fleming's realization that the boy, "to put it plainly, smelled."[29]
When he took this problem up with Bilby, the latter's response was a
nonchalant "consider the conditions under which the Eskimo live,"
adding later, "It's up to you if you want to be a reformer."

At first Fleming decided to introduce his reforms slowly, encouraging Yarley to wash his face once a day and clean his hands when he was
preparing meals. After several days he chose to take a chance and, as he
put it, "introduce Yarley to the Order of the Bath.'[30] He set to work laying out the necessary utensils including a washtub, some "carbolic soap,
towels and a sponge." He then informed Yarley that the preparations
were for him:

It came as a shock to the lad when he was told that all was for him, not for me,
and that he was going to take the first bath he ever had in his life. With some
agitation he agreed and I stood by to see that the job was well done. The knowledge that after the washing was over he would possess new clothes, the towels,
sponge, soap, etc., may have been a contributing factor to the success of the
event! At any event he came out clean and smiling as if he had been through a
great adventure, and he did not take cold.[31]

Fleming claimed that Yarley regarded him with suspicion for some
time and that the "Order of the Bath" had caused a certain stir amid the
Inuit in the area. Everyone heard about it. Fleming enjoyed both cleaning and dressing Yarley. For the first Christmas at Lake Harbour, Fleming noted that his protege "was dressed in "white man's" clothes, includ-

ing a large apron of bleached cotton made especially for the occasion by an Eskimo woman."[32] Unfortunately, we do not learn how Yarley actually felt about the bath adventure. He did, however, become an employee of the mission house and continued to work for the Anglicans in the north well into his old age.

From Fleming's perspective, the transition to Christianity required a good dose of personal and public hygiene. Sometimes lessons in hygiene became the main focus of missionary efforts, and at other times they competed with Bible stories. Cleanliness and neatness were immediate objectives, but personal salvation was the long-term goal. Many missionaries took it for granted that their hygiene programs would produce Aboriginals who were more successful students and better Christians.

A later bath narrative suggests some change from the earlier efforts of missionaries like Fleming. In her biography of Dorothy Knight, Betty Lee describes an experience similar to Fleming's but one with a considerably different outcome. Working as the only nurse in Lake Harbour, Knight cared for all the Inuit who visited the community. She used the nursing station clinic, and occasionally met patients at her home as well. A common ailment that she noticed among Inuit children was impetigo. At one point Knight decided to bathe a little girl who seemed to be suffering from both impetigo and scabies. Along with Hilda Baird, the HBC trader's wife, and her male Inuk helper, Ishawatka, she prepared the bath for the child, whose name is not made known:

> "Do you think it's her first dip?" Hilda asked as Ishwatka filled the tub.
> "I wouldn't be surprised," said Dorothy. The girl sat quietly, draped in a towel. But when the women led her to the bath, she began to sob. "Agai! Agai!"
> "Oh come on honey," said Hilda encouragingly. "I've brought my best soap!"
> "Agai!"
> Dorothy lifted the child into the water. The screams grew louder as the girl twisted in her arms, fighting to get away. "Agai!"
> "God!" said Hilda. "She's terrified!"
> Dorothy snatched the child out of the bath and wrapped the towel around her shaking body! Then she sat in the livingroom, the sobbing girl cradled in her lap. *What am I trying to do?* she asked herself glumly. *I can't put bathtubs into every Eskimo dwelling in the Arctic.* She would take the girl back to the hospital and tell her mother to wash her with a cloth from a familiar pot. She had no idea when regular bathing would become a habit among the Inuit, but she would never subject a child to the terrors of the tub again.[33]

This account differs from Yarley's narrative in significant ways. First, the boy was being trained to work at the mission house; therefore, at least for Fleming this justified even the traumatic effects of bathing. Nor did Yarley appear to be as terrified of the ordeal as the young girl.

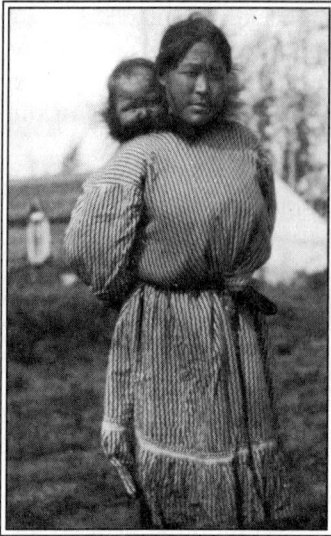

Inuit woman carrying a child at Aklavik, 1926 (Canada, Department of Interior / g-1979-001-0273)

But perhaps the most substantial difference lay in the attitude of the newcomer. According to her biographer, Dorothy Knight stopped and questioned herself. "What am I trying to do," she wondered. What was her goal? How could she expect that all of the Inuit children would suddenly be able to conform to her standards of cleanliness, when they did not have access to bathtubs? More than that though, a woman who lived after the Second World War may have found it more difficult than an earlier male visitor to take for granted her power over Aboriginal peoples. Knight certainly attempted to introduce cultural reform, but she was at times less sure of her right to demand change than the earlier missionaries, who believed they had not only an "ordained" right but a duty to try to alter consciousness.

Nonetheless, children in settlements, and in mission-run community schools, continued to face missionaries and nurses who placed as much emphasis on hygiene as they did on religion and scholarship. School medical inspections, as Mona Gleason so ably points out, became a tool used increasingly by the state to both "discipline the student body" and "legitimize medical expertise." Northern children were not immune to this surveillance. The nurse at Southampton Island in the early 1950s, Donalda McKillop Copeland was quite representative. The wife of a federally appointed welfare officer and schoolteacher, she volunteered her time in the classroom when she was not busy with her nursing duties. School hours became a combination of health lesson and medical clinic. Each student was exposed to a bodily inspection and became the subject of a health record with details on "height, weight [and] condition of skin, eyes, ears and throat."[34] After a school clinic one day she allowed her hopes to be overheard by her husband: "'What a fine thing it would be,' I sighed, 'if only we had some sort of communal wash and bath-house.'"[35] He immediately rigged up a galvanized tub in the kitchen of the school where they invited, not just the pupils, but also all of the Inuit in the community to bathe and wash their clothes.

Donalda Copeland also joined a host of southerners in complaining that hair lice constituted a common hygienic problem among the children. In each clinic she routinely soaked a "comb with cuprex, [and] thoroughly I curried each head of straight black hair."[36] If she could not remove the lice, she would cut the hair. While taboos forbade cutting the tresses of Inuit girls, Copeland would not be deterred.

Rhoda Kaujak Katsak remembered the ordeal. She felt that newcomers or "Qallunaat," as they were called by the Inuit, were always telling her people just exactly what to do. On a trip to the nurse's station in Igloolik, she faced a haircut: "The nurses, they taught us that we weren't supposed to have lice in our hair. We had never thought that lice in our hair was necessarily a bad thing."[37] The presence of vermin was an ongoing concern for nurses and missionaries, yet Rhoda was unbothered. Remembering the new rules she lived under, she felt resentful. Yet she also recalled benefits: "I have had some very good friends in my life who have been Qallunaat. There was a nurse from Montreal who was here for a while."[38] Gender relations played a role in this friendship. At least occasionally it seemed that female nurses more easily could befriend Inuit women and sometimes temper the intensity of the new bodily regimes that were being imposed.[39]

Scheduling

Newcomers rarely hesitated to reprimand their Native hosts, especially the youngest, about their inadequate standards of health and hygiene. They paraded the possibilities of the technologies of cleanliness and hygiene, the carbolic soap, Cuprex, towels, bathtubs, and other devices before northern communities. Lessons in routine, scheduling, and clock orientation were supplemented with instruction in birth, bathing, and clothing. Repetition was viewed as the key to success. Donald Marsh explained his classroom management style. He held school at the mission house, where every day involved a ritualized cleaning: "I put out a basin of water, a towel, and a comb, ready for use before each session. This became a highlight of 'school,' with grandmothers and children alike assisting each other to delouse themselves."[40] This spectacle, Marsh was convinced, produced students who were not only cleaner but "much more studious." "School lessons," as he concluded "like church sermons, were as much about hygiene and health as about religion and the three Rs."[41] They were also about establishing a routine set of practices.

Attempting to impose Western order on northern bodies could sometimes pose unique challenges. So too could the long daylight hours in the high Arctic. In *The Other Side of Eden*, anthropologist Hugh Brody recalled becoming embroiled in a struggle between some Inuit parents at Pond Inlet and newcomers, particularly schoolteachers. Like many other Arctic communities, Pond Inlet was a settlement established by the Canadian federal government and administered by southerners. It was created to encourage the Inuit to desert their traditional hunting camps and to live in prefabricated houses, attend local schools, and when ill, receive medical supervision from the nurses at the local nursing station.[42] Inuktituk was the primary language spoken, but a few of the Inuit could speak English, and they were eager for their children to learn the language. In fact, children stood at the centre of the struggle recalled by Brody. The trouble was that it was June, and in the land of the midnight sun, time began to take on a different meaning, a meaning that did not fit the schedules of southern schoolteachers. Children stayed up, gallivanted around Pond Inlet, played baseball, went on bike rides, but they often did not go to bed until breakfast time. The school hours, however, did not reflect this pattern. Pupils were expected to be in school early in the morning, and many did not meet this standard. A community meeting was called to discuss the problem. Teachers believed it was the responsibility of the parents to arouse their sleepy children. Parents, on the other hand, believed that since it was the teachers who were so vexed about the children, then they should ensure that the children were in school on time. The teachers should come to the houses to awaken their charges.[43] While the problem remained unresolved, it offers a striking example of the tension between what Brody calls "an Inuit sense of culture and the colonial enterprise."[44] Pond Inlet kids were treated as individuals who could make decisions without being coerced by adults. They carried the name of their ancestors and, as such, were treated as rational decision makers by their kin. Parents were more than willing to have their offspring attend school, but they were not about to force them to adapt to the classroom routines and discipline.

This effort to enforce strict bedtime routine, associated in Western culture with successful, healthy children, was but one of the new regimes to which Inuit children were exposed by southerners. And, as Brody reminds us, at times there was strong resistance. The summer months offered children alternatives more appealing than the classroom.

Resisting

The Pond Inlet children were not unique in their desire to assert their freedom and independence. Their efforts to challenge the newly imposed schedule were matched by those of other children who collaborated in order to talk, joke, and sometimes to downright refuse new disciplines.

In her memoirs Amy Wilson recalled a clinic that she held in Lower Post, Yukon, during one of her many stops along the Alaska Highway. Together with a doctor from Edmonton and the assistant Indian agent, she occupied the schoolhouse for the day to carry out their duties. Since no one was actually sick, the doctor spent the day extracting teeth, acting as a dentist. Amy Wilson found herself administering vaccinations and measuring weight. The scales were the most popular of attractions, as many school girls and young women wanted to try them out: "No woman bothered to take off the jacket that might weigh an extra pound or so. One, anxious for her turn, stepped on the scale with her baby slung on her back. As the weight indicator swung to 200 pounds, and then passed it, peals of laughter rang out from those crowding round. Unabashed, she stepped off the scales. She and her healthy baby made a pretty figure."[45] The unfamiliar technology provided an opportunity to joke about others' numbers with "peals of laughter" ringing out. Measurements would set in motion a new consciousness about size and appearance, just as bathing in soap and water raised new possibilities about perceiving the Westernized version of the proper body.

The significance of the "peals of laughter" heard in the school that day should not be ignored. While the newcomers approached their technologies of health—the weights, measurements, bathtubs, and soap—with seriousness and respect, Aboriginal children, like their mothers, could be much less intense about it all. Humour could be a form of resistance, or at least a response, which helped contain the threat of foreign intrusion into private Aboriginal spaces.

Another account by Jane Willis, a first-year boarding student at the St. Philip's Indian and Eskimo Anglican Residential School of Fort George, Quebec, made the same point. She remembered sitting on the grass with her Cree girlfriends and talking about white people, a subject she claimed was a favourite with her classmates. Their exposure to the "White race" was limited to Hudson's Bay Company employees and missionaries, and, as Willis joked, "What we did not know about them we made up as we went along." On the subject of hygiene and germs the girls all agreed: "Did you know that white people don't have germs like us?" "Because they're always yelling at us about *our* germs. They're so afraid of catching them. When we sneeze or cough, they always scream at us to cover our mouths so we won't spread our filthy germs around.

If they had germs, they wouldn't be afraid of ours would they?"[46] Foreign preoccupations, while powerful, provided moments of hilarity. The
girls were naturally curious about obsessions for which they found no
obvious explanation.

The administration of cod-liver oil, a frequent accompaniment of
instruction in hygiene, similarly offered moments for youthful recalci-
trance. Alice French, an Inuk student at Aklavik's Anglican All Saints Residential School in the 1930s, remembered how she and her friends were
forced each morning to gulp down the evil-tasting vitamin supplement
cod-liver oil, but she also joked about how they then enjoyed dashing "to
the toilet to spit it out" after it had been scooped into their mouths.[47]
Their pleasure soon ended when the supervisor caught word of the cod-
liver oil's final destination. Ultimately, Native youngsters were, like many
adults, in a poor position to persist in rejecting the foreign regimes that
promised better health, even as they underpinned traditional cultures.

Conclusion

While it is critical not to dismiss the valuable work of southern health care
providers in assisting at births, getting rid of vermin, battling epidemics,
diagnosing tuberculosis, and sometimes heading off real tragedies,
nurses and missionaries were at the forefront of reforms that threatened, even as they beckoned. Children and their bodies stood at the
centre of the battle waged with Native people over the regimes and rituals that would govern the most intimate parts of their lives. The history
of encounter in northern communities deeply affected Aboriginal children and childbearing practices. Bodies were not only carefully scrutinized, but they were also poked, prodded, washed, dressed, and weighed
by Euro-Canadians who frequently found them wanting. Concern was
expressed, advice freely given, and, to some extent, practices amended.
Demands for acquiescence took place within the context of colonization. There were also occasional surprising moments in the encounter
between newcomers and Aboriginals, which promised something else.
Sometimes it seemed as if the intensity of the relationship had given way
to a deeper understanding of the meaning of change. These moments
may have been few and far between, but they existed. Dorothy Knight
realized that the attempt to bathe the little girl under her care was point-
less. And Rhoda Kaujak Katsak fondly remembered befriending a nurse.
Other youngsters refused to take the newcomers entirely seriously. Such
negotiations were not inconsequent in individual lives. Yet, ultimately,
in the encounter between Whites and Natives over children's bodies,
Euro-Canadian missionaries and health workers had the upper hand.
Youthful laughter could reduce but it could not eliminate this power.

However, the survival of Aboriginal birthing rituals and the perseverance of traditional medicine makers suggests that the contest between the old and new was waged with equal determination on both sides.

Acknowledgement

I would like to thank the very skillful editorial work of both Veronica Strong-Boag and Cheryl Krasnick Warsh, as well as the generous financial support of the CRC post-doctoral fellowship in Native/Newcomer Relations with Jim Miller at the University of Saskatchewan. Thanks also to Robert Rutherdale for his helpful comments. I am very fortunate to belong to such a wonderful community of scholars.

Notes

1 See Celia Haig-Brown, *Resistance and Renewal: Surviving the Indian Residential School* (Vancouver: Tillacum, 1988); J. R. Miller, *Shingwauk's Vision: A History of Native Residential Schools* (Toronto: University of Toronto Press, 1996); and John Milroy, *"A National Crime": The Canadian Government and the Residential School System 1879–1986* (Winnipeg: University of Manitoba Press, 1999).

2 Mary-Ellen Kelm, *Colonizing Bodies: Aboriginal Health and Healing in British Columbia* (Vancouver: University of British Columbia Press, 1998), 57.

3 Kelm, *Colonizing Bodies*, 59. See also Maureen Lux, *Medicine That Walks: Disease, Medicine and Canadian Plains Native People, 1880–1940* (Toronto: University of Toronto Press, 2001), 226.

4 See, for example, Shirley Sterling, *My Name Is Seepeetza* (Vancouver: Douglas and McIntyre, 1992); Mary Lawrence, *My People, Myself* (Prince George: Caitlin, 1996); Lee Maracle, *I Am Woman: A Native Perspective on Sociology and Feminism* (Vancouver: Press Gang, 1996); and Nancy Wachowich, ed., in collaboration with Appha Agalakti Awa, Rhoda Kaukjak Katsak, and Sandra Pikujak Katsak, *Saqiyuq: Stories from the Lives of Three Inuit Women* (Montreal and Kingston: McGill-Queen's University Press, 1999).

5 There is now a considerable literature on domestic Christian missions to Aboriginals. See Kerry Abel, *Drum Songs: Glimpses of Dene History* (Montreal and Kingston: McGill-Queen's University Press, 1993); Clarence Bolt, *Thomas Crosby and the Tsimshian: Small Shoes for Feet Too Large* (Vancouver: University of British Columbia Press, 1992); Brett Christophers, *Positioning the Missionary: John Booth Good and the Confluence of Cultures in Nineteenth-Century British Columbia* (Vancouver: University of British Columbia Press, 1998); Ken S. Coates, *Best Left as Indians: Native–White Relations in the Yukon Territory, 1840–1973* (Montreal and Kingston: McGill-Queen's University Press, 1991); Peter Murray, *The Devil and Mr. Duncan: A History of the Two Metlakatlas* (Victoria: Sono Nis Press, 1985); Myra Rutherdale, *Women and the White Man's God: Gender and Race in Canada's Mission Field* (Vancouver: University of British Columbia Press, 2002); John Webster Grant, *Moon of Wintertime: Missionaries and Indians of Canada in Encounter since 1534* (Toronto: University of Toronto Press, 1984); Margaret Whitehead, "Women Were Made for Such Things: Women Missionaries in British Columbia 1850s to 1940s," *Atlantis* 14 (Fall 1988): 141–50; and Margaret Whitehead, "'A Useful Christian Woman': First Nations Women and Protestant Missionary Work in British Columbia,"

Atlantis 18 (Fall–Summer 1992–93): 142–66. On medical missions, see Jamie Scott, "Doctors Divine: Medicine and Muscular Christianity in the Canadian Frontier Adventure Tale," in *Colonies, Missions, Cultures in the English-Speaking World: General and Comparative Studies*, ed. Gerhardt Stilz (Tübingen: Stauffenburg Verlag, 2001): 13–26.

6   Embodiment as a category of analysis is beginning to receive special treatment by Canadian historians. See especially Mona Gleason, "Embodied Negotiations: Children's Bodies and Historical Change in Canada, 1930–1960," *Journal of Canadian Studies* 34, 1 (Spring 1999): 112–38. Southern Canadian reformers were also busy in Canadian cities and have received scholarly attention. See Neil Sutherland, *Children in English-Canadian Society: Framing the Twentieth Century Consensus* (Waterloo: Wilfrid Laurier University Press, 2000); and Mariana Valverde, *The Age of Light, Soap and Water* (Toronto: McClelland and Stewart, 1991).

7   Initially the Anglicans were sponsored by the Church Missionary Society head-quartered in London, England, but by the early twentieth-century the Mission Society for the Church of England in Canada based in Toronto was supporting a good portion of the northern work.

8   Sharon Richardson, "Alberta's Provincial Travelling Clinic, 1924 to 1942," in this volume.

9   For the most part, Inuit and Inuvialuit children were not taken away to residential schools until after the Second World War. Their education was attended to by missionaries in their own communities when they were not out on traplines or at the floe-edge. However, some Inuit and Inuvialuit children, especially but not exclusively orphans, were sent to schools like either of the Anglican-operated schools at Herschel Island and Aklavik, or in the Eastern Arctic, at the St. Philip's Indian and Eskimo Anglican Residential School of Fort George, Quebec. The situation differed for Indian children in the Yukon Territory, who were more likely to be sent away to residential school (usually Carcross), and had in comparison to the Inuit and Inuvialuit children more rapidly felt the negative impact of Newcomers, particularly during and after the gold rush of 1898.

10 A thorough discussion of the increased medicalization of childbirth throughout the first fifty years of the twentieth century is provided in Wendy Mitchinson, *Giving Birth in Canada 1900–1950* (Toronto: University of Toronto Press, 2002). For the north, also see "The Politics of Health in the Fourth World: A Northern Canadian Example," in *Interpreting Canada's North: Selected Readings*, ed. Kenneth S. Coates and William R. Morrison, 279–98 (Toronto: Copp Clark Pitman, 1989); and John O'Neil and Penny Gilbert, eds., *Childbirth in The Canadian North: Epidemiological, Clinical, and Cultural Perspectives* (Winnipeg: Northern Health Research Unit, University of Manitoba, 1990). On the history of nursing in Canada, the most comprehensive study is Kathryn McPherson, *Bedside Matters: The Transformation of Canadian Nursing, 1900–1990* (Toronto: Oxford University Press, 1996).

11 Patricia Jasen, "Race, Culture, and the Colonization of Childbirth in Northern Canada," in *Rethinking Canada: The Promise of Women's History*, ed. Veronica Strong-Boag, Mona Gleason, and Adele Perry (Toronto: Oxford University Press, 2002), 353–67. On northern nursing, see Judith Bender Zelmonovits, "'Midwife Preferred': Maternity Care in Outpost Nursing Stations in Northern Canada 1945–1988," in *Women, Health and Nation: Canada and the United States since 1945*, ed. Georgina Feldberg, Molly Ladd-Taylor, Alison Li, and Kathryn McPherson, (Montreal and Kingston: McGill-Queen's University Press, 2003): 161–89.

12 Winifred Marsh, ed., *Echoes from a Frozen Land: Donald B. Marsh* (Edmonton: Hurtig, 1987), 117–18.

13 Marsh, *Echoes*, 118.

14 Marsh, *Echoes*, 118.

15 Amy V. Wilson, *No Man Stands Alone* (Sidney: Gray's Publishing, 1965), 48.

16 Wilson, *No Man Stands Alone*, 49.

17 Wilson, *No Man Stands Alone*, 49.

18 Wilson, *No Man Stands Alone*, 57.

19 Betty Lee, *Lutiapik: The Story of a Young Woman's Year of Isolation and Service in the Arctic* (Toronto: McClelland and Stewart, 1975), 102–103.

20 Lilian Lucey Papers, Diocese of the Yukon Church Records, Yukon Territorial Archives.

21 Lucey Papers.

22 Wachowich et al., *Saqiyuq*, 97.

23 Wachowich et al., *Saqiyuq*, 104.

24 For a discussion about the government's sudden statistical flurry in the late 1950s, see Jasen, "Race, Culture," 360. See also John S. Willis, "Disease and Health in Canada's North," *Medical Services Journal Canada* 19 (1963): 748–49. Northern nurses were concerned about infant mortality, but they rarely attributed it to birthing practices. See, for example, Lee, *Lutiapik*, 201.

25 Minnie Hackett, "Extracts of Interest from Letters Written by Miss Hackett, of Aklavik Hospital," *Living Message*, April 1928, 135, General Synod Archives of the Anglican Church of Canada.

26 Donalda McKillop Copeland, *Remember, Nurse* (Toronto: Ryerson Press, 1960), 150.

27 Copeland, *Remember, Nurse*, 151.

28 Archibald Lang Fleming, *Archibald the Arctic: The Flying Bishop* (New York: Appleton-Century-Crofts, 1956), 66.

29 Fleming, *Archibald the Arctic*, 66.

30 Fleming was using a pun here as the Order of the Bath was a meritorious military order in British knighthood dating back to the medieval era, when induction into the knighthood involved a ritual bath to purify the spirit. My thanks to Neil Sutherland for this information.

31 Fleming, *Archibald the Arctic*, 67.

32 Fleming, *Archibald the Arctic*, 71.

33 Lee, *Lutiapik*, 102–103.

34 Copeland, *Remember, Nurse*, 74. School medical inspections in British Columbia are carefully analyzed in Mona Gleason, "Race, Class, and Health: School Medical Inspection and 'Healthy' Children in British Columbia, 1890–1930," in this volume.

35 Copeland, *Remember, Nurse*, 76.

36 Copeland, *Remember, Nurse*, 74.

37 Wachowich et al., *Saqiyuq*, 194–95.

38 Wachowich, et al., *Saqiyuq*, 199.

39 Jo-Anne Fiske makes an interesting case for the relations of friendship and concern that developed between Catholic nuns and young Carrier girls at Legic, a Catholic residential school near Vanderhoof, BC. Jo-Anne Fiske, "Pocahontas's Granddaughters: Spiritual Transition and Tradition of Carrier Women of British Columbia," *Ethnohistory* 43 (Fall 1996): 663–81.

40 Marsh, *Echoes from a Frozen Land*, 29.

41 Marsh, *Echoes from a Frozen Land*, 30.

42 Hugh Brody, *The Other Side of Eden: Hunters, Farmers and the Shaping of the World* (Vancouver: Douglas and McIntyre, 2000), 26.
43 Brody, *Other Side of Eden*, 30.
44 Brody, *Other Side of Eden*, 30.
45 Wilson, *No Man Stands Alone*, 87.
46 Jane Willis, *Geniesh: An Indian Girlhood* (Toronto: New Press, 1973), 48–49.
47 Alice French, *My Name Is Masak* (Winnipeg: Peguis, 1977), 26.

Experts

❧

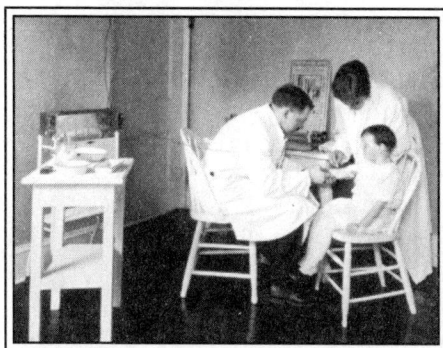

Physician Denial and Child Sexual Abuse in America, 1870–2000

CR

Hughes Evans

I n 1908, J. Taber Johnson summarized his thoughts about gonorrhea in children in a chapter of an influential textbook on gonorrhea. His confident assertions, "That coitus is not essential to gonorrheal infection is an established fact," and "An overwhelming proportion of the cases of vulvovaginitis in young girls is gonorrheal in origin and is of innocent origin" reflected the dominant view held for most of the nineteenth and twentieth centuries, that gonorrhea in children was *not* sexually transmitted.[1] By the 1970s this widely held view was beginning to come under fire as researchers recognized sexual abuse in significant proportions of their patients with gonorrhea.[2] This change led one leading child abuse advocate and researcher to reflect, "Twentieth century physicians, for the most part, have shirked, bypassed, or otherwise failed to fulfill their responsibilities toward young children with gonorrhea."[3] How and why physicians neglected to recognize sexual abuse in their young patients with gonorrhea forms the crux of this paper.

The taboo of child sexual abuse has shrouded the problem in secrecy and prevented public debate about its causes, consequences, and treatments until recently. Nevertheless, child sexual abuse has been a common and tragic constant in society.[4] Physicians in the late nineteenth and first half of the twentieth century were frequently called upon to examine and treat girls who had been sexually abused. Usually these girls visited the doctor because of symptoms caused by the abuse, not because of the abuse itself. In their discussions of the medical evaluation of these girls, however, doctors rarely mentioned the fact that their patients may have been abused. If these young girls disclosed abuse to their doctors, the doctors rarely reported it—to social or legal authorities, or in case reports in the medical literature.

Many of these girls suffered from gonorrheal vaginitis, an infection that is almost always transmitted sexually.[5] While there are many infectious causes of vaginitis, gonorrhea is among the most blatantly symp-

tomatic, causing abundant greenish pus to flow from the vagina, with
associated painful urination, swollen genitals, and often intense discom-
fort. Prior to the discovery of the gonococcus in 1879, most physicians
considered sexual transmission as the predominant method of transmission of gonorrhea in their adult patients. After the bacterial etiology
was established, physicians gathered more scientific evidence to stress the
key role sexual contact played in disease spread. They remained reluctant, however, to attribute pediatric gonorrhea to sexual transmission.

In the pre-antibiotic era, pediatric gonorrheal infections were difficult to treat and often simmered for months, causing frequent trips to
the doctor, uncomfortable symptoms, unpleasant treatments, and social
stigma.[6] Doctors struggled with ways to understand this disease. Their
research focused on several topics: hypotheses about why the pediatric
form of the disease differed from its adult counterpart, explanations of
how children acquired the disease non-sexually, the relationship between
pediatric complaints and emerging knowledge about the changing physiology of the genital tract, and treatment regimens to attempt to cure this
tenacious infection. These doctors wrote hundreds of articles about this
recalcitrant infection and often hypothesized about the mode of transmission.[7]

In spite of the frequency of this medical problem and amount of
attention given to it in the medical literature, physicians consistently
downplayed and often denied the possibility of sexual transmission,
providing other, less plausible explanations. This paper examines the
published anglophone medical literature on childhood gonorrhea and
child sexual abuse from 1870 to 2000. It argues that physicians rarely
attributed gonorrhea in their child patients to sexual abuse for myriad
reasons. This physician denial was a multifaceted phenomenon, reflecting a complex interaction among cultural, medical, scientific, and social
factors.

The STD Milieu of the Nineteenth and Early Twentieth Centuries

It is impossible to understand the importance of pediatric gonorrhea
without exploring the meaning of venereal disease in the nineteenth
and early twentieth century.[8] For most of the nineteenth century, physicians had appreciated the communicability of gonorrhea and other
venereal diseases like syphilis and had recognized the important role that
sexual contact played in spreading these infections. The great discoveries of bacteriology in the late nineteenth century offered a cogent explanation for how sexual contact could lead to disease: micro-organisms from
an infected person would pass to an uninfected partner through intimate

contact with genital secretions. They also knew that these diseases could be passed not only between men and women, but also from mothers to their unborn children, and in rare cases, from adults to children. The ravages of these diseases were legendary: blindness, infertility, mental illness, neurological impairment, fetal death, and chronic pain, just to mention a few. Doctors felt a sense of urgency to curb these horrible diseases.

In the minds of many doctors, the terrible physical consequences of venereal diseases paled in comparison to their association with moral corruption. The fact that gonorrhea was a venereal disease added a layer of heightened moral scrutiny to the diagnosis that other, non-venereal diseases did not share. The disease was commonly associated with vices such as prostitution, premarital sex, homosexuality, and adultery. Fearing the stigma and blame of such a diagnosis, patients often sought alternative explanations for their disease. Patients who acquired venereal disease without engaging in extramarital sex were called "innocent victims."

Innocent victims, then, included wives of diseased husbands who had acquired their venereal disease from a prostitute and other illicit sexual encounters, and newborn children who caught the disease as fetuses or through the birth canal. In addition, doctors also believed that nonsexual transmission was possible in some circumstances.[9] For instance, doctors argued that a patient could develop gonorrhea innocently by having contact with an object that had been infected inadvertently with gonorrheal pus. This notion provided a seemingly plausible way of explaining disease without alluding to the possibility of sexual contact. Thus, given that sexual contact was felt to be extraordinarily rare in children, almost any child who developed gonorrhea was called an innocent victim.[10]

The notion of innocent transmission provided physicians with an alternative explanation that was less morally reprehensible and legally explosive. Thus, for physicians with wealthy or socially respectable patients with this dreaded disease, innocent transmission offered a convenient and morally untainted explanation for their infection.

Nevertheless, the importance of sexual contact to the spread of gonorrhea and syphilis was so clearly understood that doctors often became moral crusaders expounding the dangers of extramarital sex.[11] The social hygiene movement flourished in the late nineteenth and early twentieth centuries and had the explicit goal of improving society by eliminating sexual immorality and promoting Christian values. Venereal disease was a prime target of these reform efforts. The social hygiene movement drew clear distinctions between who was at risk of venereal disease and who wasn't. In the social hygiene literature, then, sexually transmitted diseases were adult diseases, not pediatric. Their discussions of pediatric victims of venereal disease were limited to the devastating medical consequences of perinatal disease transmission and the deleterious moral effects on a family when the parents were promiscuous. Gonorrhea acquired through sexual abuse was rarely mentioned. Thus, despite enormous attention paid to stamping out venereal disease, the social hygiene movement virtually ignored child sexual abuse.

The Social Context of Child Protection in the Nineteenth and Twentieth Centuries

Although physical and sexual abuse of children has a long history, organized social responses to these problems are relatively recent. Issues affecting children were a major focus of many Progressive Era reforms, so it was not surprising that abused and neglected children rose to their attention in the late nineteenth century.[12] In 1874 a young, severely abused, and neglected girl in New York City named Mary Ellen Connolly was turned in to the American Society for the Prevention of Cruelty to Animals.[13] Her case received enormous attention, not only because of the horrible abuses that she had endured, but also because by taking her to an animal rights organization, the lack of an analogous organization for children was highlighted. Societies for the Prevention of Cruelty to Children quickly sprang up to replace this void. Staffed initially by concerned volunteers and then by the new profession of social workers, these forerunners of modern-day child abuse professionals took in abused children, investigated their homes and work environments, advocated for children in the legal system, and often found alternative places for these children to live.[14]

The increasing involvement of social workers and the government in family life reflected broader changes in the family as a legal unit. Although laws protecting children had existed since the colonial era, the authority of the family, and especially the father, to govern children as they chose, was largely unquestioned until the late nineteenth century.[15] With the Progressive Era reforms, social work agencies, often working under governmental auspices, began to scrutinize parental actions, and parental authority was called into question.

One consequence of increasing organizational responses to child abuse was improved public awareness of the issue. Mary Ellen's case, and others like it, garnered enormous attention in the newspapers. Child abuse, however, was generally framed as a problem affecting the lower socio-economic classes and immigrant and urban populations. As a result, this profiling of abuse reinforced preconceived opinions that it occurred primarily among newly arrived immigrants, denizens of urban squalor, and as a result of the pressures of poverty. Abuse was felt to be extremely rare in middle- and upper-class households.

The Scientific Argument: The Patient and the Organism

Given how rare child sexual abuse was thought to be, physicians naturally sought alternative explanations to sexual transmission in their young patients with this stigmatized disease. They began with the assumption that the disease *must not* be sexually acquired in most children, and developed explanations that reinforced that assumption. Borrowing on the rising popularity of pediatrics and bacteriology, they argued that the uniqueness of children, distinctive features of the bacteria, or a combination of both, made non-sexual transmission in children far more likely than sexual transmission.

The understanding of gonorrheal vaginitis in girls was enhanced by the rapidly evolving understanding of bacteriology in general. The causative organism of the disease, the gonococcus, was identified by Albert Neisser, a German dermatologist, in 1879.[16] Perhaps in part because of the moral overtones to any venereal disease, most pre-bacteriological era physicians felt that transmission was influenced not merely by sexual contagion but also by inheritance, constitution, and a variety of environmental and moral traits such as poverty, filth, intemperance, and immorality.

After Neisser's discovery, researchers recognized the infectious nature of the disease and gradually discarded the inheritance and constitutional explanatory models. They intensely studied the bacteria and its unique properties and found that it was fairly easily seen in a smear of infected pus. By combining the characteristic symptom of purulent vaginal discharge with the unique microscopic appearance, most physicians could make the diagnosis in their offices. In sexually active adults, in whom the disease was relatively common and transmission was easy, the addition of a relatively simple microscopic test that could be performed in the doctor's office improved the accuracy of the diagnosis substantially and added scientific legitimacy to the diagnosis. In children, however, obtaining the pus was technically more difficult and emotionally traumatizing. In addition, over the first half of the twentieth century, doctors discovered that some normal inhabitants of the pediatric vagina could be confused for gonorrhea.[17]

The use of culture to confirm diagnosis, while more accurate, was problematic in practice.[18] As Reith Fraser reported in 1926, "Where staining methods are inconclusive, however, cultural methods are invariably still more so."[19] The gonococcus proved to be recalcitrant to traditional culture techniques and required very specific culture media and incubation conditions that were difficult to reproduce in the office-based laboratory. Even in research settings, the organism was difficult to grow and earned the reputation of being very "fastidious." As a result, venere-ologists were forced to question the utility of culture in diagnosis and cli-nicians were left in a quandary.[20] Which diagnostic techniques should they trust: a positive gram stain combined with classic clinical symptoms, or only those patients whose cultures grew gonorrhea? By the 1920s, many researchers claimed that smear was the only practical method to use. As three researchers from the Michael Reese Hospital in Chicago con-cluded, "Our failure to isolate the organism in a certain percentage of cases in which the organism was believed to be present in direct smears, leads us to conclude that the smear method as a diagnostic procedure is preferable to the cultural method in office and dispensary work."[21] A. K. Paine, an expert in women's diseases at the Boston Dispensary, summed up the difficulty of using culture in diagnosis in his 1932 con-tribution to a special symposium on the problem on gonorrheal vagini-tis, saying,

In the absence of a reasonable explanation of how the infection in a given case could have occurred, one is justified in questioning a laboratory diagnosis of gon-orrhea which is based on a smear examination alone. Obviously the doubt aris-ing in such a case might be overcome by cultured methods. This theoretically is an easy solution of one of the problems presented by this subject but in practice seems not so simple. Technical difficulties in growing the gonococcus, plus the time and trouble involved, together with results not always conclusive have mit-igated to make the procedure less commonly employed than its theoretical dependability would seem to warrant.[22]

In other words, even as physicians were becoming increasingly com-fortable with laboratory-based diagnosis of infectious diseases, the tech-nical difficulties of applying laboratory techniques to daily practice ham-pered their ability to use the new technology.

But the problem went further than technical difficulty. Physicians had a hard time trusting the conclusions of laboratory tests. Paine com-plained that in one-quarter of their patients "we have a laboratory diag-nosis of gonorrhea but not available a reasonable explanation of how the child could have acquired this disease."[23] Paine's dilemma was a common one: should he trust the laboratory data that a child had gonorrhea when his clinical opinion was that the child could not have a sexually transmitted disease? Which was more accurate: the laboratory or clini-cal judgment?

Although physicians increasingly recognized the importance of accu-rate, laboratory-based diagnosis, they still relied heavily on traditional diagnostic techniques garnered from the history and the physical examination and clinical intuition from years of experience. Faced with seeming inconsistencies between the laboratory and their clinical conclusions, they tended to believe their own deductions rather than the laboratory. Thus, the biases built into the history and physical examination were slow to die.

When faced with laboratory evidence of gonorrhea in their patients but no convincing explanation for how their patient could have acquired it, some doctors argued that a different type of gonorrhea infected girls. A survey of pathologists and bacteriologists published in 1915 revealed that one in five experts believed that the gram negative diplococcus found in girls with clinical gonorrhea was not the "true" gonococcus.[24] In a related study, 20 per cent of the pediatricians surveyed felt that the gonococcus infecting children differed from the bacteria that infected adults. They believed that this other type resembled the gonococcus that infected adults, but that neither morphologic examination under a microscope nor culturing the offending organism would differentiate the two bacteria. Although this theory was never proven, a vocal minority of influential experts in the field promulgated this notion.

The idea of a morphological twin was not a new one to bacteriology. As bacteriologists developed more sophisticated techniques for identifying and growing microscopic organisms, they realized that many organisms once presumed to be a single entity were actually distinct bacteria with unique properties. After the turn of the century, scientists interested in gonorrhea and other sexually transmitted diseases began to report that the Neisseria gonococcus that caused genital-tract infections had several non-pathological mimickers in the genito-urinary tract.[25] If these similar-appearing bacteria could be normal flora, or non-sexually transmitted, then not all bacterial smears that looked like gonorrhea actually represented true gonococcal infection. Doctors applying this bacteriological observation to their clinical practice could and did use their own discretion to decide if what looked like gonorrhea actually was gonorrhea.

The persuasiveness of this theory lay in its seemingly plausible explanation for the difference in presentation and in transmission between adults and children. The idea of morphological similarity was powerful in part because it provided an explanation for how children could get the disease innocently while adults obtained it sexually. Scientists did not elaborate the theory to explain why this organism infected children but did not infect adults. Nor could they investigate the biological characteristics of this other type of gonorrhea more fully. The idea of an indistinguishable twin bacterium that infected girls eventually disappeared from the literature, because it lacked scientific credibility. However, its brief tenure reflects one of the ways that doctors and scientists sought to explain how children could acquire what was commonly understood to be a sexually transmitted disease.

If, on the other hand, the organism that infected women and girls was the same gonococcus, then, doctors felt, something unique about the host must explain why girls would become infected with what was typically thought of as a sexually transmitted disease. One clear difference between the infection in women and girls was that girls' vaginas became infected while in women the infection was located in the uterus and upper genital tract. Doctors following this line of inquiry hypothesized that something about the girls' genital tract altered the way they expressed infection. This potent area of scientific interest involved studying the changing vaginal environment of girls.[26] Researchers in this area noted that prior to puberty the vagina differed from the adult vagina, with different types of cells lining its walls and its own distinct bacterial and biochemical properties. These properties created a vaginal environment that was more conducive for the propagation of the gonococcus. Thus, children who were exposed to gonorrhea tended to get a vaginal infection rather than uterine involvement.

While this argument may have explained the symptoms of gonorrhea in girls, it did not explain how the gonorrhea got there in the first place. Many doctors who recognized this peculiar propensity of the vagina to allow gonorrheal growth assumed that the pediatric vagina somehow invited gonorrheal infection. They used words like *invite* and *hospitable* when describing the vagina's relationship with gonorrhea.[27] They argued that this lack of physiologic and anatomic protection against infection made casual contact with gonorrheal pus more likely. This choice of words continued in the medical literature into the 1980s.[28]

Arguments that rested on emerging information about the reproductive system of young girls reflected a growing body of knowledge in both endocrinology and pediatrics, two young fields that were gaining scientific legitimacy and clinical followings. The fact that the pre-pubertal vagina possessed a unique bacteriologic and biochemical milieu that differed substantially from that of adult women was particularly persuasive to pediatricians who embraced scientific explanations for the distinctiveness of pediatric disease. This ability to combine physiologic, anatomic, biochemical, and bacteriological knowledge to explain disease was particularly powerful in the early years of the twentieth century, when physicians were trying to shed earlier, more empirical explanations of disease.

By the 1930s the burgeoning field of endocrinology had not only helped to explain why gonorrhea caused vaginitis in children, but it also offered the first realistic treatment. Scientists realized that estrogen not only led to the major changes in the vaginal environment during puberty but also protected the vagina against gonorrheal infection.[29] Thus, estrogen treatments became the standard treatment for girls with gonorrhea. Under the influence of a variety of estrogen concoctions, the profuse purulent discharge of gonorrheal vaginitis would diminish. While not all girls were cured with estrogen, many noted a significant improvement in symptoms while taking the medicine.

The impact of finding a realistic treatment in the pre-antibiotic years was substantial. Prior to the introduction of hormonal treatments, children had been subjected to frequent douches with a variety of compounds, such as silver nitrate. These treatments were time-consuming, painful, and largely ineffective. Estrogen represented a huge improvement in therapy for these young girls. With an improved therapy at their disposal, doctors spent less time discussing modes of transmission and prevention tactics.

While estrogen treatments improved symptoms, antibiotics created cures. Penicillin in particular caused dramatic improvement. Vaginitis appeared to have been conquered.

The Fear of Spread of Infection

Prior to the advent of antibiotics, however, the contagiousness of gonorrhea incited enormous concern among doctors and officials dealing with infected children. As physicians in the State Venereal Disease Clinic in Denver, Colorado, stated, "The disease is the most infectious of all infectious diseases."[30] If children acquired gonorrhea non-sexually, then the potential for spread through casual contact was staggering. The best way to explain the non-sexual spread of gonorrhea was to invoke the theory of fomites, or infected objects that could act as inanimate vectors of disease. The idea of fomites was not new. Even prior to the advent of bacteriology, public health officials had pointed out the association between hygiene and health. But fomites were to play a crucial role in the explanation of gonorrhea infection and treatment strategies for the next century.

Doctors investigating gonorrhea in children developed a long laundry list of potential fomites. Most of these were objects that might come in contact with gonorrheal pus, either in the home, the hospital or institutional setting, or in public spaces. The objects included articles of personal hygiene like washcloths and sponges, medical equipment like bathtubs and thermometers, bed linens, and the ever popular culprit, the toilet.[31] In addition, physicians warned that the hands of an infected nurse, domestic servant, or mother could inadvertently act as fomites and spread disease to a child.[32]

The plausibility of applying the fomite theory to gonorrhea transmission was challenged by the fact gonorrhea was notoriously difficult to culture and did not survive long outside the body. It was extremely sensitive to drying and had very strict temperature and moisture requirements for growth. Not long after the gonococcus was identified, it was already well known that it did not survive long outside the body, a feature that made it a poor candidate for fomite spread. How did doctors justify this paradox? For the most part they ignored it. They rarely set out to test the usual array of proposed fomites to see if any of them carried the organism.[33] Their lack of curiosity about the credibility of the fomite argument suggested that they did not want to know if the argument held water. Fomite spread was a very handy way to explain how young children contracted a typically sexually transmitted disease.

Perhaps the most surprising fact about the fomite theory of gonorrhea spread was how long it persisted in the medical literature. One could make a persuasive argument that fomites were plausible within the explanatory framework of the late-nineteenth- and early-twentieth-century medicine and public health, but it is harder to explain how physicians continued to invoke fomites into the 1970s. For instance, one study of Alaskan children in 1971 argued that children became infected from sharing a bed with an infected parent.[34] The most recent recommendations from the American Academy of Pediatrics consider a diagnosis of gonorrhea in a pre-pubertal child "diagnostic" of sexual abuse "in virtually every case."[35] They make sexual transmission the rule rather than the exception and argue that a child with gonorrhea has been sexually abused "unless proven otherwise."[36]

The fomite theory was fuelled in large part by late-nineteenth- and early-twentieth-century reports of hospital epidemics of gonorrhea. Initial reports about these epidemics began to crop up in the medical literature in the 1870s.[37] These reports described large numbers of children acquiring a purulent vaginitis, presumed to be gonorrhea based on the clinical characteristics, after bathing together in public baths or while housed in child-caring institutions like hospitals and orphanages.[38] Epidemics of vaginitis among children led to numerous changes in institutional policies, not only in hospitals and orphanages, but also in schools and other organizations caring for children.

Hospital-based epidemics were frequently reported and were particularly problematic to control.[39] Doctors described how the infection could quickly spread through a ward of girls. These infections were difficult to contain and notoriously hard to treat. They often delayed hospital discharge and could even shut down a ward to new admissions. Many hospitals developed policies to isolate all new admissions until they were tested free of gonorrhea, and only then allow these girls on the wards.[40] For them, isolation of new female patients was "the keynote of prophylaxis."[41] Other hospitals had rules in place that required that all girls routinely undergo vaginal smears as a surveillance technique to look for gonorrhea.[42] If a girl tested positive, she would not be allowed contact with other children until her vaginal smears were gonorrhea-free for several weeks in a row.

Some communities were so concerned about the spread of gonorrhea in their hospitals that they established special wards and even special hospitals for girls with gonorrheal vaginitis.[43] The Francis Juvenile Home in Chicago opened in 1909 to care for girls with vaginitis.[44] Patients there not only underwent the prolonged treatments required to arrest their infection, but also attended a special school and received instruction in domestic science.

Whether in the hospital or in the school, these policies rarely mentioned that the girls with these diseases may have been sexually abused. Occasionally they would identify an index case—a girl who brought the disease to the institution.[45] Sometimes this girl was accused of manipulating the genitals of other girls on the ward or in the orphanage, thereby spreading the infection. The fact that this girl may have been sexually abused was never mentioned. Instead, the investigation ended, and she was castigated for her immoral behaviour.

Hospitals were not the only institution that dealt with the contagiousness of gonorrhea. Schools expressed significant concern about the impact of gonorrhea on the health of their pupils.[46] Some schools instigated policies that prohibited girls with vaginitis from attending school. Given the long course of treatment needed for these notoriously difficult to treat infections, many girls were out of school for months.[47] One physician wrote, "Perhaps the greatest compensation I had for my investigations was the bright and happy smiles of the youngsters as we handed them their notes that would readmit them to the common fellowship of the schoolroom after an absence of months and, in one case, years."[48] Other schools developed plans to test girls at school for gonorrhea, examining their underwear for the telltale discharge and then sending those girls home until a physician declared her free of disease.

In schools, contagion was also felt to be transmitted predominantly through fomites; lascivious behaviour of pupils was thought to be highly unlikely. The major fomite of concern in schools was the toilet.[49] Girls with a purulent vaginal discharge would theoretically leave a drop of pus on the toilet that could infect the next girl who went to the bathroom. Belief in the toilet seat as the source of infection was so strongly held that considerable attention was paid to the properties of the toilet that facilitated its role in spread of infection. Many physicians believed that toilets in school were too high. As a result, children slid off and on the toilet, making smearing pus on the seat more likely. In addition, the oval shape of the seat itself also facilitated leaving pus behind, so vaginitis experts called for the redesign of toilet seats. They claimed that the U-shaped seat would minimize the chance of contact between a child's genitals and any pus left behind by a prior user of the toilet. They successfully lobbied for lowering the height of toilet seats in schools and, more importantly, for the adoption of U-shaped seats in all public restrooms and schools.

The U-shaped toilet seat subtly yet powerfully underscored the belief that venereal diseases, and especially gonorrhea, could be acquired nonsexually. Like the belief that gonorrhea could spread through an institution of children in epidemic waves, school policies that excluded children with gonorrhea and changed the shape of the toilet encouraged average Americans to believe that gonorrhea in children was not sexually acquired. The blame for the disease was shifted from the potential perpetrators of sexual abuse to inanimate objects.[50] The belief in the toilet seat as fomite remained strong into the 1980s, when several studies demonstrated that "the toilet seat is a remarkably ineffective fomite."[51] Even today, the popular use of toilet seat covers reflects the widely held concern that diseases like gonorrhea can be caught from the public toilet.

Medical Expertise

There were many groups of physicians who encountered gonorrhea infections in children. The general practitioner often treated vaginal discharge in pediatric patients. Gynecologists who staffed outpatient clinics and dispensaries also saw and wrote about this problem frequently. Urologists diagnosed the disease in boys. The young field of pediatrics, which had formed in the 1880s, only a decade after the discovery of the gonorrheal bacillus, became increasingly involved in the diagnosis and treatment of gonorrhea in children.[52] And finally, physicians particularly interested in infectious diseases and the flourishing field of venereal disease research weighed in on the problem.

This plurality of experts on what was felt to be a common pediatric problem may have affected the advice that was given. It was difficult for these doctors to reach a consensus about the best ways to diagnose, treat, and prevent the disease. One gynecologist called gonorrheal vaginitis "a free lance disease," complaining "there is no uniformity in diagnostic procedure or mode of therapy, or is there any accepted plan of procedure endorsed by a single specialty."[53] Venereologist Reuel Benson agreed, saying, "For many years gonococcic infection in little girls has been a rather disreputable waif, going from the pediatrician, the gynecologist, to the urologist, asking for help and never getting it."[54] Some advocated diagnosing the disease clinically and bypassing bacteriological methods of diagnosis. Others promoted the use of vaginal smears but eschewed more technically difficult cultures. Still others argued that a combination of diagnostic techniques could be used, depending on the circumstances.

Without an identified group of experts on pediatric genital infection (or on pediatric sexual abuse), the disease remained a problem without a home. For infectious disease experts interested in gonorrhea, the pediatric manifestations were dwarfed by the adult dimensions of the problem. Gynecologists were the group that initially published the most information on vaginitis, but as the twentieth century progressed they were becoming less interested in pediatric issues; they, too, focused on their adult patients. The pediatricians who tackled the issue tended to be more interested in developing effective treatments and not in figuring out why their patients contracted the disease. Even the doctors who made vaginitis their area of expertise acknowledged that this disease was notoriously difficult to treat, and that the rewards were few. With so many opinions expressed about the etiology, diagnosis, and management of childhood gonorrhea, doctors facing this problem in their practices could feel reassured that sexual abuse was not likely in their patients.

Most doctors encountering the disease in their practices turned to major textbooks or medical journals for advice about how to treat it. As practitioners in the trenches, they were interested in applying knowledge, not creating it. They must have been heartened by the message that gonorrhea was rarely sexually transmitted in children. They could calm anxious parents, telling them that their child had caught the disease from something as anonymous and benign as a toilet seat. Goodrich Schauffler, an Oregon gynecologist, spoke to these concerns in his readership, saying, "I have often made the statement to a distracted parent that I would rather a little girl of my own be infected with vaginal gonorrhea than that she be the subject of a draining mastoid or a chronic running ear or even a chronic sinus."[55]

Doctors and Myths about Sexual Abuse

Myths about sexual abuse also influenced physicians' responses to sexual abuse allegations. In spite of their scientific and medical training, doctors have always been influenced by tacit assumptions about sexuality that pervade society. One such myth was that rape would invariably leave physical evidence of penetration. This myth of the broken hymen often led doctors to question that sexual abuse had occurred if hymenal injury was not apparent.[56]

Doctors in the nineteenth century rarely reported that hymenal examinations formed part of their practice.[57] In fact, the details of female genital anatomy were generally glossed over in medical school. As Jerome Walker noted in 1886, "Probably because the books give so little definite information as to the location and character of the hymen, and there is so little that is definite about it known to medical students, it happens that some physicians have never seen one, or have vague notions about it."[58] A few doctors, however, who worked with local institutions and social service agencies, performed hymenal examinations as part of their evaluations of girls who were either suspected of being abused or were accused of being promiscuous.[59] These doctors frequently looked for hymenal abnormalities, such as lacerations and clefts, as proof of prior sexual encounters. A child without hymenal injury—or in the terms of the time, was virginal in appearance—lacked credible evidence of sexual abuse.

Hymenal examinations do not appear to have been a routine part of the examination of children with gonorrhea. In fact, most discussions of hymens in the literature on vaginitis focused on the concern that the treatment (involving multiple vaginal washes and douches) might damage the hymen.[60] Thus, the fact that hymenal examinations were not advocated as part of the evaluation of gonorrheal vaginitis reflects the prevailing belief that the disease was rarely sexually transmitted. It may have also represented a belief that the doctor's duty was limited to treating the infection and not investigating the cause of the infection. The myth of the torn hymen was only dispelled in the 1980s when credible research began to emerge demonstrating that vaginal penetration does not always lead to permanent hymenal injury.[61]

Doctors were understandably hesitant to say that rape had occurred, without convincing physical evidence. In some ways, the issue of rape fell outside their traditional realm. Sexual assault was more a social than a medical problem. Child sexual abuse did not become medicalized until the late twentieth century, when a group of interested and experienced physicians began to call for the use of medical expertise to advocate for abused children.

Beginning in the 1980s and 1990s, physicians interested in child sexual abuse began to gather evidence to dispel these myths. Several studies of newborn girls proved that girls are always born with hymens and described normal configurations of hymens, thus setting the stage for detailed studies of the effects of abuse on girls' genitals.[62] Studies over the last ten years have demonstrated the types of injuries caused by sexual abuse as well as how well the female genitalia can heal after abuse. These studies provided resounding evidence that overturned the myth that sexual abuse always leads to a torn hymen.[63]

Doctors' attitudes about child sexual abuse often incorporated prevailing attitudes about sexuality. Thus, doctors often shrugged off sexual abuse of black children, explaining that African-Americans were inherently promiscuous and that African-American children were generally introduced to sexuality early in life.[64] Similarly, sexual abuse was felt to be more common among immigrant populations and among the poor. Pediatricians warned mothers to beware of the hands of domestic servants who could infect their young charges. One effect of applying these stereotypes was to ghettoize the issue and make it appear that middle-class American children were immune to sexual abuse. This would reinforce exactly what doctors wanted to believe—that sexual abuse was rare, and when it did exist, it could be contained.

Another recurring myth from the late nineteenth century that is still occasionally cited is that intercourse with a virgin will cure a person of sexually transmitted disease.[65] This myth recently received attention when it was offered as an excuse to explain several rapes of very young girls in South Africa.[66] Most physicians in the nineteenth and twentieth centuries also condemned this practice, citing it as an example of how ignorance and superstition led to tragic consequences. However, some physicians seemed to feel that this belief reflected such profound ignorance on the part of the rapist, that it inspired a degree of pity in addition to censure. Flora Pollack, a gynecologist at Johns Hopkins, explored this myth in great detail in 1909. In her mind, the infected man who raped a child to cure his venereal disease "has no sensual, cruel impulse as [his] motive."[67] She believed that "this superstition is so deeply rooted in the belief of men that were you to ask ten police officers, cab drivers, hucksters, etc. of the truth of it I think eight would affirm it as a *fact* and all would know of its existence."[68] This myth allowed people to place perpetrators of sexual abuse on a scale of guilt, with some rapes being more morally reprehensible than others. Perpetrators who abused children out of desperation to cure themselves of gonorrhea were wrong, but their ignorance somehow tempered their guilt.

The Special Role of Girls

Predominant attitudes about virginity and threats to it created an aura of mystery around the female genitalia. Many physicians worried that doing a genital exam, even if limited to simply inspecting the genitals, would promote masturbation and sexual curiosity in girls. That part of the body remained largely terra incognita to doctors. As late as 1958 pediatrician Edward D. Allen complained that the genitalia of girls received a cursory examination at birth and were not reevaluated until the premarital physical.

From [birth] on we throw such an aura of protection and perfection about our little girls that we have innumerable instances withheld from them some of the advances in medical knowledge and therapeutics which are their due. Not until they appear for premarital examination is further exploration of the virginal pelvis attempted, or even advised by some authorities, unless grave local symptoms occur.[69]

Not only did girls not know about their bodies, but their doctors also were woefully ill-equipped to recognize gynecologic problems in their young female patients.

Doctors worried that girls with gonorrhea would be considered "damaged goods," that they would become overly sensitized to their genitals, or that aggressive treatment would instill bad habits like masturbation. Gynecologist William Robinson warned parents about the many dire consequences of this diagnosis in his 1917 advice manual:

It has a disastrous effect on the child's *morale*; most parents, though they may love the child most affectionately, look somewhat askance at it; and continuous vaginal treatment somehow or other has a humiliating effect on the child, which begins to consider itself as an outcast, as something apart from other children.... Sixth, and this is a point not sufficiently appreciated by the profession and the laity, but it is an important point, nevertheless: vulvovaginitis in children has unfortunately a disastrous effect in *hastening the sexual maturity of the child*. Whether this is due to the congestion of the organs produce by the inflammation, or to the speculum examinations, paintings, douches, applications, tampons, suppositories, etc., the fact remains that girls who suffer from vulvovaginitis in childhood become sexually mature considerably earlier than normal girls of the same class, stratum, and climate, and their demand for sexual satisfaction is much more insistent.[70]

Girls with gonorrhea, then, were imbued with a heightened sexuality and were sometimes seen as seductresses rather than the innocent victims of their abusers.[71] One pediatrician, writing in 1967, said that girls move from victims to consensual sexual partners "probably around age nine or ten, with a few precocious exceptions."[72] Teenage girls with gonorrhea were generally assumed to be sexually precocious and that their disease was their fault.[73]

Issues of Medical Practice

Aside from the scientific and cultural issues that contributed to the lack of awareness of sexual abuse in these patients, what other factors influenced the doctors who were encountering gonorrhea in their practices? These doctors were influenced by professional issues as well as economic ones.

Routine practice did not necessarily reflect textbook advice. Busy clinicians saw their patients and relied on a combination of prior experience and knowledge accrued through textbooks, medical journals, and discussions with colleagues, to devise a management plan. In the pre-antibiotic era, when the disease was protracted and the treatment was difficult, doctors reached for the seemingly endless array of promising cures of antiseptic douches and silver nitrate preparations—in hopes of abating the irritating symptoms of the disease. The estrogen instillations of the 1930s promised better results but could have unseemly side effects from excessive hormone absorption, prompting doctors to alter or abandon this treatment. These doctors worked in the trenches, so to speak; they were not the ones creating new medical knowledge. Although they were probably discomforted by a diagnosis of gonorrhea in a child, they were likely relieved that their textbooks attributed transmission to fomites. Fomite transmission offered a stabilizing reassurance that sexual transmission did not.

Most doctors, then, did not question the truism that gonorrhea was non-sexually transmitted in children and sexually transmitted in adults.[74] These opinions about the contagiousness of gonorrhea bore the imprimatur of expert opinion and offered a scientifically legitimated alternative to the disquieting notion of sexual abuse.

Physicians may have also been influenced by the economic reality of medical practice. Physicians caring for children were paid by their parents; although the child was the patient, the parent needed to be satisfied with the care provided. That the child may have acquired gonorrhea from a family member or close family friend was information that would potentially upset the doctor's relationship with the parent. Doctors rarely stated these economic realities explicitly, but there is some evidence that economic and social forces may have influenced their practice. For instance, doctors frequently argued that gonorrhea was more common in charity patients. In a survey conducted in the 1910s about physician attitudes about vaginitis, several respondents discussed the difference between vaginitis in private and hospitalized patients, stating that gonorrhea was a rare cause of vaginitis in private patients, while in hospital (i.e., charity) patients gonorrhea accounted for 75 to 100 per cent of cases.[75] While this argument may have reflected the epidemiology of vaginitis in their practices, doctors may also have been influenced by what they wanted to believe was true. They may have been more likely to interpret a vaginal smear as gonorrhea in a charity patient and as being caused by an organism resembling gonorrhea in their private patients.

Faced with a diagnosis of gonorrhea in a child from a wealthy family, doctors were unlikely to identify a family member as the source of the disease. Private patients with gonorrhea were likely to have their infection attributed to the hands of a domestic servant or to the public toilet seat. It was rare for wealthy family members to be scrutinized as sources of the disease.

Even as economic pressures may have influenced physician behaviour, the economic realities of child sexual abuse pressured family members who suspected child sexual abuse to squelch their suspicions. If the breadwinner of the family was also the abuser, then the mother was forced to choose between protecting her children from further abuse and facing dire financial consequences like homelessness and poverty in addition to the social stigma. Although mothers increasingly entered the workplace as the twentieth century progressed, many were nevertheless financially vulnerable because of the significant role male family members played in supporting the family. Faced with destitution and social ostracism if they exposed the abuse, many families preferred to hush the abuse up and either ignore it or deal with it themselves. Therefore, financial pressures worked in different ways to discourage families from talking about abuse and physicians from inquiring about it.

The Changing Roles of Children and Their Doctors

Attitudes about gonorrhea in children were also affected by images of children at the time. The prevailing image of the child was of innocence.[76] Yet considerable research has shown that the Victorian preoccupation with sexual mores and childhood innocence was in many ways a veneer covering their fears about the dangers and allures of sexuality.[77] In the Victorian imagination, the wide-eyed innocence of childhood could be seen as a preoccupation with virginity and sexual purity. The family was the temple of virtue against the immorality of the world. The parent's role was to protect the child from the evils of society. Nevertheless, in spite of their straight-laced reputation, the Victorians spent a great deal of energy worrying about sexual risk.

The tension between child innocence and seductiveness were important undercurrents in Victorian attitudes about child-rearing and child behaviour, but these issues were not uniquely Victorian. As the twentieth century progressed, the image of the seductive child continued to play a role in the American imagination. The impact of Vladimir Nabokov's 1954 novel, *Lolita*, for instance, is hotly debated, but the very fact that the debate exists testifies to the level of concern about childhood sexuality. Historian Joan Jacobs Brumberg has examined the increasing preoccupation with sexuality in American girls over the last 150 years.[78] This recognition of children's sexual allure—sometimes covert, other times overt—meant that children were not always seen as victims when sexual abuse was suspected. When they were described as seductive or sexualized, they were blamed for inviting or allowing the abuse to occur. As one pediatrician remarked about some of his patients,

Masturbation is extremely common among the infected cases. Whether as a result of this or not, I am unable to say, but these children are many of them sexually precocious. Just how far this has gone in some instances it is impossible to know, since their precociousness makes them secretive. The usual lack of embarrassment during examination seen in a child of six has entirely disappeared in many of these children.[79]

A constant feature of childrearing throughout the last century and a half has been the parents' responsibility to both teach their children how to become accepted members of society and also to protect them from society's dangerous influences. Numerous books have documented how child-rearing has adapted over time to this ever-present tension.[80] Increasingly, over the twentieth century, parents turned to child experts for guidance in issues related to sexuality.

Pediatricians' role as child experts has changed over time. During the first half-century of pediatrics, the predominant interests in the field involved reducing infant mortality through improving nutrition, fighting diarrheal diseases, and treating life-threatening infectious diseases.[81] With the advent and incorporation of effective vaccines and then antibiotics, the thrust of pediatrics began to shift toward health maintenance and disease prevention. Pediatricians have always advocated for children, but these issues were frequently eclipsed by issues with a clear medical focus.

Several events in the twentieth century cleared the way for pediatrics to become more involved in advocacy issues. Beginning in the 1920s and 1930s, the child guidance movement began to make child-rearing more scientific. Child-rearing came under scrutiny as professionals examined the relationships between parenting styles and child behaviour and health. One of Benjamin Spock's more lasting influences was to popularize the principles of psychotherapy and child guidance and deliver them in an accessible and non-threatening form to parents. Spock epitomized the integral role that the pediatrician could play as child-rearing advisor to parents.[82]

The social activism of the 1960s primed pediatricians to play a more active role in child abuse. The elucidation of "the battered child syndrome" in the 1960s challenged pediatricians to become more aware of the ways in which children were at risk of victimization.[83] The sexual revolution of the 1960s and 1970s, combined with the feminist movement, played important roles in the emergence of a realization that child sexual abuse existed and merited attention. Feminism provided a vocabulary of sexual victimization that could be adapted to children. These forces coalesced to create interest among a growing number of pediatricians in child sexual abuse. Pediatricians finally began to question the dogma of innocent transmission of gonorrhea in children. Suzanne Sgroi, a physician in Connecticut active in the early child abuse field, almost single-handedly called on physicians to reverse their beliefs about gonorrhea in children. She castigated physicians, saying, "Physicians must not evade responsibility by telling family members that the child might have acquired the infection from a toilet seat or towel. Instead, physicians must affirm that only sexual transmission of gonorrhea occurs beyond the neonatal period."[84]

The current shaping of child sexual abuse reflects a larger trend in American society to medicalize social problems.[85] No one would argue that someone needed to address the problem of child sexual abuse, but doctors needed to be convinced that child abuse merited *their* attention. While doctors had always accepted their role in caring for the child who had been injured by abuse, or who had acquired a disease through abuse, it was not until recently that they felt ownership of the issue. But as the role of pediatrics expanded to include the psychosocial well-being of children, as well as their biological health, pediatricians began to embrace many advocacy issues. It is not surprising, then, that the involvement of pediatricians in sexual abuse came on the heels of their interest in child physical abuse, and can be seen as part of a larger interest in advocacy issues ranging from injury and poisoning prevention to gun control. And when physicians accepted the broader issue of child abuse—and not merely its symptoms—their denial of the problem began to erode.

Conclusion

In spite of the knowledge that gonorrhea was a sexually transmitted infectious disease, physicians misinterpreted the significance of gonorrhea in their young patients for well over a century. The reasons for this oversight are relatively obvious in the late nineteenth century, when the findings of bacteriology were still contested and many experts felt that fomites were responsible for disease transmission. However, as more and more knowledge about venereal diseases accumulated, it became harder to rationalize the belief in fomite transmission in gonorrheal vaginitis. Physicians' inability to recognize sexual abuse in their patients— and often their denial that sexual abuse existed—represents a very complex response to professional, scientific, social, and cultural forces that influenced their knowledge and behaviours. These forces changed over time, allowing physicians to acknowledge that some of their young charges had been sexually abused and that the doctor had an important role to play in recognizing abuse and managing its treatment. Denial of sexual abuse has not disappeared; it will probably continue to exist as long as the problem remains stigmatized. Understanding the factors that influenced physician denial, however, may help them protect their young patients from abuse.

Notes

1 J. Taber Johnson, "Sociology," in *Gonorrhea in Women*, ed. Palmer Findley (St. Louis: C. V. Mosby, 1908), 70.

2 Geraldine Branch and Ruth Paxton, "A Study of Gonococcal Infections among Infants and Children," *Public Health Reports* 60 (1965): 347–52; D. S. Folland R. E. Burke, A. R. Hindman, and W. Schaffner, "Gonorrhea in Preadolescent Children: An Inquiry into Source of Infection and Mode of Transmission," *Pediatrics* 60 (1977): 153–56; R. C. Low, T. C. Cho, and B. A. Dudding, "Gonococcal Infections in Young Children," *Clinical Pediatrics* 16 (1977): 623–26; and Suzanne M. Sgroi, "'Kids with Clap': Gonorrhea as an Indicator of Child Sexual Assault," *Victimology: An International Journal* 2 (1977): 251–67; .

3 Suzanne M. Sgroi, "Pediatric Gonorrhea and Child Sexual Abuse: The Venereal Disease Connection," *Sexually Transmitted Diseases* 9 (1982): 154.

4 There are no accurate data about just how prevalent child sexual abuse has been in American history. Current estimates are that 20 per cent of all girls and 9 per cent of all boys will be sexually abused prior to adulthood. Most of this abuse will go unreported. Kent Hymel and Carol Jenny, "Child Sexual Abuse," *Pediatrics in Review* 17 (1996): 236–50.

5 American Academy of Pediatrics, Committee on Child Abuse and Neglect, "Guidelines for the Evaluation of Sexual Abuse of Children: Subject Review," *Pediatrics* 103 (1999): 186–91.

6 See, for instance, William J. Robinson, *Woman: Her Sex and Love Life* (New York: Eugenics, 1929), 164–67.

7 Several articles have examined this body of medical literature. See Hughes Evans, "The Discovery of Child Sexual Abuse in America," in *Formative Years: Children's Health in the United States, 1880–2000*, ed. Alexandra Minna Stern and Howard Markel (Ann Arbor: University of Michigan Press, 2002), 233–59; Lynn Sacco, "Sanitized for Your Protection: Medical Discourse and the Denial of Incest in the United States, 1890–1940," *Journal of Women's History* 14 (2002): 80–104; and Karen J. Taylor, "Venereal Disease in Nineteenth Century Children," *Journal of Psychohistory* 12 (1985): 431–63.

8 The best exploration of the social history of venereal disease is Allan M. Brandt, *No Magic Bullet: A Social History of Venereal Disease in the United States since 1880* (New York: Oxford University Press, 1987). Brandt's book deals primarily with adults with venereal disease, not children, and most closely examines syphilis. Other, more recent analyses of the history of venereal disease include Peter Lewis Allen, *The Wages of Sin: Sex and Disease, Past and Present* (Chicago and London: University of Chicago Press, 2000); and Roger Davidson and Lesley A. Hall, eds., *Sex, Sin and Suffering: Venereal Disease and European Society since 1870* (London and New York: Routledge, 2001).

9 Walter M. Brunet and Robert L. Dickinson's conclusions were typical: "Gonorrhea in the adult female is practically always the result of sexual intercourse with an infected male who has gotten it from a prostitute, professional or clandestine." Brunet and Dickinson, "Gonorrhea in the Female," *Venereal Disease Information* 10 (1929): 150. They concluded that as few as 1 per cent of adult cases were not sexually transmitted.

10 Some children were felt to be promiscuous, however, and were, therefore, not entirely innocent. This was particularly true for girls who were either pubertal or almost pubertal. It was also true for certain ethnic groups, like African-Americans, who were felt to be innately promiscuous.

11   See, for instance, Prince Morrow, *Social Diseases and Marriage* (New York: Lea Bros., 1904) and Brandt, *No Magic Bullet.*

12   On the Progressive response to physical abuse, see Elizabeth Pleck, *Domestic Tyranny: The Making of Social Policy against Family Violence from Colonial Times to the Present* (New York: Oxford University Press, 1987). On the Progressive response to sexual abuse, see Linda Gordon, *Heroes of Their Own Lives: The Politics and History of Family Violence, Boston 1880–1960* (New York: Penguin, 1988).

13   On the significance of Mary Ellen's case and on the child-saving movement in general, see LeRoy Ashby, *Endangered Children: Dependency, Neglect and Abuse in American History* (New York: Twayne, 1997).

14   On the history of social work, see Roy Lubove, *The Professional Altruist: The Emergence of Social Work as a Career 1880–1930* (New York: Atheneum, 1980). On the response of social workers in the late nineteenth and early twentieth centuries to reports of incest and child abuse, see Linda Gordon, *Heroes of Their Own Lives.*

15   On the legal history of the family in American society, see Michael Grossberg, *Governing the Hearth: Law and Family in Nineteenth-Century America* (Chapel Hill: University of North Carolina Press, 1985); and Mary Ann Mason, *From Father's Property to Children's Rights: The History of Child Custody in the United States* (New York: Columbia University Press, 1994).

16   Brandt, *No Magic Bullet,* 10.

17   Grace Campbell Hardy, "Vaginal Flora in Children," *American Journal of the Diseases of Children* 62 (1941): 939–54.

18   The gonococcus was first cultured in 1885, only six years after its discovery. However, reliable and convenient culture techniques remained elusive for several decades. Mary J. Erickson and Henry Albert, "Cultivation of the Gonococcus," *Journal of Infectious Disease* 30 (1922): 268–78.

19   A. Reith Fraser, "Vulvovaginitis in Children," *Venereal Disease Information* 7 (1926): 5.

20   On the usefulness of culture versus stain, see Ruth A. Anderson, Oscar T. Schultz, and Irving F. Stein, "A Bacteriologic Study of Vulvovaginitis of Children," *Journal of Infectious Disease* 32 (1923): 452.

21   Anderson, Schultz, and Stein, "Vulvovaginitis of Children," 452.

22   A. K. Paine, "The Point of View of the Clinician," *New England Journal of Medicine* 207 (1932): 138.

23   Paine, "Point of View of the Clinician," 138.

24   J. Claxton Giddings, Charles A. Fife, and Howard Childs Carpenter, "Report of the Committee of the American Pediatric Society on Vaginitis in Children," *Transactions of the American Pediatric Society* 27 (1915): 344.

25   Anderson, Schultz, and Stein, "Vulvovaginitis of Children," 444–55; and W. L. Whittington, R. J. Rice, J. W. Biddle, and J. S. Knapp, "Incorrect Identification of *Neisseria gonorrhoeae* from Infants and Children," *Pediatric Infectious Disease Journal* 7 (1988): 3–10.

26   Examples of this type of research include, among others, Warren R. Lang, "Pediatric Vaginitis," *New England Journal of Medicine* 253 (1955): 1152–60; Charles Mazer and Fred R. Shechter, "Treatment of Vulvovaginitis with Estrogen," *Journal of the American Medical Association* 112 (1939): 1925–28; and Louis Weinstein, Maxwell Bogin, Joseph H. Howard, and Benjamin B. Finkelstone, "A Survey of the Vaginal Flora at Various Ages, with Special Reference to the Doderlein Bacillus," *American Journal of Obstetrics and Gynecology* 32 (1936): 211–18.

27 Y. M. Felman and J. A. Nikitas, "Gonococcal Infections in Infants and Children," *New York State Journal of Medicine* 79 (1979): 1064; and Mazer and Shechter, "Treatment of Vulvovaginitis with Estrogen," 1925.

28 In 1982, gynecologist Albert Altchek wrote that the childhood vagina "may be the best culture medium in the world for the gonococcus." Albert Altchek, "Brief Guide to Office Counseling: Gonococcal Vaginitis in Children," *Medical Aspects of Human Sexuality* 16 (1982): 46.

29 The literature on the use of estrogen compounds in the treatment of gonorrheal vaginitis is voluminous. See, for instance, Louis E. Goldberg, Carl I. Minier, and Ellis L. Smith, "Estrogenic Treatment of Gonorrheal Vaginitis," *Journal of Pediatrics* 7 (1935): 401–17; Robert M. Lewis and Eleanor L. Adler, "Gonorrhea Vaginitis: Results of Treatment with Different Preparations and Amounts of Estrogenic Substance," *Journal of the American Medical Association* 106 (1936): 2054–58; Mazer and Shechter, "Treatment of Vulvovaginitis with Estrogen," 1925–28; and Richard Betts Phillips, "Theelin Therapy in Vulvovaginitis," *New England Journal of Medicine* 213 (1935): 1026–29; and Richard W. TeLinde, "The Treatment of Gonococcic Vaginitis with the Estrogenic Hormone," *Journal of the American Medical Association* 110 (1938): 1633–38.

30 S. R. McKelvey, Nolie Mumey, and George K. Dunklee, "Gonorrhea in Female Children," *Venereal Disease Information* 6 (1925): 290.

31 Numerous articles provide lists of potential fomites. See, for instance, Brunet and Dickinson, "Gonorrhea in the Female," 149–69; Frederick J. Lynch, "Vulvovaginitis in Children," *New England Journal of Medicine* 202 (1930): 1251–52; and E. W. Titus and Bernard Notes, "Gonorrhea in Female Children, with Special Reference to Treatment," *Archives of Pediatrics* 50 (1933): 284–87.

32 Abraham L. Wolbarst, "On the Occurrence of Syphilis and Gonorrhea in Children by Direct Infection," *American Medicine* 18 (1912): 495. For Wolbarst, direct infection included sleeping in the bed with an infected person; handling toys, linens, or other objects that come in contact with a child's genitals; and sexual touching.

33 See Haven Emerson's remarks in the discussion section of John L. Rice, Alfred Cohn, Arthur Steer, and Eleanor L. Adler, "Recent Investigations on Gonococcic Vaginitis," *Journal of the American Medical Association* 117 (1941): 1769.

34 William B. Shore and Jerry A. Winkelstein, "Nonvenereal Transmission of Gonococcal Infections to Children," *Journal of Pediatrics* 79 (1971): 661–63.

35 American Academy of Pediatrics, "Sexually Transmitted Diseases," in *Red Book: 2003 Report of the Committee on Infectious Diseases*, ed. Larry K. Pickering, 26th ed. (Elk Grove Village, IL: American Academy of Pediatrics, 2003), 160, 162.

36 American Academy of Pediatrics, "Gonococcal Disease," In *Red Book: 2003 Report of the Committee on Infectious Diseases*, ed. Larry K. Pickering, 26th ed. (Elk Grove Village, IL: American Academy of Pediatrics, 2003), 287.

37 Epidemics of gonorrhea in hospitals and elsewhere are summarized in Alice Hamilton, "Gonorrheal Vulvo-Vaginitis in Children, with Special Reference to an Epidemic Occurring in Scarlet Fever Wards," *Journal of Infectious Disease* 5 (1908): 133–57.

38 An early report of an epidemic in a charitable institution is I. E. Atkinson, "Report of Six Cases of Contagious Vulvitis in Children," *American Journal of Medical Science* 75 (1878): 444–46.

39 Pediatricians commonly discussed hospital-based epidemics of gonorrhea. See, for instance, Aristidfes Agramonte, "Infectious Vulvo-Vaginitis in Children," *Med-*

ical Record 49 (1896): 46–47; A. C. Cotton, "An Epidemic of Vulvovaginitis among Children," *Archives of Pediatrics* 12 (1905): 106–115; and Hamilton, "Gonorrheal Vulvo-Vaginitis in Children."

40 J. Thornwell Witherspoon, "The Clinical and Social Aspects of Vulvovaginitis in Children, with an Outline of a Special Method of Treatment," *New Orleans Medical and Surgical Journal* 85 (1932): 108–112. J. Claxton Gittings et al. summarized a survey of office and hospital practices related to vaginitis in "American Pediatric Society on Vaginitis in Children," 331–53.

41 Witherspoon, "Vulvovaginitis in Children," 108.

42 J. Hubert von Pourtales, "Control and Treatment of Gonorrheal Vaginitis in Infants," *Archives of Pediatrics* 49 (1932): 121–25.

43 Vaginitis wards in hospitals are described in Rice et al., "Recent Investigations on Gonococcic Vaginitis," 1766–1769; Clara P. Seippel, "Venereal Diseases in Children," *Illinois Medical Journal* 22 (1912): 50–56; Richard M. Smith, "Vulvovaginitis in Children," *American Journal of the Diseases of Children* 6 (1913): 355–62; and Edith Rogers Spaulding, "Vulvovaginitis in Children," *American Journal of the Diseases of Children* 5 (1913): 248–67.

44 The Francis Home is described in Seippel, "Venereal Diseases in Children," 50–56.

45 See, for instance, Atkinson, "Contagious Vulvitis in Children," 445.

46 On concerns about gonorrhea in the schools, see S. H. Rubin, "The Point of View of the School Physician," *New England Journal of Medicine* 207 (1932): 142–44.

47 Ella Oppenheimer and Ray H. Everett, "School Exclusions for Gonorrheal Infections in Washington, DC," *Journal of Social Hygiene* 20 (1934): 129–38.

48 Joseph Brown, "Treatment of Gonorrheal Vaginitis in Immature Girls," *Journal of the American Medical Association* 102 (1934): 1294.

49 Nancy Tomes discusses the persuasiveness of the theory of fomite spread of disease in *The Gospel of Germs: Men, Women, and the Microbe in American Life* (Cambridge: Harvard University Press, 1998). See also Suellen Hoy, *Chasing Dirt: The American Pursuit of Cleanliness* (New York: Oxford University Press, 1995). On the purported role of toilets in transmitting gonorrhea, see Lynch, "Vulvovaginitis in Children," 1251; Frederick J. Taussig, "The Contagion of Gonorrhoea among Little Girls," *Social Hygiene* (1914–1915): 415–22; and Titus and Notes, "Gonorrhea in Female Children," 285.

50 Estelle B. Freedman made a similar argument in her examination of the popularization of the stranger as child molester myth. See Estelle B. Freedman, "'Uncontrolled Desires': The Response to the Sexual Psychopath, 1920–1960," *Journal of American History* 74 (1987): 83–106.

51 James H. Gilbaugh and Peter C. Fuchs, "The Gonococcus and the Toilet Seat," *New England Journal of Medicine* 301 (1979): 93. See also T. Elmros and P.-A. Larsson, "Survival of Gonococci outside the Body," *British Medical Journal* 2 (1972): 403–404; and Michael F. Rein, letter to the editor, *New England Journal of Medicine* 301 (1979): 1347.

52 By 1958, pediatric gynecologist Goodrich Schauffler would write, "The time is at hand when the preponderance of care in the field of the gynecologic aspects of infancy, childhood and adolescence descends upon the pediatrician and family doctor." Goodrich Schauffler, "Foreword," *Pediatric Clinics of North America* 2 (1958): 1.

53 Irving F. Stein, "A Clinical Investigation of Vulvovaginitis," *Surgery, Gynecology and Obstetrics* 36 (1923): 43.

54 Quotation is contained in the discussion following Rice et al., "Recent Investigations on Gonococcic Vaginitis," 1768.

55 Goodrich C. Schauffler, Ray Duke, S. F. Crynes, and Corlyn Schauffler, "Infection of the Immature Vagina: Observations and Results: A Study of 189 Patients," *Western Journal of Surgery, Obstetrics and Gynecology* 42 (1934): 682.

56 In a rare article on injuries from rape, a letter from Abraham Jacobi is included, in which he argues that rape does not invariably cause hymenal injury. See Jerome Walker, "Reports, with Comments, of Twenty-One Cases of Indecent Assault and Rape upon Children," *Archives of Pediatrics* 3 (1886): 336. It was more common for doctors to exclude rape if no hymenal injury was apparent. See for instance, Fred J. Taussig, "The Prevention and Treatment of Vulvovaginitis in Children," *American Journal of Medical Science* 148 (1914): 482.

57 Joan Jacobs Brumberg, *The Body Project: An Intimate History of American Girls* (New York: Random House, 1997).

58 Walker, "Reports, with Comments," 335. S. Ladson, C. F. Johnson, and R. E. Doty, "Do Physicians Recognize Sexual Abuse?" *American Journal of the Diseases of Children* 141 (1987): 411–15.

59 W. Travis Gibb, "Criminal Aspects of Venereal Diseases in Children," *Medical Record* 71 (1907): 643–46. Mary E. Odem discusses genital examinations of "promiscuous" adolescent females in *Delinquent Daughters: Protecting and Policing Adolescent Female Sexuality in the United States, 1885–1920* (Chapel Hill and London: University of North Carolina Press, 1995). Philip Jenkins discusses the role of genital evaluations in *Moral Panic: Changing Concepts of the Child Molester in Modern America* (New Haven and London: Yale University Press, 1998).

60 Lynch, "Vulvovaginitis in Children," 1252; and Titus and Notes, "Gonorrhea in Female Children," 286.

61 J. A. Adams, K. Harper, S. Knudson, and J. Revilla, "Examination Findings in Legally Confirmed Child Sexual Abuse: It's Normal to Be Normal," *Pediatrics* 93 (1994): 310–17; and David Muram, "Child Sexual Abuse: Relationship between Sexual Acts and Genital Findings," *Child Abuse & Neglect* 13 (1989): 211–16.

62 A. B. Berenson, Astrid H. Heger, and S. Andrews, "Appearance of the Hymen in Newborns," *Pediatrics* 89 (1992): 387–94; and Carol Jenny, M. L. D. Kuhns, and F. Arakawa, "Hymen in Newborn Female Infants," *Pediatrics* 80 (1987): 399–400.

63 These studies are listed in the annotated bibliography of Astrid Heger, S. Jean Emans, and David Muram, *Evaluation of the Sexually Abused Child: A Medical Textbook and Photographic Atlas*, 2nd ed. (New York and Oxford: Oxford University Press, 2000), 245–66.

64 See, for instance, Lucien Lofton, "Juveniles with Gonorrhea," *New York Journal of Medicine* 64 (1896): 456.

65 The myth that intercourse with a virgin will cure venereal disease was commonly cited. See Agramonte, "Infectious Vulvo-Vaginitis in Children," 46; Frederick W. Lowndes, "Venereal Diseases in Girls of Tender Age," *Lancet* 1 (1887): 169; and Flora Pollack, "A Report of the Women's Venereal Department of the Johns Hopkins Hospital Dispensary," *Maryland Medical Journal* 49 (1906): 289–94.

66 Rachel L. Swarns, "Child Rape Increasing at Alarming Rate in South Africa," *New York Times*, January 29, 2002.

67 Flora Pollack, "The Acquired Venereal Infections in Children: A Report of 187 Children Treated in the Women's Venereal Department of the Johns Hopkins Hospital Dispensary," *Bulletin of the Johns Hopkins Hospital* 20 (1909): 144.

68 Pollack, "Acquired Venereal Infections in Children," 143.

69 Edward D. Allen, "Examination of the Genital Organs in the Prepubescent and in the Adolescent Girl," *Pediatric Clinics of North America* 2 (1958): 21.
70 Robinson, *Woman: Her Sex and Love Life*, 166.
71 Charles Mazer and Fred R. Shechter wrote, "The persistence of vulvar irritation for many months or years centers the attention of the growing child on the generative organs and often leads to the habit of masturbation and premature heterosexual inclinations." Mazer and Shechter, "Treatment of Vulvovaginitis with Estrogen," 1925.
72 Lawrence F. Nazarian, "The Current Prevalence of Gonococcal Infections in Children," *Pediatrics* 39 (1967): 374–75.
73 Odem, *Delinquent Daughters*.
74 There were a few exceptions. Flora Pollack, for instance, argued, "The possibilities of towel, bathtub or toilet infections of gonorrhea are extremely rare, but they offer a very useful shield for the guilty individual, and they also impede justice, and make it extremely difficult to protect children from these assaults. Let it be known once and for all that gonorrhea is thus acquired only most exceptionally; and this possibility when offered in court as a defense should only be accepted after the most exhaustive examination of all the attending circumstances of the case. Gonorrhea thus acquired probably occurs in much less than one percent on all the cases." Pollack, "Venereal Infections in Children," 147.
75 Gittings et al., "American Pediatric Society on Vaginitis in Children," 334.
76 See, for instance, Harvey Green, *The Light of the Home: An Intimate View of the Lives of Women in Victorian America* (New York: Pantheon, 1983).
77 See James R. Kincaid, *Child-Loving: The Erotic Child and Victorian Culture* (New York and London: Routledge, 1992); and James R. Kincaid, *Erotic Innocence: The Culture of Child Molesting* (Durham: Duke University Press, 1998).
78 Brumberg, *Body Project*; and Joan Jacobs Brumberg, *Fasting Girls: The Emergence of Anorexia Nervosa as a Modern Disease* (Cambridge: Harvard University Press, 1988).
79 Smith, "Vulvovaginitis in Children," 358.
80 See Rima D. Apple and Janet Golden, *Mothers and Motherhood: Readings in American History* (Columbus: Ohio State University Press, 1997); Julia Grant, *Raising Baby by the Book: The Education of American Mothers* (New Haven, CT: Yale University Press, 1998); Ann Hulbert, *Raising America: Experts, Parents, and a Century of Advice about Children* (New York: Alfred A. Knopf, 2003); and Peter N. Stearns, *Anxious Parents: A History of Modern Childrearing in America* (New York and London: New York University Press, 2003).
81 On the history of pediatrics, see Alexandra Minna Stern and Howard Markel, eds., *Formative Years: Children's Health in the United States, 1880–2000* (Ann Arbor: University of Michigan Press, 2002). This book contains a useful and comprehensive bibliography about the history of pediatrics in America.
82 Ann Hulbert, "Dr. Spock's Baby: Fifty Years in the Life of a Book and the American Family," *New Yorker* 20 (May 20, 1996): 82–92; G. H. Steere, "Freudianism and Child-Rearing in the Twenties," *American Quarterly* 20 (1968): 759–67; A. M. Sulman, "The Humanization of the American Child: Benjamin Spock as a Popularizer of Psychoanalytic Thought," *Journal of the History of the Behavioral Sciences* 8 (1973): 258–65; and Nancy Pottisham Weiss, "Mother, the Invention of Necessity: Dr. Benjamin Spock's *Baby and Child Care*," in *Growing Up in America: Children in Historical Perspective*, ed. N. Ray Hiner and Joseph M. Hawes (Urbana: University of Illinois Press, 1985), 283–303.

83 C. H. Kempe, F. N. Silverman, B. F. Steele, W. Droegemueller, and H. K. Silver, "The Battered Child Syndrome," *Journal of the American Medical Association* 181 (1962): 17–24. On the medical history of child physical abuse, see Margaret A. Lynch, "Child Abuse before Kempe: An Historical Literature Review," *Child Abuse & Neglect* 9 (1985): 7–15.

84 Suzanne M. Sgroi, "Childhood Gonorrhea," *Medical Aspects of Human Sexuality* 16 (1982): 124.

85 See, for example, Anne Hendershott, *The Politics of Deviance* (San Francisco: Encounter Books, 2002).

"Living Symptoms"

Adolescent Health Care in English Canada, 1920–1970

∝

Cynthia Comacchio

D uring the opening decades of "Canada's Century," as Canadians were impelled to come to terms with modernity, a number of voices joined in chorus to identify a "youth problem." Adolescents embodied the nation's potential. By simple virtue of having reached a certain life stage during a tumultuous time, they became another of the myriad "social problems" that demanded the attention of reform-minded, or otherwise just anxious, Canadians.[1] Medical doctors were significant constituents among those authorized to address the often-overlapping "social problems" of the day. As they successfully professionalized and took the reins of a burgeoning child welfare movement, doctors became interested in the care and training of adolescents. Yet population health surveys for this entire period consistently demonstrated that young Canadians between the ages of twelve and twenty-four years enjoyed the soundest health and lowest mortality rates of all age groups. Why, then, did doctors increasingly espouse a systematic, regulatory health supervision for this "critical" sector?

This essay considers the medicalization of adolescence in English Canada between 1920 and 1970. As demonstrated in Mona Gleason's essay on school medical inspection in British Columbia, and Margaret Tennant's on the New Zealand children's health camps movement, "modern" health inspection and education were as reflective of persistent ideas about class, gender, and race as they were of emergent medical and psychological theories. During this half-century, doctors, and those concerned more specifically with "mental hygiene"—psychologists, psychiatrists, educators, and social workers—formulated a body of shared ideas and approaches to the all-encompassing "health" of the young. This process of theorizing a modern adolescence owes much to the rise of "modern experts" and its concomitant, their active participation in family life and in the expanding state. The new experts helped to devise age-defined regulatory policies and programs premised on a typology of ideal traits that defined what was normal in each life stage. Modernity's age-consciousness was reflected in universal age-grading in schools, and in new measuring systems for "age-appropriate" physical and mental development and behaviour, such as the Intelligence Quotient (IQ) testing that came into common use in classrooms by the interwar years.[2]

The principal objective of this study is to consider the intersections of medical discourses with wider public concerns about the nature of modern adolescence: how they reveal, beneath the clinical interest in the physiological and emotional terrain of this life stage, a variety of middle-class, race-and-gender based ideals about the very role that "modern experts" should play in training "the rising generation" in appropriate notions of citizenship. The question of timing and "progress" is also important. Despite sustained and growing multidisciplinary interest and pioneering efforts, the field was not securely established in the United States until 1951.[3] In Canada, the time lag between the early stirrings of medical interest and the formalization of a new specialty dedicated to the end of adolescent health is even more pronounced: 1970 marks the inauguration of the Canadian Paediatric Society's Standing Committee on Adolescent Medicine, its first official recognition of a field that has yet to become a certified sub-specialty. What explains the doctors' evident inability to "capture" their target clientele by devising ways and means of supplying the very health care whose necessity they argued for so long and hard, with little variation in theme and substance? What national factors have contributed to this differential trajectory?

What Wilfrid Laurier designated as Canada's Century also dawned as the Century of the Child, a historic moment in which children came to be conceptualized as national assets whose well-being concerned the state as much as their parents. Infant mortality became the focus of international child welfare campaigns fuelled by shared anxieties about declining birth rates, the often-appalling conditions of urban working-class life, and social degeneration. These acquired urgency with sensationalized reports about the number of young men classified as unfit for service during the First World War and, of course, modern warfare's horrific casualties. Although eugenic principles were a common current in child welfare discussions, Canadian doctors generally warned against a strict eugenic understanding of child health, which would lead only to "the sacrifice of the unfortunate, not the unfit."[4] Many argued that environmental reform remained crucial to the overall improvement of health. Most of all, the medical profession contended, Canadians had to be educated about their personal responsibility for health and fitness. At the same time, a growing public respect and their own energetic profession-

alization gave modern medicine a key role in "the program of any civilized state which wishes to preserve its power and government from century to century."[5]

Also an effective spur to medical leadership was the ongoing process
of specialization. In 1914, there were only two pediatric specialists in
Canada, both located in Toronto. In 1929, there were forty-eight in all
Canada. When the Society for the Study of Diseases of Children was
established in 1922, the limited number of pediatricians in the country
obliged its founders to embrace all doctors interested in child health. The
pre-eminent Canadian pediatrician through the first half of the twentieth century, Alan Brown, chief of Toronto's Hospital for Sick Children,
urged his fellows to take the lead in "all matters pertaining to problems
of child life" as "the highest authority" on the subject.[6] Pediatrics was
increasingly an important part of general medical service for a paying
middle-class clientele, as the profession relentlessly, and with some success, urged parents to seek regular medical advice. As was the case in
infant care, however, because general practitioners attended the majority of children of all ages, adolescent health was never exclusively the
domain of the limited number of child specialists.[7]

Theories about adolescence circulated before the early twentieth
century, but it was during those years that young people increasingly
became objects of scientific study. As child welfare became a leading
reform objective throughout the Western world, the boundaries between
medicine and psychology were especially permeable. Doctors and social
scientists drew up new measures of the normal—consequently the
deviant—that reflected both their own status concerns and related fears
about a North American/Western European social milieu that seemed to
be destabilizing under the combined pressures of industrialization,
urbanization, and mass immigration. Within a fundamentally racist
"recapitulationist" framework derived from evolutionary theory, they
contended that research on "lower species," such as women, children and
"the races," disclosed the means to sure progress for their own "better
stock"—or at least suggested ways to prevent the troubling "others"
from impeding it. Borrowed from cultural anthropology, recapitulation
theory, with its premise that individual human development and human
evolution are parallel trends, was a major influence on early-twentieth-
century theories about child development.[8]

Just as doctors began to involve themselves in childrearing matters
that were only vaguely related to physical health, so their definition of
adolescent health would soon embrace much more than the physiological changes of that life-stage. The publication of American psychologist
G. Stanley Hall's authoritative *Adolescence: Its Psychology and Its Relation
to Physiology, Anthropology, Sociology, Sex, Crime, Religion, and Education*

[1904] encouraged this expansion of medical interest. An evolutionary psychologist who adhered to the recapitulation model, Hall identified puberty as a time of moral, sexual, and psychological upheaval, during which young people were vulnerable to the temptations of the adult world but ill-equipped to handle them in a recognizably mature, adult, civilized fashion. Under the careful direction of their more evolved elders, they would eventually make the evolutionary leap themselves. While emphasizing the psychological dimensions of this life-stage, Hall defined them as fundamentally biological.[9] Thus it was a psychologist rather than a physician who probably issued the first call for specialized medical attention to adolescent health. The experts agreed that the interrelations of mental and physical health were more acute during this emotion-dominated period than in any other life-stage. Just as expert supervision of adolescent health was critical, so too was attention to its "mental hygiene." Yet, as Alan Brown lamented, "the importance of an early recognition of mental disturbances arising during the period of adolescence demands a broader and more comprehensive handling of the subject than most medical schools are today prepared to give." Until physicians were sufficiently trained in psychology, its practitioners would be called upon "to give most valuable assistance to the department of paediatrics."[10]

The child welfare campaign's focus on young children during the interwar years prompted closer attention to the differences in the health needs of children, adolescents, and adults—not coincidentally, just as the "flaming youth" of the 1920s were being subjected to mounting public criticism. As adolescence became a more distinct life-stage, with its own identifying socio-cultural attributes, it naturally drew more "expert" notice and commentary. Such developments followed upon, and were directly influenced by, many of those unfolding in the United States. Hall's writings on youth, and those of such key American reform figures as Jane Addams, were well known and often cited in the pages of Canadian publications on medicine and social welfare, and in newspapers and mass-distribution magazines—without fail, as though their findings were directly applicable to the Canadian situation—and reached a wide audience of experts and "ordinary," largely middle-class readers.[11] The experts' insistence on the importance of parent education also justified extending vigilance into the passage that awaited childhood's end. For doctors and other "child-savers," the invention of a modern adolescence was a logical extension of the movement to save infant lives and regulate child nurture and training according to perceived national goals.[12]

For the better part of the century following Hall's landmark publication, those concerned with adolescence as field of study and site of practice tended to conflate puberty, or the physical manifestations of adolescence, with the life-stage itself.[13] Adolescence became a condition of "physical and mental anarchy" fraught with nervous disorders and all their imagined ill effects. Doctors and psychologists drew a direct line of causation between the "rapid physical and mental growth" of those years and their characteristic "emotional confusion." Many adolescents consequently found themselves thrust, without adequate preparation, into a "hostile world" of adult customs. Anxiety and alienation were the inevitable—indeed the "natural"—outcome, so that it was "not to be wondered that so many…break down physically or mentally, but the wonder is that so many survive the ordeal with the little health supervision and health knowledge they receive."[14] This normative disease-model framework made adolescence a state of disequilibrium caused by the bodily changes triggered by sexual maturation. Just as the liminal nature of adolescence explained many of its characteristics, organic and otherwise, it also provided an opportune moment for medical intervention. The bodies of adolescents thus became objects for adult regulation and control, in the interests of their safe passage to the ultimate human developmental/evolutionary stage of civilized adulthood.[15]

Supported by scientific theories that construed adolescence as a form of organically based psychosis, doctors argued for both medical supervision of adolescent health and its necessary corollary, health education. It did not matter that there were no illnesses or "defects" found to be endemic to the age group, and that its general health status was excellent. The supervision that physicians prescribed, like their "scientific" regimen for younger children, was all-embracing. Every part of the adolescent's life, from family relations through friendship, courtship, schooling, recreation, and work, harboured threats to physical and mental health that could negatively affect the young person's present health status, while also threatening his or her future. Expressed in myriad contemporary discussions about public health, national welfare, and "racial hygiene," this futurist orientation also demanded "the protection of parenthood" through medical supervision of the entire adolescent experience. The singular objective had to be the "stabilization of youth during this important period," for so much depended upon "the rising generation."[16] Despite their steadfast recurrence, however, views of adolescence as a dangerous time were generally balanced, often in the same discussion, by hopeful theories hinging on the power of education. This was an expansive concept that embraced not only knowledge about the bodily changes affecting young people, but also "constructive education in citizenship and the ideals of national and individual life."[17] Training the young in a regimen to care for their own bodies is an integral part of their socialization into particular cultural milieus, in this case that of adulthood, just as is their training in civic duties. The two were considered mutually supportive and essential to the attainment of "national health."[18]

Although biology remained central to all medical/social constructions of modern adolescence, it was most emphatically so in regard to young women. Hall saw women as perpetually adolescent, their psychology determined by gender, their "formation" never complete, never attaining the same level as that of the fully evolved male.[19] A 1904 advice manual written by a female physician and purporting to be "The Twentieth Century Book for Every Woman" stressed that the young woman owed "much of her beauty and power" to the "regular healthy performance" of menstruation.[20] There was also little of the distinctly modern in one doctor's declaration, in 1920, that "nothing in the whole range of life can compare in importance with the potential powers of reproduction" of the adolescent girl. Amid a postwar celebration of maternalism, even as more girls attended high school and pursued higher education and careers than ever before, earlier medical concerns about the potential for "intellectual development" to undermine "the physical development of our girl life at a time when every attention should be given it" took on extra resonance.[21] With the evolved male as reference point within this medical model, advice to young men centred on preservation of health in the name of ideal manliness, the kind of masculine virility signified by "vim," "push," "pluck" and "stick-to-it-iveness," the identifying traits of the "wholesome manly boy."[22]

Adolescence was understood, paradoxically, as both a period of sexual maturation—and often discussed only as such—and one of sexual limbo. Late-nineteenth-century social purity campaigns had succeeded in bringing sexual matters into the public forum; by the interwar decades, Freudian ideas about the centrality of sexuality to human experience were gradually becoming accepted. Yet sexuality posed a special danger to adolescents simply because they were not adults: all things associated with autoerotic practices, same-sex attraction, indeed, youthful sexual experimentation of any kind, continued to be strictly proscribed. The physical consequences were made inseparable from mental and moral deterioration, which, for good measure, were causally linked to social degeneration, even devolution.[23] Sex was an adult domain, as evidenced in public discourses about the "flaming youth" of the 1920s, who gave tangible form to Canadian fears that the "modern age" had given rise to a "revolution in morals" that right-thinking adults could not countenance.[24] The war had called into question traditional middle-class sexual mores, had "loosened things up," recalled one young man who was in high school when it ended: "the girls were more free, permissive, the men more daring."[25] It is impossible to know whether

premarital sex was actually increasing as a result of these shifts in attitudes and behaviour among the younger generation. Whatever the
quantitative reality, youthful sexuality was much in the air during the
interwar years. Entire books were devoted to "the petting convention of
modern adolescence," characterized by some as the "chief diversion of
the young." Most ominously, many of the adolescents "in danger"
appeared to be "on the road to becoming sexual perverts."[26] D. A.
Thom, psychiatrist and author of a popular advice manual for parents
of adolescents, warned that heterosexuality would never be "accomplished in a normal way" if it were not "accomplished" during that critical life-stage, except by means of "some technical interference...only
after much conflict, failure and illness."[27] Finally, venereal disease scares
originating during the Great War made sex education more important
than ever before, in that these scourges represented both "the greatest
single public health problem of modern times" and also "foul and sin-
ister manifestations of our failure to attend to the organized study and
care of our growing young people."[28]

Although they gave a passing nod to Freud-inspired modern attitudes, interwar doctors and psychologists alike tended to look to the
dark side of the adolescent "sex impulse." Because of the adolescent's
emotionality, impulsiveness, and overwhelming "sex consciousness," it
was feared that making sex "normal"—giving it expert sanction, so to
speak—would promote a fundamental immorality that could only lead
to individual breakdown and its inevitable corollary, social disintegration.
They were ambivalent as to whether boys or girls were more endangered or sources of danger. Girls certainly continued to draw public
admonition about sexual danger, and they might pay the higher price
in unwed pregnancy, but boys were also seen to be threatened by sex outside of lawful, heterosexual—by definition, adult—marriage. And even
though sexual awakening was biologically determined, modern society
appeared to present both sexes with an incredible new range of sexual
"traps." The notorious Arthur Beall, employed by the Ontario education
department as "lecturer on eugenics and personal hygiene," used hyper-
bole, melodrama, and foreboding to deliver his fundamentally anti-sex
message to great numbers of adolescent boys across the province during the first three decades of the twentieth century. Among the "traps,"
Beall named "the deadly cigarette, degrading dime novels, unclean
moving pictures, indecent dances."[29] Although understated by comparison, the eminent social hygiene reformer Peter Sandiford similarly
warned a Hamilton audience in 1922 to pay attention to "all that society holds out to the boy and girl of the later 'teens—the beauties and the
dangers of the dance—the use and abuse of card games—and of the
cigarette craze."[30]

According to concerned observers, then, "modern trends" were clearly implicated in this modern predicament. The "revolutionary nature of the change in attitude to sex" was believed to be attributable to changes in gender ideals among the young. The traditional concepts of manly chivalry and protectiveness, underlying the prescript that all girls should be treated as sisters, had been subverted. The modern boy, however, would not demand more from a girl "than he is given reason to believe he can get." Just as had generations before them, girls had to accept the responsibility of understanding "where harmless relationships leave off and practices leading to sexual intercourse begin."[31] Thus the double standard that demanded sexual purity and self-control of women, while making them the irresistible sirens at the root of many a man's downfall, remained curiously unmodified within the contemporary medical/psychological value system. Doctors also continued to worry that "for the most part, our girls remain in ignorance of their danger, from the shrinking on the part of the parents from talking frankly to them."[32] On the critical subject of sexuality, as in many others pertaining to the youth problem, medical mediation appeared a viable means of breaching an intergenerational barrier made all the higher because of the very different adolescent experiences that divided the younger generation and its parents.

The subtext of these pervasive nervous discussions about adolescent sexuality did not actually concern that life-stage so much as it did "normal" adult sexuality, which was believed to be seriously, perhaps irrevocably, compromised if the young were not taught the sort of respect for "the sex impulse" that would make celibacy their choice until "maturity" saw them safely married off. There was nothing especially modern about this particular concern, but the times made it appear all the more urgent, as youth seemed to flaunt openly what they had once at least attempted to carry off discreetly. Moreover, in the aftermath of war and upheaval, young Canadians needed a "definite training" in sex hygiene in order to become "not only citizens who are longer lived and who are free from disease, but contented, happy units in a well balanced state."[33] Given the magnitude and intensity of fears about adolescent sexuality, sex education was easily the issue that drew the most attention from doctors and youth-watchers of the interwar years, a trend that would remain constant, despite changing historical contexts, throughout the period considered here.[34] Supporters of school-based sex education, among whom doctors were a significant component, acknowledged that physiological principles should be the starting point, but stressed above all a sound "training in right habits and proper attitudes" and the cultivation of "ideals of purity, reverence for parents and parenthood."[35] The outcome would manifest in the "unborn generations of Canadians," ensuring that they, in turn, would become "citizens ennobling their country."[36] Parents were urged to educate themselves, or to rush their children to properly trained physicians lest they do inestimable harm by "conducting their own campaign."[37] Yet the much-favoured simple and direct school-based approach to sex education would never be that simple, nor would it be readily accomplished. Fervent discussion on the part of medical and education authorities, social hygiene organizations, and youth groups, as faithfully reported in the professional and popular press, was not transformed into regular sex instruction for students of any age on any systematic basis during the interwar years, or for some time following.

Notwithstanding the well-documented shortcomings of sex education programs in Canada during the first half of the twentieth century, doctors found much support for their early commitment to the regulation of adolescent health through the school. The preventive public health programs inaugurated in Canadian schools between 1880 and 1914 gained support from growing commitment to disease prevention, but also to practical concerns about the state's role in health care delivery. Urban health departments in Canada, the United States, and Great Britain introduced school medical inspection in the early 1900s, just as the Canadian infant mortality campaign got underway.[38] As was also the case in that campaign, the nature and scope of school health programs varied widely, even within provinces, with notable discrepancies between urban and rural areas.[39] The most populous, urbanized, and industrialized province, Ontario boasted the most developed and comprehensive system, here as elsewhere in public health matters. Doctors, or much more commonly, nurses, were employed by school boards and municipal health boards to assess pupil health periodically, and to carry out basic health instruction oriented to the child's age. No treatment was offered. Children were sent home with explicit directions to their parents to call their own physicians—a class-based assumption that every family had one at hand for regular consultation, even though the very existence of school inspections suggested that this was often not the case.[40] By 1914, most Canadian urban school systems were committed to these measures, and some initiatives were being undertaken for rural and outpost areas.[41]

The 1920s saw the formation of a medical consensus that adolescent health was "a stimulating new field of endeavour worthy of our best efforts," and that school inspection and education programs constituted the most practical and efficient approach. Action toward those ends was painstakingly slow. In addition to the perennial budgetary issues, later exacerbated by Depression constraints, a large part of the problem lay with professional jurisdiction, an issue of internal politics that plagued all contemporary public health programs. There was much trepidation among doctors as to what teachers and school nurses should properly advise about health, and what should be the strict domain of the medical practitioner. Doctors were determined that "the health of the pupil really belongs with the family physician." Their commitment to maintaining clear bounds between public and private health care, between lay and professional health instructors, and within the ranks of medicine itself, meant that even the advocates of high school health programs—like those who promoted well baby clinics—wanted health supervision but generally opposed "routine physical examinations" in the schools. They reasoned that providing the actual service was less important than impressing young people with the understanding that an annual health examination was "very necessary," so that they would continue the practice once school days were over.[42]

The gendered nature of the health education curriculum is also notable. Describing an "experiment" at Winnipeg's Daniel McIntyre Collegiate Institute initiated in 1920, supervising nurse K. E. Dowler indicated how health instruction was presented within the regular domestic science course for tenth grade girls. The mode of delivery supported the medical view that girls needed health training because of their special vulnerability at that age, and also because everything under the rubric of health was properly a womanly concern and an essential component in training for marriage and motherhood. The young women under her supervision were weighed and measured, taught "the signs of positive health," and urged "to seek medical examination to find out if they are free from physical defects." Health talks, health literature, and lessons in nutritious meal preparation were the program's core. Each student also kept a daily personal "health rule record," which was checked regularly by the nurse. "It is a hard thing to keep health rules but a good and jolly game, I am much better and less nervous since trying to keep the rules faithfully," noted one participant. Another young woman remarked that she had been "a girl who had no colour and what colour I had, I had to put on myself." As a result of learning about and following the health rules, she had achieved "natural colour" and "smiled a lot more." Much was made of such personal testimonials to the benefits of health education. The nurse-teacher was gratified by "the splendid evidences of health improvement, in weight, in appearance, in class standing; and the gain toward the close of each year in cheerfulness, improved discipline and happiness."[43] Dowler did not mention any corresponding course for boys, nor did she hint that such a course might be just as valuable to them.

Other high schools made more systematic attempts to incorporate health education into their regular curriculum. Based on both "the new philosophy in education and the needs and hazards involved in health guidance of the 'teen age students," the "consultative health service" at St. Catharines Collegiate Institute and Vocational School (Ontario) was organized in 1929. The program was believed to give the school's 1400 students "a rare opportunity to express themselves on an adult level." Their desire for independence would help them to accept responsibility for their own "health adjustment," even to the extent of securing a physical examination from the family physician—albeit "through their parents." Classroom teachers were considered integral to this health program, their day-to-day and year-to-year relationships with students providing a "splendid opportunity of observing in the pupils any deviation from the normal."[44] Teachers and nurses consequently performed a surveillance role that was critical to medical regulation. By keeping an eye on adolescents, and keeping in touch with parents, they were widening the net containing the youth problem. As long as neither ventured into the doctors' territory, their participation was urged and applauded.

Under the auspices of the provincial health department's Health Education Division, with the intention of encouraging school boards to arrange their own inspection programs in high schools, an "experiment in health teaching" was carried out in Ontario during the academic year 1931–32. High schools representing "a wide variation in economic and social life," both rural and urban, were visited by public health doctors, nurses, and dentists. Their inspections revealed that, by the time they reached high school, 60 per cent of children had decayed permanent teeth, more than 10 per cent had vision defects, and in every classroom, one or more suffered from impaired hearing.[45] Prompted by these results, Burlington High School was one of the first in Ontario to inaugurate regular medical inspection in 1931. Examination by a doctor was restricted to entering students, and repeated only for those who revealed defects and those involved in school sports, while a public health nurse visited periodically for consultation and "health talks." It was asserted that "no infringement is made on the rights of the family physician," through strict adherence to the rule of directing those needing medical attention to their family doctor. Most of the service's cost was met by the school board, but students were required to contribute 50 cents each, a not inconsiderable sum for many families during hard economic times. The Burlington experiment was held to be a successful model of delivering medical supervision to adolescents. Similar provisions were made in 1939 under the auspices of the Dominion Youth Training Program, designed to deal with the problem of the Depression's "idle youth."[46]

The health supervision and teaching of high school students was meant to build on the foundation ideally established in the elementary schools, where adolescents should have been introduced to proper health habits, which should have been reinforced in the home by committed, properly trained parents. Most doctors recognized that such ideals were largely that, given the persistence of regional and urban/rural differences in public health delivery, and the inconsistency of delivery even in areas believed to be well-served. Just as important, during a time when fee-for-service medical care made it a luxury for many Canadian families, if regular physician consultation for the younger, more vulnerable age groups was problematic, it was even less likely to be a familial priority for their older siblings who had safely negotiated the "danger zone" of childhood. Doctors who at least tacitly understood this, and saw that health inspection in the schools was probably the sum total of medical attention for many children, also saw the importance of extending these services through the child's entire school career. Despite the recognized class and "race" differences within the new high school cohort, the benefits were believed to be universal. They could be passed on to younger siblings in deprived homes, often the "inferior" homes of immigrants, where "health habits" were either entirely neglected or negated by superstition and outmoded tradition. The adolescent could serve as an intermediary between the "Old World ways" of parents and the "Canadian" ways of the children. Regardless of "race," inspection and instruction would enhance the health status of "the vast majority" who would enter "the industrial world where health is an important factor in finding a job and in keeping one." And because "the vast majority" would also become parents, "surely no better opportunity exists than to use this period of receptivity and interest to start pre-parent education."[47] Here was another chance to upgrade the childrearing skills of immigrants and the working class, the principal targets of child welfare campaigners.[48]

Medical discourses reveal that "normal youth" status was determined in accordance with the values and customs of the white, Canadian-born, Anglo-Celtic middle class. By the end of the nineteenth century, laws proscribing child labour and establishing mandatory elementary schooling to age fourteen defined childhood's end, or at least legislated a period that was protected under the name of childhood. Yet for many farm and working-class children, full-time labour, usually by the fourteenth birthday, marked the obligatory entry into the adult world.[49] The children of immigrants in the nation's industrial towns often contributed vital wages to fragile family economies.[50] In addition, it was reasoned that most adolescents were not academically inclined, an estimated 70 to 90 per cent leaving school at fifteen, not as a result of economic pressures, but their state of adolescence: their "innate restlessness" made them eager to depart the classroom. This considerable proportion of young people could not be reached—or contained—in the schools. Conse-

quently, "untrained, uncultured, and undersized," they would reproduce all their class disadvantage, physically and morally, in future generations.[51]

Committed to educating the young about their personal responsibility for health, doctors ascribed little significance to health indicators
that reflected their subjects' material, class-designated environment.
While doctors argued the necessity of adolescent health supervision to
the formation of healthy, productive workers, the actual health problems of young workers, pertaining to class and labour, were not integral to medical discourses of the time. What was specifically adolescent
health care for the better part of this period was what was delivered
through the high school, even though its advocates knew they were missing many of their most important "targets." When the discussion did turn
to "child labour," doctors were vague about the relationships among
health, class, age, and the nature of work: "the damage done to the
child from excessive work may be difficult to detect until he has been
engaged at it for a period of years." It was noted that young workers were
"seldom given any follow up care" after leaving the domain of school
inspectors, explaining away "the difficulty of getting figures for a large
number of cases." And, consistent with the larger medical discourse
about adolescence, medical concerns explicitly tied to the life stage of
these workers referred to emotional or psychological more than physical problems. Thus doctors worried about the "striking phenomenon"
of their "rebellion against authority," a phenomenon otherwise regarded
as normal among adolescents, though perhaps only within their own
social group, whose experience was the chief reference point of normality. Among young workers, they contended, "Monotony in this period of
life will kill the best instincts of the future citizen, and very often leads
to Bolshevistic tendencies, or sometimes to the vicious characters so
often encountered in city life." They might, moreover, embrace views "sufficiently warped to drag down hundreds or even thousands."[52]

For working girls, biological destiny overrode any concerns about
rebellion and Bolshevism. Where they were vague about the health pressures of long hours and heavy physical labour for young men, doctors
worried about the impact of fatigue and other work-related health threats
on the more fragile physical and nervous systems of women in this "delicate" age group, especially considering that they might lead to "permanent derangement of health and difficulty in childbearing." The "fundamental fact" determining women's place in industry was that "nearly
every woman is a potential mother." Young working women were believed
to be even more prone to all manner of "breakdowns" than were their
more affluent sisters. Concerns about physical health and worker efficiency were also closely connected, at times masking anxieties about

production with those about reproduction. The 1908 royal commission on the working conditions of female telephone operators, the majority of whom were young single women, concluded that "the breaking point of the operator's health is not far from the breaking point of efficient work." Moral health was also a particular problem of working girls: at the common wage rate of seven dollars per week or less, overstepping the bounds into casual prostitution appeared a real danger, rendering working girls the "social wreckage" of the nation.[53] When war-inspired interest in the correlates of worker health, productivity, and "national efficiency" inspired government forays into "industrial hygiene" during the First World War, a few attempts were made in industrial centres, starting with Ontario, to instigate factory medical inspections that included physical examinations for workers. There is no suggestion that the youth of workers was a specific concern, however, or that the particular health needs and deficiencies of adolescent workers were given special consideration.[54]

During the Great Depression, especially in rural and sparsely settled areas, local school and health boards had great difficulty even paying teachers and public health nurses, much less establishing new high school health inspection services. While public health advocates argued that the service was well worth providing, the municipal authorities who bore the brunt of the cost were not easily persuaded. The simple facts that the preventable illness rate within this age group was relatively low, and absenteeism due to medical causes likewise, also inhibited general implementation.[55] Where diagnostic public health programs such as clinics, home visits, and school inspections were already in place, their avowed benefits could not overcome the reality that follow-up treatments were left to patients—in this case, their parents—to pursue and pay for. An Ontario health department survey of twelve cities revealed a delay of a year or more in securing the necessary medical attention in 45.5 per cent of such cases, across all age groups, due primarily to inability to pay for treatment.[56] Even school boards that had adopted health instruction programs appeared to be "carrying along in the high school much as they do in elementary schools," with little attention to the special needs of adolescents for a specially designed program of health education.[57] In 1940, after twenty years of hopeful discussion among doctors, public health workers, and educators, most Canadian cities still did not carry out any health inspection or instruction in their high schools.

By the time that the Second World War commenced, the results of the child welfare campaign were making themselves felt: infant and maternal mortality rates were declining, communicable diseases were being checked with mass immunization and the new sulphonamides, and maternal and child health divisions were in place in every provincial health department, assisted by the federal health department and such national agencies as the Council on Child and Family Welfare and the Health League of Canada. When war exigencies once again made "national health" a condition for victory, the focus readily shifted to new initiatives on behalf of young people. As they had been in 1914, Canadians were shocked to learn from early recruitment statistics that 43 per cent of young men who had applied for service were rejected for health reasons. This news was taken (once again) as irrefutable proof that "the health standard of the young men and women of Canada is far below the level which the efficiency and happiness of the country demand." At its annual meeting in 1942, the Canadian Public Health Association (CPHA) formally resolved that, in order to train "useful citizens" during this time of international crisis, instruction in healthful living had to be "intelligently given in all the schools of Canada."[58] Despite "general recognition" that an adequate school health service would go far to remedy health defects in "the young manhood and womanhood of the nation," and despite the fact that 30 per cent of the adolescent age group attended high schools, the majority of these were not covered by any such program. The CPHA urged "a considerable extension in secondary school health services," to include mandatory physical examination of all pupils on entrance and at regular intervals thereafter, and "the inculcation of correct attitudes and habits."[59]

Under the pressures of war, governments were inclined to take up the cause on behalf of youth, the nation's major resource for military duty, vital war production, and other home front services. Provincial health ministers "very wisely" asked municipalities to reconsider the long-delayed implementation of high school health inspection, not only in order that their students might efficiently serve the nation, but also "to assure the mental and physical health of the next generation."[60] The National Physical Fitness Act (1943) proposed to "make it possible to give advantages only enjoyed by the few before the war, to all Canadians in the postwar period." Its goals were to extend physical education in schools, universities, and other institutions, including "industrial establishments," and to coordinate sports nationwide. In promoting health, loyalty, and cooperation, the act was supposed to be integral to a home front campaign that called upon each citizen to accept the "prime duty" of "an all-out effort to win the war" and to "get himself in good physical condition."[61] For all practical purposes, the school-age population was most amenable to such intervention, constituting a ready laboratory for training, measurement, and regulation. In the end, the plan's initiatives had scarcely begun when the federal government's wartime fervour gave way under the pressures of postwar reconstruction.

Another of the public/medical worries about youth recirculated from the Great War years involved the perceived war-induced loosening of sexual morality and its foremost physical repercussions: the spread of venereal diseases and increased rates of prostitution and unwed pregnancy. Venereal diseases were the "internal enemies of any nation," and every effort had to be extended to "enlist every responsible citizen in the war against this unseen but dangerous enemy."[62] K. J. Backman, director of Venereal Disease Control for Manitoba, noted the "alarming fact" that the increase was chiefly in the younger age group, many of whom were only in their teens. These were the "khaki kids" who "hang around barracks and railway stations or go soldier hunting in juke joints and dance halls," caught up in "the vast social dislocation of a country at war and without any organized constructive part to play in that country's war effort." When he and other concerned observers spoke of these young people, they were primarily, if not exclusively, discussing young women. A Winnipeg juvenile court judge reported that girls ranging in age from twelve to seventeen were "regular hangers-on at military camps or railway stations, picking up soldiers and spending a day or night at one of the hotels." There was evidently a "serious increase" in the numbers aged thirteen to fifteen reported missing from home, while the proportion of infected girls in the fourteen to seventeen age range had apparently risen 50 per cent over the year 1941–1942. Victoria's welfare officer announced that the number of unmarried mothers in that city alone increased from 70 in 1941 to 114 in 1942; 49 of the latter were under twenty-one, the youngest a child of twelve. Doctors inflamed a veritable moral panic about the wartime degeneration of youth, especially girls, whose participation in the seeming wave of juvenile delinquency was largely related to sexual misdemeanours.[63] In reality, the distribution of illegitimate births by age did not change to any considerable extent between 1931 and 1951; during those twenty years, it actually declined for the group under age twenty.[64]

A wartime survey of youth organizations by the Canadian Youth Commission (CYC) revealed the paucity of programs aimed specifically at young people and their resulting dissatisfaction with the *status quo*. Its summary, *Youth and Health* (1946), emphasized that "in the development of a bold constructive health program for Canada, the understanding and support of the new generation is an essential condition of success." Although the majority polled strongly supported health education—especially sex education—and "more comprehensive," compulsory physical examinations in the high schools, their highest priority was affordable medical care for all Canadians. The CYC called for health insurance jointly underwritten by federal and provincial governments—the foremost recommendation of the participating 3000-member Canadian Association of Medical Students and Interns—along the lines of the National Health Insurance Bill under consideration by the Mackenzie King Liberal government. The bill was scuttled over the usual federal–provincial jurisdictional questions. Like many other war-born initiatives, the CYC saw few of its recommendations materialize once the emergency ended.[65]

If nothing concrete was achieved in spite of hopeful beginnings, postwar Canada saw adolescence entering a new stage of medical—and public—consciousness. More than ever, doctors were insisting that this "dynamic period" demanded "fuller exploitation" by health workers, in case "a priceless opportunity" to ensure adult success were squandered. Among those leading the call to "exploit" adolescence were the pediatricians, perhaps grasping the moment to capitalize on their interwar gains in persuading parents of the importance of pediatric consultation and regular well-baby care.[66] Echoing Alan Brown a generation prior, one doctor declared that "the problems of adolescent and physical maturation do...belong in the field of the paediatrist; not only because he has watched over the individual through the period of infancy to that of adolescence and, like any other physician, is sorry to lose his patients, but even more definitely because his is the only really interested medical group who have tackled, though fitfully and sometimes with a poor technique, the emotional problems of that particular age group." He was concerned that this age group might end up "deprived of the expert care which they need and to which they are entitled."[67] Although by no means as successful in Canada as in the United States, the pediatricians' drive for recognition did see the formation of the Canadian Paediatric Society from the Canadian Society for the Study of Diseases of Children in 1951.[68] Ultimately, the impassioned views of specialists and generalists alike took little account of the scarcity of pediatricians in Canada during the 1940s, and none of the fact that the central problem of health care was the scarcity of regular medical attention of any kind for a significant number of Canadians of any age.

In the early postwar years, amid a renewed celebration of the "normal" family with its traditional male breadwinner, dependent wife, and children, the trend toward state-supported expert intervention in private lives received new impetus. The federal government's Health Grants Act of 1948 provided funds to the provinces to expand their public health services. By 1950, most towns were served by some form of public health nursing, while new county health units looked after a growing number of previously neglected rural and less-populated areas across the country.[69] Although the historic regional, class, "race," and gender differentials were by no means erased, more Canadians enjoyed better living standards than ever before.[70] New medical research supported the view that, through such related factors as improved nutrition, access to medical care, and overall better health, better economic times were contributing to an increase in the physical size of adolescents as well as an earlier age of sexual maturation. Studies conducted at ten-year intervals between 1936 and 1956 among Saskatoon public school children, nine to fourteen years of age, showed that both boys and girls were taller and heavier in 1956 than were their earlier counterparts. Within the 1956 cohort, those classified "upper socioeconomic" were also taller and heavier than all the others. Data from the IQ testing in widespread use during those decades also demonstrated the "greater mental age" of the 1956 cohort. Researchers believed that such combined physical and mental advancements had led to an earlier age at puberty as well. Subjective observations supported the data: they were currently obliged to provide gowns to Grade 6 girls for physical examinations because of their breast development, something rarely necessary before 1946. Many Grade 7 boys, at the age of thirteen, were also showing physical signs of sexual maturation, and it was "not uncommon for their mothers to express concern over the extent and earliness of their sexual development and the fact that their sons are now shaving regularly." The researchers consoled parents, and doubtless themselves, by surmising that, "fortunately" any increase in "sexual urge" had been accompanied by "greater mental maturity."[71] Adolescents seemed to be responding bodily to socio-economic changes, providing a physical measure of rising living standards.

But earlier physical maturity was also interpreted as another of the "problems" of adolescents in a rapidly changing world, as the watershed 1964 Royal Commission on Health Services (known as the Hall Commission). The commissioners found that their age group "perhaps more than any of the other groups is profoundly affected by the social changes of our time." While the traditional familial and community responsibilities of adolescents had been reduced in some respects, in others they faced heightened expectations, "resulting in stresses which cannot fail to be reflected in the health status of this group."[72] By this time, the ideas of psychoanalyst Erik Erikson, as detailed in his landmark 1959 publication, *Identity and the Life Cycle*, were pointing to the complications inherent in the prolonged "psychosocial moratorium" that signified contemporary adolescence, which kept young people infantilized and restrained in a lengthy transition to adulthood through which they were often powerless to navigate successfully on their own.[73] The statistical evidence nonetheless confirmed that this generation was physically in better health than any before. But many of the old concerns regarding the youthful propensity for destructive "habits" and emotional instability persisted, intensifying within the troubling context of a youth-led counterculture, another historical explanation superimposed on seem-ingly immutable adolescent biological imperatives. The unrelenting media spotlight on teenagers since the Second World War ensured that a corresponding expansion of public, medical, and state attention was effected on behalf of an age group more demographically significant, healthier—and wealthier—than ever before.

In regard to school health programs, the difficulties that had marked the earliest years of such "experiments" continued, despite this new inter-generational anxiety, and despite steady improvements in the political/economic framework of health care, which would culminate in universal medicare in 1968. Doctors still had misgivings about encroach-ments on their professional territory and about the inadequacy of non-medical efforts, their doubts perhaps worsened by this rapidly increas-ing state involvement. In 1965 a national survey of teacher training programs, intended "to provide a better understanding of the overall emphasis on health education in Canada," found that health was taught in all provincial high schools with the exception of Newfoundland; only New Brunswick and Ontario continued to Grade 12, while the majority had no compulsory health program after ninth grade.[74] Still the Cana-dian Medical Association contended that the "psychological and bio-logical aspects" of adolescence should be taught only by well-trained physicians, "rather than a teacher who has only a limited basis of knowl-edge upon which to found his teaching." Since it was clearly difficult to have physicians deliver entire high school health courses, the association recommended that "well motivated and knowledgeable physicians" should at least be "intimately involved" in the design of such courses.[75] If the perennial emphasis on citizenship training as a vital part of health education had become less emphatic, it remained an important sub-text: doctors still maintained that the health curriculum should teach young people both what they needed to know to maintain a high stan-dard of health, and also about "mature living in our society."[76]

There is much that is familiar, as well, in the priority given to par-ticular adolescent health issues during the 1960s. It is clear that sexu-ality burns straight through the twentieth century as the foremost source of adult dread regarding youth. In the midst of a "sexual revolution," the importance of instruction in human sexuality was easily "the most discussed educational topic" of the 1960s.[77] In the face of youth rebel-lion and sexual revolution, adolescents' own views finally began to be heard, as the "helping professions" and the state agencies actively solicited youth participation in discussions—"speak-ins," in contem-porary lingo—about their needs and concerns. A Montreal symposium on sex education convened by medical professionals, educators, and social workers, with an invited contingent of high school participants, suggested just how little satisfied young people were with the current state of things. Formal instruction in sexual matters not only started too late, but, committed to starting from first principles, was often not age-appropriate as a result: "At 16 we learn what happened to us when we were 12," one young man complained. Teenagers also objected to the values imposed by their "square" elders, preferring to regard their sexuality as "natural" and seeing no reason, for example, why pregnant girls should be ostracized and not permitted to attend school freely and openly. They strongly advocated the dissemination of contraceptive information from earliest puberty, and freer access to contraceptive devices, which doctors still very much controlled and generally hesitated to prescribe to unmarried young women, especially minors, without parental consent.

Among the specific health concerns of the sixties generation, smoking and the recreational use of drugs ranked close behind sexual matters in order of priority, both for medicine and society at large. The tobacco evil had long been a target of temperance and social purity advocates; by the early 1960s, there was a considerable body of scientific evidence to associate smoking with rapidly increasing rates of lung cancer and coronary heart disease. In 1962, a Calgary survey, among the first to measure the smoking habits of high school students, found that 46.4 per cent of boys and 33.1 per cent of the girls were regular smokers. The majority had smoked their first cigarette between the ages of twelve and fifteen years.[78] Recognizing the peer group's powerful conforming influence, and that teenagers were "tired of adults telling them what to do," the University of Saskatchewan's Social and Preventive Medicine team initiated a student-directed program in smoking education for the province's junior high and high schools.[79] The federal government also took the stand that "teenage leaders are a resource that can prove very useful to the field of health education" in its national "Smoke-In" of 1965, which drew together seventy-five delegates from high schools for three days of discussion with experts and government health officials.[80] The students themselves were cynical about the outcome. As one young woman expressed it, "Although the conference was very interesting and informative and encouraged a great deal of personal participation, little concrete value in the form of a nation wide attack on smoking was achieved." A male participant was even more pessimistic: because "propaganda" had made smoking seem "a natural part of growing up," teenagers were unlikely to be influenced by fear of the long-term ill effects of smoking.[81] The continued, and increasing, incidence of teenage smoking since the mid-1960s, despite the barrage of anti-smoking educational campaigns and restrictive legislation, sustains their observations.[82]

Teenagers also embraced drug use as "the thing to do," not only as an age-group pastime, but as a fundamental part of the rebellious "tune in, turn on, drop out" ethic associated with the youth-led counterculture percolating through the Western world. With growing intensity, doctors contended that illicit drug use among Canadian youth was "high enough to cause serious concern," a concern that their views helped to sustain, since doctors were naturally regarded as the leading experts on drugs and their health effects. Thanks to vigorous media coverage, anxious discussion by "professionals in close contact with youth," the climbing number of drug-related court cases, and, probably most significant, the fact that young users "flaunted their drug practices," Canadians were persuaded that drug use was now "a part of youth culture in this country."[83] While clearly not an accurate measure of actual use, the numbers dominating government reports and disseminated by the mass media gave the situation crisis proportions. Between 1967 and 1968, for example, arrests for marijuana use jumped 300 per cent; the median age at time of arrest was a parent-chilling seventeen years. The situation across the land was perceived to be grave enough for public health and educational authorities in larger centres such as Toronto, Vancouver, Winnipeg, Montreal, and Ottawa to initiate school programs about the dangers of drug use, especially the popular street drugs such as LSD, marijuana, and amphetamines.

What made the drug scene so morbidly fascinating was the fact that the use of drugs for non-medicinal purposes—for "kicks"—by young, white, otherwise "ordinary" and "normal" people, really was a shocking new phenomenon. No longer drawn from the historic "underclass," often racially defined, drug-users were the children of the affluent, respectable, middle class. They were also well-educated, in decided contrast to the socially disadvantaged youths who were the subjects of earlier reports about adolescent drug abuse.[84] If the problem was new, the explanation was the familiar one that tied the biological "upheavals" of adolescence to those of intense societal change, making both, in effect, a process of anomie. Doctors explained teenage drug use in terms of maturational difficulties, which, exacerbated by institutional flux, fostered the growth of such malignant subcultures. Like parents and other reasoning adults through the generations, doctors could "only speculate on why teenagers adopt these bizarre practices," but they believed that it had everything to do with their life stage. As adolescents, like generations before them, they were "just experimenting and hoping to gain the acceptance of the peer group." The doctors who dealt with much of the negative outcome of recreational drug use had to take into account "the probability that the cultural milieu of the patient may approve and indeed encourage drug use."[85]

Public anxiety about the widespread use of psychoactive drugs prompted the Trudeau government's establishment of the Commission of Inquiry into the Non-Medical Use of Drugs (known as the LeDain Commission) in 1970. The Canadian Medical Association, not surprisingly, presented the most extensive brief to the commission, asserting that, while the problems of young people were not "solely medical" in nature, "medicine has a vital integral part to serve in the necessary approach to their solution."[86] Federal Minister of Health and Welfare John Munro argued that the whole debate about the non-medical use of drugs was "losing sight of its essential problem," and becoming moralized to the degree of castigating an entire generation for the practices of a minority, by depicting drug use as a "retrograde step in personal and societal development"—a case of devolution, in effect. The most efficacious response, he believed, was the expansion of the street clinic "in the neighbourhood of its primary clientele," its staff perhaps more closely resembling it than did "regular health personnel," as in one case he described in which "the central doctor [had] shoulder-length hair and a headband and serape."[87] But neither education nor even the harsh sentences handed to first-time teenage drug users appear to have been effective. Drugs were a symbol of the defiance of a particular generation that, having latched onto the "generation gap" as its explanation for many of its cultural innovations, was not going to be regulated by family, church, school, state, or medicine, nearly as much as its predecessors had allowed. The door opened during the 1960s would not be so easily closed.[88]

Although seemingly a constant of recorded history, adult fascination with the lives—actually the lifestyles—of the young reflects cultural as much as generational, age-based perspectives. What is seen to typify adolescence at particular historical moments reveals much about the pressing concerns of "society," that is, a sector of adults whose status carries considerable political and economic weight. Adolescents become, in Erik Erikson's apt description, "living symptoms" of all that represents social malaise.[89] Not long after early twentieth century, Canadians were told that "the child is not a little man," they were advised that the adolescent was "a being in the process of constant physical formation, the features of which are so delicate that the same care is required to reach the proper stage of adult life as was needed to save that life in infancy."[90] The particular medical concerns of the day matched, and gave substance to, wider social concerns about a life stage often conflated with a "youth problem." Although adolescents were ostensibly among the healthiest of all Canadians throughout this entire half-century, they were believed to need regular medical attention because of a litany of age-specific problems, often defined in moral rather than scientific terms. When discussion of the problems considered "inherent in this mysterious developmental process called adolescence" turned to socio-cultural influences, these were typically grafted onto the biological stem without really affecting the explanation. Thus, adolescence was "characteristic of and created by our form of civilization." Yet if "hectic modern times" shared a large part of the blame, there was little doubt that the young person's inability to cope with problems peculiar to the age group was a manifestation of the peculiar biology of adolescence.[91] Despite some dissension among experts, this Hall-inspired perspective held firm. No less an authority than J. Roswell Gallagher, credited with establishing adolescent medicine in the United States, argued that "adolescents are no more enigmatic than any other people." But Gallagher also recognized that "adolescence puts the result of heredity and environment and childhood training to a severe test."[92] While historicizing psychoanalytic concepts, Erikson also depicted adolescence as an identity crisis sparked by a "physiological revolution."[93] A 1970 text intended for use in medical schools still proclaimed adolescence to be distinguished by "a restlessness of body and a discontentment of mind...brought about by biological changes."[94]

Until very recently, medical interest in adolescence manifested itself primarily in the form of high school programs of health supervision and education. Much as was the case across the broadly defined child welfare campaign, the bounds delineated by commitment to privatized medical care and physician dominance over nurses and "lay volunteers" made education the favoured approach. Educational efforts were conceivably easier to deliver and more efficacious for this age-group: doctors could target the clients directly, though much attention was given to parental involvement in preparing the young for adulthood, especially for marriage and parenthood, which were supposed to be the "normal" outcome of adolescence. As growing numbers entered high school, making it the common experience of teenagers, just as primary schooling had earlier defined a modern childhood for the younger set, the framework was conveniently in place, requiring little extra state investment. Medical supervision of the adolescent gradually became institutionalized in an expanding secondary school system that was itself the most convenient means of containing the youth problem. For the most part, it remained there until the 1960s. At that conjuncture, just as state medicine was becoming established, the "youth rebellion" made the "youth problem" appear so acute as to merit the creation of a network of what might be called "extramural," diagnostic, educational, and treatment facilities to meet the needs of young Canadians.

Canadian doctors, like their American colleagues, demonstrated an early and steadfast interest in adolescence as a life stage requiring special—if not specialized—medical attention and health care provision. Yet Canadian efforts remained almost exclusively school-centred until the 1970s. A 1985 survey of Canadian paediatricians did not count a single doctor who concentrated on adolescent medicine. At the beginning of the twenty-first century, adolescent medicine remains peripheral, and has not yet established itself as a certified subspecialty of pediatrics.[95] What helps to explain this differential history are national differences in training and certification practices, in health care delivery and funding, and especially in numbers, both in terms of population and the proportion of physicians to population.[96] At the end of the period considered here, Canadian pediatricians were caring for about 700,000 children, or just over one-tenth of the child population, with one active pediatrician for every 8575 children. In the United States in 1970, there were roughly twice as many pediatricians, or one for every 4446 American children. There are also national differences in training and practice that suggest why adolescent medicine as a subspecialty has been so slow to take off in Canada. As the number of general practitioners declined during the late twentieth century, American pediatricians increasingly acted as a type of family doctor, as well as filing the traditional role of personal physicians to children. According to doctors themselves, in order to provide American-type pediatric care effectively, Canada would need ten times as many pediatricians as we have, in short, over four thousand more immediately.[97]

If the formalization of adolescent medicine has yet to be achieved, steps toward that end have been taken nonetheless. In 1970, the Canadian Paediatric Society established its Adolescent Medicine Committee as an advisory and advocacy group on the "medical, psychological, and social challenges of the development and transition from childhood to adulthood," with emphasis on fostering "the adolescent's capacity to take responsibility for himself or herself."[98] At its General Council meeting in 1977, noting that "adolescent children in Canada meet special problems and needs with regard to their development," the Canadian Medical Association submitted an official request to make adolescent medicine a certified subspecialty to the Royal College of Physicians and Surgeons of Canada. The timing, however, was unfortunate: the RCPSC was in the process of issuing a moratorium on accrediting subspecialties due to the high costs associated with the examination process.[99] Efforts were solidified, however, with the creation of the Canadian Association for Adolescent Health/Association canadienne pour la santé des adolescents (CAAH/ACSA) in 1993, a multidisciplinary nationwide organization that promotes adolescent participation in its activities, thereby encouraging self-advocacy.[100] The RCPSC recently reopened the files that closed in the late 1970s, and the Canadian Paediatric Society is once again working toward having adolescent medicine recognized in the very near future. If the twentieth century saw the invention of a modern adolescence and the steady development of medical interest in this age group, the twenty-first appears to herald a new partnership among medicine, other professions, and community groups dedicated to the concerns of youth, and members of "the rising generation" itself.

Acknowledgements

Thanks are owed to the Social Sciences and Humanities Research Council of Canada, the Hannah Institute for the History of Medicine, and the Research Office, Wilfrid Laurier University, for ongoing and much-appreciated support of the larger project of which this is a part.

Notes

1 Contemporary commentaries include, for example, H. Dobson, "Youth: Scapegrace or Scapegoat," *Social Welfare* (July 1929): 228; Editorial, "Hygiene of Recreation," *Canadian Practitioner* (June 1924): 309; and T. R. Robinson, "Youth and the Virtues," *Social Welfare* (October 1928): 9. These anxieties are explored more fully in C. R. Comacchio, "Dancing to Perdition: Adolescence and Leisure in Interwar English Canada," *Journal of Canadian Studies* 32, 3 (Fall 1997): 5–27. Although used occasionally in the media during the interwar years, the term *teenager* does not seem to have come into popular usage until the 1950s; on developments after the Second World War, see M. L. Adams, *The Trouble with Normal: Postwar Youth and the Making of Heterosexuality* (Toronto: University of Toronto Press, 1997). On similar European developments regarding "modern youth," see K. Alaimo, "Shaping Adolescence in the Popular Milieu: Social Policy, Reformers, and French Youth, 1870–1920," *Journal of Family History* 17, 4 (1992): 420; W. S. Haine, "The Development of Leisure and the Transformation of Working-Class Adolescence in France," *Journal of Family History* 17, 4 (1992): 451. Among the seminal works on the historical experience of adolescence are M. Childs, *Labour's Apprentices* (Montreal and Kingston: McGill-Queen's University Press, 1993); H. Hendrick, *Images of Youth* (London: Oxford University Press, 1990); J. Kett, *Rites of Passage: Adolescence in America* (New York: Basic Books, 1977); D. Linton, *Who Has the Youth Has the Future* (Cambridge, MA: Harvard University Press, 1990); J. Modell, *Into One's Own: From Youth to Adulthood in the United States* (Berkeley: University of California Press, 1988); J. Neubauer, *The Fin-de-Siècle Culture of Adolescence* (New Haven, CT: Yale University Press, 1992); J. Springhall, *Coming of Age: Adolescence in Britain, 1860–1960* (London: Oxford University Press, 1986); and R. Wegs, *Growing Up Working Class: Youth in Vienna, 1870–1920* (Philadelphia: University of Pennsylvania Press, 1989). Specifically on adolescent health in the United States is the recent study by H. Munro Prescott, *A Doctor of Their Own: The History of Adolescent Medicine* (Cambridge, MA: Harvard University Press, 1998). There is no historical overview of twentieth-century Canadian adolescence, although several studies touch on some portion of it for certain periods, e.g., V. Strong-Boag, *The New Day Recalled* (Markham: Penguin, 1988); and, more recently, B. Bradbury, *Working Families* (Toronto:

McClelland and Stewart, 1993); K. Dubinsky, *Improper Advances* (Chicago: University of Chicago Press, 1993); J. Taylor, *Fashioning Farmers* (Regina, SK: Canadian Great Plains Research Centre, 1994); S. Morton, *Ideal Surroundings* (Toronto: University of Toronto Press, 1995); D. Owram, *Born at the Right Time: A History of the Baby Boom Generation* (Toronto: University of Toronto Press, 1996); and C. Strange, *Toronto's Girl Problem* (Toronto: University of Toronto Press, 1995).

2 Alaimo, "Shaping Adolescence," 419–21; see also H. P. Chudacoff, *How Old Are You? Age Consciousnes in American Culture* (Princeton: Princeton University Press, 1989); and P. Fass, "Testing the IQ of Children," in *Childhood in America*, ed. P. S. Fass and M. A. Mason (New York: New York University Press, 2000), 307–12. See, in this volume, Mona Gleason, "Race, Class, and Health: School Medical Inspection and 'Healthy' Children in British Columbia, 1890 to 1930," and Margaret Tennant, "Complicating Childhood: Gender, Ethnicity, and 'Disadvantage' within the New Zealand Children's Health Camps Movement."

3 Munro Prescott, *A Doctor of Their Own*, 1–6. The book traces the American trajectory of specialization in adolescent medicine from the early 1950s, particularly with the establishment of the Boston Children's Hospital Adolescent Unit in 1951 under the foremost adolescent specialist of the time, J. Roswell Gallagher; see especially chap. 2, 37–75.

4 During the period of the *Military Service Act*, 68 per cent of applicants were rejected as unfit for service. The ill health of these young men resulted from "our life before the war." Similar worries surfaced in Britain and the United States. See Editorial, "Social Hygiene," *Social Welfare* 7, 3 (1924): 48. The statistics were referred to constantly in health discussions; see, for example, Canada, *House of Commons Debates* (March 3, 1930), 221–22 (Mr. E. G. Garland, MP for Bow River). On eugenic concerns, see, for example, P. H. Bryce, "The Scope of a Federal Department of Health," *Canadian Medical Association Journal* 10, 1 (1920): 3; A. Meyer, "The Right to Marry: What Can a Democratic Civilization Do about Heredity and Child Welfare?" *Canadian Journal of Mental Hygiene* 1, 2 (1919): 145; and H. MacMurchy, "The Parents' Plea," *Canadian Journal of Mental Hygiene* 1, 3 (1919): 211. See also MacMurchy's reports on "The Feeble-Minded in Ontario," in Ontario, *Sessional Papers*, Board of Health Annual Reports, 1907–15, and her larger study, *Sterilization? Birth Control?* (Toronto: King's Printer, 1934). On eugenics in Canada, see A. McLaren, *Our Own Master Race: Eugenics in Canada, 1885–1945* (Toronto: McClelland and Stewart, 1990).

5 H. MacMurchy, "The Medical Inspection of Schools," *Canadian Medical Association Journal* 3, 2 (1913): 111; also A. Brown, "The General Practitioner and Preventive Paediatrics," *Canadian Public Health Journal* 21, 6 (1930): 268.

6 A. Brown, "The Relation of the Paediatrician to the Community," *Canadian Public Health Journal* 10, 2 (1919): 54–55; also Brown, "The General Practitioner," 267–68; and Canadian Medical Association, "Report of the Committee on Economics: Appendix, Presentation of the Canadian Society for the Study of the Diseases of Children," *Annual Report* (1945), 66–67. Similar views are expressed in Editorial, "The Health of The Child," *Canadian Medical Association Journal* 2, 7 (1912): 704; and B. F. Royer, "Child Welfare," *Canadian Public Health Journal* 12, 8 (1921): 293. See also J. H. Ebbs, "The Canadian Paediatric Society: Its Early Years," *Canadian Medical Association Journal* 126, 12 (1980): 235. The society was founded at a conference at Toronto's Hospital for Sick Children, June 1922; Brown was its first vice-president. For a general overview of the specialty's development, see S. Halpern, *American Pediatrics: The Social Dynamics of Professionalism, 1880–1980* (Berkeley: University of California Press, 1988).

7 Munro Prescott, *A Doctor of Their Own*, 184, notes that, even as the 1990s closed, only 50 per cent of American and Canadian medical schools had an adolescent medicine division, and that budgetary cuts were obliging many institutions to phase out even those that existed, or to combine them with other departments.

8 N. Lesko, "Denaturalizing Adolescence: The Politics of Contemporary Representations," *Youth and Society* 28, 2 (December 1996): 147–48. On early twentieth-century child psychology in Canada and the United States, see T. Richardson, *The Century of the Child: The Mental Hygiene Movement and Social Policy in the United States and Canada* (Albany, NY: State University of New York Press, 1989); for developments after the Second World War, see M. Gleason, *Normalizing the Ideal: Psychology, Schooling and the Family in Postwar Canada* (Toronto: University of Toronto Press, 1999).

9 A number of historians have dealt capably with his tremendous influence in foregrounding a view of adolescence that would suffer little contestation through much of the twentieth century: see Kett, *Rites of Passage*, 218–19; Lesko, "Denaturalizing Adolescence," 144–47; Munro, *A Doctor of Their Own*, 6–8; Adams, *The Trouble with Normal*, 43–47; and D. Randall, *Kipling's Imperial Boy: Adolescence and Cultural Hybridity* (New York: Palgrave, 2000): 9–10. The definitive biography remains D. Ross, *G. Stanley Hall: The Psychologist as Prophet* (Chicago: University of Chicago Press, 1983).

10 A. Brown, "Toronto as a Paediatric Centre," *Canadian Medical Monthly* 5, 6 (June 1920): 205. Munro, *A Doctor of Their Own*, 14, notes that the Commonwealth Fund actively promoted this "cross-training" in medicine and psychology. This was a charitable organization established by the Harkness family to support medical research, during the 1930s.

11 On Addams's influence, see C. L. James, "Practical Diversions and Educational Amusements: Evangelia Home and the Advent of Canada's Settlement Movement, 1902–09," *Historical Studies in Education* 10, 1–2 (Spring/Fall 1998): 49–51.

12 On the subject of changing views on childhood, and the development of child welfare movements, see N. Sutherland, *Children in English Canadian Society: Framing the Twentieth-Century Consensus* (Toronto: University of Toronto Press, 1976; Waterloo: Wilfrid Laurier University Press, 2000); Richardson, *Century of the Child*; C. R. Comacchio, *"Nations Are Built of Babies": Saving Ontario's Mothers and Children, 1900–40* (Montreal and Kingston: McGill-Queen's University Press, 1993), especially chap. 2; and K. Arnup, *Education for Motherhood: Advice for Mothers in Twentieth-Century Canada* (Toronto: University of Toronto Press, 1994).

13 Adams, *The Trouble with Normal*, 43–47; G. S. Hall, *Adolescence: Its Psychology and Its Relations to Physiology, Anthropology, Sociology, Sex, Crime, Religion and Education*, vol. 1 (New York: D. Appleton, 1904), xvi–xvii, 438–39; and Munro Prescott, *A Doctor of Their Own*, 24–25.

14 D. V. Currey and A. G. Nicolle, "Development of a Health Program in the Secondary School," *Canadian Public Health Journal* 31 (April 1940): 176; also, Editorial, "School Health Supervision in Secondary Schools," *Canadian Public Health Journal* 31 (April 1940): 199. See the psychiatrists' viewpoint on the "mental, social and moral difficulties" of adolescence in W. T. B. Mitchell, "The Clinical Significance of Some Trends in Adolescence," *Canadian Medical Association Journal* 22, 30 (February 1930): 182–87. Similar views are found in D. A. Thom, *Normal Youth and Its Everyday Problems* (New York: D. Appleton, 1932), ix; also, A. Goldbloom, "Problems of the Adolescent Child," *Canadian Medical Association Journal* 43, 4 (October 1940): 336–39.

15 Lesko, "The Denaturalization of Adolescence," 150; on this model and its context, see also A. James and A. Prout, *Constructing and Reconstructing Childhood: Contemporary Issues in the Sociological Study of Childhood* (London: Falmer, 1990).
16 Editorial, "Hygiene of Recreation," *Canadian Practitioner* 49, 6 (June 1924): 309.
17 Mitchell, "Some Trends in Adolescence," 182–87.
18 Similar themes are discussed in Gleason, "Race, Class, and Health," and Tennant, "Complicating Childhood," both in this volume.
19 Hall, *Adolescence*, vol. 2, 624.
20 M. R. Melendy, "Becoming a Woman," in *Vivilore: The Pathway to Mental and Physical Perfection* (Toronto: J. L. Nichols, 1904), 300. Melendy was a Chicago physician and "lecturer on the diseases of women and children," according to the book's jacket biography.
21 W. F. Roberts [minister of Public Health, New Brunswick], "The Reconstruction of the Adolescent Period of Our Canadian Girl," *Social Welfare* (January 1920): 100; similar views are expressed in A. F. Hodgkins, "Recreation for Woman and Girls." *Canadian Public Health Journal* 14, 7 (July 1923): 314–17. See also J. Brumberg, "Chlorotic Girls, 1870–1920: A Historical Perspective on Female Adolescence," *Child Development* 53 (1982):1468–77; Brumberg, *The Body Project: An Intimate History of American Girls* (New York: Random House, 1997); G. Elder, "Adolescence in the Life Cycle," in *Adolescence in the Life Cycle*, ed. G. Elder and S. E. Dragastin (New York: Cambridge University Press, 1974), 1–3; and B. Hanawalt, "Historical Descriptions and Prescriptions for Adolescence," *Journal of Family History* 17, 4 (1992): 341–44. The best Canadian account of adolescent girls remains Strong-Boag, *The New Day Recalled: Lives of Girls and Women in English Canada, 1919–1939* (Toronto: Copp Clark Pitman, 1988), especially chap. 1, 7–41; and Strong-Boag, 21–22, notes that the percentage of girls fifteen to nineteen in high school surpassed that of boys for each census year 1921 to 1941. On the influence of medical views about education for girls, see also Mitchinson, *The Nature of Their Bodies: Women and Their Doctors in Victorian Canada* (Toronto: University of Toronto Press, 1991), especially chap. 2, 83–87.
22 L. A. Banks, *A Manly Boy: A Series of Talks and Tales for Boys* (Toronto: William Briggs, 1900), 2. On gender constructions and health inspection/education, see Gleason, "Race, Class, and Health," and Tennant, "Complication Childhood," both is this volume.
23 On early-twentieth-century sex education, see M. Bliss, "Pure Books on Avoided Subjects: Pre-Freudian Sexual Ideas in Canada," in *Studies in Canadian Social History*, eds. M. Horn and R. Sabourin (Toronto: McClelland and Stewart, 1974), 338–51; C. Sethna, "Men, Sex and Education: The Ontario Women's Temperance Union and Children's Sex Education, 1900–20," *Ontario History* 88, 3 (September 1996): 186–206; and for the postwar period, Adams, *The Trouble with Normal*, 107–35; M. Gleason, *Normalizing the Ideal*, 72–3; Owram, *Born at the Right Time*, 261; and Sethna, "We Want Facts, Not Morals: Unwanted Pregnancy, The Toronto Women's Caucus, and Sex Education," in *Ontario Since Confederation: A Reader*, ed. E. A. Montigny and L. Chambers (University of Toronto Press, 2000), 409–28.
24 Strong-Boag, *The New Day Recalled*, discusses courtship briefly, 81–83; on the modernization of courtship in the United States, see B. Bailey, *From Front Porch to Back Seat* (Baltimore: Johns Hopkins University Press, 1988).
25 Reminiscences of J. Foran, who grew up on a farm in Southern Ontario, from D. Read, ed., *The Great War and Canadian Society: An Oral History* (Toronto: New Hogtown Press, 1978), 213–14. See also the testimony about adolescent immoral-

ity, drinking, and dancing at Ottawa Collegiate Institute, given at the Royal Commission: Ottawa Collegiate Institute Inquiry, January 6, 1927, Evidence, 2, 11–15, B-72, Box 1, RG 18-88, Public Archives of Ontario. The commission is also discussed in Comacchio, "Dancing to Perdition."

26 G. Pringle, "Is the Flapper a Menace," *Maclean's*, June 15, 1922, 19; M. J. Exner, *The Question of Petting* (New York: American Social Hygiene Association, 1926); F. E. Williams, *Adolescence: Studies in Mental Hygiene* (New York: Appleton-Century, 1932), 54; and Thom, *Normal Youth*, 69–70. See also some of the material published during the interwar years by various social hygiene organizations, such as [n.a.] *The Wonderful Story of Life: A Mother Talks with Her Daughter Regarding Life and Reproduction* (Washington, DC: Government Printing Office, 1921); Helen W. Brown, *Sex Education in the Home* (New York: American Social Hygiene Association, 1933); O. Davies, *The Story of Life: As Told to His Sons and as Told to Her Daughters* (Naperville: J. L. Nichols, 1922); G. L. M. McElligott, *Ourselves: A Few Facts for Young Men* (Birmingham: British Social Hygiene Council, 1935); Valeria H. Parker, *Social Hygiene and the Child* (New York: American Social Hygiene Association, 1939); John Robertson, *What Every Lad Should Know about Sex* (London: Peoples League of Health, 1935); these and others are in the Public Health Nursing Division Records, RG10-30-A-1, 7.02–7.03, Public Archives of Ontario.

27 Thom, *Normal Youth*, 60–63. Nearly twenty years later, Gallagher's view was more tolerant toward adolescent experimentation, but he still considered homosexuality aberrant; see Dr. J. R. Gallagher, *Your Son's Adolescence* (Boston: Little, Brown, 1951), 104.

28 G. Bates, "The Venereal Disease Problem," *Canadian Journal of Public Health* 13, 4 (April 1922): 265–69; Bates, who headed the Social Hygiene Council of Canada (founded 1921) presented this paper to the Hamilton Social Hygiene Council. Also L. A. Hamilton, "Educational Opportunities," *Canadian Public Health Journal* 12, 2 (February 1921): 59–64; W. H. Roberts, "The Venereal Problem in Large Towns and Small Cities," *Canadian Public Health Journal* 11, 9 (September 1920): 63–5. On VD scares during the First World War, see Sethna, "Men, Sex and Education," 193–202; and J. Cassel, *The Secret Plague: Venereal Disease in Canada, 1838–1939* (Toronto: University of Toronto Press, 1987), 24–45.

29 A. Beall, file 4.1, Historical Pamphlets and Bulletins, Department of Health, RG 10-30-A.1-4.08, Public Archives of Ontario, 1. Sethna discusses Beall's work thoroughly in "Men, Sex and Education," 191–97.

30 P. Sandiford, "The School Programme and Sex Education," *Canadian Public Health Journal* 13, 3 (March 1922): 60–61.

31 Thom, *Normal Youth*, 42, 68–79.

32 Edna Guest, "Problems of Girlhood and Motherhood," *Canadian Public Health Journal* 13, 5 (May 1922): 193–95. Oral testimony from the time suggests that there may have been some truth to this medical worry; see the memories of Helen Gloucester, who was hospitalized at Toronto General to deliver her first child during the war, when her doctor discovered that she "didn't know which way the baby was coming;" in Read, ed. *The Great War and Canadian Society*, 62; see also Strong-Boag, *The New Day Recalled*, 15, 86–89; and the recollections of Montreal housewives about the interwar years in D. Baillargeon, *Making Do: Home and Family in Montreal during the Great Depression* (Waterloo: Wilfrid Laurier University Press, 1998).

33 Bates, "The Venereal Disease Problem," 269.

34 Already by 1911, the Vancouver Medical Association was recommending the teaching of "sex hygiene" to high school pupils, though Vancouver doctors soon

concluded that it was impossible to deal adequately with this subject in a course of lectures delivered by a physician at the close of a high school course; see T. G. Hunter and C. H. Gundry, "School Health Practices: Ritualistic or Purposeful?" *Canadian Journal of Public Health* 46, 1 (January 1955): 59–64.

35 Roberts, "Venereal Problem in Large Towns and Small Cities," 65.

36 Beall, file 4.1, 3, Historical Pamphlets and Bulletins, Department of Health, RG 10-30-A.1-4.08, Public Archives of Ontario.

37 Thom, *Normal Youth*, 21; see also Sandiford, "The School Programme and Sex Education," 59–63.

38 Sutherland, *Children in English Canadian Society*, 40–48.

39 The most horrendous example of the gap between rhetoric and practice was the Native residential schools, where both health conditions and the paltry government resources dedicated to inspection and treatment prompted the first federal medical superintendent of Indian health, Peter Bryce, to call their existence "a national crime"; see J. B. Waldram, D. A. Herring, T. K. Young, *Aboriginal Health in Canada: Historical, Cultural and Epidemiological Perspectives* (Toronto: University of Toronto Press, 1995), 157. Bryce, a public health activist in many areas, published *The Story of a National Crime: An Appeal for Justice to the Indians of Canada* in 1922. He was unable to win government support for his program of school health nurses, health instruction, and fitness.

40 As late as 1940, about one third of Canadian families were classified "medically indigent" because their family income was less than the $1000 per year, which would allow for basic medical attention; see Canadian Youth Commission, "Appendix C: Some Special Studies and Reports," *Youth and Health* (Toronto: Ryerson Press, 1946), 60.

41 Sutherland, *Children in English Canadian Society*, 55; S. L. Jean, "Promoting Health through the Schools," *Canadian Nurse* 32 (July 1936): 307–10. On school health inspection/education, see Gleason, "Race, Class, and Health," in this volume.

42 Currey and Nicolle, "Development of a Health Program," 182.

43 K. E. Dowler, "Co-relating Health Education in a City Secondary School," *Canadian Nurse* 25 (1929): 624–27. On gender and health education, see Gleason, "Race, Class, and Health," and Tennant, "Complicating Childhood," in this volume.

44 Currey and Nicolle, "Development of a Health Program," 183. The school served the city of St. Catharines and part of Lincoln County.

45 Ontario Department of Education, *Health: A Handbook of Suggestions for Teachers in Public and Private Schools* (Toronto: Ryerson, 1938), 1–2. A similar survey of rural Manitoba youth found that 70 per cent of the total exhibited "one or more remediable defects or conditions about which they needed medical advice"; see Canadian Youth Commission, *Youth and Health*, 60.

46 A. H. Speers, "High School Medical Inspection in Burlington, Ontario," *Canadian Public Health Journal* 32, 12 (December (1941): 608–10. It was also noted that students entering from rural schools, many of whom had had no previous medical supervision or health education, presented the most defects. In Manitoba, 3000 students were given physical examinations and talks on social hygiene under the program, which also taught an "outline of health" as part of its mandatory citizenship course. As in every province where young people signed on, the Manitoba participants were all referred to their own doctors for treatment, and "no attempt was made by the visiting physician to suggest such treatment in any case"; see Editorial. "A New Health Venture in Manitoba," *Canadian Pub-*

lic Health Journal 31, 4 (April 1940): 204. The Manitoba initiative was declared "very successful."

47 Currey and Nicolle, "Development of a Health Program," 175–77.

48 Editorial, "School Health Supervision in Secondary Schools," *Canadian Public Health Journal* 31, 4 (April 1940): 190.

49 Sutherland, *Children in English Canadian Society*, 165. In 1891, 13.8 per cent of children between the ages of ten and fourteen were "officially" employed in industry; by 1921, the percentage was 3.2. The drop was even more precipitous in agriculture (at least by official count), from 11.4 to 1.9 per cent. Bradbury, *Working Families*, is the only monograph treatment of the family economy in Canada; S. Morton, *Ideal Surroundings*, 97–98, notes that, in 1931, only 25 per cent of children over fifteen in Halifax were in school, and only 12 per cent of children in single-parent households. See also N. Sutherland, "We Always Had Work to Do," *Labour/Le Travail* 25 (1990): 105–41, and the childhood memories in Sutherland, *Growing Up: Childhood from the Great War to the Television Age* (Toronto: University of Toronto Press, 1998); also "Canadian and International Child Labour Conventions," March 1924, file 38, v. 8, Canadian Welfare Council, Library and Archives Canada.

50 Memorandum re: Night Employment of Children in Ontario, March 9, 1925, Provincial Secretary L. Goldie to C. Whitton, executive director, file 38, v. 29, Canadian Welfare Council. See also the reminiscences in I. Abella and D. Millar, *The Canadian Worker in the Twentieth Century* (Toronto: Oxford University Press, 1978), especially "Interview with Anonymous Ukrainian Women," 109–12; the excerpt from R. England, *The Central European Immigrant in Canada* (Toronto: Macmillan, 1929), 107–108; and the testimony before the Royal Commission on Industrial Unrest. *Canada: Royal Commission on Industrial Unrest* (Ottawa: King's Printer, 1919), 82–83; 1211–22.

51 "The Christian's Attitude to Preparation for and Motives in the Choice of His Life Work: Summary of General Discussion," Proceedings of the 7th Manitoba Boys Parliament, 1928, 10, Tuxis Collection, University of British Columbia Archives; and C. L. Roman, "Sacrifice and Burnt Incense," *Social Welfare* (August 1924): 224.

52 A. B. Chandler, "The Relation of Child Labour to Child Health," *Canadian Journal of Public Health* 12, 7 (July 1921): 397.

53 J. Martin, "The Married Woman in Industry," *Canadian Public Health Journal* 43, 3 (1919): 380; Martin, "The Four Ages of Woman: How Far Is Industrial Subjugation of the Sex Involved in Certain Phases of Feminism," *Canadian Public Health Journal* 43, 4 (1919): 186–88; R. Asals, representing the Women's Labour League of the Trades and Labour Council, Regina, Testimony to the Royal Commission on Industrial Unrest (1919); see also the excerpt from the *Report of the Social Survey Commission*, Toronto (1915), 114–19, in I. Abella and D. Millar, eds., *The Canadian Worker in the Twentieth Century* (Toronto: Oxford University Press, 1978). Strange, *Toronto's Girl Problem*, discusses the Social Survey Commission's findings in some detail.

54 H. Michell, "A Study of the Efficiency of Canadian Labour," *Industrial Canada* (June 1928): 183; O. A. Cannon, "Health Opportunities in Industry," *Canadian Public Health Journal* 21, 1 (1930), 2–3. See also Dominion of Canada, Honorary Advisory Council for Scientific and Industrial Research, *Survey of General Conditions of Industrial Hygiene in Toronto* (Ottawa: Privy Council of Canada, 1921), 3; Editorial, "Industrial Fatigue," *Canadian Medical Association Journal* 15 (1925): 737; R. M. Hutton, committee secretary, "Industrial Hygiene in Cana-

dian Factories," *Industrial Canada* (June 1920): 80–83; A. Mitchell, "The Scope of Medical Services in Industry," *Canadian Public Health Journal* 30, 11 (November 1939): 521; and F. S. Parney, "Division of Industrial Hygiene," *Canadian Public Health Journal* 23, 4 (April 1939): 149.

55 Editorial, "The Revolt of Youth," *National Home Monthly* (June 1934): 3; D. L. M. McLeachy, "The Effect upon Young People of the Economic Depression and Unemployment," *Child and Family Welfare* (November 1935): 15; Ritchie, "The Plight of Youth," *Social Welfare* (June 1934): 50; and "Youth Tells," *Maclean's*, December 15, 1933, 8. Concerns about idle youth are explored further in Comacchio, "Dancing to Perdition," 23–26.

56 J. T. Phair, "Effectiveness of Child Health Programs in Ontario by Survey Methods," *American Journal of Public Health* 30, 1 (1933): 127.

57 Editorial, "School Health Supervision in Secondary Schools," *Canadian Public Health Journal* 31, 4 (April 1940): 190.

58 Editorial, "Health Training in Schools," *Canadian Public Health Journal* 33, 4 (April 1942): 178–79.

59 Editorial, "A Public Health Charter for Canada," *Canadian Public Health Journal* 33, 7 (July 1942): 345, 353. On the changes to child and youth health education during the Second World War, see Tennant, "Complicating Childhood," in this volume.

60 Editorial, "The Health of Secondary School Pupils," *Canadian Public Health Journal* 33, 9 (September 1942): 464.

61 I. Eisenhardt, director, National Physical Fitness Plan, "Physical Fitness in Canada," *Health* (Spring 1945): 9–12. The act was part of the proposed health insurance act, but the need for action in this field persuaded the minister, Ian Mackenzie, to move on it. See also V. S. Blanchard, "School Health Problems," *Canadian Public Health Journal* 36, 6 (September 1945): 217–22.

62 W. Clarke, director, American Social Hygiene Association, "They Are in Danger," *Health* (March 1941): 12–14. Clarke was speaking before the Vancouver Social Hygiene Council on "Social Hygiene Day."

63 C. Smith, "Teen Age Tragedy," *Health* (Autumn 1945): 10–14. See also C. Sethna, "Wait till Your Father Gets Home: Absent Fathers, Working Mothers and Delinquent Daughters in Ontario during World War II," in *Family Matters: Papers in Post-Confederation Canadian Family History*, ed. E. A. Montigny and L. Chambers (Toronto: Canadian Scholars Press, 1998), especially 22–23. Adams, *The Trouble with Normal*, 108, points out that the actual number of teenagers affected by VD was greatly exaggerated, amounting to no more than 10 per cent of the whole.

64 [n. a.] *The Liberty Study of Young Canada* (Toronto: Canadian Marketing Analysis, Ltd., 1955), Chart 13, 17. The percentage of mothers under twenty in 1931 was 38.8; for 1941, 29.9; for 1951, 33.

65 Canadian Youth Commission, *Youth and Health*, 14–20. The CYC was established by the federal government in April 1943 "with the avowed object of studying the main problems of young people" ranging in age from fifteen to twenty-four years. The health committee was under the direction of Brock Chisholm, former director of medical services for the Canadian Army, now deputy minister of health.

66 J. F. Webb, "Horizons in Child Health Supervision," *Canadian Public Health Journal* 50, 12 (December 1959): 494. Munro Prescott, *A Doctor of Their Own*, discusses the "new paediatrics" of the era after the Second World War in light of these expansionary tendencies; the first Adolescent Health Clinic was established

under the auspices of Boston Children's Hospital in 1951. The decidedly small number of Canadian pediatricians during this time seems to have made for efforts more rhetorical than real on this side of the border.

67 R. R. Struthers, "Recent Advances in Child Hygiene," *Canadian Public Health Journal* 35, 3 (March 1944): 116–17.

68 For their part, general practitioners argued that adolescents were their own "natural" customers, in that many had watched over them since birth and were eager to make "lifetime patients" of them and their own future children; see [editorial-n.a.], "Babies: Life Patients," *Canadian Doctor* 10 (October 1937): 27–32.

69 J. R. Mayers, "A School Health Service in a New Ontario Health Unit," *Canadian Public Health Journal* 52, 9 (September 1960): 372–74; Mayers describes services provided by the Norfolk District unit, including high school inspection. Ontario, Department of Health, *Annual Report*, 1950, 6, 79, 81.

70 Several Canadian studies are devoted to an understanding of the post–Second World War family and the baby boom experience: Owram, *Born at the Right Time*, pays careful attention to the domestic ideals of the 1950s over the first three chapters of his study, and devotes a chapter to "The Fifties and the Cult of the Teenager," 136–58. Focusing on the relationship between a newly influential child psychology and the "normal" family, Gleason's *Normalizing the Ideal* discusses how, in the midst of postwar anxieties after the upheaval of depression and war, psychology came out of the university laboratory and into the homes of ordinary Canadians, 3–82; Adams's *The Trouble with Normal* pays specific attention to the postwar discourses surrounding "normal youth" within the context of a renewed obsession with heterosexual marriage, hence a corresponding obsession with sex education for teenagers. K. Dubinsky, *The Second Greatest Disappointment* (Toronto: Between the Lines, 1999), although not devoted exclusively to the post–Second World War years, also emphasizes the 1950s as a golden age of heterosexuality. See also the essays in J. Parr, ed., *A Diversity of Women* (Toronto: University of Toronto, 1995), and Parr, *Domestic Goods* (Toronto: University of Toronto Press, 1999), which considers the rise of consumer culture within the context of postwar affluence, domesticity, and the developing welfare state.

71 G. Binning, "Earlier Physical and Mental Maturity among Saskatoon Public School Children," *Canadian Public Health Journal* 49, 1 (January 1958): 16–17. A survey of London (Ontario) high school students in grades 10 to 13, undertaken between September 1967 and January 1969, likewise found significant height and weight increases in comparing contemporary data with those of a 1939 study. The rate of increase in the previous study (comparing 1923 and 1939) was much smaller than that occurring in the thirty years since 1939, strongly suggesting that the physical gains were directly related to the improved material basis of life during the war and since; see R. G. Sennett and D. M. Cram, "Cross-Sectional Percentile Height and Weight Norms for a Representative Sample of Urban, School-Aged Ontario Children," *Canadian Public Health Journal* 60, 12 (December 1969): 465–70. The original study was N. Keyfitz, *A Height and Weight Survey of Toronto Elementary School Children, 1939* (Ottawa: Dominion Bureau of Statistics, 1942).

72 Royal Commission on Health, R. Kohn, *Life and Health of Canadians* (Ottawa: Queen's Printer, 1964), 43. In reference to age-specific death rates, for the ten-to-fourteen group, these declined from 1.4 per 100,000 in 1931 to 0.4 in 1963; for the fifteen-to-nineteen group, from 2.1 to 0.8 in that period; Table 13, 129.

73 E. H. Erikson, *Identity and the Life Cycle* (New York: W. W. Norton, 1959), 17–18, 94–96; on Erikson's influence as "the foremost theorist of human development

of the latter part of the 20th century," see J. E. Cote and A. L. Allahar, *Generation on Hold: Coming of Age in the Late 20th Century* (Toronto: Stoddart, 1994), 70–75.

74 British Columbia doctors criticized routine medical examinations and immunizations in schools—easily taken care of by family physicians—as major drains on the time of public health employees, who could be better occupied in other community services. The provincial health and education departments were compelled to cancel certain routine procedures and to clarify the respective roles of health and education personnel; see K. Benson and A. Beattie, "A New Approach to the School Health Program," *Canadian Public Health Journal* 55, 9 (September 1964): 371–77; and J. M. Marshall, "Teacher Preparation in Health and Health Education in Canada," *Canadian Public Health Journal* 57, 10 (October 1966): 458. Marshall's survey found that all the provinces granted relatively low priority to teacher preparation in health education.

75 Canadian Medical Association, "Report of the Committee on Maternal Welfare, 1967," *Canadian Medical Association Journal* 97, 9 (September 1967): 676–77.

76 Canadian Medical Association, "Report of the Committee on Physical Education and Recreation," *Canadian Medical Association Journal* 91, 9 (September 1964): 522–23.

77 G. Szasz, "Sex Education and the Public Health Nurse," *Canadian Public Health Journal* 60, 11 (November 1969): 429–34; and A. M. Juhasz, "Sex Knowledge of Prospective Teachers and Graduate Nurses," *Canadian Nurse* 63 (1967): 48–50.

78 T. J. Wake and F. R. Laughlin, "Socio-psychological Aspects of Cigarette Smoking," *Canadian Journal of Public Health* 6, 4 (July/August 1970): 301–305. The survey covered 6206 pupils in grades 10 to 12, with an average age of seventeen. Boys were much heavier smokers: 5.5 per cent smoked twenty or more cigarettes per day; only 1.1 of girls were in that category, while 36.7 per cent of boys and 60.6 per cent of girls smoked one to four per day only.

79 J. A. Jones, G. W. Pipe, and V. L. Matthews, "A Student-Directed Program in Smoking Education," *Canadian Public Health Journal* 61, 3 (May/June 1970): 253–56. The program was initiated by the University of Saskatchewan's Department of Social and Preventive Medicine in 1968.

80 Wake and Laughlin, "Socio-psychological Aspects of Cigarette Smoking," 302; Canada, National Health and Welfare, *Canadian Youth Conference on Smoking and Health: Summary Report* (Ottawa: Department of National Health and Welfare, 1965), 22.

81 "A Brief Submitted by the Ontario Department of Health to the Ontario Legislative Assembly's Select Committee on Youth," 1965, file 4.9, box 4, Ministry of Health, RG 10-161-4.01–4.09, Provincial Archives of Ontario. The brief recommended that a provincial youth conference on health be convened; Canada, *Canadian Youth Conference on Smoking and Health*, 11.

82 "Laws on Age of Smoking," *News Bulletin of the Canadian Paediatric Society* (November 1994): 1.

83 Canadian Medical Association, "Non-Medical Use of Drugs with Particular Reference to Youth," *Canadian Medical Association Journal* 101, 12 (December 1969): 73–87.

84 J. R. Unwin, "Illicit Drug Use among Canadian Youth," *Canadian Medical Association Journal* 98, 2 (February 1968): 402–408.

85 V. Gellman, "Glue-Sniffing among Winnipeg School Children," *Canadian Medical Association Journal* 98, 2 (February 1968): 410–14.

86 Canadian Medical Association, "Non-Medical Use of Drugs," 74.

87 J. Munro, "What Society Must Do to Solve Problem of Drug Use among Young," *Canadian Medical Association Journal* 103, 11 (November 1970): 1091–96; this was a speech presented before the BC Medical Association. See also L. P. Clement and W. R. Solursh, "Hallucinogenic Drug Abuse," *Canadian Medical Association Journal* 98, 2 (February 1968): 407–10.

88 Canadian Medical Association, "How Total Community Should Confront Today's Drug Abuse Problem," *Canadian Medical Association Journal* 101, 11 (November 1969): 9–11; and R. G. Smart and M. S. Goodstadt, "Trends in the Prevalence of Alcohol and Other Drug Use among Ontario Students, 1977–83," *Canadian Public Health Journal* 76 (May/June 1985): 157–60. Smart and Goodstadt present the findings from four surveys conducted between 1977 and 1983, intended to monitor alcohol and drug use among Ontario students in grades 7, 9, 11, 13. They found that, between 1981 and 1983, the non-medical use of stimulants increased significantly. Owram, *Born at the Right Time*, 200–202, argues that anti-drug campaigns not only failed, but backfired, because they were received as yet another instance of state (or adult) repression of youthful pleasure and creativity.

89 E. H. Erikson, *Identity, Youth and Crisis* (New York: W. W. Norton, 1968), 102.

90 Chandler, "The Relation of Child Labour to Child Health," 399.

91 Thom, *Normal Youth and Its Everyday Problems*, 18.

92 J. R. Gallagher, *Your Son's Adolescence* (New York: 1949; also Gallagher, *Medical Care of the Adolescent*, 2nd ed. (New York: Appleton-Century-Crofts, 1966), 12.

93 Erikson, *Identity and the Life Cycle*, 94.

94 W. A. Daniel, *The Adolescent Patient* (St. Louis: C. V. Mosby, 1970), 19. The authoritative text by I. N. Kugelmass, *Adolescent Medicine: Principles and Practice* (Springfield, IL: Charles C. Thomas, 1975), opens with the declaration that "Adolescent life is a revolt against the rules of Nature," 3.

95 Munro Prescott, *A Doctor of Their Own*, 117; Dr. J. R. Roswell, "The Origins, Development and Goals of Adolescent Medicine," *Journal of Adolescent Health Care* 3, 1 (1982): 57–63. The American Society for Adolescent Medicine was established in 1968, and the first international symposium on adolescent health care was held in 1974 in Helsinki, Finland.

96 In 1967, there were 875 pediatricians in Canada, of whom 769 identified themselves as "active." Most continued the historic trend of practising in larger centres, with 82.4 per cent located in the metropolitan areas in which 48 per cent of Canadians live. Of the total of 769 pediatricians, 271 were in Ontario, 250 in Quebec; there was only 1 in Prince Edward Island. Only 1 paediatrician in all Canada, located in Ontario, declared a sub-specialty in psychiatry; see P. Banister, "Too Many Children or Too Many Pediatricians?" *Canadian Medical Association Journal* 103, 7 (July 1970): 157–59.

97 Banister, "Too Many Children or Too Many Pediatricians?" 159.

98 Adolescent Medicine Committee, Canadian Paediatric Society, "Family Friendly Adolescent Health Care," *Paediatrics & Child Health* 2, 5 (1997): 356–57.

99 Canadian Medical Association, General Council Proceedings, 1977, Resolution 77–46, 133. The RCPSC is the national body responsible for setting the standards for postgraduate medical education and for certifying specialist physicians and surgeons. In 1990, the Canadian Paediatric Society added an Adolescent Health Section to its roster, expanding the existing committee's mandate to serve as a Canadian forum for the multidisciplinary discussion of adolescent health issues, and to work toward the formulation of uniform health care standards for that age group. I am indebted to Kerry Guglielmin, Canadian Medical Association policy review coordinator, for this information.

100 The association publishes, four times a year, *Pro-Teen* in English and *Pro-Ado* in French, and holds an annual national meeting and various regional meetings. Members of the adolescent health section of the Canadian Pediatric Society have registration fees waived for CAAH membership. It is centred at Sainte-Justine Hospital in Montreal; see its website, http://www.acsa-caah.ca. The association was founded, and its constitution was written, by a group of Canadian professionals in the field of adolescent health.

The Iconography of Child Public Health

Between Medicine and Reform

◌

Janet Golden

D uring the interwar period in the United States, the links between child public health, biomedicine, and social welfare grew more tenuous. Child public health programs, once a central part of both medical and welfare efforts, operated within an increasingly restricted mandate. They fit in neither the world of pediatric medicine, which was evolving into an office-based specialty, nor the hospital, which had begun eschewing its role as a health care site for the poor in favour of a more middle-class clientele.[1] At the same time, the rejection of maternity insurance, the cessation of federal support for the Sheppard-Towner Maternity and Infancy Protection Act in 1929, and the curtailment of child-focused social welfare initiatives in the opening years of the Great Depression severed ties between health and welfare reformers, as the latter began to work on obtaining federal support for new income-based programs.[2] Yet many programs endured on the local level, attempting to provide children with an array of services aimed at preserving their health and improving their standard of living.

This article is a case study of one of those local efforts, based on an analysis of glass lantern slide images. I argue that the images comprise a distinct photographic genre that developed in the Progressive Era and expanded during the interwar years. Child public health imagery imported stylistic conventions from two earlier genres—reform photography (sometimes termed documentary social realism) and medical photography—but was a genre all its own. As a result, child public health photographs present to American historians a tableau that might be titled "the path not taken."[3] They have been little studied. However, if we pay attention to the inclusiveness of child public health images and incorporate them into our histories, we can recapture and interpret more fully the brief period in which the trajectories of hospital development, urban public health initiatives, and social welfare programs overlapped at the local level even as they began to disengage at the level of national social policy.

The 276 glass lantern slides collected by Howard Childs Carpenter (1878–1955) are housed at the College of Physicians of Philadelphia and fully described in the College's publication, *Fugitive Leaves*.[4] Some document particular child health efforts Carpenter was associated with, but the collection as a whole ranges over many subjects. The majority of the lantern slides (195 of 276) are made from photographic images, while others are of paintings, posters, cartoons, architectural drawings, and graphs (see table 1). The images portray child public health as it was conceived of by numerous public and private health, medical, and welfare organizations operating in the United States. They also display the lives of children more generally—including images of Native American and foreign youngsters, paintings of the Madonna and child, and a few portraits of leaders of the child public health movement.

The Carpenter Lantern Slides and the Iconography of Child Public Health

Carpenter founded the Department for the Prevention of Diseases (DPD) at the Children's Hospital of Philadelphia in 1914.[5] In many ways, it was a quintessential progressive reform program, aiming to apply the skills of an array of professionals—physicians, nurses, and health educators—to the task of preventing disease in order to avoid the less efficient job of curing or caring for those who fell ill. The slide collection carefully documents the work of the DPD and includes images that appeared in the hospital's annual reports. Yet the collection as a whole moved well beyond the confines of the clinics and the neighbourhood.

The iconographic conventions of child public health are relatively straightforward. The most common subjects are the child, the mother, and the health care provider. Stylistically, the images tend to be didactic, and they often include captions. The settings range broadly from the clinic to the home, and from the urban slum to the rural barn. Among the topics presented are infant feeding, household safety, food science, and the environmental threats to health. The thematic sweep is characteristic of the genre.

Images in the Carpenter Collection came from state and local boards of health (including those in Michigan, Illinois, Kansas, and from the Bureau of Child Hygiene of the New York City Department of Health) and from at least one federal agency: the United States Department of Agriculture. Carpenter also acquired images from voluntary health, medical, and educational organizations, including the American Association for Study and Prevention of Infant Mortality, the American Social

Hygiene Association, the National Council for the Prevention of Blindness, the National Association for the Study and Prevention of Tuberculosis, the American Medical Association, the Boy Scouts of America, and the National Educational Association. Other slides were apparently purchased from professional supply houses, such as those depicting milk production, distributed by the International Harvester Corporation.[6]

Viewed individually, the lantern slides present images that resemble those typically defined as medical or reform photographs. There are classic medical scenes of physicians ministering to patients in the clinic, and street scenes typical of documentary social realism that expose viewers to the harsh realities of slum life. When considered as a single entity, however, Carpenter's collection presents a coherent, if anachronistic, vision different from each of these categories. The images do not show the technical/scientific/institutional world of medicine nor do they represent the political and increasingly fragmented world of social reform. Instead, the collection demonstrates in visual terms Carpenter's faith that health created welfare, that saving children saved society, that the neighbourhood (rather than the hospital or the legislative chamber) was the appropriate site for intervention, and that the mother was the key figure in achieving the desired transformation in the lives of children.

Carpenter used his slides to reach out to the public and to professionals. He exhibited the images when he delivered a keynote address on "Health Teaching" at the opening of a new building of the Children's Hospital of Philadelphia.[7] In that setting, the slides were viewed by dignitaries and members of the public sympathetic to the work of the hospital—an audience similar to the viewers of reform photographs. Mothers and children visiting the DPD clinic and classes comprised a second and perhaps more important audience for the lantern slides. Notes in the collection indicate that two sets of images had been grouped and labelled, presumably to use in instructing patients. One group bore the handwritten title "Infant Hygiene," the other "Care of the Baby." Other child health programs no doubt had similar compilations of images, ready for use in educating clinic patients.[8]

Reform Photography and Child Public Health Photography

In the 1880s Jacob Riis, the muckraking photojournalist and reformer, began giving lantern-slide lectures on "The Other Half–How It Lives and Dies in New York," inaugurating what would become a popular method of arousing moral indignation among middle-class Americans sympathetic to both the plight of the poor and the goals of progressive reformers.[9] Other investigators followed Riis's lead, exploring the back streets of America's growing cities to plumb the depths of poverty and shoot candid pictures of immigrant ghettos. The photographic exposé became so popular that businesses were soon packaging and selling lantern slides for use in public lectures. A New York optical company, for instance, marketed a set of two hundred images titled "The Dark Side of New York" to "exhibitors and lecturers."[10] By the twentieth century, as social justice and social welfare crusades grew more focused, photographers working for various organizations would aim their cameras at specific targets. The National Child Labor Committee, for example, sent photographer Lewis Hine to record scenes of children employed in southern textile mills.[11]

Photography became central to the reform cause in the late nineteenth century, and the images bequeathed from that era allow us to see not only what cities and the poor "looked like" but also to interpret the ways in which outsiders gazed at the poor. According to scholar Peter Bacon Hales, the photographic conventions employed within reform photography at the turn of the century encompassed four elements: (1) human subjects; (2) environmental cues that were "at best both boldly graphic and symbolic"; (3) a direct stare into the camera lens "to invoke contact between the viewer and the slum subject"; and (4) signs of "dynamic life."[12] Other common stylistic devices included side-by-side images contrasting the real and the ideal, images depicting the subject before and after intervention, and scenes in which the subject and the reformer posed together. The growing iconographic complexity reflected the numerous intentions of the photographs: to educate, to inspire, to stimulate reform, and to promote donations.[13]

In reform photographs, street urchins, mill girls, and slag-heap boys stared at the viewer with a nonchalance that underscored the hard lessons already learned. Their toughness (and ultimate vulnerability) conveyed a warning: without proper supervision and sufficient schooling—in short, without proper social intervention—the youngsters would fall prey to criminal influences and contribute to the breakdown of the social order. Paradoxically, documentary social realism invoked as well a small sense of reassurance, instructing the audience that the problems being witnessed could be remedied.[14]

Child health images encapsulated a similar duality—presenting viewers with both a threat and a promise. Unlike reform images, however, they emphasized the latter. The subjects of many child public health images were very young and seemed intrinsically more vulnerable and less threatening than the older children displayed in reform photographs. Moreover, the infants and children in child public health scenes typically appeared under the care of physicians, nurses, and health

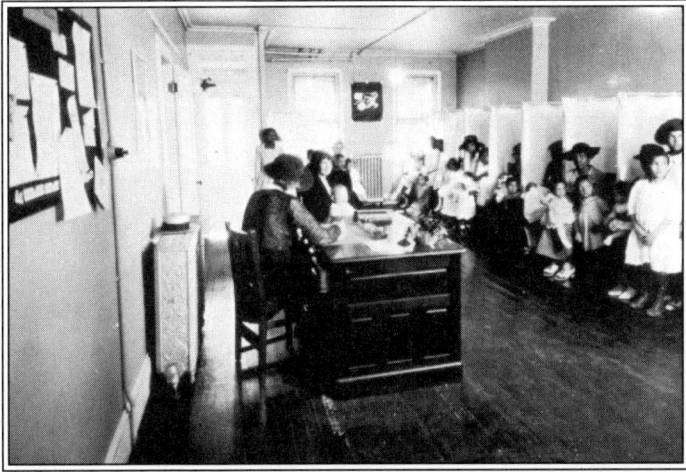

Figure1. Clinic scene, Department for the Prevention of Diseases, Children's Hospital of Philadelphia (DPD) (Carpenter Collection)

teachers, seeming to be contained and cared for, unlike the youth in the reform photographs who appeared to be fending for themselves on the street or the factory floor. Figure 1, a classic clinic scene from the DPD, illustrates the ways in which child public health imagery attempted to both assure and inspire viewers. The small waiting room filled with mothers and children appears quiet and orderly. Behind a desk sits a woman who will presumably direct the waiting patients to the consulting rooms. The scene telegraphs a message of control and, like many medical photographs, shows the patients as passive recipients of professional care. But it is different from reform photography because the mothers and children do not stare into the camera.

Child health images and documentary social realism employed different aesthetic vocabularies. While the former sometimes scrutinized their subjects directly, most images (and particularly those involving children) eschewed the confrontational gaze. In child public health images, the viewer stands back to watch as adults carefully tend to their flock of children. In one of the images children are photographed in the classroom, smiling at the camera as they brush their teeth. Another image of a street scene presents girls in white dresses and boys in white shirts and ties, all wearing large pointed hats with the cross of St. George and standing aside a papier-mâché dragon in what appears to be an anti-tuberculosis parade. In figure 2, mothers stand with their babies in front of a welfare station and the image is captioned—although a portion of it appears to be missing. Neglected and unaccompanied children, by contrast, are shown to be at risk. Carpenter collected a series

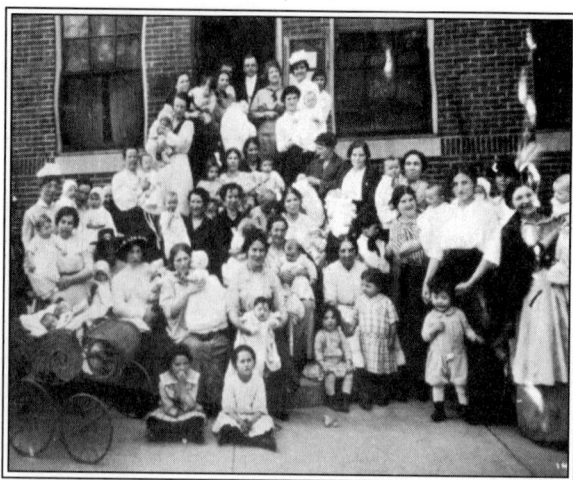

Figure 2. Mothers and babies at a Welfare Station (Carpenter
Collection)

of slides from the Brooklyn Street Railway that displayed, in sequence,
children roller skating near the trolley car, falling under the wheels, and
being carted off to the hospital. In these images, it is not the city or
even the trolley that is dangerous, but the child who had not been taught
to play safely and was left without adult supervision.

The country as well as the city appears as a dangerous place. As
large-scale public works projects and investments in urban sanitation
made cities healthier places in the early twentieth century, the high rates
of mortality and morbidity in rural areas became more visible, as did the
links between the two.[15] Despite the fact that Carpenter's clinic served
an urban population, his slide collection had numerous images of rural
life. A few showed children walking barefoot down dirt roads, but the
majority depicted milk and food production. There were lantern slides
of dirty and clean milking sheds and of sickly and healthy cows. The link
between rural health practices and urban life could not have been clearer
to an audience taught to value milk as a food for children. The focus on
modern technology also appeared in images of clean and dirty kitchens,
of new and old-fashioned butter churns, and in schematic drawings of
modern plumbing.

The only pictures in which Carpenter is identified as the photographer present the neighbourhood surrounding the Children's Hospital
of Philadelphia. One bears a handwritten label "dirty alley" and gives the
address; the other names the street, and notes "filth and dirt." The Carpenter lantern slides are clearly derivative of reform photography, particularly the documentary style used to disclose poor housing condi-

tions.[16] But they lack the emotional power of the images taken by skilled reform photographers working within the conventions of "street scene" imagery. In Carpenter's slides there are no ragged children with dirt-smeared faces starring into the camera; neither image contains a single human figure. Instead, the subject is the street itself, clearly in need of a thorough cleaning.

In the lexicon of public health advocates, the environment was a distinct entity that contained numerous threats. The unventilated tenement, the flies that entered through unscreened windows, the milk kept unrefrigerated on a table—each imperilled the health of the child. Where the reform photographer depicted the slum neighbourhood as the source of deprivation, child public health advocates saw the many threats in each individual dwelling. Indeed, public health activists viewed the home as a vector of disease, a place in which ill health was too often nurtured by the ignorance of its inhabitants. Two slides exemplify this theme. One, entitled "Latimer as the Nurses Found Him," shows an infant in a cramped hovel, lying swaddled on a bed as a sibling watches over him. Nearby (and barely discernable in this image) is a mother in a wheelchair and another child. In a second slide, titled "Latimer after a Month of Proper Feeding," a plump, healthy Latimer is sitting erect, holding his bottle. Before-and-after images were standard reform fare, and public health advocates evidently imported the technique from reform imagery into that employed.[17] Used in the service of child public health, images such as those of Latimer and his family provided vivid testimony about the work of the hospital and the clinic and a thinly veiled criticism of conditions just outside their walls.

The visual taxonomy employed by reformers typically referenced victims and saviours, including child workers and street urchins, settlement house visitors and poor families, and public health nurses and mothers. Child public health imagery incorporated another pair: disease carriers and the public health crusaders who attacked and vanquished them. Numerous public health slides illustrate rats and flies, the leading villains on the public health enemies' list. In one image boys in knickers stand before an unidentified woman (possibly a health teacher) with their rat traps, ready to vanquish that urban menace. Even more prominently represented in Carpenter's collection is the fly. There are slides of fly bottles, built to trap the "germs with legs," slides of various species of flies, and slides meant to teach mothers to be wary of the perils posed by flies.[18] Figure 3, captioned "A Day in the Life of a Fly," illustrates its migration from the garbage pile to the baby's face. The final image reads, "Swat that fly....Scientists say it is deadlier than the tiger or the cobra."

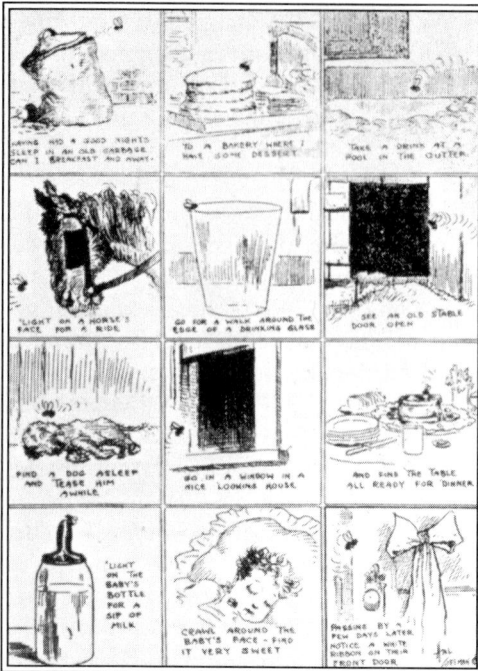

Figure 3. "A Day in the Life of a Fly" (Carpenter Collection)

Many of the lantern slides are captioned, attesting to their intended use as educational material and distinguishing them from reform or medical images. One clinic picture shows a physician examining a child—a typical medical image. Yet its caption clearly indicates it was not meant to advertise medical science but to instruct families. It reads, "These mothers take their children for a thorough physical examination after any acute illness. Do you? For a thorough examination, clothes must be removed." Another captioned image, which Carpenter apparently acquired from the Pennsylvania Tuberculosis Association (which used this scene in its exhibits for schoolchildren), is of a downtrodden street vendor. Reformers might deploy the image to convey the hard life of an immigrant entrepreneur, to celebrate the dignity of labour, or to invoke pity that a day of work did not yield enough money to feed a family that evening. Public health reformers used the image to engender disgust that the food being sold was uncovered and thus vulnerable to flies and dust. There is no mistaking the intended message; the caption reads, "Street Dust and Germs Cover This Man's Food. Don't Buy from Him. Candy, Cake, Bread Should Be Kept under Glass Cases." The vendor is not a victim but a victimizer.

Reform imagery had a submerged yet still palpable theme of poverty as the cause of many social problems, including high rates of infant mortality and childhood disease. Although far from radical in their approach to social inequality, reformers at least conceded its significance, and their images sometimes had a voyeuristic quality meant to reveal the hidden lives of the poor. Reformers peered into hovels to underscore the need for tenement house reform and also to reveal the lives hidden in the back alleys. Child public health leaders also knew what poverty meant in terms of death and disease among the young, but their concerns lay with the results of impoverishment—the failure to buy proper food, or ignorance about how to rear children—and they appeared, perhaps not intentionally, to censure families for their poverty.

The line between educating mothers and berating them often blurred in the Carpenter images, as it did within the broader child public health movement. Charles V. Chapin, a leading spokesman for the modern public health crusade argued, "It has now been demonstrated beyond a doubt that the chief cause of a high infant death rate is the ignorance of mothers."[19] With a similar message, a cartoon image obtained from the Illinois Department of Health introduced the "Seven Deadly Sins Committed by Ignorant Parents Against Their Babies." Among them were "the wrong food," "shoes too small," and "bulky wet irritating diapers." There were no suggestions as to how parents might overcome the economic obstacles to replacing the "wrong" items with the right ones. One of Carpenter's images was of an anti-tuberculosis poster titled, "Which Way Are You Going?" One side showed the way to a good health and a long life; the other consumption and early death. In instructing tenement residents to screen their windows, mothers to keep milk in iceboxes, and poor families of the need to purchase nourishing food it illustrated how middle-class families met these goals and poor families did not. Middle-class children were drawn playing tennis in the "clean open air," while their poorer counterparts played marbles on a wooden floor while their mother swept the dust away.

As the images conveyed, the champions of child public health believed that children could be sprung from the trap of sickness and set free to become good workers and good citizens not by remaking society but by educating mothers and providing health services. Issues of income were not addressed. It was a narrow yet ultimately optimistic vision, and one that set public health apart from the increasingly political agenda of reformers. The source of much optimism within the child public health community was the expanding therapeutic and institutional base of organized medicine, which also endowed many of the stylistic conventions of the iconography of child public health.

Medical Photography and Child
Public Health Photography

As Daniel M. Fox, Christopher Lawrence, and other scholars explain, physicians had a long tradition of using the camera to record unique morbid phenomena and characteristic clinic findings, of making pictures of themselves and their patients, of documenting life on the wards, and of enshrining operating theatres as temples of science. The conventions of public health photography—images of children, of poor people waiting in clinics, of environmental filth and slum housing, and of visiting nurses at work—were not the core images that represented and advertised the medical profession and its workplaces to the public.[20]

A number of lantern slides in the Carpenter collection fit the definition of medical photography. Figure 4 shows a child being measured at a time when weighing and measuring became the core of well-child care.[21] Figure 5 shows a doctor giving a dose of diphtheria toxin-antitoxin, one of the first preventive vaccines in pediatric medicine.[22] The images are of medicine in broad strokes, reifying medical science and its practitioners. The doctors and nurses appear kindly and adept, their eyes focused on the patient, not meeting the gaze of the photographer. Such scenes were emblematic in the twentieth century, assuring viewers that the ethic of caring would never be outstripped by the science of curing.

The Carpenter collection has hardly any purely clinical images or those that celebrate science. Among the few are an X-ray of a child with rickets, a photograph of cells in a petri dish bearing a handwritten label (invisible to the viewer) that says "washing water free from contamination," a diagram of fetal circulation, and three sagittal-section views of a newborn child. Similarly, the lantern slides show little in the way of medical technology—defined as tools for diagnosing, treating, or preventing illness. There are no operating rooms and only a few bits of hospital equipment, among them simple items such as hospital beds and examining tables. Scientific implements and remedies are also sparsely represented. There is an anovea lamp, which gave "sun bath" treatments for rickets, a stethoscope, a scale, and a few illustrations of devices meant for home use, including a steam atomizer and a croup kettle.

For the most part, medical photographs of hospitals, clinics, and medical offices portrayed them as places of cleanliness and light, order and efficiency—as settings in which scientific authority and professional skills were brought to bear on the problems of suffering individuals. Child health imagery incorporated clinic scenes, but also peered into the worlds that medicine had yet to fully invade and conquer. Thus, a critical theme in the Carpenter collection is the need to convey the discoveries of modern medicine, the techniques of sanitary science, and the

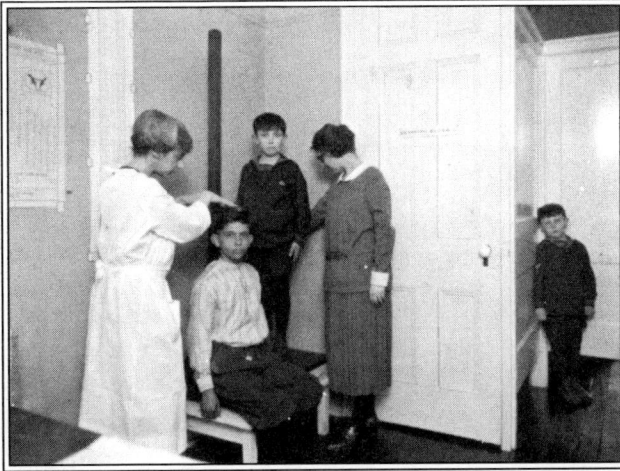

Figure 4. Child being measured (Carpenter Collection)

wisdom of health teaching to those at the farthest remove from those advantages.

Characteristic of medical photographs were images of various illnesses; child public health photographs, by contrast, depicted the conditions causing disease. One lantern slide offers an image of a slovenly woman sitting with a baby in her lap as she drinks from its bottle. At the bottom the caption reads, "Don't taste the milk from the bottle. Mothers who love their babies often give them diseases." Warnings about cow's milk also appear in the images, including a drawing of a cat licking the top of a milk bottle. By the cat's tongue are the words "measles, scarlet fever, tuberculosis, diphtheria, typhoid and septic sore throat." Despite the references to medical diagnoses, the message is clearly intended for mothers needing to protect the health of their children.

A key distinction between medical and child public health imagery is the array of practitioners shown. Public health photography celebrated the work of public health nurses as well as doctors. Clearly secondary subjects in most medical photographs, nurses took centre stage in many child public health images and sometimes shared the spotlight with public health educators. Unlike medicine, child public health was a field that was shown as dependant upon its female workforce. Not surprisingly then, there are more photographs of female physicians in child public health photographs than in traditional medical photographs. In the United States, the percentage of female physicians peaked in 1910 at 6 per cent, and a vastly disproportionate share of them engaged in what historian Regina Morantz-Sanchez termed "social medicine" for reasons of both choice and necessity.[23]

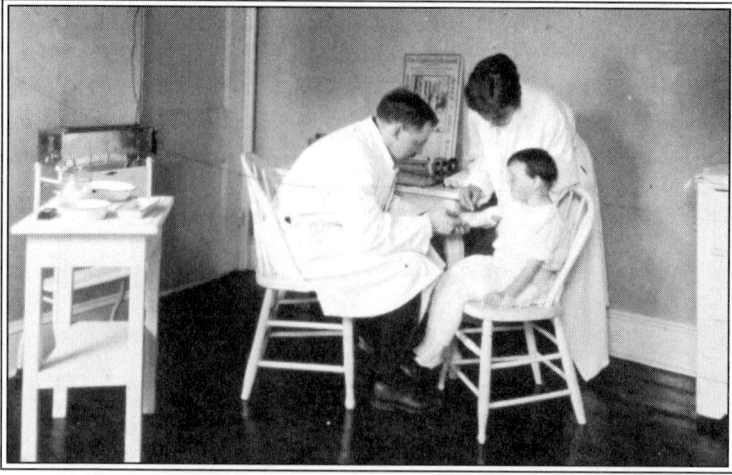

Figure 5. Diphtheria vaccination (Carpenter Collection)

The composition of the various departments of the Children's Hospital of Philadelphia suggests how gender structured career opportunities. Between 1915 and 1920, the DPD staff was largely male. In the 1920s, however, the number of female physicians in the department increased to three (of nine physicians), and by 1930 the staff was entirely female (five physicians) with the exception of Carpenter. The outpatient departments of the hospital were staffed entirely by male physicians.[24] The images in his collection therefore provide equivocal information. They show a greater number of health workers, including physicians, than would be found in a collection of medical photographs from the same period. Yet they do not document the actual situation, because they present a disproportionately large number of images of male physicians. Possibly Carpenter deliberately misrepresented the staffing patterns at the clinic in an attempt to impart status to what was clearly becoming less valued work within hospital medicine.

A similar deception may have occurred in terms of the race of patients in both the Carpenter collection and in other child public health photographs. Lantern slides of the DPD show very few African-American children and mothers visiting the clinics. One image in which they are present shows an African-American woman having her blood pressure checked; figure 1, described earlier, shows what appears to be a racially segregated waiting room. For the most part, Carpenter's images show only Euro-American youngsters and mothers, and it is unclear whether this is an accurate portrayal of the patient population at the DPD or a collection of images shaped to appeal to the interests of supporters.

The purpose of the lantern slides was not to give an accounting of what child health practitioners and practice looked like or to show whom they served. They were meant to function as educational tools and as propaganda. Seeing their links with and derivations from medical photography and reform photography makes clear how child public health advocates adapted and used familiar imagery to their own purposes. They promised science—to be applied by professionals and taught to mothers. They presented the domain of science as vast, incorporating the home, the street, the school, the countryside, and the city. And they showed the practitioners of science to be numerous—with doctors at the helm of the metaphorical ship of health, with nurses and health teachers serving as the crew.

A Vanished World

Medical photographs from the interwar years introduced scenes that we continue to associate with medicine. Comparisons among doctor–patient images of the 1920s and those of a later vintage reveal a common thread. In Eugene Smith's famous 1948 *Life* magazine pictures of a country doctor and in more recent photographs of physicians at the bedsides of AIDS patients we see echoes of past medical photographs. All of them display the caring and skilful physician beside the patient in scenes that are reassuringly familiar because the work of healing continues. Similarly, modern photojournalism retains the stylistic conventions of an earlier era. The youthful newsboy boldly facing the camera in the early twentieth century has been replaced by the equally young and bold drug dealer (who stands, perhaps, at the same corner). And urban neighbourhoods and rural hallows continue to be shown as decrepit and in some instances menacing, implicitly demanding attention from those who would make a better world for their inhabitants.

Child public health imagery, however, presents a world that has largely vanished. There are no modern equivalents of the boys with fly bottles and rat-trap boxes setting out to vanquish what in retrospect seem to be trivial enemies. Certainly, physicians still treat infants and children in public clinics, visiting nurses still instruct patients in their homes, and health educators still endeavour to teach personal and family hygiene. Yet the expansive vision of child public health, which linked medical intervention to measures such as urban sanitation, after-school health classes, and more abundant clinic care, has narrowed. While some of the images from the Carpenter collection present aspects of medicine and welfare that are familiar, collectively the lantern slides show a world that is no more.

When scholars neglect to study images such as those in the Carpenter collection, they implicitly and maybe correctly acknowledge that broadly imagined child public health work in the 1920s was not the foundation of the medical system we have today. Nevertheless, in discarding depictions of what became, in retrospect, small historical detours, historians lose the chance to interpret the full course of the journey. The similarities and differences among the genres of medical photography, reform photography, and child public health photography testify to the links among these endeavours as well as displaying some of the reasons for their ultimate unravelling. Like the written record of this era, the visual account helps explain how, as medicine and social welfare evolved into distinct disciplines, child public health was pushed to the periphery of each.

Table 1. Types of images in the Carpenter lantern slide collection

Photographs	195
Drawings, prints, lithographs	28
Paintings	20
Posters	17
Cartoons	9
Charts and graphs	5
Other	2
Total	276

Acknowledgement

I would like to thank Rima Apple, Jeffrey Brosco, Robert Joy, Naomi Rogers, Eric Schneider, Arleen Tuchman, and Russell Viner for their helpful comments on earlier drafts of this paper. All images reproduced in this paper come from the Carpenter slide collection of the College of Physicians of Philadelphia. I would like to thank Joan Zoref for her assistance with the photographs.

Notes

1 On the shifting role of pediatrics, see Thomas E. Cone, Jr., *History of American Pediatrics* (Boston: Little Brown, 1979), and Sydney A. Halpern, *American Pediatrics: The Social Dynamics of Professionalism, 1880–1980* (Berkeley: University of California Press, 1988). On the transformation of the hospital, see Charles E. Rosenberg, *The Care of Strangers: The Rise of America's Hospital System* (New York: Basic Books, 1987), and Rosemary Stevens, *In Sickness and in Wealth: American Hospitals in the Twentieth Century* (New York: Basic Books, 1989). On child public health, see

Richard A. Meckel, *Save the Babies: American Public Health Reform and the Prevention of Infant Mortality, 1850–1929* (Baltimore: Johns Hopkins University Press, 1990). For a comparative perspective, see Deborah Dwork, *War Is Good for Babies and Other Children: A History of the Infant and Child Welfare Movement in England, 1898–1918* (London: Tavistock, 1987), and Cynthia R. Comacchio, *Nations Are Built of Babies: Saving Ontario's Mothers and Children, 1900–1940* (Montreal: McGill-Queens University Press, 1994).

2   On child welfare in the Progressive era and after, see Linda Gordon, *Heroes of Their Own Lives: The Politics and History of Family Violence, Boston, 1880–1960* (New York: Viking, 1988), 59–81; Linda Gordon, *Pitied but Not Entitled: Single Mothers and the History of Welfare, 1890–1935* (Cambridge: Harvard University Press, 1994); Michael B. Katz, *In the Shadow of the Poorhouse: A Social History of Welfare in America* (New York: Basic Books, 1986), 113–45; Molly Ladd-Taylor, *Mother-Work: Women, Child Welfare, and the State, 1890–1930* (Urbana: University of Illinois Press, 1994), 74–103, 167–96; Robyn Muncy, *Creating a Female Dominion in American Reform, 1890–1935* (New York: Oxford University Press, 1991), 38–65; James T. Patterson, *America's Struggle against Poverty, 1900–1980* (Cambridge: Harvard University Press, 1981), 20–34; and Walter I. Trattner, *From Poor Law to Welfare State: A History of Social Welfare in America* (New York: Free Press, 1974), 96–135, 179–247. For contemporary perspectives, see Robert Hunter, *Poverty: Social Conscience in the Progressive Era* (New York: MacMillan, 1904); and John Spargo, *The Bitter Cry of the Children* (New York: Macmillan, 1906).

3   On medical photography, see Daniel M. Fox and Christopher Lawrence, *Photographing Medicine: Images and Power in Britain and America since 1940* (New York: Greenwood Press, 1988); Janet Golden and Charles E. Rosenberg, *Pictures of Health: A Photographic History of Philadelphia Health Care, 1862–1945* (Philadelphia: University of Pennsylvania Press, 1991); and Rick Smolen and Phillip Moffitt, *Medicine's Greatest Journey: One Hundred Years of Healing* (Boston: Bullfinch Press, 1992). Fox and Lawrence discuss their decision to focus on medicine rather than public health; Golden and Rosenberg incorporate some public health images (including some from the Carpenter collection analyzed in this article).

4   Janet Golden, "The Howard Childs Carpenter Slide Collection, *"Fugitive Leaves,"* 3rd ser., 2 (1987): 5–6.

5   Information about the DPD can be found in Jeffrey P. Brosco, "Sin or Folly? Child and Community Health in Philadelphia, 1900–1930" (PhD dissertation, University of Pennsylvania, 1994); Charles V. Dorwarth, "The Establishment of a Department of Preventive Medicine in a Hospital Teaching Children," *Archives of Pediatrics* 34 (1917): 206–10; Haven Emerson, *Philadelphia Health and Hospital Survey* (Philadelphia: Philadelphia Health and Hospital Survey Committee, 1930), 263–65, 430–33, 689–92; "Ignorance Given as Disease Cause," *Philadelphia Inquirer*, December 16, 1921; and the annual reports of the Children's Hospital of Philadelphia. For a general history of the Children's Hospital of Philadelphia, see Samuel X. Radbill, "The Children's Hospital of Philadelphia," *Philadelphia Medicine* 70 (1974): 352–67. Biographical information on Carpenter can be found in Samuel X. Radbill, "Memoir of Howard Childs Carpenter," Radbill Papers, College of Physicians of Philadelphia; Philadelphia Pediatric Society, "Special Meeting, May 18, 1933" (pamphlet); Joseph Stokes, Jr. "Memoir of Howard Childs Carpenter (1878–1955)," *Transactions and Studies of the College of Physicians of Philadelphia*, 4th ser. 24 (1956): 41–42; "H. C. Carpenter, Pediatrist, Dies," *Philadelphia Inquirer*, April 8, 1955; and *New York Times*, April 8, 1955.

6 Other sources of slides in the collection include the National Exhibits Company, Providence, RI; John F. Sweeny and Son, High Class Lantern Slides, New York, NY; J. A. Glenn, Albany, NY; Flotz, Washington, DC; Victor Animatiograph Company, Davenport, IA; and the Standard Slide Corporation, New York, NY.

7 According to the article "Ignorance Given as a Disease Cause," *Philadelphia Inquirer*, his talk included "a series of slides showing the results attained from disease prevention methods, how poor mothers and children were taught to visualize prevention means through pictures, and the remarkable results."

8 Carpenter's colleague William Bradley, medical director of the nearby Starr Centre clinics, gave lectures on "Care of the Baby," "How To Feed the Baby," and "The Fly and the Baby," using lantern slides. See Starr Centre Association, Minutes of the Milk and Medical Committee, February 1, 1912, series 3, folder 87, box 5, Center for the Study of the History of Nursing, University of Pennsylvania.

9 Maren Stange, *Symbols of Ideal Life: Social Documentary Photography in America, 1890–1950* (New York: Cambridge University Press, 1989).

10 Peter Bacon Hales, *Silver Cities: The Photography of American Urbanization* (Philadelphia: Temple University Press, 1984), 221. On using images in exhibit posters, see Evart G. Routzahn and Mary Swain Routzahn, *The ABC of Exhibit Planning* (New York: Russell Sage Foundation, 1918), 50, 69. Note that I have distinguished between health teaching directed at particular audiences and health education that had a broader reach and used newer media including radio after the 1920s and, later, film.

11 John R. Kemp, *Lewis Hine: Photographs of Child Labor in the New South* (Jackson: University Press of Mississippi, 1986); James Guimond, *American Photography and the American Dream* (Chapel Hill: University of North Carolina Press, 1991), 57–98; Judith M. Gutman, *Lewis Hine and the American Social Conscience* (New York: Walker, 1967); Judith M. Gutman, *Lewis Hine: Two Perspectives* (New York: Grossman, 1974); and Alan Trachtenberg, *Reading American Photographs: Images as History, Mathew Brady to Walker Evans* (New York: Hill and Wang, 1989), 164–230.

12 Hales, *Silver Cities*, 247–48.

13 The use of the lantern slide lecture to arouse moral indignation, and the adoption of the technique by Philadelphia reformers, particularly the Octavia Hill Association, is described in Frederic M. Miller, Morris J. Vogel, and Allen F. Davis, *Still Philadelphia: A Photographic History, 1890–1940* (Philadelphia: Temple University Press, 1983), 121–22. For a description of social investigators seeking candid glimpses of the poor in back alleys, see Hales, *Silver Cities*, 163–217; Stange, *Symbols of Ideal Life*, 1–87; Alan Thomas, *Time in a Frame: Photography and the Nineteenth-Century Mind* (New York: Schocken Books, 1977), 136; and Trachtenberg, *Reading American Photographs*, 164–230.

14 Stange, *Symbols of Ideal Life*, 47–87. Susan Sontag notes that many photographers were enraptured by "melancholy objects" and created a "habit of seeing" she labels "detached." Susan Sontag, *On Photography* (New York: Farrar, Straus & Giroux, 1973).

15 Samuel H. Preston and Michael R. Haines, *Fatal Years: Child Mortality in Late-Nineteenth-Century America* (Princeton: Princeton University Press, 1991) 97–102, 150–54, 166–67.

16 Similar images of Philadelphia can be found in George W. Norris, *The Housing Problem in Philadelphia* (Philadelphia: J. J. McVey, 1913), and in the photograph collections of the Philadelphia Housing Association and the Octavia Hill Association, located at the Urban Archives, Temple University, Philadelphia.

17 Thomas, *Time in a Frame*, 143–44. Of course, before-and-after images long pre-
    dated photography. Thomas notes that J. T. Barnardo, an evangelical preacher
    and medical student, raised funds for his juvenile mission in London using
    before-and-after images.

18 Naomi Rogers, "Germs with Legs: Flies, Disease, and the New Public Health,"
    Bulletin of the History of Medicine 63 (1989): 599–617.

19 Charles V. Chapin, "How Shall We Spend the Health Appropriation?" *American
    Journal of Public Health* 3 (1913): 202–208. A broader discussion of the "new pub-
    lic health"—the application of scientific knowledge to social problems through,
    among other things, popular education—can be found in Barbara Gutman
    Rosenkrantz, *Public Health and the State: Changing Views in Massachusetts, 1842–1936*
    (Cambridge: Harvard University Press, 1972), 128–76. See also Karen Buhler
    Wilkerson, *False Dawn: The Rise and Decline of Public Health Nursing, 1900–1930*
    (New York: Garland, 1989).

20 Fox and Lawrence, *Photographing Medicine*; Stanley Burns, *Early Medical Photog-
    raphy in America* (New York: Burns Archive, 1983); George Rosen, "Early Medical
    Photography," *Ciba Symposium* 4 (1942): 1344–55; and Daniel M. Fox and James
    Terry, "Photography and the Self-Image of American Physicians, 1880–1920," *Bul-
    letin of the History of Medicine* 52 (1978): 435–457. Physicians could, of course, be
    reform photographers or child public health photographers. Allies from the
    City Health Department, for example, accompanied Jacob Riis on his sojourns
    through the slums of New York. See Hales, *Silver Cities*, 163–217.

21 Jeffrey P. Brosco, "Weight Charts and Well Child Care: How the Pediatrician
    Became the Expert in Child Health," *Archives of Pediatrics and Adolescent Medicine*
    155 (2001): 1385–89.

22 On diphtheria, see Evelynn Maxine Hammonds, *Childhood's Deadly Scourge: The
    Campaign to Control Diphtheria in New York City, 1880–1930* (Baltimore: Johns
    Hopkins University Press, 1999).

23 Regina Markell Morantz-Sanchez, *Sympathy and Science: Women Physicians in Amer-
    ican Medicine* (New York: Oxford University Press, 1985), 271–72.

24 Children's Hospital of Philadelphia, *70th Annual Report* (Philadelphia: Children's
    Hospital of Philadelphia 1926), 10; *75th Annual Report* (Philadelphia: Children's
    Hospital of Philadelphia, 1931), 12; and Brosco, "Sin or Folly," 125.

Institutions

ଔ

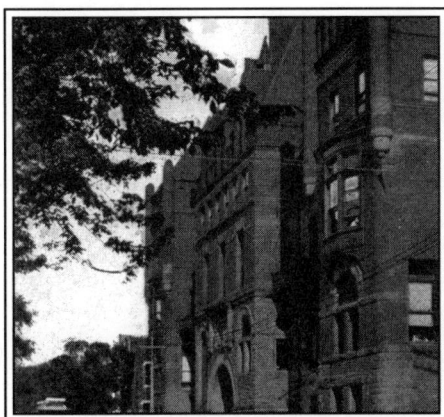

La contribution de l'Hôpital Saint-Paul et de l'*Alexandra Hospital* à la lutte contre les maladies contagieuses infantiles à Montréal, 1905–1934[1]

CR

Marie-Josée Fleury et Guy Grenier

A u tournant du XXe siècle, près de la moitié des décès au Québec sont rapportés parmi la population infantile et sont attribués aux maladies infectieuses[2]. Les villes et les quartiers défavorisés sont les lieux les plus touchés par ces dernières, l'industrialisation des centres urbains s'étant trop souvent accompagnée d'une détérioration de l'environnement (entassement et qualité inadéquate des habitations) et d'une insuffisance des services sanitaires (égouts, aqueducs, collecte des déchets et inspection des aliments par exemple)[3]. Montréal possède spécifiquement l'un des taux les plus élevés de mortalité infantile des villes d'Occident. Alors qu'actuellement le taux de mortalité infantile se situe autour de 9 pour 1 000, il est au début du XXe siècle de plus de 150 pour 1 000 pour l'ensemble de la province et de plus de 250 pour 1 000 dans les grands centres urbains[4]. Les maladies infectieuses (typhoïde, tuberculose, diphtérie, rougeole, rubéole, scarlatine et coqueluche), les désordres intestinaux (diarrhée, entérite et dysenterie) et les maladies dites «d'enfance» (débilité congénitale, sclérème et ictère – jaunisse) étaient répertoriés comme les principales causes de mortalité des enfants.

C'est afin de remédier à cette situation que se développent, au tournant du siècle, une politique de santé publique et une infrastructure institutionnelle visant à sauvegarder la force de travail de la communauté et à rehausser le pouvoir politique de l'État et de la médecine[5]. Dans ce contexte et grâce à l'avancement des sciences, les premiers hôpitaux permanents et/ou publics pour le traitement des maladies contagieuses sont introduits : l'Hôpital de la Marine du Québec (1834), subventionné par le gouvernement et destiné prioritairement aux traitements des émigrants atteints de maladies contagieuses; l'Hôpital des contagieux du *Montreal General Hospital* (1868–1893) financé surtout par des fonds privés; et l'Hôpital civique des variolés (1874–1885) créé à l'initiative du bureau de santé de Montréal.[6] L'établissement de ces hôpitaux témoigne de la volonté des pouvoirs publics et des médecins d'enrayer les épidémies et de consolider leurs interventions et leurs expertises dans ce domaine. Goulet et Keel ont d'ailleurs démontré, pour les années 1896–1905, la popularité de l'Institut Pasteur (en France) auprès du corps médical québécois comme lieu d'apprentissage des derniers développements de la science bactériologique[7]. Ces médecins auraient constitué, à leur retour, une relève critique pour le déploiement des institutions scientifiques au Québec.

L'organisation d'hôpitaux pour traiter les maladies contagieuses infantiles avait d'autant plus d'intérêt qu'il n'existait au Québec que peu d'institutions spécialisées pour soigner les enfants. Les hôpitaux consacrés aux traitements des enfants sont surtout mis en place à partir du début des années 1900 : le *Children's Memorial Hospital*[8] est érigé en 1903 et l'Hôpital Sainte-Justine[9] en 1907. À Montréal, les premières *Gouttes de lait,* qui sont des endroits destinés à la distribution de lait stérilisé et où un certain suivi médical est assuré pour les nouveau-nés, ne sont aussi établies que durant la première décennie du XXe siècle[10]. Et d'après Baillargeon, ces dernières ne se sont véritablement imposées qu'à partir des années 1930 comme lieu de consultation des enfants auprès de la population féminine[11]. Au tournant du siècle, peu de services sont donc accessibles pour les enfants qui sont malades, et la pratique de ne mettre sur pied des hôpitaux temporaires qu'au moment de grandes épidémies demeure toujours la plus courante.

Malgré l'importance que peut représenter la mise en œuvre des hôpitaux pour traiter les maladies contagieuses infantiles sur les plans médico-scientifique et socio-organisationnel, l'historiographie s'est peu intéressée au rôle de ces derniers[12]. À partir de l'étude de deux hôpitaux publics établis pour soigner la population infantile de Montréal, infectée par les maladies contagieuses, l'Hôpital Saint-Paul et l'*Alexandra Hospital,* nous chercherons à mieux comprendre quelle a été la contribution de ces institutions à la lutte contre les épidémies. Nous postulons que parallèlement à l'amélioration de l'hygiène publique, l'introduction de ces hôpitaux a constitué l'une des premières pierres de la prise en charge des maladies contagieuses infantiles par les pouvoirs publics et les médecins montréalais au début du siècle.

Nous verrons que tout en étant des établissements consacrés au traitement des maladies contagieuses infantiles, l'Hôpital Saint-Paul et l'*Alexandra Hospital* ont soutenu la formation, l'accumulation et la diffusion des connaissances en bactériologie. L'analyse de l'organisation des services médicaux et du fonctionnement de ces hôpitaux atteste de leur importance dans la prise en charge des maladies contagieuses et de leur efficacité à répondre à la demande de la population. L'étude du déroulement des activités de l'Hôpital Saint-Paul et de l'*Alexandra Hospital* démontre aussi la volonté de leur administration de leur donner un statut hautement scientifique, en les modelant selon les meilleurs modèles d'hôpitaux américains et européens spécialisés dans les soins des maladies contagieuses, et en articulant leurs services médicaux selon l'avancement des techniques et des savoirs les plus efficaces dans ce champ de spécialisation. Cependant, l'histoire de ces hôpitaux met aussi en évidence les limites de la science médicale et des centres hospitaliers de l'époque à endiguer les maladies contagieuses. Tout comme aujourd'hui, mais dans un contexte bien différent, le développement de l'Hôpital Saint-Paul et de l'*Alexandra Hospital* – comme nous le verrons – a été également restreint par des considérations purement économiques et administratives.

Saint-Paul et Alexandra : des hôpitaux modernes au centre d'un projet d'éradication des maladies contagieuses infantiles

Au tournant du siècle, une lutte plus effective contre les maladies contagieuses s'organise dans un premier temps sur le plan municipal, puis à partir de la création du Conseil d'hygiène du Québec (1887), de plus en plus au niveau provincial[13]. Parallèlement, un intérêt plus marqué envers la santé des enfants est notoire. Cet intérêt nouveau pour la lutte contre la mortalité infantile s'explique par la montée à la fin du XIXe siècle des nationalismes[14]. À titre d'illustration, mentionnons la mise à la disposition de la profession médicale d'un laboratoire provincial où il est possible de commander des examens diagnostiques en 1896; l'établissement en 1903 de la vaccination obligatoire; l'ouverture de la division des maladies contagieuses au Conseil d'hygiène de la province en 1905; l'engagement au niveau municipal d'infirmières hygiénistes, qui ont joué un rôle essentiel dans les domaines de la prévention des maladies infantiles et de l'éducation des mères[15]; et la création des *Gouttes de lait* qui organisation aussi contribué significativement à ces dernières[16], etc. Au tournant du siècle, la pédiatrie tend aussi à s'organiser au niveau de l'enseignement universitaire et à l'intérieur de structures hospitalières. Par exemple, la loi médicale de 1909 introduit la pédiatrie au nombre des disciplines du programme de cinq ans des facultés de médecine de la province de Québec[17].

　　C'est dans ce contexte et résultant d'un taux catastrophique de mortalité due aux épidémies que l'Hôpital Saint-Paul[18] et l'*Alexandra Hospital* sont édifiés, en 1905 et en 1906 respectivement, afin de traiter les maladies contagieuses infantiles[19]. Le Bureau de santé de Montréal avait hésité sur la pertinence soit de subventionner l'ensemble des hôpitaux de la ville (pour qu'ils possèdent chacun un service pour les maladies contagieuses); soit de fonder un seul hôpital (qui desservirait l'ensemble de la population de la métropole)[20], soit de financer deux hôpitaux, respectivement pour les communautés francophone et anglophone[21]. Ces deux dernières options, qui permettaient une concentration des ressources, avaient notamment comme avantage de favoriser la recherche et l'enseignement clinique. Finalement, le clivage confessionnel et linguistique, omniprésent à l'époque, est venu justifier la prise de décision de la création de deux hôpitaux pour contagieux.

Pour administrer et diriger les services médicaux de l'Hôpital francophone, l'Hôpital Notre-Dame est choisi[22]. Ce dernier avait déjà géré, entre les années 1894 et 1895, un établissement consacré aux maladies contagieuses, l'Hôpital civique, établi à la suite d'une épidémie de scarlatine survenue en 1893[23]. Le maire et le président du comité des finances et de la commission d'hygiène de la ville de Montréal sont membres du bureau d'administration de l'Hôpital Notre-Dame en ce qui regarde la gestion financière et médicale de l'Hôpital Saint-Paul[24]. Pour sa part, l'*Alexandra Hospital* est dirigé par un bureau de gouverneurs composé de représentants du *Montreal General Hospital*, du *Royal Victoria Hospital* et du *Western Hospital* et de donateurs particuliers[25]. Ces gouverneurs (Edward Seaborne Clouston[26], James Ross[27] et Jeffrey Hale Burland[28]) étaient tous des membres influents de la communauté anglophone.

Les deux nouveaux hôpitaux pour contagieux ont une capacité d'hospitalisation assez importante avec 100 lits chacun à leur ouverture. Dans les années 1920, 33 places s'ajoutent à l'Hôpital Saint-Paul, situé en face du parc Lafontaine sur la rue Plessis. À la même période, l'*Alexandra Hospital*, situé sur la rue Charron dans le quartier Pointe-Saint-Charles, voit son nombre de lits passer à 165. L'implantation d'une structure hospitalière d'une telle capacité d'accueil, et pouvant intervenir dans le traitement d'une diversité de maladies contagieuses démontre la volonté des autorités d'abaisser la mortalité infantile due aux épidémies.

Les hôpitaux de Saint-Paul et d'Alexandra sont consacrés surtout à l'étude et au traitement de quatre maladies contagieuses : la diphtérie, la scarlatine, la rougeole et, à partir de 1907, l'érysipèle. Toutefois, les autorités du Service de santé de la ville de Montréal peuvent utiliser les pavillons de ces hôpitaux pour le traitement de toute autre maladie contagieuse qu'elles jugent prioritaire de combattre[29]. Ainsi en 1918, 220 personnes atteintes de la grippe espagnole sont hospitalisées ou à Alexandra ou à Saint-Paul[30]. De même, ces hôpitaux servent en 1927 au traitement de 144 personnes touchées par la fièvre typhoïde[31]. Par ailleurs, ils reçoivent chaque année des enfants atteints d'autres maladies contagieuses ont la varicelle, la coqueluche, les oreillons, la poliomyélite et la rubéole.

Bien que l'Hôpital Saint-Paul soit administré par des catholiques francophones et l'*Alexandra Hospital* par des anglo-protestants, ces hôpitaux acceptent tout patient envoyé par la municipalité de Montréal, indépendamment de sa nationalité ou de sa religion[32]. Les pourcentages de Canadiens français, de Canadiens anglais et ceux des autres nationalités admis dans ces établissements connaissent d'ailleurs d'importantes fluctuations au fil des années, variant sans doute en fonction des quartiers frappés par les maladies contagieuses. À titre d'exemple, en 1917, 61 % des 2 366 malades admis à Saint-Paul et à Alexandra sont des Canadiens français[33]. Quatre ans plus tard, ils ne forment que 27 % des 2 781 patients admis durant l'année, soit moins que le nombre total de patients d'origine juive (17 %) ou de nationalités diverses (17 %) réunis[34].

Même si leur clientèle est formée presque exclusivement d'enfants, les hôpitaux Saint-Paul et Alexandra reçoivent également chaque année un certain nombre d'adultes. Nous savons que des mères ont ainsi été admises à l'*Alexandra Hospital* en même temps que leurs enfants[35]. Le personnel hospitalier (tel qu'infirmières, conducteurs d'ambulances, préposés, et étudiants en médecine) infecté par une maladie contagieuse est également traité dans les deux hôpitaux. En 1909, l'*Alexandra Hospital* a ainsi traité 17 de ses employés qui avaient contacté la diphtérie, la scarlatine, la rougeole ou l'érysipèle au cours de l'année[36].

L'Hôpital Saint-Paul et l'*Alexandra Hospital* ont majoritairement accueilli une clientèle montréalaise pauvre, dont les frais d'hospitalisation étaient couverts par la municipalité. Une preuve d'indigence était exigée des familles qui voulaient y faire soigner gratuitement leurs enfants. À quelques reprises, des villes (Outremont, Saint-Lambert, Montréal-Nord, Westmount, Verdun et Maisonneuve) se sont aussi prévalues de leurs services moyennant une indemnisation. La ville de Westmount a ainsi été l'une des premières municipalités à signer une entente avec l'Hôpital Saint-Paul, ce qui témoigne du fait que la communauté anglophone de l'Île de Montréal reconnaissait la qualité des soins donnés par l'Hôpital Notre-Dame. Les deux hôpitaux pour contagieux ont de plus traité une clientèle qui était en mesure de payer. L'*Alexandra Hospital* et l'Hôpital Saint-Paul possédaient respectivement 25 et 10 lits privés pour le traitement de cette clientèle[37]. Pour les décennies 1900–1920, les montants perçus par Saint-Paul pour cette catégorie de patients varient entre 500 $ et 3 500 $ par année. Ainsi, sur un total de 732 enfants hospitalisés à l'Hôpital Saint-Paul en 1910, 659 étaient des patients de type public, 28 étaient de type privé, et 45 venaient de municipalités environnantes[38]. Pour la même année, la clientèle de l'*Alexandra Hospital* comprenait 731 patients de type public, 34 étaient de type privé, et 35 qui venaient de l'extérieur de Montréal[39]. Ces hôpitaux publics ont donc majoritairement desservi une clientèle démunie.

Des institutions hospitalières répondant aux exigences de l'asepsie

Saint-Paul et Alexandra sont des hôpitaux modernes qui respectent, par leur aspect architectural et leur fonctionnement interne, les conceptions véhiculées par la révolution pasteurienne; tout y est conçu afin de minimiser les risques de la contagion[40]. S'inspirant du modèle de l'Hôpital des enfants-malades de Paris, ils sont en ce sens composés de trois pavillons assurant la ségrégation des malades[41]. Le premier est établi principalement pour le traitement de la diphtérie. Le deuxième sert surtout à soigner les patients atteints de scarlatine, une maladie responsable de plus de 40 % des hospitalisations à Saint-Paul et à Alexandra durant cette période. Le troisième est consacré à la rougeole et, à partir de 1907, à l'érysipèle. À partir de 1913, la quasi-totalité des cas de rougeole est dirigée à l'*Alexandra Hospital*, tandis que l'Hôpital Saint-Paul reçoit la majorité des cas d'érysipèle[42]. Ce troisième pavillon a sans doute également accueilli les autres maladies contagieuses que les médecins de la municipalité jugeaient prioritaires de contrôler. En 1932, un pavillon de l'*Alexandra Hospital* est ainsi consacré au traitement des cas de coqueluche[43].

Dans chacun de ces pavillons, les murs, les serviettes et les rideaux, voire même les cahiers et les feuilles de service, sont de la couleur associée à la maladie contagieuse. Aucun objet ne peut se transmettre d'un pavillon à un autre sans passer par un stérilisateur. Suivant cette même ligne de pensée, les infirmières[44] et autres employés sont aussi isolés dans leur pavillon respectif : «Les gardes-malades ne devaient fréquenter que les autres infirmières de leur pavillon et ne manger que dans leur propre vaisselle[45]». Les bureaux de l'administration et les départements destinés aux employés étaient aussi complètement isolés des pavillons où l'on traitait les maladies contagieuses.

Les deux hôpitaux possèdent des chambres d'isolement complètement vitrées servant à l'accueil des patients[46]. À l'Hôpital Saint-Paul, sur une capacité d'accueil de 100 lits, 24 – soit huit par pavillon – sont destinés à cet usage. Les médecins y traitent les malades qui sont dans un état critique (croup ou dédoublement de maladies contagieuses par exemple) et les patients dont les problèmes de santé n'ont pas été identifiés. Cet isolement permet également de mieux préciser le diagnostic, les premiers symptômes de certaines maladies, comme la scarlatine et la diphtérie, étant similaires[47]. La recherche du signe de Koplik (présence de taches rouges avec un point blanc-bleuâtre au centre sur la face interne de la muqueuse des joues et des lèvres), qui permet de dépister une rougeole trois ou quatre jours avant son éruption, est une pratique courante à l'Hôpital Saint-Paul. L'isolement d'un jeune malade admis pour diphtérie après la découverte de ce signe a ainsi permis d'éviter une épidémie de rougeole parmi les diphtériques[48].

Les autres chambres sont conformes à l'hygiène moderne. Les chambres communes, généralement de six lits en fer émaillé, qui disposent de lavabos et de tous les autres meubles de toilette, sont notamment larges et bien aérées. Les chambres semi-privées (à deux lits) et privées, qui couvrent environ 10 % de la capacité d'accueil de l'hôpital, sont pourvues «de tout ce qu'un malade peut désirer : sonnettes électriques, téléphones, éclairage, thermomètres, etc.»[49]. Enfin, la permission de recevoir des visiteurs n'est accordée qu'aux patients qui sont gravement malades ou encore mourants, cela afin de ne pas augmenter les risques de contagion. Ces visiteurs doivent se soumettre à de multiples précautions visant à enrayer les germes : ils passent notamment par une chambre de déshabillage, sont désinfectés (par un système d'arrosage), et revêtent une blouse blanche. Le médecin et le personnel soignant doivent également se vêtir d'une blouse de toile avant de pénétrer dans la chambre du malade et, après chaque visite, plongent leurs mains dans des solutions antiseptiques[50].

Des hôpitaux pourvus d'un personnel important et compétent

L'administration interne (telle qu'achats du ménage et de la nourriture, tenue des livres de compte et direction du personnel de soutien, etc.) et la direction des soins infirmiers et du service de pharmacie de l'Hôpital Saint-Paul ont été déléguées aux Sœurs Grises de Montréal (ou Sœurs de la Charité), suivant ainsi le même modèle d'organisation qu'à l'Hôpital Notre-Dame. D'ailleurs, avant 1908, année marquant la nomination d'une sœur au titre de supérieure générale de Saint-Paul, ces fonctions relevaient des sœurs de l'Hôpital Notre-Dame. Les Sœurs Grises ont été près d'une vingtaine à œuvrer à l'Hôpital Saint-Paul. Des étudiantes en soins infirmiers, évaluées aussi à près d'une vingtaine pour les décennies 1910–1920, auraient complété les soins donnés à Saint-Paul par les sœurs. Les élèves infirmières ont constitué une source importante de main d'œuvre bon marché pour les hôpitaux de l'époque, fournissant les soins de base aux patients[51]. À partir des années 1930, des infirmières laïques seront de plus en plus embauchées à l'Hôpital Notre-Dame; ainsi, on en dénombre 9 en 1930, et 31 en 1934. On ignore cependant leur nombre pour l'Hôpital Saint-Paul. Le rôle critique des religieuses dans le déroulement des activités de l'Hôpital Saint-Paul, comme pour les autres hôpitaux francophones du Québec, souligne l'importance des dimensions spirituelle et charitable dans l'organisation des hôpitaux jusqu'aux années 1960, même si au fil du XXe siècle, la vocation scientifique de l'hôpital tend à l'emporter sur sa vocation spirituelle et charitable[52]. Les religieuses-infirmières intègrent par ailleurs ce mouvement en structurant dès le début du XXe siècle les conditions de leur formation[53].

À l'*Alexandra Hospital*, comme dans les autres hôpitaux anglo-canadiens, la direction des domestiques, les services infirmiers et la formation des gardes-malades sont sous la responsabilité d'une surintendante. Comme l'a noté Cohen,[54] les surintendantes ont joué un rôle important dans la professionnalisation des infirmières dans les hôpitaux anglophones en cultivant une complémentarité idéologique et professionnelle avec les médecins. Ainsi, Miss Grace Fairley, surintendante des infirmières de l'*Alexandra Hospital* de 1912 à 1919, a été la première présidente de la *Graduate Nurse Association of the Province of Quebec*[55]. Devant la difficulté de trouver des infirmières, l'*Alexandra Hospital* utilise en 1906 les infirmières en formation dans les trois autres hôpitaux anglophones de Montréal[56]. En 1918, une école d'infirmières est finalement fondée à l'Hôpital[57].

Le Bureau médical de l'*Alexandra Hospital* est formé de médecins du *Montreal General Hospital*, du *Royal Victoria Hospital* et du *Children's Memorial Hospital*. Son président, le Dr Alexander Dougall Blackader est considéré comme le premier pédiatre canadien[58]. Il a été en effet le premier à donner, à l'Université McGill en 1881, un cours sur les maladies de l'enfant. En 1888, il est membre fondateur de l'*American Paediatric Society*,[59] une organisation qu'il présidera en 1892. Il a également été le premier président, en 1922, de la *Canadian Society for the Study of Diseases of Children*, qui deviendra en 1951 la *Canadian Paediatric Society / Société canadienne de pédiatrie*[60]. Le Dr Blackader a aussi présidé, à partir de 1892, le Bureau médical du *Montreal Founding and Baby Hospital*, une institution dédiée aux soins des bébés et des enfants trouvés. De plus, il a été médecin en chef du *Children's Memorial Hospital* et directeur, jusqu'à sa mort en 1932, du *Canadian Medical Association Journal*[61]. Le secrétaire du Bureau médical, le Dr Harold Beveridge Cushing a pour sa part été l'un des fondateurs du *Children's Memorial Hospital*, institution dont il a été le médecin en chef de 1905 à 1938. Il a également été vice-président de l'*American Paediatric Society* et médecin à l'Hôpital Shriner de Montréal[62]. Dès 1906, un médecin visiteur est attitré pour chacun des pavillons. Celui du pavillon réservé à la scarlatine, jusqu'en 1914, est le Dr John McCrae, auteur en 1915 du poème «*In Flanders Fields*» récité lors des cérémonies du jour du Souvenir[63]. Tout comme à l'Hôpital Saint-Paul, l'*Alexandra Hospital* fait appel également à des spécialistes (ophtalmologistes, oto-rhino-laryngologistes, chirurgiens)[64].

À l'Hôpital Saint-Paul, les services donnés par les Sœurs Grises sont complétés par l'emploi d'un surintendant general, à partir de 1909, et d'une équipe médicale. Le surintendant général est responsable de l'application des règlements de l'hôpital et de l'exécution des décisions respectives du Bureau d'administration et du Bureau médical de Notre-Dame concernant Saint-Paul. Il a aussi la tâche d'exercer une surveillance générale sur l'administration interne de l'hôpital et de prendre les mesures appropriées afin d'en assurer le bon fonctionnement[65]. L'équipe médicale de Saint-Paul est sous la responsabilité d'une figure marquante, le Dr Joseph-Arthur Leduc, dont l'importance des activités scientifiques et cliniques témoigne de son rôle sur la scène médicale québécoise. En plus d'avoir été nommé directeur médical de Saint-Paul de 1905 à 1934, ce dernier a en effet été professeur (émérite en 1949) à la Chaire des maladies contagieuses de l'Université de Montréal dès 1911. Il s'est aussi occupé du dispensaire et du département de pédiatrie de Notre-Dame, et des Services des maladies contagieuses de la crèche d'Youville et de l'Hôpital Sainte-Justine. À la fermeture de Saint-Paul en 1934, il deviendra chef de service à l'Hôpital Pasteur (hôpital des contagieux affilié à l'Hôpital Saint-Luc). Il a en outre été consultant à l'Institut Bruchési, membre de la Commission des Infirmières de l'Université de Montréal, de l'Union nationale française, de l'Union médicale du Canada et de la Société médicale de Montréal[66]. La famille du Dr Leduc était propriétaire de la plus importante chaîne de pharmacies francophones du début du XXe siècle[67], et a joué un rôle de pionnier en matière de médecine préventive. En 1899, le grand-père du Dr Leduc, en compagnie du Dr G. Archambault, avait fondé l'Institut vaccinal de Montréal[68]. Cet institut restera la propriété des pharmacies Leduc & Leduc jusqu'en 1942, moment où le Dr J.-A. Leduc le cédera à l'Institut de microbiologie et d'hygiène de Montréal, fondée quatre ans auparavant par le Dr Armand Frappier[69].

Le Dr Leduc s'est rendu, à plus d'une reprise, aux États-Unis et en Europe pour parfaire sa formation en bactériologie et en pédiatrie. Mentionnons qu'au tournant du siècle, le savoir médical au Québec était de type presque exclusivement périphérique, c'est-à-dire importé des États-Unis et d'Europe[70]. Jusque dans les années 1920, la formation des médecins des facultés de médecine de Montréal et de Laval ne fournissait guère les éléments didactiques encourageant une spécialisation médicale. La plupart des praticiens de la santé désireux de se perfectionner devaient s'inscrire dans une institution étrangère. C'est ainsi qu'avant de prendre en charge ses nouvelles fonctions à l'Hôpital Saint-Paul, le Dr Leduc a effectué un stage au *Boston City Hospital* (qui était considéré comme un modèle pour l'organisation et le traitement de ces maladies en Amérique)[71], et au *Massachusetts General Hospital*, pour perfectionner ses connaissances en pédiatrie. En complétant aussi des études à Boston (Harvard), à New York et à Paris, il s'est enrichi de plusieurs nouvelles théories et méthodes de guérison.

La structure médicale des hôpitaux pour contagieux se complexifie progressivement au cours des années, ce qui atteste d'une spécialisation et d'une médicalisation accentuées des services. Les changements de la structure médicale à l'Hôpital Saint-Paul confirment cette tendance. En plus de la fonction de directeur médical, un poste d'interne est établi à Saint-Paul à partir de 1906. En 1919, ils sont quatre à occuper cet emploi. Les internes constituaient le pivot des activités médicales quotidiennes de l'hôpital. Ils examinaient notamment les nouveaux patients dès leur arrivée, et coordonnaient leurs traitements. Ils ont aussi assumé les responsabilités relatives aux services de laboratoire, jusqu'au début des années 1910. Après cette période, un médecin assistant se spécialise dans ce travail et dans les techniques d'anesthésie. À partir de 1926, le nombre d'internes tend à s'accroître puisque l'internat est maintenant obligatoire pour les étudiants de 5e année de l'Université de Montréal.

Des médecins assistants sont aussi distribués dans les différents pavillons des hôpitaux des contagieux. À l'Hôpital Saint-Paul, ils faisaient leurs services tous les jours à des heures fixes. En l'absence du Dr Leduc, l'un des assistants prenait la direction de l'hôpital; à partir des années 1910, ils sont trois à exercer cette fonction. Un médecin résident est enfin nommé à Saint-Paul en 1927, et s'occupe particulièrement de l'admission des malades[72]. En l'absence du chef de service ou de ses assistants, ce dernier a la responsabilité de la direction médicale de l'hôpital. En outre, des médecins de famille ont été admis à l'intérieur des murs des hôpitaux pour contagieux comme conseillers du médecin interne; ils n'étaient pas autorisés à prescrire ni à administrer un traitement, quel qu'il soit. Cependant, les patients privés ont pu être soignés par les médecins de famille.

Des centres hospitaliers à la fine pointe des connaissances de l'époque et effectuant de la recherche et de l'enseignement clinique

Les hôpitaux Saint-Paul et Alexandra étaient des lieux idéaux d'investigations cliniques, permettant d'effectuer des recherches en bactériologie, en épidémiologie et en sérothérapie. Ils disposaient, pour ce faire, des ressources en spécialistes et en équipements des facultés de médecine. De plus, la clientèle des deux hôpitaux était majoritairement publique, donc incapable de choisir le type d'interventions lui étant octroyées. Pour l'Europe du XIXᵉ siècle, Foucault a démontré comment l'expérimentation médicale sur les pauvres à l'hôpital pouvait par la suite être appliquée en toute sécurité sur la clientèle privée[73]. Les patients servaient, en ce sens, de matériel de recherche clinique. Nous pouvons fortement postuler qu'il en a été de même à l'Hôpital Saint-Paul et à l'*Alexandra Hospital*, comme dans toute autre institution comparable de cette période au Québec.

À partir du début des années 1910, une évolution dans la capacité des hôpitaux pour contagieux de diagnostiquer les maladies est aussi observable. En font foi les rapports annuels des deux hôpitaux qui, dans leur classification des maladies, ne font plus mention, de la catégorie des «cas douteux». Il existe par ailleurs une rubrique intitulée «cas non traités» dans laquelle peu de patients sont classés. Au cours des années, cette tendance s'accentue; on dénote une augmentation importante des activités de laboratoire (analyses chimiques et bactériologiques) reliées à l'anatomopathologie, effectuées à l'Hôpital Saint-Paul et à l'*Alexandra Hospital*, ce qui témoigne d'un développement accru des techniques de diagnostic et d'une pratique généralisée de ces analyses auprès d'une clientèle de plus en plus nombreuse. Par exemple, 378 examens microscopiques sont réalisés à l'Hôpital Saint-Paul en 1909. En 1915, ce nombre grimpe à 1 267, en 1920 à 2 126, et en 1926 à 5 850. Les analyses de laboratoire, qui étaient de 2 713 en 1916, atteignent le chiffre de 7 081 en 1921. Le nombre total des examens (analyse de l'urine et du sang, culture de la gorge, test Shick par exemple) pratiqués à l'*Alexandra Hospital* atteindra le chiffre de 17 422 au cours de l'année 1926[74]. Les rapports annuels de l'*Alexandra Hospital* indiquent en outre le nombre d'autopsies pratiquées, contrairement à ceux de l'Hôpital Notre-Dame, ce qui semble confirmer la thèse selon laquelle cette dernière pratique n'était pas fréquente dans l'hôpital francophone durant le premier quart du XXe siècle[75].

Pour soigner les quatre principales maladies contagieuses présentes à l'Hôpital Saint-Paul, la thérapeutique utilisée s'est inspirée du savoir et des techniques élaborés au plan international. La diphtérie semble avoir été la maladie qui a le plus bénéficié des découvertes biologiques de la fin du XIXe siècle[76]. Le sérum antidiphtérique[77] (agent curatif), la toxine-antitoxine et l'anatoxine de Ramon (méthodes préventives), la réaction Schick (méthode de dépistage des individus susceptibles de contracter la diphtérie consistant en une injection sous la peau de faibles doses de toxine diphtérique[78]) la trachéotomie et l'intubation ont tous été employés à Saint-Paul et à l'*Alexandra Hospital*[79]. En ce qui concerne l'emploi et la diffusion des méthodes de tubage et de sérothérapie pour traiter la diphtérie, notons que l'Hôpital Saint-Paul a particulièrement joué un rôle de chef de file par rapport aux hôpitaux québécois de l'époque[80]. À partir de 1910, la trachéotomie n'est presque plus appliquée. L'intubation, qui est jugée comme une procédure moins complexe et comportant moins de risques pour le patient, est plutôt mise de l'avant. Dans les années 1920, l'antitoxine est administrée par intraveineuse, une technique plus efficace que l'ancienne méthode d'injection subcutanée ou intramusculaire[81]. La clé de l'élimination de la diphtérie sera toutefois l'immunisation avec l'anatoxine, mise au point par le médecin français Ramon en 1918. Des séances d'immunisation seront inaugurées à partir de 1926 par l'École d'hygiène sociale appliquée de Montréal[82].

Dès son apparition sur le marché, le sérum antiscarlatineux est également prescrit pour diagnostiquer ou soigner la scarlatine ou comme agent prophylactique. Par exemple, en 1926 on en donne à 75 gardes-malades effectuant leur stage à l'*Alexandra Hospital* afin de les immuniser contre la scarlatine. Trois semaines après leur entrée dans le service des maladies contagieuses, seulement 9 % des infirmières contractèrent une scarlatine bénigne, comparativement à 15 % précédemment et d'une façon beaucoup plus sévère[83]. Le sérum avait aussi un effet bénéfique pour la prévention ou le traitement des complications habituelles causées par la scarlatine : otite, mastoïdite, adénite cervicale, arthrite et néphrite. Cette découverte abaissera encore plus le taux de mortalité par la scarlatine, ainsi que le nombre d'opérations chirurgicales. En 1926, seulement 13 opérations de la mastoïde ont été pratiquées à l'*Alexandra Hospital*, comparativement à 30 l'année précédente[84]. Les élèves infirmières reçoivent également de l'antitoxine diphtérique[85]. Pour traiter la rougeole, les médecins de Saint-Paul et d'Alexandra ont surtout employé le sérum de convalescent[86]; un sérum antistreptococcique (soit le sérum monovalent de Marmorek, soit le sérum polyvalent de Travel) était plutôt employé pour soigner l'érysipèle[87]. Un traitement à base de morphine et de chloral (le Paveral) a aussi été mis à l'essai contre la coqueluche[88].

L'Hôpital Saint-Paul a de plus été à l'avant-garde concernant le régime des nourrissons en décourageant les médecins de les sous-alimenter, comme le préconisait alors l'école française[89]. Saint-Paul a ainsi été perçu comme un hôpital moderne de grande efficacité, comme en font preuve ces citations tirées de *La Presse* :

C'est dans cet hôpital que durant 29 ans le docteur Leduc et toute une phalange de médecins dont plusieurs sont devenus des sommités combattirent efficacement les maladies contagieuses. Si la diphtérie et la scarlatine ne créent plus les terreurs d'autrefois (l'incidence des décès est à son plus bas minimum de nos jours) disons-nous bien qu'on le doit à Saint-Paul, creuset clinique de grande valeur où la science a toujours trouvé des compétences pour aller sans cesse de l'avant[90].

L'immunisation préscolaire aujourd'hui obligatoire; la vaccination et combien d'autres formules qui ont réduit au minimum les dangers de la diphtérie et de la scarlatine notamment, c'est au travail d'un Leduc et de son équipe qu'on doit la création de cet appareil défensif contre la contagion[91].

Certes, les essais cliniques réalisés à l'*Alexandra Hospital* et à l'Hôpital Saint-Paul durant les premières décennies du XXe siècle n'étaient pas soumis à des protocoles rigoureux (groupes de contrôle par exemple) tels qu'appliqués actuellement. Ces essais cliniques témoignent cependant, pour l'époque, de l'existence d'une volonté réelle des médecins de comprendre et de traiter le plus efficacement possible les maladies contagieuses.

La recherche à l'Hôpital Saint-Paul et à l'*Alexandra Hospital* s'accompagnait d'une fonction d'enseignement clinique, afin d'assurer une relève en médecins et en infirmières spécialisés dans le domaine des maladies contagieuses. Ainsi, Saint-Paul était un hôpital universitaire, affilié à l'Université de Montréal[92]. Par petits groupes, les étudiants en médecine de cette université y faisaient des stages d'une durée d'un mois[93]. À partir de 1917, les étudiants de 5e année de l'Université y suivent un stage d'un mois[94]. Plus tard, en 1926, les étudiants en médecine se voient désormais contraints de suivre un stage d'une ou de deux années dans les différents services de l'Hôpital Notre-Dame, y compris Saint-Paul[95]. Pour sa part, l'*Alexandra Hopital* a ouvert ses portes aux étudiants en médecine de l'Université McGill dès l'année scolaire 1909–1910[96]. Cet hôpital est l'un des six hôpitaux anglophones de Montréal où, par petits groupes, les étudiants de 4e et de 5e année de McGill iront acquérir une formation clinique en pédiatrie durant les décennies 1910 et 1920. Après 1932, l'enseignement de la pédiatrie sera concentré au *Children's Memorial Hospital.* L'*Alexandra Hospital* restera cependant le lieu où sera donné l'enseignement clinique des maladies contagieuses[97].

Par ailleurs, à partir de la fin de la décennie 1900, les élèves infirmières de l'Hôpital Notre-Dame effectuaient à Saint-Paul un stage d'une durée de 5 à 6 mois. En 1921, 16 étudiantes y sont enregistrées sur un total de 56 inscrites à l'École de Notre-Dame[98]. De plus, l'Université de Montréal et les écoles d'infirmières de – l'Hôtel-Dieu de Montréal, de la Miséricorde, de Sainte-Jeanne d'Arc, du Sacré-Coeur de Cartierville, de Saint-Jean-de-Dieu, du Sanatorium Prévost, de Saint-Joseph de Lachine, de l'Hôpital Saint-Jean de Saint-Jean d'Iberville, du Sacré-Cœur de Hull[99], de l'Hôpital de la Providence de Montréal-Est et de l'Hôpital Normand et Cross[100] de Trois-Rivières – ont envoyé des étudiants à l'Hôpital Saint-Paul pour parfaire leur formation dans les soins à donner aux malades contagieux. Les futures infirmières y suivaient un stage de deux mois. Elles étaient encadrées par une élite médicale souvent spécialisée dans les meilleures écoles américaines et européennes. Cohen a démontré, en cette matière, le rôle-clé joué par les Sœurs Grises de l'Hôpital Notre-Dame dans la modernisation du sciences infirmières au Québec[101].

L'*Alexandra Hospital* reçoit pour sa part les élèves des diverses écoles d'infirmières anglophones de la province, comme celles du *Royal Victoria Hospital*, du *Montreal General Hospital*, du *Children's Memorial Hospital*, du *Homeopathic Hospital*, du *Saint-Mary's Hospital*, du *Women's General Hospital*, du *Lachine General Hospital*[102], du *Verdun Protestant Hospital*[103], du *District Hospital*[104] de Sweetburg et du *Sherbrooke General Hospital*[105]. Sa réputation dépassait les frontières du Québec puisque des élèves infirmières venant d'écoles de l'Ontario (*Belleville General Hospital*[106], *Great War Memorial Hospital*[107] de Perth, *Saint Vincent de Paul Hospital* de Brockville, *Cornwall General Hospital* et *Hôtel-Dieu Hospital*[108] de Cornwall) de Nouvelle-Écosse (*Highland View Hospital*[109] d'Ambert) et du Nouveau-Brunswick (*Soldiers Memorial Hospital*[110] de Campbellton) y suivaient également ment un stage à partir des années 1920. Près de 1500 élèves infirmières y ont appris les théories et les méthodes à la fine pointe des connaissances entre 1924 et 1933[111].

Les médecins de Saint-Paul et d'Alexandra ont ainsi favorisé une intervention active auprès de la clientèle et, semble-t-il, indépendamment de l'état de la thérapeutique disponible. Cette situation a sans doute contribué, pour l'époque, à consolider le savoir et les techniques en matière de traitement des maladies contagieuses.

Limites de la science médicale et de l'efficacité des hôpitaux au début du XXe siècle

Malgré ces progrès, d'importantes lacunes existaient quant à la prophylaxie et aux traitements des maladies contagieuses durant le premier tiers du XXe siècle. Mis à part l'anatoxine de Ramon, peu de sérums donnaient en effet des résultats d'une efficacité générale ou étaient d'un emploi assez simple pour en répandre l'utilisation et la production. Par exemple, la difficulté de fabrication du sérum antiscarlatineux en limitait l'emploi. Avant la décennie 1940, qui marque l'avènement des antibiotiques (dont pénicilline, érythromycine et sulfamide) et le renouvellement de la scène thérapeutique, peu de vaccins sont également ajoutés à celui empiriquement appliqué contre la variole depuis 1798[112]. Bien qu'au tournant du siècle, la plupart des bactéries propres aux différentes maladies contagieuses aient été identifiées, le microbe responsable de la rougeole restait aussi encore inconnu, même si l'on supposait fortement son existence.

La diphtérie, la scarlatine, la rougeole et l'érysipèle étaient parfois associées à d'autres maladies, contagieuses ou non (telles que le rachitisme, la tuberculose, l'herpès et la pneumonie, etc.) qui pouvaient compliquer le traitement. L'*Alexandra Hospital* a ainsi reçu plusieurs patients atteints à la fois de la scarlatine et de la rougeole durant l'année 1926.

L'emploi du sérum contre la rougeole a prévenu l'expansion de cette infection[113]. Par contre, le sérum antidiphtérique donnait des résultats beaucoup moins satisfaisants quand la diphtérie était associée à une autre maladie contagieuse. Le nombre d'accidents sérieux reliés à l'injection massive de ce sérum aurait été considérable[114]. Plusieurs traitements demeuraient également expérimentaux. Le traitement de l'érysipèle variait ainsi beaucoup d'un médecin à un autre : «les uns se contentaient de laisser le malade au lit et de prescrire une légère diète; les autres employaient des moyens locaux : des enveloppements, des pommades antiseptiques, des injections, la méthode Bier, la photothérapie, l'air chaud; d'autres encore préconisaient un sérum antistreptococcique, soit le sérum monovalent de Marmorek, soit le sérum polyvalent de Travel[115]».

L'étude des taux de mortalité est aussi significative de l'efficacité d'un hôpital à traiter les maladies. À Saint-Paul, le taux général de mortalité était, tout au long de la période considérée, autour de 8 à 10 %. Il a notamment été de 4.5 % en 1906, de 8.2 % en 1916, et de 9.7 % en 1927[116]. Ce taux de mortalité est comparable à celui de l'Hôpital Notre-Dame, de l'Hôtel-Dieu de Montréal et de l'Hôpital général de Montréal, lequel se situe autour de 7.5 %[117]. Le taux de mortalité était cependant moindre si l'on en soustrayait du décompte les patients décédés avant 48 heures de présence à l'hôpital. Il était ainsi d'environ 3.5 %. Notamment, il a été de 2.6 % en 1906, de 3.6 % en 1916 et de 3 % en 1925[118]. Cette dernière façon de comptabiliser la mortalité avait toutefois le défaut de soustraire du taux global certains décès qui pouvaient fort bien être la conséquence d'erreurs diagnostiques et thérapeutiques, de négligence dans les soins ou d'opérations chirurgicales manquées. Mais comme il arrivait fréquemment que les enfants entrent moribonds à l'hôpital, il s'avérait important que l'on identifie le taux de mortalité avant et après 48 heures de séjour à l'hôpital. En 1927, 22 des 41 patients décédés de diphtérie à l'*Alexandra Hospital* étaient ainsi décédés moins de 48 heures après leur admission à l'hôpital malgré des injections massives d'antitoxine par intraveineuse[119]. L'hospitalisation des malades dès les premières heures d'identification de la maladie était considérée, de fait, comme déterminante dans la guérison d'un patient. Les enfants les plus malades en point étaient généralement ceux qui provenaient des crèches[120]. Aussi, les médecins ont-ils insisté, à plus d'une reprise, sur l'importance d'une hospitalisation rapide des individus atteints de maladies contagieuses. Au début du XXe siècle, la négligence et l'ignorance de la population et de certains médecins à diagnostiquer les maladies contagieuses infantiles expliqueraient, selon les autorités médicales du Service de santé de Montréal, encore le recours trop souvent tardif à l'*Alexandra Hospital* et à l'Hôpital Saint-Paul[121]. Il ne faut cependant pas négliger le fait que plusieurs familles, sans être indigentes, ne pouvaient payer les coûts prohibitifs associés à l'époque à l'hospitalisation.

Enfin, les efforts pour juguler les épidémies ont été contrecarrés par le fait qu'il n'existait pas de telles institutions pour la population adulte. D'ailleurs, cette situation a certainement eu des répercussions sur le destin même des enfants qui s'avéraient ainsi plus susceptibles de contracter des maladies contagieuses. Pour la population adulte, la pratique d'ériger des hôpitaux temporaires seulement durant les périodes d'épidémie était encore en vigueur. Les hôpitaux généraux se sont néanmoins mobilisés, à maintes reprises, lors des épidémies, même si leurs règlements interdisaient l'hospitalisation de tels malades. Durant les décennies 1880–1920, les maladies infectieuses et les traumatismes accidentels ont notamment été les principales causes rapportées de mortalité à l'Hôpital Notre-Dame[122]. La fièvre typhoïde et la tuberculose y ont également constitué, à l'exception des cas d'alcoolisme, les deux maladies les plus fréquentes.

Les aléas techniques et administratifs ayant mené à la fermeture de l'Hôpital Saint-Paul

La construction et la prise en charge d'un hôpital pour contagieux par l'Hôpital Notre-Dame n'allaient pas être sans retombées sur ses propres services[123]. Certaines années, «le nombre de patients à l'Hôpital Saint-Paul atteignait presque 50 % de la population totale de l'Hôpital Notre-Dame[124]». La gestion financière de Saint-Paul, qui représente l'un des services les plus importants de l'Hôpital Notre-Dame en termes du nombre d'admissions de patients, a entraîné notamment un retard de près de vingt ans dans la construction de ses nouveaux pavillons sur la rue Sherbrooke[125].

Une analyse des dépenses réalisées à l'Hôpital Saint-Paul (1905–1934), classées sous différentes rubriques (besoins ménagers, domaine médical, transports, salaires, réparation et dettes et comptes divers), souligne par ailleurs l'investissement fort limité effectué dans le domaine médical, lequel comprend les dépenses relatives au laboratoire, à la pharmacie, à l'instrumentation, aux services des rayons X et à la sérothérapie. En fait, de toutes les rubriques considérées, seul le service des transports a engendré des dépenses moins importantes que ce dernier. Par exemple, en 1910, les rapports annuels de l'hôpital signalent que seulement 420 $ auraient été alloués au service de la pharmacie; ce montant augmente à 2 256 $ en 1917 et redescend à 1 764 $ en 1924. La situation est encore plus dramatique en ce qui concerne l'instrumentation : seulement 47 $ sont rapportés comme dépense en 1910, 458 $ en 1917, et

1 151 $ en 1924. Une correspondance en date du 30 novembre 1927 indique en cette matière que «les docteurs Simard et Charbonneau se sont plaints des conditions dans lesquelles se faisaient les autopsies à Saint-Paul, qui ne permettaient pas de recueillir ou conserver suffisamment de pièces utiles pour l'enseignement. Cette situation aurait entraîné l'autorisation de transporter de l'Hôpital Notre-Dame à Saint-Paul le matériel nécessaire lorsqu'une autopsie à cet endroit était jugée nécessaire»[126]. Quant aux allocations accordées pour les rayons X, elles n'apparaissent dans les rapports annuels qu'à partir de la décennie 1920; 719 $ sont notamment consacrés à ce service en 1921 et 660 $ en 1924. Nous pouvons donc affirmer, qu'en raison des faibles moyens financiers dont disposait l'hôpital, la médecine telle qu'elle se pratiquait à l'Hôpital Saint-Paul est demeurée, comme à l'Hôpital Notre-Dame, «à mi-chemin entre une médecine anatomo-clinique qui conserve une grande importance et une médecine de laboratoire qui tarde à se développer[127]».

Plus chanceux, l'*Alexandra Hospital* pouvait compter sur le soutien financier des membres de la communauté anglophone de Montréal. À titre d'exemple, le colonel Jeffrey Hale Burland et l'homme d'affaires James Ross ont ainsi versé, d'une façon récurrente jusqu'à leur décès, des dizaines de milliers de dollars aux divers hôpitaux anglophones dont ils ont été gouverneurs, y compris l'*Alexandra Hospital*. Néanmoins, cet hôpital allait connaître également, dans ses débuts, des déficits qui allaient nuire à son expansion. Ainsi, en 1909, le Dr Thomas Roddick, président du bureau des gouverneurs, suggérait la création de deux pavillons supplémentaires, le premier pour l'érysipèle, le second pour les patients atteints d'infections mixtes[128]. Cette suggestion allait cependant rester lettre morte.

La situation financière difficile de Saint-Paul et d'Alexandra poussera, à plus d'une reprise, la direction des hôpitaux à se concerter pour exiger que la ville de Montréal augmente le financement alloué pour leur fonctionnement. Ainsi, au début de 1907, dans une requête conjointe, les administrateurs des deux hôpitaux demandent que leur allocation annuelle passe de 15 000 $ à 30 000 $[129]. Leurs demandes recevront un accueil favorable de la part du maire de Montréal : l'allocation générale de 15 000 $ par année en 1905, qui couvre les frais de fonctionnement et de construction de l'hôpital, atteint ainsi 35 000 $ à partir de 1911[130]. La même année, l'allocation pour le supplément d'hospitalisation de 1.00 $ par patient et par jour – sur un total de 25 patients envoyés par jour par la municipalité – sera augmentée à 2.00 $ par patient et par jour pour un total de 35 patients; ce supplément passera à 2.50 $ en 1924[131], puis à 3.30 $ en 1929[132]. Les montants reçus pour le supplément d'hospitalisation ont fluctué de 6 000 $ à 17 000 $ par année pour les décennies 1910 et 1920.

Par ailleurs, le bureau d'administration de l'Hôpital Notre-Dame exige en 1916 un tarif uniforme de 2.00 $ par jour pour tout contagieux provenant d'une autre municipalité que Montréal[133]. Ce montant passe à 3.00 $ en 1921[134] puis à 4.00 $ en 1924, en plus des frais d'ambulance, de médicaments et de sérums[135]. On décide également d'augmenter les prix des chambres privées[136]. Néanmoins, les revenus perçus par l'Hôpital Saint-Paul en provenance d'autres sources que la ville de Montréal (clientèle privée et de municipalités avoisinantes, dons, frais de laboratoire et certificats de décès) restent dérisoires.

Certains problèmes se rapportant à la construction de l'Hôpital Saint-Paul (comme imperméabilité insuffisante de ses foundations et la déficience de son système de chauffage) marquent aussi d'une façon récurrente son fonctionnement, perturbant spécifiquement ses services médicaux[137]. Dès 1905, on signale que l'eau s'infiltre dans ses fondations[138]. Dans les années 1910, l'infrastructure de l'Hôpital Saint-Paul se dégrade d'une façon telle que des réparations importantes s'avèrent essentielles comme en témoigne une correspondance : «Trois ou quatre pieds d'eau dans les caves toute l'année, et jusqu'à la cheville dans les tunnels, chaque printemps, entretiennent une humidité et des fraîcheurs malsaines, et font que l'hygiène laisse beaucoup à désirer. La santé de nos gardes-malades, religieuses et laïques, en souffre d'autant et ce serait une faute contre la justice de n'y pas prendre garde. L'expérience de tous les jours laisse voir les lacunes de l'hôpital qui n'a pas encore toutes les pièces convenablement requises pour le service[139]». Tous les pavillons de Saint-Paul sont pratiquement remis à neuf[140]. Cependant, dès le milieu des années 1920, l'hôpital fait encore face aux mêmes difficultés. C'est pour remédier définitivement à cette situation, et afin d'éviter d'autres restaurations coûteuses, qu'un projet de construction d'un nouvel édifice à la fine pointe de l'innovation technologique et scientifique dans le domaine des maladies contagieuses est alors préconisé par les autorités de Notre-Dame. L'augmentation considérable des taux d'hospitalisation exigeait aussi l'élaboration d'un tel projet (d'une moyenne de 14.4 par jour en 1906, comparativement à 103 par jour en 1921).

Le nouvel hôpital pour contagieux envisagé par Notre-Dame afin de remplacer Saint-Paul comprenait quatre étages pouvant loger environ 284 malades, dont plus du quart en stage d'observation et d'isolement complet[141]. Il avait été planifié en fonction des plus récents modèles d'hôpitaux pour traiter les maladies contagieuses; une délégation de l'Hôpital Saint-Paul s'était rendue à Boston et à Providence pour étudier et inspecter certains de ces hôpitaux[142]. À la fin des années 1920, des démarches avec la ville de Montréal sont effectuées afin de concrétiser le projet, mais elles s'avèreront malheureusement infructueuses. En

1934, le contrat octroyé à Notre-Dame pour le fonctionnement de Saint-Paul n'est donc pas renouvelé, la Ville de Montréal ayant plutôt décidé d'accorder ses subventions à l'Hôpital Saint-Luc, lequel ouvrira un service pour les maladies contagieuses. Les rapports annuels nous signalent dès lors que les malades ont été transportés à l'Hôpital Pasteur, annexe de l'Hôpital Saint-Luc, et que les bâtiments de Saint-Paul sont demeurés vacants[143]. De plus, le personnel œuvrant dans ce dernier a majoritairement été transféré à l'Hôpital Pasteur, qui de 1934 à 1975, sera sous la surintendance médicale du Dr J. Henri Charbonneau[144]. L'enseignement clinique des maladies contagieuses était par ailleurs donné désormais à l'Hôpital Sainte-Justine, où un pavillon d'isolement d'une capacité de 60 lits avait notamment été ouvert en 1932[145]. Des services de neurologie, de dermato-syphilligraphie et de pédiatrie sont établis dans les anciens locaux de l'Hôpital Saint-Paul jusqu'à leur démolition en 1955 en vue de la construction du pavillon Lachapelle de l'Hôpital Notre-Dame, achevé en 1960[146]. À la fin des années 1970, l'ancien Hôpital Pasteur, désormais baptisé Centre Hospitalier J.-Henri Charbonneau, sera transformé en centre hospitalier de longue durée[147]. Pour sa part, l'*Alexandra Hospital* cessera d'admettre des contagieux en juin 1968[148].

Conclusion

Par le financement de l'Hôpital Saint-Paul et de l'*Alexandra Hospital*, la municipalité de Montréal démontrait sa volonté d'intervenir pour enrayer quelques-unes des plus importantes causes de mortalité infantile dans la population de la ville. Pour le début du siècle, il s'agissait d'un projet original, qui s'opposait à la pratique traditionnelle d'ouvrir des hôpitaux pour traiter les maladies contagieuses seulement en période d'épidémie. L'implantation d'hôpitaux pour soigner les enfants répondait aussi à un réel besoin, puisque cette population disposait de peu de services hospitaliers. Les représentants de la municipalité ont joué un rôle actif dans l'organisation des hôpitaux, siégeant par exemple aux délibérations des bureaux administratif et médical de l'Hôpital Notre-Dame lorsqu'il était question de l'Hôpital Saint-Paul. Ils n'ont pas hésité, à plus d'une reprise, à augmenter leurs subventions à Saint-Paul et Alexandra, ce qui leur a permis de mieux répondre à la demande sociale et de conserver majoritairement une clientèle de type public.

Les gouverneurs et les médecins des principaux hôpitaux anglophones de Montréal, ceux de l'Hôpital Notre-Dame ainsi que les Sœurs Grises, se sont associés à ces projets, en organisant des hôpitaux d'une capacité d'hospitalisation importante et d'une efficacité répondant aux standards de l'époque. Leurs démarches sont en ce sens significatives de l'intérêt d'instituer des hôpitaux modernes. L'architecture et le fonctionnement des meilleurs hôpitaux américains et européens dans le traitement des maladies contagieuses ont été scrutés avant d'édifier Saint-Paul et Alexandra; leurs directeurs médicaux ont été formés dans les meilleures écoles de l'époque; les religieuses-infirmières et les surintendantes se spécialisent dans les soins donnés aux malades contagieux. Saint-Paul et Alexandra sont des institutions qui se consacrent au traitement, mais aussi à la formation et à la recherche clinique. Ils possèdent un statut d'hôpitaux universitaires. Ces différentes fonctions leur ont permis de jouer un rôle actif dans la lutte contre les maladies contagieuses infantiles à Montréal : soignant les enfants, formant une relève en médecins et en infirmières spécialisés dans ce domaine, expérimentant et consolidant les méthodes de diagnostic et de traitement, et conscientisant la population à l'importance d'hospitaliser et de traiter dans les plus brefs délais les enfants atteints de maladies contagieuses.

L'implantation de l'Hôpital Saint-Paul et de l'*Alexandra Hospital* atteste de l'intérêt d'une élite de se donner plus d'outils en vue d'enrayer la mortalité infantile par maladies contagieuses. Ces projets s'insèrent dans un dispositif institutionnel plus vaste, établi à partir de la fin du XIXe siècle, visant à améliorer l'état de santé générale de la population. La marche pour juguler la mortalité relative aux épidémies s'est donc faite sur différents fronts à la fois. Sur le plan médical, la consolidation d'une infrastructure hospitalière et d'une expertise médicale s'est avérée souhaitable. Sur le plan sanitaire, un ensemble de mesures prophylactiques (telles que les Gouttes de lait, l'inspection médicale des écoles[149], et les infirmières visiteuses[150]) ont graduellement été développées pour améliorer le milieu environnant et éduquer la population[151]. Les limites de la science médicale entre les années 1905–1934 exigeaient d'autant plus l'installation d'une ingénierie sanitaire (système d'adduction d'eau et d'ébouage, purification de l'eau potable[152]).

L'effort des gouvernements et des médecins sera recompense, puisqu'on assiste dans les premières décennies du XXe siècle à une diminution substantielle des taux de mortalité. Ainsi, le taux de mortalité générale de 377 par 100 000 de population en 1896 sera de 236 en 1917, soit une diminution de 37.4 %. Durant cette période, les taux de mortalité reliés à la diphtérie et à la scarlatine enregistrent aussi une diminution de 85 % pour cette première maladie, et de 59 % pour la seconde[153]. Quant au taux de mortalité infantile à Montréal, de 301.5 par 1000 naissances en 1900, il sera de 42.2 en 1946[154]. L'*Alexandra Hospital* et l'Hôpital Saint-Paul, dont les fonctions sont reprises par l'Hôpital Pasteur (annexe de l'Hôpital Saint-Luc) après sa fermeture, ont été parmi les dispositifs qui ont permis, entre les années 1905 et 1934, de mieux contrôler les maladies contagieuses infantiles à Montréal. Leur influence sur le cours des épidémies hors des murs de la ville, sur l'organisation et le développement médical des hôpitaux du Québec, ainsi que les liens entre la construction de ces hôpitaux permanents et les besoins de l'enseignement clinique au début du XXᵉ siècle ne sont cependant que peu connus. L'histoire de l'Hôpital Pasteur et de l'*Alexandra Hospital* après 1934 est également méconnue. Les exemples de l'Hôpital Saint-Paul et de l'*Alexandra Hospital* révèlent ainsi l'intérêt de mieux cerner l'évolution des structures hospitalières mises en place dans la province au tournant du XXᵉ siècle pour contrer les maladies contagieuses, ainsi que de comparer l'évolution et l'impact du dispositif hospitalier et clinique avec celui établi dans d'autres provinces et pays.

Notes

1 Les auteurs remercient M. Othmar Keel et les deux évaluateurs anonymes du *Bulletin Canadien d'histoire de la médecine/ Canadian Bulletin of Medical History* pour leurs commentaires et suggestions ainsi que Magali Marc qui a procédé à une première correction du manuscrit. Nous voudrions par ailleurs dédier cet article à la mémoire de notre collègue, Céline Déziel, qui nous a malheureusement quitté récemment.

2 MartinTétreault, *L'état de santé des Montréalais de 1880 à 1914*, mémoire de MA, Université de Montréal, 1979, p. 102.

3 Terry Copp, *Classe ouvrière et pauvreté, les conditions de vie des travailleurs montréalais 1897–1929* (Montréal : Boréal Express, 1978), p. 88.

4 Jacques Bernier, *La médecine au Québec. Naissance et évolution d'une profession* (Québec : Les Presses de l'Université Laval, 1989), p. 146.

5 Pour un historique du développement des services d'hygiène publique au tournant du siècle, il est suggéré de se référer à Michael Farley, Peter Keating et Othmar Keel, «Les origines de l'action publique dans le domaine de la santé au Québec : Une critique du modèle explicatif par l'intervention de l'Etat à partir de la Révolution Tranquille», *Communication au Congrès de l'Association canadienne d'histoire de la science, de la médecine et de la technologie*, Kingston, 1984; James I. Gow, *Histoire de l'administration publique québécoise de 1867–1970* (Toronto et Montréal : L'Institut d'administration publique du Canada et Les Presses de l'Université de Montréal, 1986; Hervé Anctil et Marc-André Bluteau, *La santé et l'assistance publique au Québec, 1886–1986* (Québec : Santé Société, édition spéciale,1986); Michael Farley, Peter Keating et Othmar Keel, «La vaccination à Montréal dans la seconde moitié du XIXᵉ siècle : pratiques, obstacles et résistances» dans *Sciences et médecine au Québec. Perspectives socio-historiques*, dir. Marcel Fournier, Yves Gingras et Othmar Keel (Québec : Institut québécois de recherché sur la culture, 1987); Michael Farley, Othmar Keel et Camille Limoges, «Les commencements de l'administration montréalaise de la santé publique (1865–1885)», dans *Science, Technology and Medicine in Canada's Past : Selections from Scientia Canadensis*, dir. Richard A. Jarrel et James P. Hull (Thornhill : Sciencia Press, 1991) : 269–308; Benoit Gaumer, Georges Desrosiers, Othmar Keel et Céline Déziel, «Les services de santé de la ville de Montréal. De la mise sur pied au démantèlement», *Cahiers du Centre de recherches historiques (Écoles des Hautes Études en Science Sociale)*, 12 (avril 1994) : 131–158; Denis Goulet, Gilles Lemire et Denis Gauvreau, «Des bureaux d'hygiène municipaux aux unités sani-

taires. Le Conseil d'hygiène de la province de Québec et la structuration d'un système de santé publique 1886–1926», *Revue d'histoire d'Amérique française* 49, 4 (Printemps 1996) : 491–520; François Guérard, *Histoire de la santé au Québec* (Montréal : Boréal, 1996); François Guérard, «La formation des grands appareils sanitaires, 1800–1945» dans *L'institution médicale, Atlas historique du Québec*, dir. Normand Séguin (Sainte-Foy : Les Presses de l'Université Laval, 1998) : 75–106; Georges Desrosiers, Benoit Gaumer et Othmar Keel, *La santé publique au Québec. Histoire des unités sanitaires de comté : 1926–1975* (Montréal : Les Presses de l'Université de Montréal, 1998); George Desrosiers, Benoit Gaumer, François Hudon et Othmar Keel, «Les renforcements des interventions gouvernementales dans le domaine de la santé entre 1922 et 1936 : Le Service provincial d'Hygiène de la province de Québec», *Bulletin canadien d'histoire de la médecine/Canadian Bulletin of Medical History* 17,1 (2001) : 205–240; et Benoit Gaumer, Georges Desrosiers et Othmar Keel, *Histoire du Service de santé de la ville de Montréal* (Québec : Les éditions de l'IQRC, 2002).

6   Denis Goulet et André Paradis, *Trois siècles d'histoire médicale au Québec. Chronologie des pratiques et des institutions* (Montréal : VLB éditeurs, 1992).

7   Denis Goulet et Othmar Keel, «Les hommes-relais de la bactériologie en territoire québécois et l'introduction de nouvelles pratiques diagnostiques et thérapeutiques (1890–1920)», *Revue d'histoire de l'Amérique française* 46, 3 (1993) : 417–442.

8   Jessie Boyd Scriver, *The Montreal Children's Hospital: Years of Growth* (Montréal: McGill Queen's University Press, 1979).

9   Rita Desjardins, *Hôpital Sainte-Justine, Montréal, Québec (1907–1921)*, mémoire de MA, Université de Montréal, 1989. Du même auteur : *L'Institutionnalisation de la pédiatrie en milieu franco-montréalais, 1880–1980. Les enjeux politiques, sociaux et biologiques*, thèse de doctorat, Université de Montréal, 1999.

10   J.-E. Dubé, «Les débuts de la lutte contre la mortalité infantile à Montréal. Fondation de la première Goutte de lait», *Union Médicale du Canada* 65 (1936) : 879–891.

11   Denyse Baillargeon, «Fréquenter les Gouttes de lait. L'expérience des mères montréalaises 1910–1965», *Revue d'histoire de l'Amérique française* 50, 1 (1996) : 29–68. Également de Baillargeon, «Gouttes de lait et soif de pouvoir. Les dessous de la lutte contre la mortalité infantile à Montréal, 1910–1953», *Bulletin canadien d'histoire de la médecine/Canadian Bulletin of Medical History* 15,1 (1998) : 27–57.

12   Pour une bibliographie assez exhaustive de l'histoire de la médecine et de la santé au Québec, il est suggéré de se référer à Peter Keating et Othmar Keel, «Introduction», dans *Santé et société au Québec, XIXe-XXe siècle*, dir. Keating et Keel (Montréal : Boréal, 1995) : 9–34; François Guérard, «Ville et santé au Québec. Un bilan de la recherche historique», *Revue d'Histoire de l'Amérique française*, 53,1 (1999) : 19–46; et Également de François Guérard, «L'histoire de la santé au Québec : filiations et spécificités», *Bulletin canadien d'histoire de la médecine/Canadian Bulletin of Medical History* 17, 1–2 (2000) : 55–72.

13   Denis Goulet et Othmar Keel, «Généalogie des représentations et des attitudes face aux épidémies au Québec depuis le XIX siècle», *Anthropologie et Société*, 15 (1991) : 205–228.

14   Pour un aperçu des liens entre la lutte contre la mortalité infantile et le nationalisme canadien-français, voir le texte de Denyse Baillargeon, «Entre la "Revanche" et la "Veillée" des berceaux: Les médecins québécois francophones, la mortalité infantile et la question nationale, 1910–1940» dans le présent ouvrage.

15 Yolande Cohen et Michèle Gélinas, «Les infirmières hygiénistes de la Ville de Montréal : du service privé au service civique», *Histoire sociale/Social History* 22, 44 (novembre 1989) : 219–246.

16 Denyse Baillargeon, «Fréquenter les Gouttes de lait» et «Gouttes de lait».

17 Rita Desjardins, *Hôpital Sainte-Justine, Montréal, Québec (1907–1921)*, mémoire de MA, Université de Montréal, 1989.

18 L'Hôpital Saint-Paul est ainsi dénommé en l'honneur de l'Archevêque de Montréal, Mgr Paul Bruchési, qui avait fortement soutenu ce projet.

19 Voir à ce sujet Goulet et Paradis, *Trois siècles d'histoire*, p. 131 et 133.

20 J. A. Lesage, «Le projet d'hôpital pour les maladies contagieuses à Montréal», *Union Médicale du Canada* 30, 3 (Mars 1901) : 176.

21 Archives de l'Hôpital Notre-Dame, *Procès-verbaux du Bureau d'administration de l'Hôpital Notre-Dame*, 22 décembre 1902. Nous avons consulté les procès-verbaux des années 1900–1934.

22 Pour un historique de l'Hôpital Notre-Dame : Lucie Deslauriers, *Histoire de l'Hôpital Notre-Dame, 1880–1924*, mémoire de MA, Université de Montréal, 1985; Denis Goulet, François Hudon et Othmar Keel, *Histoire de l'Hôpital Notre-Dame de Montréal, 1880–1980* (Montréal : VLB éditeur, 1993); et François Hudon, *L'Hôpital comme microcosme de la société : Enjeux institutionnels et besoins sociaux à l'Hôpital Notre-Dame de Montréal, 1880–1960*, thèse de doctorat, Université de Montréal, 1997. Pour un historique de l'Hôpital Saint-Paul, voir : Marie-Josée Fleury, *L'Hôpital Saint-Paul (1905–1934) et sa contribution à la prévention et à la lutte contre les maladies contagieuses*, mémoire de MA, Université de Montréal, 1993.

23 Goulet et Paradis, *Trois siècles d'histoire*, p. 258.

24 Goulet, Hudon et Keel, *Histoire de l'Hôpital Notre-Dame*, p. 88–89.

25 Maude Abbott, *History of the Medicine in the Province of Quebec* (Montréal : McGill University Press, 1931), p. 85; et Goulet et Paradis, *Trois siècles d'histoire*, p. 132.

26 Edward Seaborne Clouston a été directeur de la Banque de Montréal. En plus de l'*Alexandra Hospital*, il a fait partie du Conseil d'administration de six autres hôpitaux de Montréal. Carman Miller, «Edward Seaborne Clouston», *Dictionnaire biographique du Canada, XIV* (Québec, Toronto : Les Presses de l'Université Laval/ University of Toronto Press, 1998), p. 239–242.

27 Theodore D. Regehr, «James Ross», *Dictionnaire biographique du Canada, XIV* (Québec, Toronto : Les Presses de l'Université Laval/ University of Toronto Press, 1998), p. 977–980.

28 Peter Keating, «Jeffrey Hale Burland», *Dictionnaire biographique du Canada, XIV* (Québec, Toronto : Les Presses de l'Université Laval/ University of Toronto Press, 1998), p. 173–174.

29 Archives de l'Hôpital Notre-Dame, *Procès-verbaux du Bureau d'administration de l'Hôpital Notre-Dame*, 12 novembre 1907.

30 *Rapport du Service de santé de la Cité de Montréal, 1918*, (Montréal : 1919), p. 23.

31 *Rapport du Service de santé de la Cité de Montréal, 1927*, (Montréal : 1928), p. 63.

32 Archives de l'Hôpital Notre-Dame, *Procès-verbal du Bureau d'administration de l'Hôpital Notre-Dame*, 3 mars 1903.

33 *Rapport du Bureau municipal d'hygiène et de statistique de Montréal, 1917* (Montréal : 1918), p. 43.

34 *Rapport du Service de santé de la Cité de Montréal, 1921* (Montréal : 1922), p. 35. Les rapports annuels du service de santé de Montréal ne font pas de distinction entre les gens d'origine israélite et ceux dont le judaïsme était la religion.

35 *Rapport sur l'état sanitaire de la cité de Montréal, 1909* (Montréal : 1910), p. 33–34.

36 *4th Annual Report of the Alexandra Hospital for Infectious and Contagious Diseases, 1909* (Montréal : 1910), p. 12.

37 *Rapport du service de santé de la cité de Montréal, 1923* (Montréal : 1924), p. 55.
38 *30ᵉ Rapport annuel de l'Hôpital Notre-Dame, 1910* (Montréal : 1911), p. 110
39 *5th Annual Report of the Alexandra Hospital, 1910* (Montréal : 1911), p. 8.
40 Une description détaillée ainsi des photographies de ces hôpitaux se retrouve dans le *12ᵉ rapport annuel du Conseil d'hygiène de la province de Québec, 1905–06* (Québec : 1906), p. 41–51.
41 Pour un tableau plus détaillé des hôpitaux pour enfants, voir le texte d'Annmarie Adams et de David Theodore, «The Architecture of Children's Hospitals in Toronto and Montreal, 1875–2010», dans le présent ouvrage.
42 *Alexandra Hospital for Infectious and Contagious Diseases, 8th Annual Report, 1913* (Montréal : 1914), p. 6.
43 *Alexandra Hospital, 27th Annual Report, 1932* (Montréal : 1933), p. 12.
44 J.-A. Leduc, «L'infirmière préposée à la garde des contagieux», *La garde-malade canadienne-française* 1,1 (janvier 1928) : 45–47.
45 Lucie Deslauriers, «L'Hôpital Saint-Paul», *Bulletin*, 6 (31 juillet 1979): 13.
46 *Alexandra Hospital for Contagious Diseases, 21th Annual Report, 1926* (Montréal : 1927), p. 10.
47 Catherine Braithwaite, Peter Keating et Sandi Viger, «The Problem of Diphteria in the Province of Quebec: 1894–1909», *Histoire sociale/Social History* 29, 57 (mai 1996) : 71–95.
48 J.-A. Leduc, «Le signe de Koplik- son importance pour le diagnostic précoce de la rougeole», *Le Journal de médecine et de chirurgie*, 6, 1 (janvier 1911): 11–13.
49 *26ᵉ Rapport annuel de l'Hôpital Notre-Dame, 1906* (Montréal : 1907), p. 125.
50 J.-A. Lesage, «Le traitement de la sclarlatine, hygiène, sérothérapie», *L'Union médicale du Canada*, 32, 1 (janvier 1903) : 33–39.
51 André Petitat, *Les infirmières de la vocation à la profession* (Montréal : Boréal, 1989).
52 Yolande Cohen, «La contribution des sœurs de la Charité à la modernisation de l'Hôpital Notre-Dame 1880–1940, *The Canadian Historical Review*, 77, 2 (June 1996) : 185–220. Sur la formation des infirmières francophones, il est également suggéré de consulter Yolande Cohen, Jacinthe Pépin, Esther Lamontagne et André Duquette, *Les sciences infirmières. Genèse d'une discipline* (Montréal : Les Presses de l'Université de Montréal, 2002).
53 Yolande Cohen, «La modernisation des soins infirmiers dans la province de Québec (1880–1930). Un enjeu de négociation entre professionnels», *Sciences sociales et santé* 13, 3 (1995) : 11–32.
54 Yolande Cohen, *Profession infirmière. Une histoire des soins dans les hôpitaux du Québec* (Montréal : Les Presses de l'Université de Montréal, 2000), p. 54–55. Également, Yolande Cohen et Louise Bienvenue, «Émergence de l'identité professionnelle chez les infirmières professionnelles, 1890–1927», *Bulletin canadien d'histoire de la médecine/Canadian Bulletin of Medical History* 11, 1 (1994) : 119–151.
55 Édouard Desjardins, Ellen C. Flanagan et Suzanne Giroux, *Heritage : History of the Nursing Profession in Quebec from the Augustinians and Jeanne Mance to Medicare* (Montréal : The Association of Nurses of the Province of Quebec, 1971), p. 167; Louise Bienvenue, «Le rôle du Victorian Order of Nurses dans la croisade hygiéniste montréalaise (1877–1925)», mémoire de MA, Université du Québéc à Montréal, 1995, p. 141.
56 *1st Annual Report of the Alexandra Hospital, 1906* (Montréal : 1907), p. 8.
57 Goulet et Paradis, p. 438.
58 Scriver, *The Montreal Children's Hospital*, p. 96.
59 En 1896, l'*American Paediatric Society* a tenu son 8ᵉ congrès à Montréal. Goulet et Paradis, *Trois siècles d'histoire*, p. 353.

60 Desjardins, *L'institutionnalisation de la pédiatrie*, p. 377–383.

61 *The Canadian Medical Association Journal* 34, 5 (May 1932): 519–524.

62 Scriver, *The Montreal Children's Hospital*, p. 136.

63 John F. Prescott, «John McCrae», *Dictionnaire biographique du Canada*, *XIV* (Québec, Toronto, Presses de l'Université Laval/University of Toronto Press, 1998), p. 739–740.

64 *5th Annual Report of the Alexandra Hospital, 1910* (Montréal : 1911).

65 Goulet, Hudon et Keel, *Histoire de l'Hôpital Notre-Dame*.

66 J. Henri Charbonneau, «In Memoriam, Joseph-Arthur Leduc (1877–1955)», *L'Union médicale du Canada* 85, 2 (février 1956) : 117–118.

67 Johanne Collin et Denis Béliveau, *Histoire de la pharmacie au Québec* (Montréal : Musée de la pharmacie du Québec, 1994), p. 228.

68 Goulet et Paradis, *Trois siècles d'histoire*, p. 261.

69 Pierrick Malissard, *Quand les universitaires se font entrepreneurs. Les laboratoires Connaught et l'Institut de microbiologie et d'hygiène de l'Université de Montréal*, thèse de doctorat, Université du Québéc à Montréal, 1999, p. 42–44. Voir également, Armand Frappier, *Un rêve, une lutte. Autobiographie*, (Sillery : Presses de l'Université du Québec, 1992) p. 112–113.

70 Marcel Fournier, Annick Germain, Yves Lamarche et Louis Maheu, «Le champ scientifique québécois : Structure, fonctionnement et fonctions», *Sociologie et sociétés* 7, 1 (mai 1975) : 119–132.

71 *24ᵉ Rapport annuel de l'Hôpital Notre-Dame, 1903–1904* (Montréal : 1904), p. 19.

72 *47ᵉ Rapport annuel de l'Hôpital Notre-Dame, 1927* (Montréal : 1928), p. 12.

73 Michel Foucault, *Naissance de la clinique* (Paris : Les Presses universitaires de France, 1963).

74 *Alexandra Hospital for Contagious Diseases, 21st Annual Report, 1926* (Montréal : 1927), p. 18.

75 Goulet, Hudon et Keel, *Histoire de l'Hôpital Notre-Dame*, p. 151.

76 Pierre Lereboulet, «Le traitement actuel de la diphtérie», *10ᵉ Congrès de l'Association des médecins de langue française de l'Amérique du Nord, Québec, 1928* (Québec : 1929) : 101–111.

77 Sur l'introduction au Québec du sérum anti-diphtérique, Braithwaite, Keating et Viger, «The Problem of Diptheria», p. 71–95.

78 Pierre Lereboullet et George Schreiber, «Les maladies des enfants en 1913», *Journal de médecine et de chirurgie* 9, 1 (janvier 1913) : 1–23.

79 Daniel Longpré, «Historique de la diphtérie», *L'Union médicale du Canada* 62, 4 (avril 1933) : 365–369.

80 J. Henri Charbonneau, «In Memoriam», p. 117–118.

81 *Alexandra Hospital for Contagious Diseases, 21st Annual Report*, 1926 (Montréal : 1927) p. 11.

82 Gaston Lapierre, «Prophylaxie de la diphtérie», *10e Congrès de l'Association des médecins de langue française de l'Amérique du Nord, Québec, 1928* (Québec : 1929) : 112–117. C'est également à l'École d'Hygiène sociale et appliquée que le Dr J.-Albert Baudouin a réalisé, en 1926, les premières expérimentations du vaccin BCG (Bacille Calmette et Guérin) contre la tuberculose.

83 Harold B. Cushing et Daniel Longpré, «Le sérum antiscarlatineux, ses usages», *L'Union médicale du Canada*, 55, 1 (janvier 1926) : 8–14.

84 *Alexandra Hospital for Contagious Diseases, 21st Annual Report*, 1926 (Montréal : 1927) p. 10.

85 *Alexandra Hospital for Contagious Diseases, 22nd Annual Report, 1927* (Montréal : 1928), p. 11.

86 *Alexandra Hospital for Contagious Diseases, 19th Annual Report, 1924* (Montréal : 1925), p. 8.

87 «Le sérum antistreptoccoccique dans le traitement de l'érysipèle», *L'Union médicale du Canada* 41, 4 (avril 1912) : 225–226.

88 P. Del Vecchio, «La coqueluche- quelques considérations pratiques», *L'Union médicale du Canada* 49, 3 (1920) : 606–311.

89 Charbonneau, «In Memoriam», p. 117–118.

90 Roger Champoux, «Derrière de vieux murs», *La Presse*, 1 octobre 1952.

91 Roger Champoux, «Un médecin a vu naître et mourir un grand hôpital», *La Presse*, 3 octobre 1952.

92 Denis Goulet, *Histoire de la Faculté de Médecine de l'Université de Montréal, 1843–1993* (Montréal : VLB éditeur, 1993), p. 132.

93 Céline Déziel, *L'enseignement clinique à l'Hôpital Notre-Dame de 1880 à 1924*, mémoire de MA, Université de Montréal, 1992, p. 71.

94 Desjardins, «Hôpital Sainte-Justine», p. 149.

95 Denis Goulet, *Histoire de la Faculté*, p. 198–202.

96 *McGill University, Annual Calendar for Session 1909–1910 with Pass Lists for Session 1908–1909* (Montréal : 1909), p. 298.

97 David Sclater Lewis, *Royal Victoria Hospital. 1887–1947* (Montréal : McGill University Press, 1969), p. 182.

98 *41ᵉ Rapport annuel de l'Hôpital Notre-Dame*, 1921, p. 44.

99 *47ᵉ Rapport de l'Hôpital Notre-Dame*, 1927, p. 44.

100 «Historique de la sixième école de gardes-malades canadienne-française : Hôpital des docteurs Normand et Cross aux Trois-Rivières», *La garde-malade canadienne-française*, 1, 6 (juin 1928) : 20–21.

101 Cohen, «La modernisation», p. 11–32.

102 *Alexandra Hospital for Contagious Diseases, 19th Annual Report, 1924* (Montréal : 1925), p. 17.

103 *Alexandra Hospital for Contagious Diseases, 23th Annual Report, 1928* (Montréal : 1929), p. 15.

104 *Alexandra Hospital for Contagious Diseases, 22th Annual Report, 1927* (Montréal : 1928), p. 10.

105 *Alexandra Hospital for Contagious Diseases, 28th Annual Report, 1933* (Montréal : 1934), p. 11.

106 *Alexandra Hospital for Contagious Diseases, 19th Annual Report, 1924* (Montréal : 1925), p. 17.

107 *Alexandra Hospital for Contagious Diseases, 21th Annual Report, 1926* (Montréal : 1927), p. 15.

108 *Alexandra Hospital for Contagious Diseases, 27th Annual Report, 1933* (Montréal : 1934), p. 11.

109 *Alexandra Hospital for Contagious Diseases, 19th Annual Report, 1924* (Montréal : 1925), p. 17.

110 *Alexandra Hospital for Contagious Diseases, 27th Annual Report, 1933* (Montréal : 1934), p. 12.

111 *Alexandra Hospital for Contagious Diseases, 27th Annual Report, 1933* (Montréal : 1934), p. 12.

112 Michael Farley, Peter Keating et Othmar Keel, «La vaccination à Montréal dans la seconde moitié du XIXᵉ siècle : Pratiques, obstacles et résistances» dans *Sciences et médecine*, dir. Fournier, Gingras et Keel, p. 87–115.

113 *Alexandra Hospital for Contagious Diseases, 21st Annual Report, 1926* (Montréal : 1927), p. 11.

114 G. Lapierre, «État actuel de la prophylaxie de la diphtérie», *Les Annales médico-chirurgicales de l'Hôpital Sainte-Justine* 1, 1 (mai 1930) : 28–50.

115 «Le sérum antistreptoccoccique dans le traitement de l'érysipèle», *L'Union médicale du Canada* 41, 4 (avril 1912) : 225.

116 *Rapports annuels de l'Hôpital Notre-Dame*, 1905–1934.

117 Goulet, Hudon et Keel, *Histoire de l'Hôpital Notre-Dame*, p. 217–218.

118 *Rapports annuels de l'Hôpital Notre-Dame*, 1905–1934.

119 *Alexandra Hospital for Contagious Diseases, 22*nd *Annual Report, 1927* (Montréal : 1928), p. 6.

120 *Alexandra Hospital for Contagious Diseases, 21st Annual Report, 1926* (Montréal : 1927), p. 10.

121 A. E. Laberge, «Diagnostic des maladies contagieuses», *L'Union médicale du Canada* 49, 1 (janvier 1920) : 11–25.

122 Denis Goulet et Othmar Keel, «Santé publique, histoire des travailleurs et histoire hospitalière : Sources et méthodologie», *Bulletin du Regroupement des chercheurs-chercheuses en histoire des travailleurs et travailleuses du Québec* 16, 2–3 (1990) : 47–48 et 67–80.

123 Sur le financement de l'Hôpital Notre-Dame, voir François Hudon, *L'Hôpital comme microcosme*.

124 Deslauriers, *Histoire de l'Hôpital Notre-Dame*, p. 125.

125 *30ᵉ rapport annuel de l'Hôpital Notre-Dame, 1910* (Montréal : 1911), p. 24–25.

126 Archives de l'Hôpital Notre-Dame, *Correspondance*, 30 novembre 1927.

127 Goulet, Hudon et Keel, *Histoire de l'Hôpital Notre-Dame*, p. 158.

128 *4th Annual Report of the Alexandra Hospital for Infectious and Contagious Diseases, 1909* (Montréal : 1910), p. 8

129 Archives de l'Hôpital Notre-Dame, *Procès-verbal du Bureau d'administration de l'Hôpital Notre-Dame*, 10 janvier 1907.

130 *31ᵉ rapport annuel de l'Hôpital Notre-Dame*, 1911 (Montréal : 1912), p. 33.

131 *Alexandra Hospital for Contagious Diseases, 19*th *Annual Report, 1924* (Montréal : 1925), p. 9–10.

132 Archives de l'Hôpital Notre-Dame, *Procès-verbal du Bureau d'administration de l'Hôpital Notre-Dame*, 19 décembre 1929.

133 Archives de l'Hôpital Notre-Dame, *Procès-verbal du Bureau d'administration de l'Hôpital Notre-Dame*, 10 janvier 1907.

134 Archives de l'Hôpital Notre-Dame, *Procès-verbal du Bureau d'administration de l'Hôpital Notre-Dame*, 27 avril 1921.

135 Archives de l'Hôpital Notre-Dame, *Procès-verbal du Bureau d'administration de l'Hôpital Notre-Dame*, 19 novembre 1924.

136 Archives de l'Hôpital Notre-Dame, *Procès-verbal du Bureau d'administration de l'Hôpital Notre-Dame*, 28 août 1915.

137 Archives de l'Hôpital Notre-Dame, *Procès-verbal du Bureau d'administration de l'Hôpital Notre-Dame*, 9 juin 1920.

138 Archives de l'Hôpital Notre-Dame, *Procès-verbal du Bureau d'administration de l'Hôpital Notre-Dame*, 20 juin 1905.

139 Archives de l'Hôpital Notre-Dame, *Correspondance, Lettre de la mère générale des sœurs grises au surintendant de l'Hôpital Saint-Paul, 18 mars 1913.*

140 *45ᵉ Rapport annuel de l'Hôpital Notre-Dame*, 1925 (Montréal : 1926), p. 50.

141 Archives de l'Hôpital Notre-Dame, *Procès-verbal du Bureau d'administration de l'Hôpital Notre-Dame*, 21 mars 1930.

142 Archives de l'Hôpital Notre-Dame, *Procès-verbal du Bureau d'administration de l'Hôpital Notre-Dame*, 12 septembre 1929.

143 *Rapports annuels de l'Hôpital Notre-Dame,* 1930–1934.

144 Diplômé de l'Université de Montréal en 1927, le Dr Charbonneau a complété des études à Londres, à Paris, à Strasbourg et à Boston. De 1952 à 1963, il a été directeur du département de pédiatrie de l'Université de Montréal. Il a aussi été président de la Société canadienne de pédiatrie en 1958–59. *L'Union médicale du Canada* 104, 11 (novembre 1975) : 1730–1732.

145 Desjardins, *L'institutionnalisation de la pédiatrie,* p. 344.

146 Deslauriers, «L'Hôpital Saint-Paul», *Bulletin,* 6 (31 juillet 1979).

147 Depuis 1998, suite à la fusion de différents établissements, le Centre Hospitalier J.Henri Charbonneau est l'un des pavillons du Centre hospitalier de soins de longue durée Lucille-Teasdale.

148 *Rapport du service de santé de la ville de Montréal, 1968–1969* (Montréal : 1969), p. 93.

149 Desjardins, *L'institutionnalisation de la pédiatrie,* 1999, p. 87–93.

150 Denyse Baillargeon, «Les rapports médecins-infirmières et l'implication de la Métropolitaine dans la lutte contre la mortalité infantile, 1909–1953», *Canadian Historical Review* 77, 1 (mars 1996) : 33–61; Bienvenue, *Le rôle du Victorian Order of Nurses,* p.141; et Cohen et Gélinas, «Les infirmières hygiénistes», 219–246.

151 Denis Goulet et Othmar Keel, «Généalogie des représentations», p. 205–228.

152 Ginette Gagnon, *L'aqueduc de Montréal au tournant du siècle (1890–1914) : l'établissement de la purification de l'eau potable,* mémoire de MA, Université de Montréal, 1998.

153 J.A. Baudouin, «Prophylaxie des maladies contagieuses», *L'Union médicale du Canada* 49, 1 (janvier 1920) : 28–41.

154 Adélard Groulx, «Extrait d'une conférence prononcée au dîner-causerie des fonctionnaires municipaux au Ritz Carlton», *Bribes d'histoire,* le 30 avril 1947.

The Architecture of Children's Hospitals in Toronto and Montreal, 1875–2010

∾

Annmarie Adams and
David Theodore

T his paper explores more than a century of changing ideas about the health of Canadian children through the architecture of three urban hospitals: one in Toronto, the Hospital for Sick Children (founded in 1875; known as the "Victoria" Hospital for Sick Children until 1912), and two in Montreal, the Children's Memorial Hospital (founded in 1903, its name changed to the Montreal Children's Hospital in 1954), and Hôpital Ste-Justine (1907). Hospital architecture is complex and multi-layered. What do visual sources concerning hospital design tell us about the history of children's medicine?

This question is not as straightforward as it appears, for the architectural history of the Canadian children's hospital since its beginning in the late nineteenth century sometimes contradicts and sometimes reinforces the more familiar stories of the emergence of pediatric specialties, the profound changes to the health, welfare, and education of Canadian children, and the history of the general hospital. For example, in their chapter Grenier and Fleury characterize the building of Montreal's two contagious disease hospitals, the Alexandra Hospital and l'Hôpital Saint-Paul, as a progressive moment in the struggle to control or even eradicate infectious disease among children. The architecture of the buildings, however, is evidence of more conservative, or at best ambivalent, attitudes towards understanding the causes of disease and promoting scientific explanations of health and illness: even the pavilion-plan layouts of the buildings rely on an outdated miasma theory of disease.[1] Furthermore, as Stephen Verderber and David J. Fine have argued in their study of the general hospital, revolutions in hospital design tend to come from experienced architects attacking the problem of health care for the first time, rather than from hospital design specialists or medical advisers.[2] Thus changes in the architecture of the children's hospital are perhaps more influenced by changes in architectural practice than they are by evolving structures of medical practice, childhood reform movements, or the reorientation of the hospital from a charitable to a scientific institution.

Moreover, research using architectural sources into the history of the general hospital in the important half-century from 1890 to 1940 reveals something different from the canonical story told from the textual sources by historians such as Charles Rosenberg, Rosemary Stevens, Morris J. Vogel, and more recently Guenter B. Risse.[3] Scholars of individual Canadian hospitals, too, such as J. T. H. Connor, David Gagan, Rosemary Gagan, Denis Goulet, and James de Jonge have followed the international lead in describing how the hospital made a concerted, smooth transition from charity to science, from a marginal benevolent institution to a vital medical centre.[4] But in fact architectural evidence shows a resistance to the idea of a modern, scientific medical centre. It was not until the postwar era that modernist design in the exterior image of the hospital was used to promote the modern hospital. In the interwar period, conservative, historicist exteriors were used to comfort patients and visitors, please patrons, and solidify the social status of the institution. There was a self-conscious use of architectural forms to perpetuate and symbolize traditional spatial and social orders, perhaps as a defence against fears about urbanization and industrialization.[5]

Like their counterparts throughout the Western world, acute-care Canadian children's hospitals have their roots in late-Victorian child rescue movements, beginnings the children's hospital shares with other non-medical institutions such as orphanages, schools, and day nurseries.[6] This makes the children's hospital stand out from other specialist hospitals. As historian Lindsay Granshaw has noted about specialist hospitals in Britain, most were set up "not by lay philanthropists but by medical men."[7] Pediatrics as a specialty has its origin neither in connection to particular diseases or organs (like tuberculosis) nor in the application of specific technologies (such as surgery or radiology), but rather in a meliorist program for the social reform of childhood.[8] In turn, specialist children's hospitals have their origins in benevolence, not medical specialization.

The early proponents of Canadian children's hospitals, then, worked towards an identity that differs from other acute-care hospitals, specialist and general, for social reasons, and differs from social institutions for medico-scientific reasons. But throughout the century, sick children have been fittingly accommodated outside of the specialist hospital. Infants are often housed with mothers in women's hospitals, older children in wards in general hospitals, in convalescent and chronic care homes, and in non-acute-care institutions such as Shriners' hospitals. Communities with many general hospitals—Winnipeg, Calgary, Halifax, and Vancouver—typically have only one autonomous children's facility. Thus the task of making broad conclusions about the history of children's hospitals is further complicated by their relative rarity.

For pediatric architecture, the twentieth century ended remarkably close to where it began, with Canadian sick children cared for in both general and specialized facilities. During the interwar and post–Second World War periods, however, young patients in Montreal and Toronto mostly went to separate, specialized institutions. A range of architectural types also flourished, expressing conflicting benevolent and scientific mandates for the children's hospital. Indeed, these buildings illustrate a continuous tension between romantic, playful, special places designed for children, and more hard-edged, scientific, "serious" spaces, modelled on the acute-care general hospital. A home for children or an institution devoted to science? This is the central, continuing dichotomy of the Canadian children's hospital in the twenty-first century.

The Victorian Hospital

The accommodation for children within the nineteenth-century general hospital illustrates how and why separate, purpose-built pavilions for children were considered unnecessary in Montreal as the century drew to a close. At the Royal Victoria Hospital (RVH), opened in 1893, for example, young patients were integrated with adults in the rather sprawling, pavilion-plan structure built on the southern slopes of Mount Royal.[9] Apart from a dedicated children's surgical ward in a short extension behind the general surgical wards, young patients were accorded few special spaces, diagnostic or therapeutic, in the new building.[10]

In fact, the RVH as planned was a generalized machine for healing. The most prominent features of the design by British architect Henry Saxon Snell were the large, open "Nightingale" wards, which housed surgical and medical patients on either side of a central administration block, to which they were minimally connected. The ward itself functioned as an instrument by which patients could be carefully positioned in space, according to the gravity of their condition, rather than by their age or gender. As Lindsay Prior (and many Victorian hospital architects) has noted, the key dimensions of the ward were the distances between beds, the heights of ceilings, and the relationship between windows and beds.[11] Also fundamental to its efficient operation was the spatial relationship between the patients' beds and the nurses' station or desk.

Early photographs show the general layout of these huge rooms. White metal beds were arranged along the exterior walls of the long and narrow wards.[12] Most photos show a less-than-ideal arrangement by which more than one bed was positioned between windows. The circu-

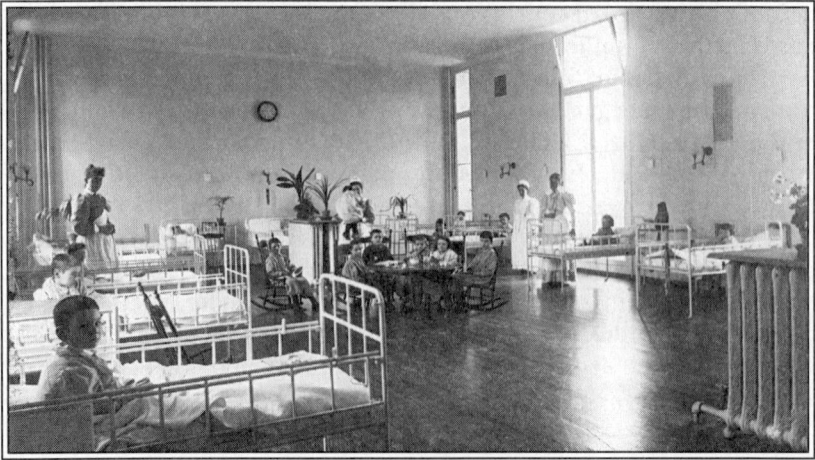

Figure 1. Children's ward, Royal Victoria Hospital, 1894 (II-105910, Notman Photographic Archives, McCord Museum of Canadian History, Montreal)

lation area in the centre of the ward, defined by the ends of the beds, was typically peppered with rocking chairs, as well as desks and tables for nurses. The gigantic central radiators, topped with marble slabs, became makeshift tables.[13] A large round institutional clock hung at the south end of the wards. Nearly every extant photo shows the space embellished with plants, perhaps in an effort to soften the room's institutional appearance.

Few photographs have survived illustrating the spaces occupied by children at the Royal Victoria; fortunately, one includes children and staff.[14] William Notman's stunning 1894 photograph (figure 1) reveals one end of a pavilion-style ward, with four adult women, twelve beds, and seventeen children. The clock, plants, and marble-topped radiators are identical to those found in the adult wards, as shown in images like the 1912 photo of the men's typhoid Ward N. Indeed, Ward N was converted to the children's ward in 1919.[15] Not surprisingly, Notman photographed the children's ward with its windows open, pointing out the fundamental concern with fresh air and ventilation. What differentiates this photo from images of other adult hospital wards is the recreational use of the space between the radiators. Notman's photo shows six children, seated in small rockers, enjoying tea at a table specially scaled for them with a tiny tea service.

It is important to keep in mind that the typical North American hospital of the 1890s was a marginal custodial institution, essentially a charity for the sick poor.[16] Parents who could afford medical care at home would never send their children to a hospital, at least until after the First World War. Effective therapy, or even accurate diagnosis, was rare. As Deborah Dwork has noted, "Hospitals were important in that

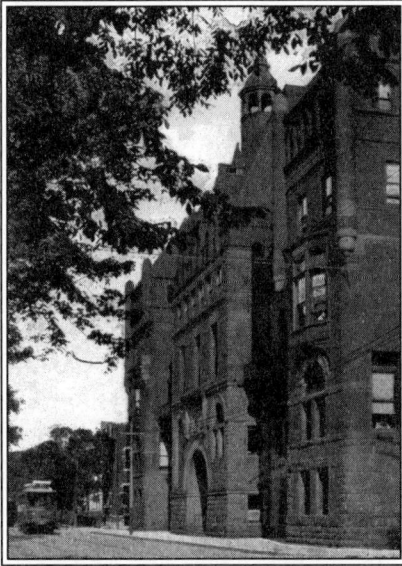

Figure 2. HSC exterior, postcard with streetcar (courtesy of Annmarie Adams, Medicine by Design)

they served as a training-ground for clinical practice and fostered research into the physiology and pathology of children. But they did not, in themselves, affect or even influence the gross morbidity or mortality rates of children as a whole."[17] In the RVH's first annual report (1894), the administration reported admissions of "1570 patients; of these 1345 were discharged, 776 cured, 401 improved, 97 unimproved, 71 not treated, 84 died, and 141 remained." This first group included 861 males, 709 females; 1017 Protestants, 501 Catholics, 52 other religions. The average stay per patient in 1894 at the RVH was 29.3 days and daily cost per patient, $1.42. As there is no separate reporting of children, it is impossible to know how many children were accommodated by this general hospital.[18] In the architectural drawings, historic photographs and the patient statistics of the urban, general teaching hospital, children are not accorded special attention. In particular, the visual evidence suggests that from the time the hospital opened in 1893, children were treated spatially like the other patients, except, crucially (as we will see), they were given opportunity and places for play.

Toronto's sick children were more visible in the cultural landscape of the city. They occupied a purpose-built facility for children as early as 1891. Designed by Frank Darling and S. G. Curry, who had designed the Toronto Home for Incurables a decade earlier, the "Victoria" Hospital for Sick Children (HSC, figure 2) was a large Romanesque-revival block, located amid the city's tenements on College Street.[19] Its steeply pitched roofs, like those of the Royal Victoria in Montreal, lent the institution an

aristocratic air, conjuring up the obvious associations of European cas-
tles, but also resembling the elaborate railway hotels constructed across
Canada at this time, such as the Chateau Laurier in Ottawa and the
Chateau Frontenac in Quebec City.[20]

Founded in 1875, Toronto's Hospital for Sick Children was typical
of other pioneering institutions in that it combined the needs of medical science with an equally strong drive for social and moral amelioration, dependent on benevolent, middle-class women. The first hospital
for children in the world was the Hôpital des enfants malades in Paris
in 1802. London's celebrated Hospital for Sick Children in Great
Ormond Street opened in 1852.[21] The first American hospital for children opened in New York in 1854.[22] By 1890, according to historian
David Charles Sloane, there were twenty-two children's hospitals in the
United States. Most of these early buildings, like the HSC in Toronto,
relied on domestic ideology to express this dual mission, appearing to
be a "big house" that would provide poor, sick children with both protection and a surrogate family atmosphere.[23] This semblance of domesticity, accomplished largely through the hospital's massing, roof type,
materials, scale, historicist imagery, plan, and furniture, also related it
to reform buildings like settlement houses. These, too, were controlled
by women and were intended to improve the lives of working-class kids
through educational initiatives.[24]

Victorian hospitals such as the RVH and HSC were part of a worldwide explosion of medical building construction;[25] however, they also
arose from obvious civic, philanthropic, and political motives. Both commemorated Queen Victoria's silver jubilee in 1888; both were conceived
as gifts to their respective cities; and both were intended to express ties
to Britain. In general terms, the plan (figure 3) of the HSC was similar
to the RVH; it was an *E*-shaped mass with a central entry on the north,
and open wards reaching south. Smaller wards were located along the
College Street elevation, separated by pantries and doctors' rooms. The
only feature in the plan that distinguished the hospital for children from
that for adults was, significantly, an outdoor playground for convalescent
children in the middle arm of the *E* on the second floor. Play and fresh
air were thus fundamental to its mandate.[26]

The Modern Hospital

It was mostly due to the complications of observing and isolating children in regular wards that the need for separate children's pavilions
was articulated. The influential German pediatricians Carl Rauchfuss in
1877, and a half-century later Emil Freer in 1928, cited the need to isolate patients with infectious diseases as the compelling reason for sepa-

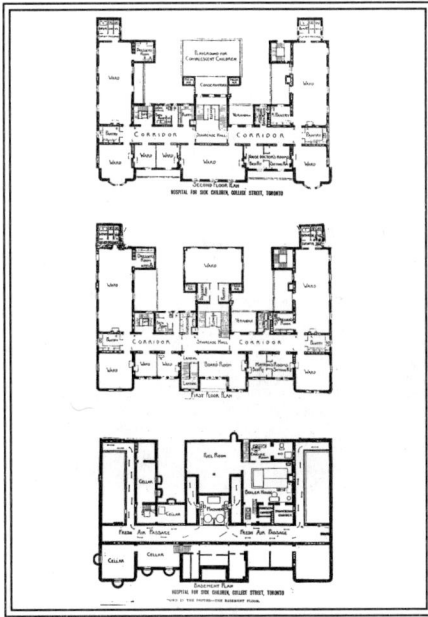

Figure 3. Basement, first floor, and second floor plans of the "Victoria" Hospital for Sick Children (courtesy of Noah Schiff). The plan of the HSC was similar to general hospitals of the era. It was an *E*-shaped mass with a central entry on the north, and open wards reaching south. An outdoor playground on the second floor distinguished the hospital for children from that for adults.

rate children's hospitals.[27] On the other hand, the practicalities of infant feeding and social expectations about mothering militated against this isolationist approach, dictating instead that adults and infants be accommodated together. The support for the specialist children's hospital thus developed only slowly. As late as 1910, hospital architect Charles Butler would still claim "the Children's Hospital as a separate institution is a recent development in the United States."[28] Five years later, pediatrician Henry Dwight Chapin wrote against the hospitalization of infants, arguing, "The best conditions for the infant thus require a home and a mother." "I do not believe," he wrote, "that the multiplication of infant's hospitals through the country should be encouraged."[29]

Edward Stevens and Frederick Lee, specialized hospital architects with offices in both Boston and Toronto, designed several early children's hospitals and were important figures in the development of the type in the first decade of the twentieth century. In his influential book *The American Hospital of the Twentieth Century*, Stevens addressed this tricky question of the separation of children in the general hospital. Noting the need to isolate them from the general patient population because of the relative high frequency of communicable diseases among the young, Stevens recommended a special observation ward for children, separated from other patients by screens. At the same time, however, Stevens reminded readers that sick children, unlike most adults, benefited from the company of others. A glass screen separating every three

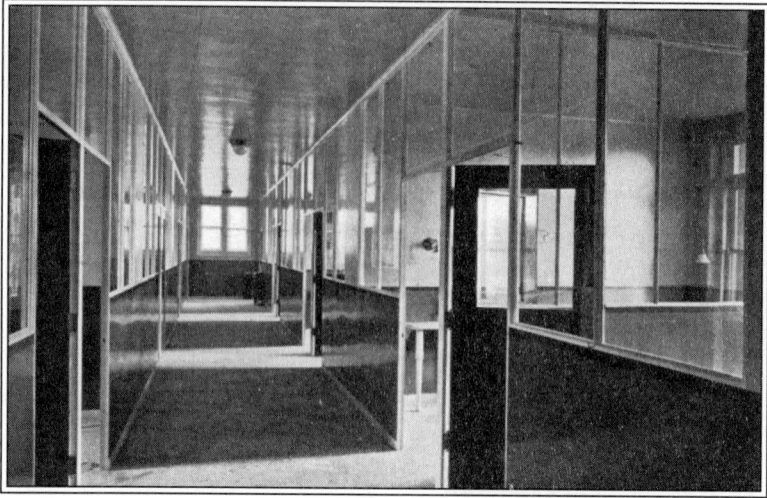

Figure 4. View down the interior corridor of the Isolation Pavilion, Hospital for Sick Children, Toronto (Stevens and Lee, *American Hospital of the Twentieth Century*, 247)

to four beds, in wards not larger than sixteen to twenty beds, was ideal in his opinion.[30]

In a typically immodest way, Stevens considered his own firm's design for a new isolation pavilion, added to the Toronto Hospital for Sick Children in 1912, a model children's hospital, perhaps because it was based on the Pasteur Hospital in Paris, which had impressed him in 1907.[31] Indeed the separation of patients by plate glass partitions was known among hospital designers and consultants as "the Pasteur principle." At the Paris hospital, patients were isolated from each other and from visitors, who communicated with patients from special open balconies, built across the long sides of these mostly rectangular buildings.

The interior of Stevens and Lee's pavilion in Toronto shows the influence of the Pasteur Hospital. A photograph (figure 4) of the HSC published in *The American Hospital of the Twentieth Century* shows a view down the interior corridor of the isolation pavilion. The dividing walls (between corridor and rooms, and between rooms and rooms) are plate glass held by a system of metal framing, extending from floor to ceiling. The overall aesthetic was one of transparency, lightness, and modularity, architectural qualities associated with modernism, and a stark contrast to the thick, masonry walls of Darling and Curry's 1891 chateau-esque building.[32]

A second, particularly scientific feature of these early-twentieth-century children's hospitals was the provision of space intended for the pasteurization of milk. Stevens included a photograph of the pasteurizing room in Toronto in his book, as well as the plan of the children's hospital he designed for Halifax. The Toronto hospital, according to Stevens, had the most "complete" plant for the pasteurization of milk for an institution of its size, providing milk for the hospital as well as for outpatient distribution.[33]

Apart from these two decidedly modern features (cubicles and milk rooms), however, purpose-built hospitals for children in the first half of the twentieth century provided few technologies or medical spaces different from those of the general hospitals, reflecting the ambiguous relationship of pediatrics to the scientific ambitions of other medical specialties.[34] Pediatrician Alton Goldbloom, for example, describes Montreal's Children's Memorial Hospital (CMH) in 1920 as "inactive," isolated" (especially in winter), with "few facilities for special treatment."[35] Milk rooms were widely distributed outside of children's hospitals.[36] Infant care did require some specialized machinery, notably the incubator.[37] But this technology was used as often in general hospitals as in children's hospitals. And historian of medicine Joel D. Howell warns that the existence of a technology does not determine how, where, or when it is used.[38] Still Goldbloom soon resigned his post at the Montreal General Hospital, believing that "the future of pediatrics in Montreal lay not in the children's departments of the large hospitals, but in the Children's Hospital," which was gradually becoming "something more than a hospital for crippled children."[39]

Despite some up-to-date features, then, the architecture of the CMH was far from modern. The ensemble was composed of temporary, unheated huts; it had one operating room; its X-ray department was lagging; the outpatient department was difficult to access; and its school for crippled children suffered from competition from the neighbouring Shriners' Hospital. At the CMH, even scientific nursing, an indispensable part of the modern medical centre, lagged behind.[40] The CMH training school closed in the 1934 as part of a modernization of the nurses' educational program at the McGill teaching hospitals.[41] Not until 1931 did the CMH have a distinct nurses' residence, and not until the 1950s did nurses have their own building.[42]

Indeed, the central ideas behind the design of buildings at the Children's Memorial Hospital in Montreal until the Second World War emphasized lingering, somewhat outdated notions of social reform and maternal benevolence, founded on a nostalgic view of childhood, rather than serving the hospital's newfound scientific orientation. Perhaps the most romantic aspect of the hospital was its site (figure 5). Located across the street from the current Montreal General Hospital and just to the west of the Shriners' Hospital for Crippled Children (designed by Montreal architects J. M. Miller and Hugh Vallance, 1924), the CMH occupied the wooded slopes of Mount Royal.[43] As such, it resembled other public

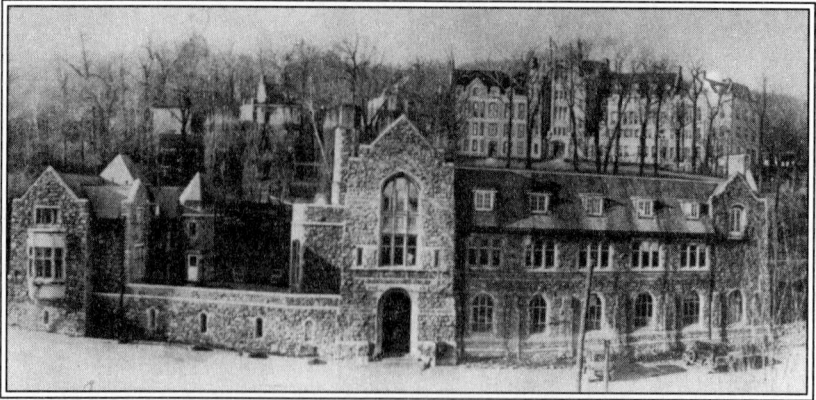

Figure 5. View from Cedar Avenue of Children's Memorial Hospital, 1932–1933 (MCH Archives)

institutions ringing the Olmsted-planned picturesque park, notably McGill University, convents, and cemeteries, and the Royal Victoria Hospital. The site thus fulfilled part of its benevolent vocation, as the hospital was intended to enhance the healing of sick poor kids by removing them from the crowded and damp quarters in which they lived, to the low-density and fresh air of Mount Royal. As Denise Lemieux has shown in her study of childhood in Quebec literature, this vocation stemmed both from concerns about sanitary conditions of the poor and from a dream of a mythic childhood located somewhere in Quebec's rural origins.[44]

A major difference between the RVH and the CMH was in the significance accorded to exterior spaces.[45] Whereas the immediate surroundings of the RVH had served only as a picturesque frame to the hospital itself, exterior spaces at the Children's Memorial actually functioned as outdoor wards for patients. Photos show children dressed for both summer and winter weather outside in beds, and nurses taking the temperature of patients in the gardens. Some images are clearly of special events, like the shot of Commencement Day that appeared in the hospital's annual report of 1912; others, however, such as one of a nurse with three beds on a walkway outside the hospital (figure 6), are more ambiguous. In both cases, however, the images underline the importance of the exterior forested spaces to the workings of the CMH in this period, perhaps a consequence of the continuing struggle by the children's hospital against tuberculosis.

Outdoor spaces were also a distinctive design feature of the CMH master plan. The general arrangement of the site, as drawn by architects David R. Brown and Hugh Vallance, was for a series of fourteen pavil-

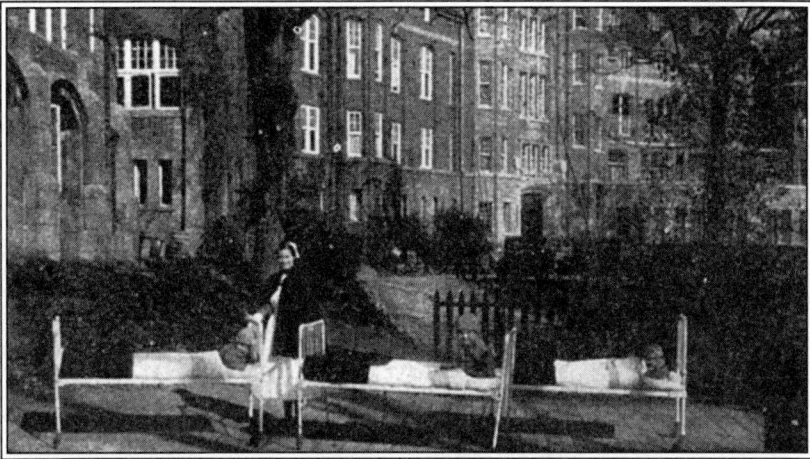

Figure 6. CMH nurse and patients on walkway (MCH Archives)

ions linked by walkways, forming a loop from Cedar Avenue. Directly accessible from the street were the James Carruthers Outpatient Building (1920) and the School (1916). Further up the hill, at the end of a circular driveway, were the administration building, the Sarah Maxwell Memorial, and the Arnott Cottage (1913). Smaller buildings on the site included the Kiwanis Hut (1924), the Kinmond Cottage (1925), the Judah Memorial Pavilion (1926), a hut for twenty boys with tuberculosis (1928), the Forbes building (1931), the George G. Foster Hut (1932), and the Hazel Fountaine Brown Pavilion (1935). Surprisingly, the corridor rooftops also served as wards (figure 7),[46] and tents that functioned as wards were scattered throughout the grounds.[47] A perspective drawing of this unusual corridor-type hospital space was published on the back of the CMH annual report in 1919, in the hope that a benefactor would subsidize this "corridor leading from the upper storey of the Hospital to the mountain park...[for] the open-air treatment of little children suffering from deforming diseases" (figure 8).

Orthopedics was a second important focus of children's hospitals, though this expertise sometimes did little to make the institutions appear to be modern and scientific. Interior photographs of the CMH physiotherapy department (figure 9) show hut-like rooms with visible structure and (sometimes) exposed plumbing. While these images may have been taken for the purpose of fundraising (and thus emphasize the building in need of repair), they also illustrate just how bucolic the buildings were. In fact, the photographs resemble images of overseas hospitals during the First World War, both for their emphasis on rehabilitation and for the flimsy, ephemeral appearance of the architecture.

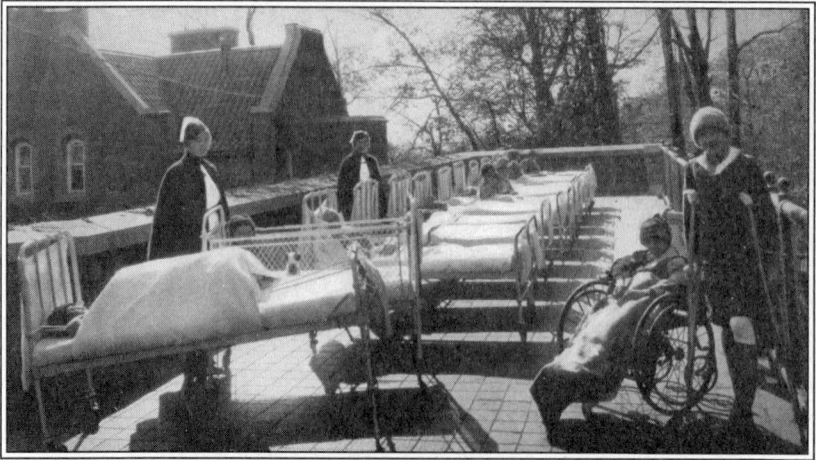

Figure 7. Nurses and patients on roof ward called the "Carruthers corridor" (MCH Archives)

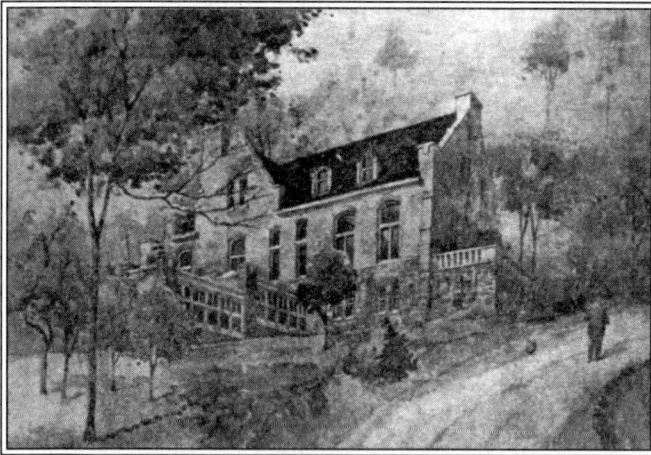

Figure 8. Fundraising advertisement for a proposed Infantile Paralysis
Pavilion, CMH Annual Report 1919 (MCH Archives)

Perhaps the continuing significance of outdoor space in the architectural evolution of the CMH also derives from its rather ad hoc beginnings. Like many others devoted to women and/or children, the institution first occupied a rented house, in 1903. Renovations to it cost four hundred dollars, financed by a sale of homemade goods by Montreal school children. From January 1904 to May 1905, 122 patients and 195 outpatients were treated there. The patients admitted to the ad hoc quarters suffered from tuberculosis (46), rickets (17), infantile paralysis (5), other paralysis (6), and other diseases (48). The cost of patient care

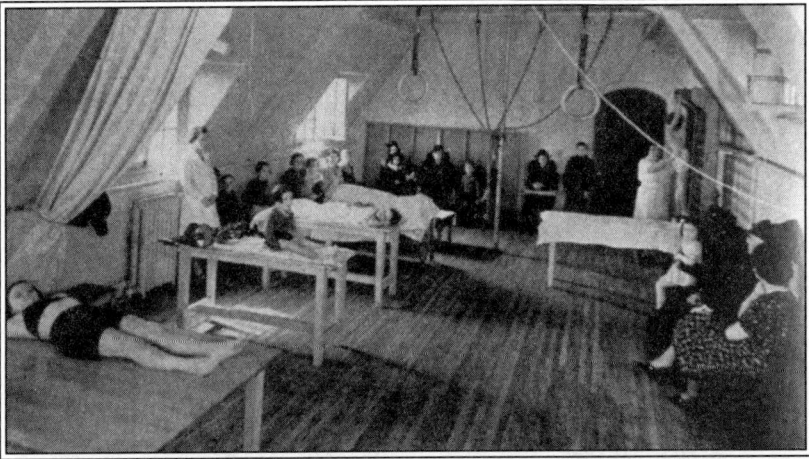

Figure 9. Patients, staff, and visitors in the physiotherapy ward, CMH, ca. 1942 (MCH Archives). Hut-like rooms with exposed structure and plumbing at the Children's Memorial Hospital in Montreal resemble temporary, wartime hospitals.

was twenty-eight cents per day, or about 20 per cent as much as the daily patient cost at the RVH a decade earlier.[48]

Under a new director, in 1936, the CMH attempted to modernize on the model of the technology-oriented research and teaching hospital. In a clear bid to associate the modern children's hospital with modern architecture, the ensuing fundraising campaign publicized images (figure 10) of a proposed addition to the hospital designed by emerging hospital specialist J. Cecil McDougall in a self-consciously modern idiom. The annual reports at this time, too, show a clear transition in style and tone from an earlier romantic view of childhood disease, to the more officious, scientific business management style associated with the general hospital.

In short, the hospital's architecture can be read as evidence of the difficulty experienced by the CMH in asserting itself as a centre of research and teaching. This difficulty paralleled the struggle for academic recognition of pediatrics as a specialty. For example, Harold Beveridge Cushing did not convince McGill University to create a Department of Pediatrics until 1937, the same year the Canadian specialty board was created.[49] Although he was appointed to the faculty in 1902, pediatrics did not appear in his academic title until 1920.[50] Simultaneously, minor adjustments occurred in the accommodation of children at the growing RVH, indicating the increasing importance of children as a special patient group; in 1919, the children's medical ward was relocated to Ward N, where it remained for the next four decades.[51]

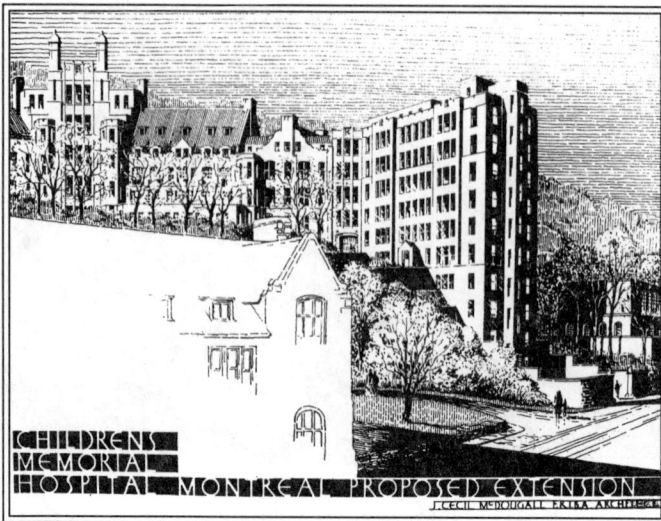

Figure 10. Fundraising perspective, proposed CMH hospital, ca. 1939 (MCH Archives). This proposed addition to the Children's Memorial Hospital, Montreal, in 1936, by emerging hospital architect J. Cecil McDougall, was a clear bid to associate the modern children's hospital with modern architecture.

The French-speaking medical schools from the beginning, by contrast, enthusiastically supported Hôpital Ste-Justine.[52] As a result, its architectural form derived from several large-scale building campaigns, unlike the rather piecemeal development of the CMH. Following its equally modest beginnings in houses, the new *H*-shaped, 300-bed Ste-Justine opened in April 1914; a six-floor north wing was added in 1921–1922, including accommodation for private patients, electrotherapy, radiotherapy, isolation, dispensaries, a laundry, and heating furnaces; and in 1925–1927 a new south wing (of eight storeys) was constructed and a fifth floor added to the centre block (figure 11). One hundred and fifty rooms for nurses were built then, too. In 1932, a nurses' home, laboratories, and laundry were added. All four buildings were designed by Montrealer Joseph Sawyer, architect of a number of hospitals such as the first general hospital for women in Canada, Montreal's Women's General Hospital (1927), with its name changed to the Herbert Reddy Memorial Hospital in 1946, and the Hôpital Notre-Dame de la Merci (1932), as well as schools, churches, and other important Catholic institutions.[53]

Hôpital Ste-Justine represented the ultimate in a scientific children's hospital; its design couldn't have differed more from the architecture of the Children's Memorial. Whereas the anglophone hospital presumed

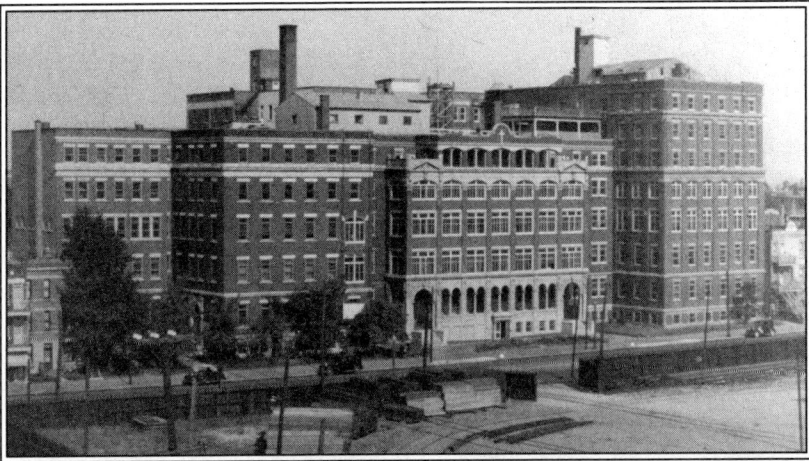

Figure 11. Ste-Justine, exterior, ca. 1935 (Ste-Justine Archives). The design of Hôpital Ste-Justine was remarkably cohesive, deriving from four large-scale building campaigns and a single architect, Montrealer Joseph Sawyer.

that poor families would benefit from its lofty location, Ste-Justine was sited on north St. Denis Street, "where the population mainly comprises families of workmen."[54] Whereas the CMH was made up of a dozen or so small pavilions, terraced into the mountain, Ste-Justine was an integrated urban mass. And the francophone hospital included all the features associated with the modern institution: operating rooms, X-ray department, laboratories, and dietetics. It was categorized as Class A by the American College of Surgeons.[55]

The relationship of pediatrics to other specialties, especially obstetrics, at Ste-Justine was more clearly delineated than in the CMH.[56] In the course of expansion in 1928, Ste-Justine added a maternity ward and *crèche* to the new north wing. The service continued throughout the 1930s, with forty beds, forty bassinets, and three doctors. The CMH opened a ward for infants in 1914, but obstetrics/gynecology remained the responsibility of the Royal Victoria, an arrangement cemented by the construction of Stevens and Lee's Royal Victoria Montreal Maternity Hospital in 1925–1926.[57] By contrast, at Hôpital Notre-Dame, the general hospital associated with Ste-Justine, pregnant women were not admitted unless they had a life-threatening condition.[58]

Historic photographs of the CMH and Hôpital Ste-Justine give further insight into the differing personalities of the two institutions. Not surprisingly, official images of the CMH, like the hand-tinted postcard of 1912 (figure 12) and Notman's photograph of the hospital in 1913, emphasize its romantic forms and domestic references.[59] The upward angle of the postcard image, for example, sets off the varied rooftop

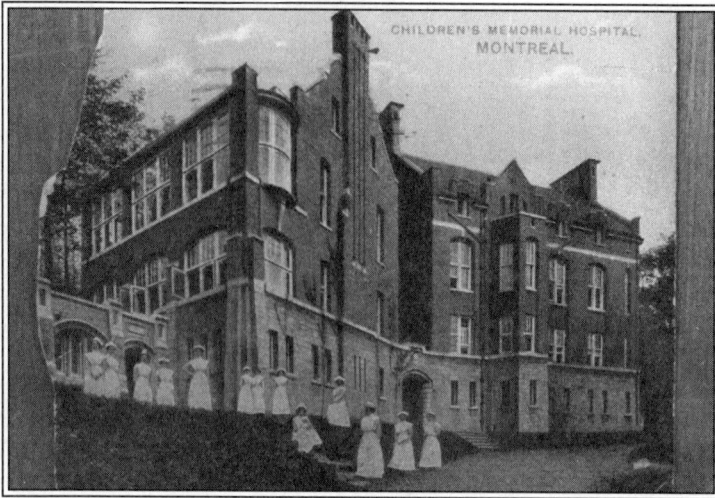

Figure 12. Children's Memorial Hospital, postcard ca. 1912 (MCH Archives)

elements of the building—gable-end chimneys, dormers, curved oriel window, and expressed parapets—features we associate with domestic rather than institutional design. The angle also showcases the hospital's bay window and fine brick detailing. The CMH's small scale, too, is reinforced by the relatively informal postures of the nurses shown in the postcard. One even sits on the ground in her starched, white uniform. The same sort of images can be seen in an extant photo album belonging to Rose Wilkinson, a nurse at the CMH, which is filled mostly with snapshots of staff members and patients. These are intimate images (figure 13) of groups huddled together, often smiling and touching, resembling family photographs. Photographs (figure 14) of Ste-Justine's patients, on the other hand, are typically more formal, emphasizing the hospital's scientific, institutional character.[60]

Comparing the design of Ste-Justine and the CMH also speaks eloquently of the differences between French and English children's hospitals in Montreal during the first half of the twentieth century. Although, as Grenier and Fleury point out, the causes of the development of twin systems are rooted in intractable linguistic, religious, economic, and administrative cleavages, the architectural comparison should dispel the notion that francophone hospitals were somehow less scientific, or more backward, than their anglophone counterparts. This presumption was most clearly articulated by art historian Shelley Hornstein, who suggested in an article published in 1991 on the architecture of Montreal's nineteenth-century teaching hospitals that the religious (French) and secular (English) institutions were in constant competition for the

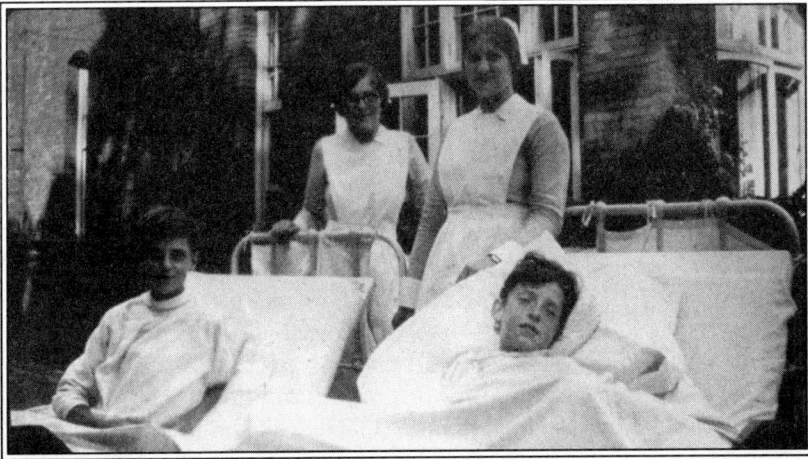

Figure 13. Snapshot of nurses and patients, from Nurse Rose Wilkinson's photo album (MCH Archives)

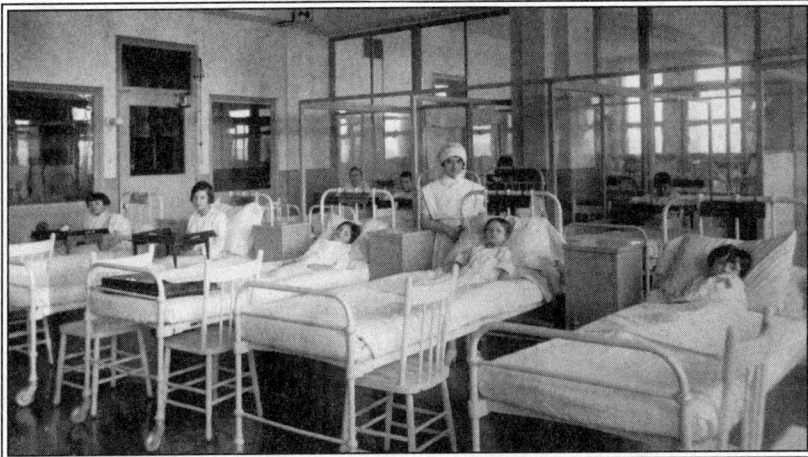

Figure 14. Interior view of ward, Hôpital Ste-Justine (Ste-Justine Archives)

domination of Mount Royal. It sets the original Montreal General Hospital and the Hôtel-Dieu in opposition, describing the English system and its buildings as "an architecture of domination," while she reads the French hospital, mostly due to its convent-derived form, as a "zone of passivity." As further support for her thesis on the competitive nature of hospital building between Montreal's supposed two solitudes, Hornstein also reads the siting of these two buildings as a case of straightforward one-upmanship, remarking that nineteenth-century teaching hospitals in Montreal literally "leapfrog[ged] up its hills" in a competition "waged for the administration of life or the conquest of death."[61] Twentieth-century children's hospitals, as should be clear by now, recount a different story.[62]

The International-Style Hospital

The planned modern addition publicized in the CMH 1936 fundraising campaign (see figure 10) was never constructed. In 1956 the CMH moved to a downtown site, surrounded by busy city streets, which had been home to hospitals since 1880. The move to downtown was prompted by a series of events that had more to do with changes in hospital administration than a careful consideration of the architectural needs of a children's hospital.[63] Most important, the Montreal General Hospital (MGH) had decided to move to a new site on the mountain just across Cedar Avenue from the CMH. Rather than follow the prewar plan to rebuild on the mountain, the CMH took over the Western Division of the MGH on Tupper Street.

The new hospital aspired to be everything the old one was not: urban, modern, and scientific. Even the name was changed to the Montreal Children's Hospital (MCH) in 1954, since the idea of commemorating Queen Victoria's benevolence by then seemed outdated.[64] Typical of North American hospitals built following the war, the new Montreal Children's Hospital (figure 15) more closely resembled an office building than a house. McDougall, of McDougall, Smith, and Fleming, by now Montreal's architect of choice for anglophone hospitals, was familiar with the terrain. Twenty-five years earlier he had designed a ten-storey Private Patients Pavilion (1932) here for the Western Division of the MGH.[65]

For the MCH, McDougall kept the Private Patients Pavilion and added two relatively stark, undecorated towers, which he accommodated by demolishing the remaining 1880 pavilion of the original Western Hospital and a 1907 addition. The new hospital had a 385-bed capacity versus 173 in the old, mostly in public wards in the new thirteen-storey west tower. With the extra beds, the MCH planned to raise the upper age limit for patients from thirteen to sixteen.[66] The old nurses' home, built for the Western Hospital in 1921, was converted into an interns' residence. The second, east tower, connected by a tunnel under Essex Street, was a new home for 165 nurses.

The new MCH, then, consisted of both old and new buildings. Two exemplary postwar children's hospitals in Canada made a more thorough break with the past. The Toronto Hospital for Sick Children (figure 16) opened an eleven-storey tower on University Avenue, south of its old College Street location, in 1951. It was the work of the prolific hospital specialists (and consultants) Govan, Ferguson, Lindsay, Kaminker, Maw,

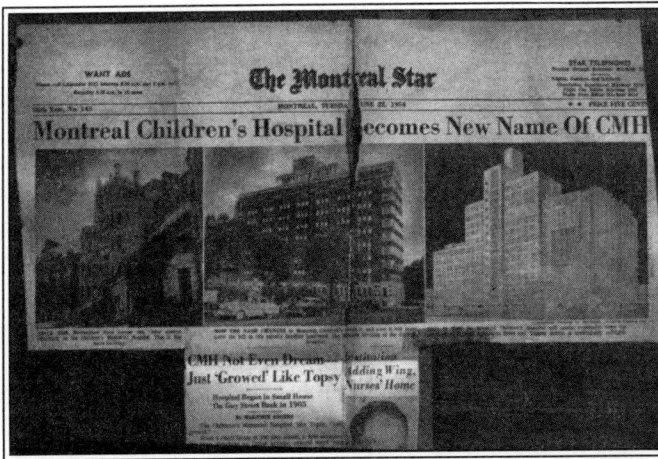

Figure 15. MCH 1955 towers (*Montreal Star*, October 22, 1954). This image shows three stages of the hospital's development: the mountainside hospital, the new downtown site before the 1955 towers were built and a rendering of the proposed 1955 towers.

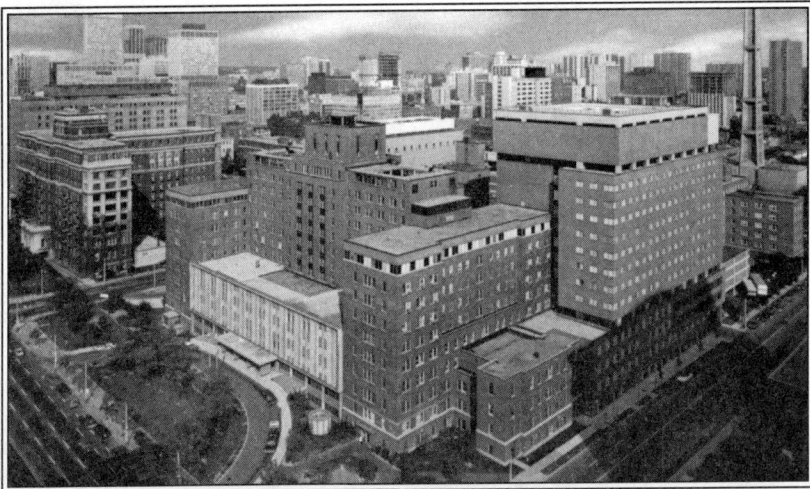

Figure 16. Hospital for Sick Children, University Avenue, Toronto, ca. 1970 (courtesy of Annmarie Adams, Medicine by Design). This postcard shows the 1951 building and later additions at the rear.

Langley, and Keenleyside. And in 1957, fifty years after its founding, Ste-Justine opened a thirteen-storey, 133,500 square-foot, 800-bed facility (figure 17) with a bold double *Y*-shape plan (figure 18) on Côte Ste-Catherine near the Université de Montréal, conceived in a modern style by Ernest Cormier, recently opened on the north flank of Mount Royal.[67]

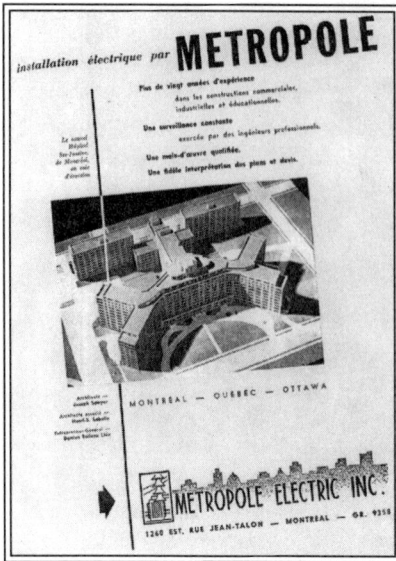

Figure 17. Model of Hôpital Ste-Justine,
advertisement for Metropole Electric,
Inc. (*Architecture-Bâtiment-Construction*,
1953)

Planning for some of these postwar children's hospitals began in the 1930s, under the guidance of established experts; for instance, the architect of the new Ste-Justine was the same Joseph Sawyer who designed all of the earlier hospital on the old site. But by the time they opened in the 1950s, both architecture and hospitals had new mandates. Hospitals were no longer charities for the poor, but much larger-scale health centres for all, offering scientific medicine based in, or at least closely connected with, universities. U.S. Surgeon General Thomas Parran, who in 1945 described the modern hospital as a "complex technical machine, employing the latest scientific diagnostic aids, preventative and curative measures, and professional skills, outlined the new mission."[68] This agenda, backed by increased state funding and the growth of private medical insurance plans, sparked an era of hospital construction across North America.[69]

General hospitals operated under a three-part mission: research, patient care, and teaching. Children's hospitals adopted this orientation. And like the general hospital, the children's hospital refused to take on chronic care or contagious diseases.[70] But pediatric institutions also tried to extend and legitimate their expertise in infant care, orthopedics, and rehabilitation. Newspaper reports described the focus of activities at the new MCH as "preventative medicine, treatment of acute ailments, and correction and assistance of handicapped patients."[71] With this new scientific mission, children's hospitals took on more importance as *centres* for social reform. Historians have shown how before 1945, children in Canada were reformed through ideas of middle-class

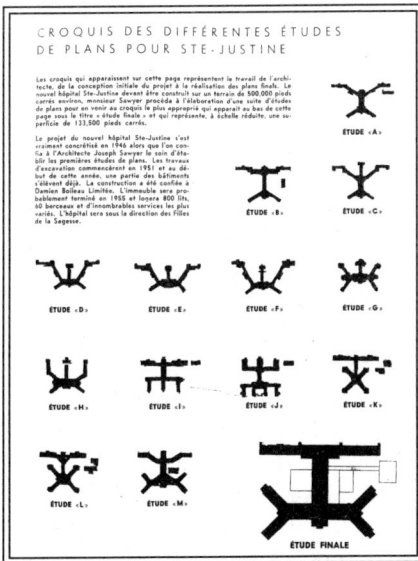

Figure 18. Plan studies, Hôpital Ste-Justine (*Architecture-Bâtiment-Construction*, 1953). Designed by Joseph Sawyer, the new Hôpital Ste-Justine featured a bold, modernist double *Y*-shape plan.

"nurturing," ideas controlled and regulated by emerging scientific experts such as pediatricians, and dispersed at home (for example, in advice books for parents) and in public institutions such as schools (for example, with regular dental clinics).[72] But it was only after the Second World War that the children's hospital, with its clinical and research services, was renewed as an active social agency important to all, rather than a custodial resort for children already marginalized by poverty and illness, and thus came to dominate the efforts to improve children's—and through them, the nation's—health.

Architectural production itself had likewise changed. A coherent and self-proclaimed modern architecture was ready to serve the new scientific hospital. Known under the rubric of the International Style, postwar architecture placed an emphasis on rational plans, often based on Taylorist motion studies and the Fordist factory as the model of production. This functional planning was housed in unadorned, boxy forms, marked by an abundance of windows, often arranged in repetitive horizontal strips. Such stripped-down elevations were often thought to create a desirable neutral or minimalist environment. Superintendent Joseph H. W. Bower, for instance, boasted that the new HSC "is utilitarian in design and little attempt has been made at architectural embellishment."[73] Historian Jonathan Hughes points out that although these principles were initially developed for tight urban conditions, they were used on non-urban sites, too.[74] Thus although McDougall originated plans for modernist towers on the CMH's mountain location, he had little trouble adapting them for downtown.[75] Hospitals could now openly use architecture to convey and communicate the modern, scientific interiors—modern in layout, technology, and organization—rather than to disguise them in historicist exteriors. Hospital experts in the postwar era made rigorous attempts to define the hospital as scientific and progressive, not simply custodial. Architectural modernism was a key factor in expressing these scientific goals both with an appropriately rational-looking architecture, and through the implementation of planning changes such as centralized kitchens and record-keeping that radically changed the habits of all hospital users, employees, and patients.

Ste-Justine's founder, Justine Lacoste-Beaubien, lobbied for a new hospital that would proclaim Ste-Justine as a thoroughly modern institution, which would be involved in research and medical education as well as treatment. She wanted to keep Ste-Justine autonomous, while forming closer links, physically and administratively, with the Université de Montréal. Some of the medical staff opposed the move to Côte Ste-Catherine. The community-based hospital had always prided itself on being accessible to its traditional clientele: the French-speaking working-class population of northeast Montreal. And Beaubien herself hesitated to give any direct control of hospital activities to the university. She argued, however, that hospitals were no longer charities, but rather health centres that could offer the best possible care to children of all classes only by a tighter relationship with the university. That association is a prominent feature in contemporary photos (figure 19), such as one taken from an airplane during construction. In other interior photos, the main university building, with its iconic tower, is clearly visible through the windows, a picturesque and authoritative backdrop to formal and casual activities within the hospital.[76]

In addition to the need to expand and grow, these hospitals were justified by the imperative to keep up to date with technology. Ste-Justine incorporated new non-medical technology. It had a four-story underground bomb shelter, capable of protecting 20,000 people. Beaubien ordered three landing pads on the roof for helicopter ambulances.[77] Built-in systems included ceiling panels for radiant heat (rather than hot water radiators) derived from a system in a children's hospital in France, and an elaborate electronic communications network that could pipe music into the nurses' and employee residences.[78] Many of the innovative ideas came from Soeur Noémi de Montfort, Beaubien's assistant and overseer of the project, who had visited over 160 hospitals in North America.[79]

Toronto's new Hospital for Sick Children, too, flourished a manifold array of medical technology. The hospital installed the latest equipment, including diagnostic and therapeutic tools, confirming the hospital as the desired location for medical treatment. A pneumatic tube sys-

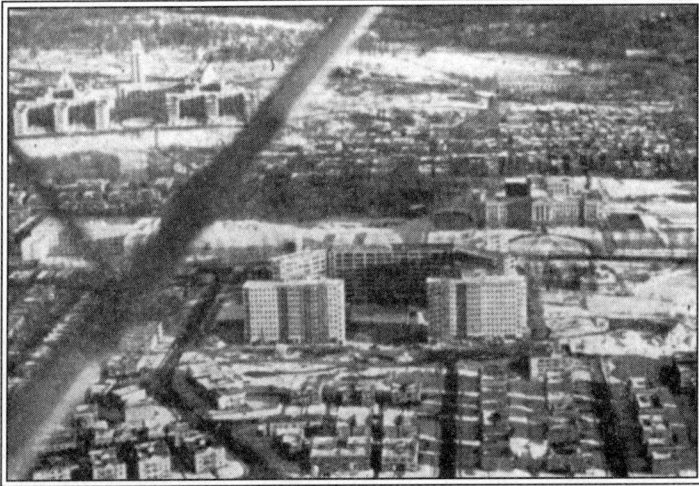

Figure 19. View through airplane window of the Université de Montréal (in the background) and Hôpital Ste-Justine (*Architecture-Bâtiment-Construction*, 1953)

tem could rapidly send documents and objects such as X-rays or medicine to twenty-five stations throughout the hospital. A central supply piped oxygen and suction to ducts beside every bed. In addition, each crib was equipped with a "germicidal" ultraviolet lamp.[80]

The HSC also used new construction technology. Since the building was erected in a hospital zone, the engineers developed a system of welding the structural steel frame (instead of riveting) that minimized noise during construction.[81] The hospital had 635 beds, but the steel structure could accommodate 200 more. Following standard skyscraper construction, whereby the entire load of the building is borne by a grid of columns, the interior partitions were independent of the main structure, so floor layouts could be easily changed, although the position of corridors and large spaces were restricted by the location of columns and elevators. This structure was thought to ensure future flexibility, a concept foremost in the twentieth-century planners' "intentions." Indeed, innovations in medical practice—for example, in 1957 the MCH performed the first open-heart surgery on a child in Canada—created a strong belief in the future of scientific medicine. Hospital experts imagined that the hospital could only continue to flourish.

Interior planning was based on the model of the acute-care adult hospital. In one of the first books on hospital design to appear after the Second World War, Charles Butler and Addison Erdman give equivocal advice to planners. They suggest that separate cubicles and isolation rooms are required for children's wards because children's diseases are

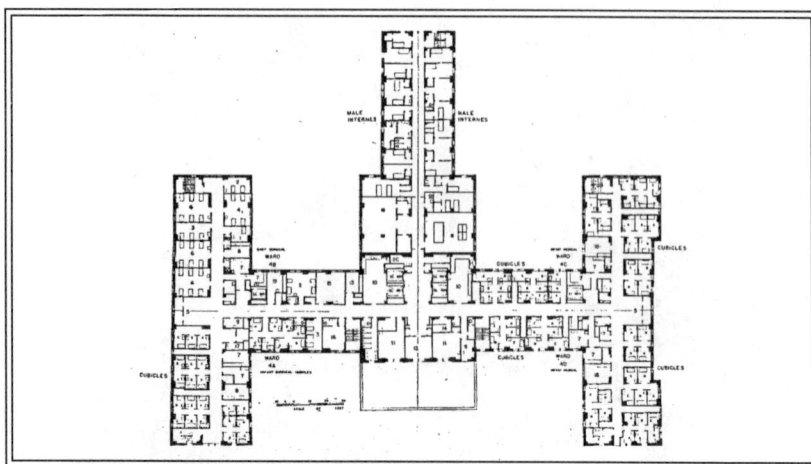

Figure 20. HSC fourth floor plan, 1951 (*Journal Royal Architectural Institute of Canada*, 1951). This plan of the fourth floor of Toronto's Hospital for Sick Children, designed in 1951, illustrates the continuing combination of public wards and private rooms.

often infectious. But children are also prone to loneliness and fear, and are thus better off in eight-bed wards rather than private rooms.[82] The plans of the HSC show private and semi-private wards on floors eight and nine. Intended for paying patients, these wards mark the diminished role of charity in the hospital's mission and reinforce the notion that the hospital was now a desired treatment centre for all children, rich and poor. Administrators were quick to point out that the difference between public and private wards was only in the degree of privacy and allotment of space, not in the quality of care.[83] As the plan of the fourth floor shows, even among the public wards (figure 20) there were a large number of private rooms, used to isolate children with contagious diseases.

The planners also instituted a rudimentary "pad and tower" vertical structure. Patient wards occupied floors four through ten. "All other services, such as operating rooms, routine and research laboratories, X-ray, together with administrative facilities, dining rooms and other general services are located on the lower floors."[84] This configuration of low service building and high ward towers reigned almost unquestioned as the form of progressive hospital design for twenty years.[85] Although the pad and tower concept, known in Britain as the "matchbox on a muffin," worked well for the zoning of hospital functions, the form came not from a close analysis of how the hospital was organized, but instead clearly copied contemporary urban office towers.[86] The quintessential pad and tower office building, however, opened after HSC: the 1952 Lever House, a Manhattan corporate headquarters designed by Skidmore Owings & Merrill. This chronology shows the interpenetration of ideas in modern architecture and modern hospital planning; architects did more than merely dress hospitals in the latest architectural fashions.[87]

Ironically, it is difficult to read from exterior or interior photographs of these three postwar hospitals that they were specifically designed as environments for children.[88] During this period the romantic and domestic imagery of early children's hospitals gave way to the bureaucratic image of a universalist, modernist architecture. In the postwar era of self-conscious progress, of plans for technological, physical, and (especially in Quebec) social modernization, the children's hospital lost a distinct architectural and urban identity, appearing virtually indistinguishable from hospitals for adults, and from other buildings such as office buildings or hotels.

The Postmodern Hospital

Later developments in children's hospitals saw a retreat from these extremes toward more patient-centred, comforting (as opposed to clinical) environments. Curing sick children remained the business of medicine, but the conception of the hospital visit as an orderly industrial process disappeared. Postmodern hospitals returned again to a belief that children's health is a family affair.

In architecture, postmodernism has a specific meaning different from its familiar connotations in cultural studies and philosophy. It describes some of the work by the generation of architects who came of age after the era of functional rationalism and the International Style. Postmodernist designs are often modern buildings in structure, organization, and planning, but decorated with playful features, such as colourful quotations of historical details. While many tout postmodernism as a return to traditional urban design principles, others deride the superficial application of glittery ornament and the embracing of the vacuous glitz of popular culture. In *Learning from Las Vegas*, a powerful 1972 architectural manifesto, Robert Venturi and Denise Scott Brown even suggest that architects must look to mundane buildings like hot-dog stands and gas stations as ideals.[89]

Postmodernism and children's hospitals make an intriguing duo because of the widespread belief that children's hospitals should have animated, distracting, colourful environments.[90] If hospitals such as the HSC a hundred years earlier used historicist imagery to reassure and comfort children and their families, postmodern hospital architects include whimsical references to the past and to popular culture to divert and entertain them. A premier example is the Atrium Patient Tower at the Hospital for Sick Children in Toronto, designed by the Zeidler Roberts Partnership/Architects (figure 21). In 1993, this 572-bed, eight-storey addition replaced all wards and inpatient services in the 1951 facility. It has 96 beds and four nursing stations on each typical floor, arranged, as the name implies, around a central atrium (figure 22).

The atrium as a hospital space appeared in the late 1980s. Verderber and Fine claim that it became an appropriate form as "providers sought new forms of prestige, new types of patients, and increased market share," referring to the rise of corporate hospitals at this time in the United States.[91] In the publicly funded Canadian system, however, the atrium is also fashionable, serving two important purposes. First, the atrium gives hospitals a grand public interior space. Earlier children's hospitals, as we have seen, had no interior spaces intended to encourage the general public to visit. Second, the bustling grand space provided by the atrium in hospitals since the 1980s provides a distraction for hospitalized children, taking its cues from psychological studies that suggest children need to be diverted when ill. And true to postmodernism, the hospital atrium refers to a building type outside its immediate architectural vocabulary: the shopping mall. The inclusion of shops, a fountain, and a 750-seat, twenty-four-hour cafeteria is supposed to make a trip to the hospital seem ordinary and familiar to children.

The atrium also has a more direct predecessor in earlier health care projects of Zeidler Roberts. The office gained international attention for the McMaster University Health Sciences Centre, which opened in Hamilton in 1972. It remains the acme of the modernist desire for functional and technological flexibility, achieved through the incorporation of "interstitial space," a system of expanded subfloors filled with mechanical, electrical, and communication services.[92] The plans of the pediatric units of that modern hospital already reveal the seeds of the ideas of the postmodern Atrium Tower: playrooms and wards arranged around interior courts.[93] More recent Zeidler Roberts projects use the same galleria device. At the Walter C. Mackenzie Health Sciences Centre in Edmonton, the teaching hospital for the University of Alberta, two five-storey, glass-enclosed atria separate the three hospital wings, and are meant to provide clear orientation for visitors and a soothing garden atmosphere. Zeidler Roberts are masterful designers of malls, too. Opened in 1977 in the heart of Toronto, and covering two city blocks, their design for Eaton Centre features a huge 900-foot-long galleria with more than 300 shops on five levels.[94] The point is, the atrium is a versatile architectural idea, which can be used to create soothing transitional spaces for adults or active, animated diverting spaces for kids.

Second, the atrium provides a clear orientation system for the hospital. That is, it helps visitors with "wayfinding," literally with finding their way from the front door to other services. The Atrium Tower entrance is emphatically marked by a semi-circular car drop-off, a large glass

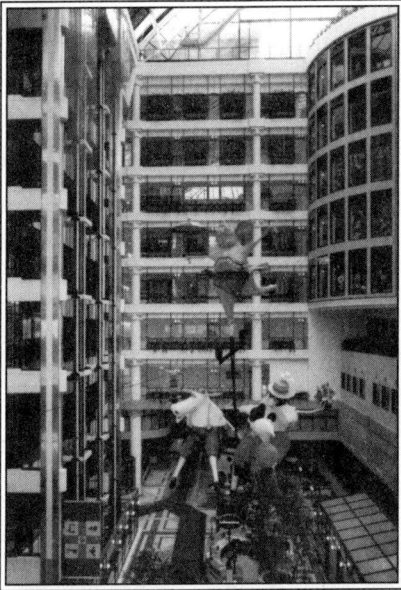

Figure 21. Entrance to the HSC Atrium tower, postcard (courtesy of Annmarie Adams, Medicine by Design).

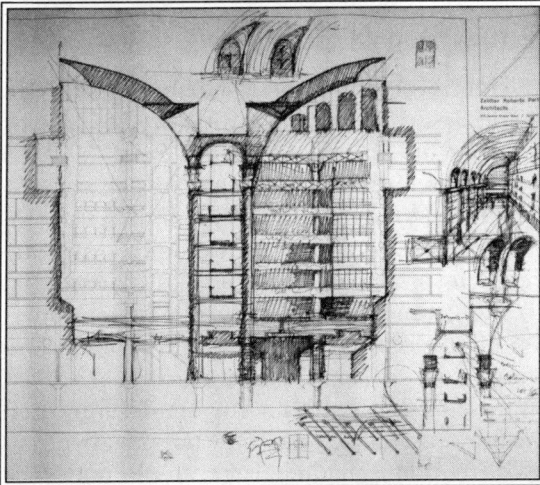

Figure 22. Proposed cross-section of the Atrium Patient Tower at the Hospital for Sick Children, Toronto, including interior perspective and details, sketched on black-line print of 1982 (courtesy ZGPA Architects)

entrance canopy, and a bridge that connects the atrium with laboratories in the Elizabeth McMaster Building across the street (figure 21). Inside, visitors are led down a "main street." Vertical circulation for the public consists of a set of clearly visible elevators and stairs set in the middle of the atrium (figure 22). On the upper floors corridors are attached to the atrium, allowing natural light in and users to look out onto the activity below. The system thus does away with the long, dark corridors found in many postwar hospitals.

The Atrium Tower is postmodern in that it adds a new spatial sequence to hospitals, derived from the experience of the mundane shopping mall. The issue of postmodernism in architecture, however, is more familiar as a debate about how buildings look, that is, the question of applying decoration that quotes historical ornament. The tower quotes pre-modern styles. Both the inside walls of the atrium and the exterior façades recall art deco or art nouveau motifs.[95] Such decoration is often derided as arbitrary, a showy gesture that only adds to the feeling of being in a shopping mall, and raising the question, Why is the illusion of going to a shopping mall an appropriate experience for sick children?[96] If the atrium is a successful wayfinding tool, its merit as an entertainment device is more complex to evaluate. Its use as a diversionary tactic suggests that hospitalization is too stressful and traumatic for patients, especially little patients, to confront; and that medical science and health care need to be disguised before they are acceptable to children. In this sense the Atrium Tower is a step backwards to earlier children's hospitals that, functionally indistinguishable from adult facilities, depended on sentimental ideas of childhood to create an identity and justify the need for a separate children's institution.

The Imaginary Hospital

Montreal is once again facing these same questions about children's health care facilities. For the first time, McGill University has lent its name to a hospital. The new McGill University Health Centre (MUHC) is the result of a voluntary 1998 merger between five of McGill's associated teaching hospitals: the Royal Victoria Hospital, Montreal General Hospital, Montreal Chest Institute, Montreal Neurological Institute, and the Montreal Children's Hospital.[97] The MUHC plans to abandon all but one of its existing buildings and move to a new $1.1 billion super-hospital facility in 2010.[98] After a century of separation, children and adults could once again be part of the same teaching facility.

Some of the strongest dissatisfaction with the current decentralized model of the university health centre is generated by the uneasy physical links among all services surrounding children. For example, under the current "far-flung MUHC arrangement," if a newborn requires surgery, the baby is transported to the MCH, perhaps accompanied by the father, while the mother must remain at the RVH Maternity Pavilion. An MUHC Foundation publicity campaign claims, "On the new one-campus Glen site, a simple wheelchair ride could reunite the entire family."[99]

Not everyone thinks the re-integration of children into the general hospital in Montreal is a good one. Planning for the inclusion of children in the MUHC was rocked by the resignation of MCH Executive

Director Patricia Sheppard in January 2000.[100] She left out of concern that pediatrics was not being given enough autonomy within the MUHC structure. The result, she fears, could be a real lowering in the quality of care the hospital can deliver to children. Sheppard and others (like Beaubien at Ste-Justine fifty years earlier) are mostly apprehensive about diminished administrative authority, about losing control over such things as budgets, medical appointments, and operating room schedules. But that anxiety includes the possible lack of specific child-oriented facilities and architectural identity in the super-hospital. In its latest presentations, the MUHC has begun to discuss separate emergency and other services for children. But if the MCH keeps its name and has its own pavilion, why should it move to the new site with the adult hospitals? The problem of designing for children thus threatens to undermine the whole "one-hospital one-site" super-hospital concept.

The Université de Montréal has similar plans for a new super-hospital. In 1996 its main teaching hospitals merged into the Centre hospitalier de l'Université de Montréal (CHUM). But Ste-Justine declined to join the administrative merger. The French-speaking children's hospital will thus not be part of the proposed $1.1 billion facility originally set to open in 2010 in the Rosemont district, ironically just across from Ste-Justine's former St. Denis Street location.[101] The difference between the futures proposed for Ste-Justine and the MCH illustrates the continuing difficulty of housing children's health care: what is best for the little convalescents, separate or attached?

At a colloquium entitled "Healing by Design: Building for Health Care in the 21st Century" held in September 2000 in Montreal, and organized by the MUHC, hospital administrator Bruce King Komiske was asked to speak about current trends in the design of children's medical centres.[102] It is not surprising he recommended a "separate but attached" model. Children's health centres must now offer the same range of specialized medical expertise as the adult hospitals, from surgery to psychiatry; but simultaneously they must conform to the idea that, because of the uniqueness of childhood development, medical workers must understand special psychological needs and distinct physiology. Children's hospitals, that is, have to deal with the artificial limits of cultural ideas of childhood; a set of medical conditions specific to children, such as congenital and chronic diseases, and the high incidence of respiratory problems; and maintain services such as neurology and oncology parallel to those in adult hospitals.

In Canada there are many approaches to negotiating the "separate-but-attached" model. Children's hospitals such as Ste-Justine, the BC Children's Hospital, and Izaak Walton Killam in Halifax have joined with other hospitals to become facilities for children and mothers; the

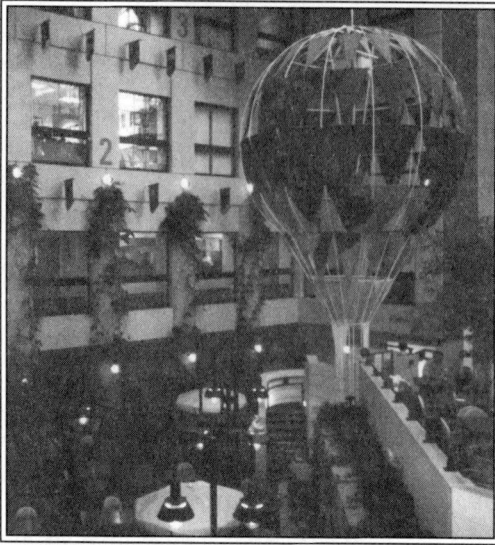

Figure 23. Lobby of the
St. Louis Children's Hospital,
Missouri (courtesy of David C.
Sloane). The spaces of recent
American hospitals, like the
St. Louis Children's Hospital,
Missouri, are designed to
divert and entertain patients
and visitors.

Children's Hospital of eastern Ontario and the HSC in Toronto are now part of a network of pediatric services; and the Winnipeg Sick Children's Hospital and the Alberta Children's Hospital have merged within larger medical centres.[103] Many of these institutions have undergone name changes in response to this "move away from bricks-and-mortar definitions of health care."[104] Like management mergers in other economic sectors, it is difficult to know whether these transformations cut costs, or improve care or patient outcomes. But taken together, they reverse the twentieth-century trend, based on the notion that sick children have special medical and social needs, towards separate buildings for pediatric care.

Komiske illustrated his talk with recent facilities in the United States, including the Hasbro Children's Hospital in Providence, Rhode Island; St. Louis Children's Hospital, Missouri (figure 23); and the Maria Fareri Children's Hospital in Westchester, New York. The site is easily big enough to contain the footprints of the five existing hospitals (figure 24). Yet the ambitious project will require a very large hospital: schematic architectural images released so far describe a building sixty-seven metres high and five blocks long on Glen Yard, a 17.5 hectare plot of old railway land.[105] The main feature of Komiske's model institutions is a complete denial of their function as hospitals. He advises incorporating regional, non-health-related themes, such as the imagery of a village, or the provision of a real zoo, sailboat, or train. "A great children's hospital should be designed so that it does not look institutional," he said.[106] In these hospitals, as in the Toronto Atrium Tower, the lobby is key, pro-

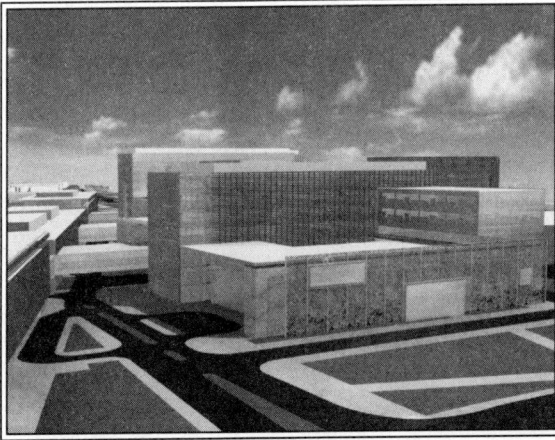

Figure 24. Architectural perspective showing the facilities for children at the proposed McGill University Health Centre. The new building connects directly to a research and care facility for adults (courtesy of MUHC Planning Office)

viding direction and diversion, and allowing children and parents to forget that they are in a hospital. A colourful, playful, childlike atmosphere seems intuitively valuable, yet there is little scientific study to show that offering children a hospital dressed up as a Disney theme park actually improves patient outcomes. Moreover, such interior decoration can detract from the search for architectural solutions to real design problems, disguising rather than defining children's experiences. Finally, what's best elsewhere in the world may not meet the requirements of Canadian children's hospitals, especially in light of the 1984 Canada Health Act, which guarantees Canadians universal, free access to insured health care. Komiske for instance, draws some funny conclusions. He says good design is important because in the year following the opening of the Hasbro Children's Hospital, the hospital's market share increased 20.5 per cent and emergency visits increased 25 per cent.[107] The measurable result of his "good design" is thus not better care but more patients and bigger profits.

One important trend in children's health services that continues to affect the design of children's health care in the twenty-first century is the concept of patient-centred care. This approach involves trying to reduce the number of hospital workers a sick child encounters, and making more provisions for keeping patients together with their families. Such changes have been successfully incorporated at the Atrium Tower. There the design of rooms was carefully studied through the construction of full-scale mock-ups. In the final building, all rooms are private, and include a daybed so a parent can spend the night in the room.[108] Likewise, the trends to reduce the length of patient stays, to use digital communication tools for long-range consultation, and to involve families in hospital care (sometimes called open visiting) change design by placing a greater emphasis on outpatient and ambulatory clinical facilities than on ward design.[109] (More children than ever are now admitted to hospitals, albeit for shorter stays.)[110] On the other hand, some crucial changes in the design of the postmodern hospital are due to social rather than architectural or medical practice. For instance, a revolution in nursing education and shifting workforce patterns has made irrelevant one of the critical architectural problems of the postwar hospital: the nurses' residence and its relationship to administrative, medical, and service spaces.

Faced with the ongoing difficulty of simultaneously providing spaces for the latest scientific medical care and research, and spaces that reflect our cultural ideas about sick and healthy children, debates over the image, location, and arrangement of Canadian children's hospitals continue. Few details of the new MUHC or the CHUM designs have been determined. In the case of the MUHC, it is even hard to confirm whether children will be treated in the same facility as adult patients, even if they occupy the same site. In public presentations, the MUHC initially talked about a campus of separate low-rise pavilions as the architectural form of the super-hospital. This rhetoric was perhaps meant to allay fears that a university medical centre would be a gigantic, imposing, unfriendly megastructure.[111] But in fact, the ambitious project will require a very large hospital. The faith in medical progress and the hopes for medical technology still eclipse the attempt to design environments that specifically support children's experience.

Acknowledgements

The authors are grateful to CIHR, the Hannah Institute for the History of Medicine, and FCAR for their generous support of this research; to two anonymous reviewers for their insightful comments; to Peter Gossage for direction in the history of Canadian families and childhood; to Celine Lemercier for research on Ste-Justine; to Susan Bronson and Jan Schotte for research on the Montreal Children's Hospital; and to Noah Schiff and David C. Sloane for sharing their unpublished research on children's hospitals. Most of the visual evidence included here was obtained from the collections of the Royal Victoria Hospital and the Montreal Children's Hospital. We are particularly indebted to Jack Charters (MCH), Martin Entin, and the late Brenda Cornell (RVH) for access to this material.

Notes

1 On the significance and development of pavilion-plan hospitals, see Jeremy Taylor, *The Architect and the Pavilion Hospital: Dialogue and Design Creativity in England 1850–1914* (Leicester: Leicester University Press, 1997).

2 The relationship of trends in health architecture and mainstream architectural design is explored in Stephen Verderber and David J. Fine, *Healthcare Architecture in an Era of Radical Transformation* (New Haven: Yale University Press, 2000).

3 Charles Rosenberg, *The Care of Strangers: The Rise of America's Hospital System* (New York: Basic Books, 1987); Rosemary Stevens, *In Sickness and in Wealth: American Hospitals in the Twentieth Century* (New York: Basic Books, 1989); Morris J. Vogel, "The Transformation of the American Hospital, 1850–1920," in *Health Care in America*, ed. Susan Reverby and David Rosner (Philadelphia: Temple University, 1979), 105–16; and Guenter B. Risse, *Mending Bodies, Saving Souls: A History of Hospitals* (New York: Oxford University Press, 1999).

4 J. T. H. Connor, *Doing Good: The Life of Toronto's General Hospital* (Toronto: University of Toronto Press, 2000); David Gagan, "For 'Patients of Moderate Means': The Transformation of Ontario's Public General Hospitals, 1880–1950," *Canadian Historical Review* 70 (1989): 151–79; David Gagan and Rosemary Gagan, *For Patients of Moderate Means: A Social History of the Voluntary Public General Hospital in Canada, 1890–1950* (Montreal: McGill-Queen's University Press, 2002); Denis Goulet, François Hudon, and Othmar Keel, *Histoire de l'Hôpital Notre-Dame de Montréal, 1880–1980* (Montreal: VLB Éditeur, 1993); and James de Jonge, "Metamorphosis of a Public Institution: The Early Buildings of the Kingston General Hospital," *Society for the Study of Architecture in Canada Bulletin* 22 (September 1997): 74–82. J. T. H. Connor, "Hospital History in Canada and the United States," *Canadian Bulletin of Medical History* 7 (1990): 93–104, and S. E. D. Shortt, "The Canadian Hospital in the Nineteenth Century: An Historiographic Lament," *Journal of Canadian Studies* 18 (Winter 1982–84): 3–14, complain that Canada lacks synthetic and comprehensive studies of hospital development.

5 On the ways historicist hospitals functioned as modern institutions, see Annmarie Adams, "Modernism and Medicine: The Hospitals of Stevens and Lee, 1916–1932," *Journal of the Society of Architectural Historians* 58 (March 1999): 42–61.

6 On the impact of social reform movements on Canadian childhood, see Cynthia R. Comacchio, *"Nations Are Built of Babies": Saving Ontario's Mothers and Children 1900–1940* (Montreal: McGill-Queen's University Press, 1993); Joy Parr, ed., *Childhood and Family in Canadian History* (Toronto: McClelland and Stewart, 1982); and Patricia T. Rooke and R. L. Schnell, eds., *Studies in Canadian Childhood: A Canadian Perspective* (Calgary: Detselig Enterprises, 1982).

7 Lindsay Granshaw, "'Fame and Fortune by Means of Bricks and Mortar': The Medical Profession and Specialist Hospitals in Britain, 1800–1948," in *The Hospital in History*, ed. Lindsay Granshaw and Roy Porter (London: Routledge, 1989), 202.

8 On the unique characteristics of pediatrics as a specialty, see Sydney A. Halpern, *American Pediatrics: The Social Dynamics of Professionalism, 1880–1980* (Berkeley: University of California Press, 1988), 9–12.

9 On the history of the Royal Victoria Hospital, see D. Sclater Lewis, *Royal Victoria Hospital 1887–1947* (Montreal: McGill University Press, 1969).

10 Lewis, *Royal Victoria Hospital*, 22, 26.

11 Lindsay Prior, "The Architecture of the Hospital: A Study of Spatial Organization and Medical Knowledge," *British Journal of Sociology* 39 (1988): 86–113.

12 Robson claimed in a letter dated April 20, 1895 to Chipman, in the possession of the RVH, that 30 beds were intended, "but we have had 32 on account of the pressure."

13 Undated specs for hot water heating apparatus, in the possession of the RVH, call for radiators to be covered by a Tennessee marble slab 1.5 inches thick.

14 There are also two photographs of Ward N in use as the Children's ward (after 1919), one showing patients and nurses in the McGill University Archives (PR023775) and one of the empty ward in the possession of the RVH.

15 Lewis, *Royal Victoria Hospital*, 182.

16 See note 2.

17 Deborah Dwork, "Childhood," in *Companion Encyclopedia of the History of Medicine* vol. 2 (London: Routledge, 1993), 1074.

18 *Royal Victoria Hospital Annual Report* 1 (1894), 8.

19 Kelly Crossman, *Architecture in Transition: From Art to Practice, 1885–1906* (Montreal: McGill-Queen's University Press, 1987), 12.

20 This resemblance is noted by Noah Schiff in "'The Sweetest of All Charities': The Toronto Hospital for Sick Children's Medical and Public Appeal, 1875–1905" (master's thesis, University of Toronto, 1999).

21 Charles West founded the hospital in a house. The 120-bed facility designed by E. M. Barry was erected in 1872–77 on the same site. See Harriet Richardson, ed., *English Hospitals 1660–1948* (Swindon: Royal Commission on the Historical Monuments of England, 1998), 110–11. On the origins of children's hospitals in Britain, see Elizabeth M. R. Lomax, *Small and Special: The Development of Hospitals for Children in Victorian Britain* (London: Wellcome Institute for the History of Medicine, 1996).

22 See Jacalyn Duffin, *History of Medicine: A Scandalously Short Introduction* (Toronto: University of Toronto Press, 1999), 317. Janet Golden claims that the first permanent pediatric facility in the United States was the Children's Hospital of Philadelphia in 1855, in Janet Golden, ed., *Infant Asylums and Children's Hospitals: Medical Dilemmas and Developments 1850–1920; An Anthology of Sources* (New York: Garland, 1989), n.p.

23 David Charles Sloane, "Caring for the Children: The Emergence of the Modern Children's Hospital, 1890–1930" (unpublished paper, 2000), 18.

24 For a discussion of domestic ideology as an expression of an overtly feminist material culture, see Annmarie Adams, *Architecture in the Family Way: Doctors, Houses, and Women, 1870–1900* (Montreal: McGill-Queen's University Press, 1996), 158–60. On the architecture of settlement houses, see Deborah Weiner, *Architecture and Social Reform in Late-Victorian London* (Manchester: Manchester University Press, 1994).

25 Planners were preoccupied with this rapid increase in health care facilities. Surgeon Albert J. Ochsner and architect Meyer J. Sturm reported in their book *The Organization, Construction and Management of Hospitals* (Chicago: Cleveland Press, 1907), 19, that in Prussia alone the number of hospitals almost tripled between 1876 (1,502) and 1900 (3,900).

26 Schiff has also noted the strategic location of the first-floor board room, which permitted a view of the entry from the room, while those in the board room remained invisible from the entry; see Schiff, "Sweetest of All Charities," 122. The plans were published in *The Hospital for Sick Children, College Street, Toronto: The Lakeside Home for Little Children; History of These Institutions* n.a, n.p. (Toronto, 1891), 63, 68, 74.

27 See Edward Seidler, "An Historical Survey of Children's Hospitals," in *The Hospital in History*, ed. Lindsay Granshaw and Roy Porter (London: Routledge, 1989), 181–97.

28 See Charles Butler, "Planning of Children's Hospitals," *Brickbuilder* 19 (August 1910), 180.

29 Henry Dwight Chapin, "Are Institutions for Infants Necessary?" *Journal of the American Medical Association* 64, 2 (January 1915): 1–3, reprinted in Golden, ed., *Infant Asylums and Children's Hospitals*, 175–77.

30 Edward Fletcher Stevens, *The American Hospital of the Twentieth Century*, 3rd ed. (New York: Dodge, 1928), 210.

31 Stevens's description of the Pasteur Institute is included in Edward F. Stevens, "The Contagious Hospital," *Brickbuilder* 17 (September 1908): 183–84. See also Edward F. Stevens, "Admitting Department of Buffalo Children's Hospital," *Modern Hospital* 14 (April 1929): 346, which may be the only article he wrote on children's hospitals. For a general description of the Hospital for Sick Children in Toronto, see Max Braithwaite, *Sick Kids: The Story of the Hospital for Sick Children in Toronto* (Toronto: McClelland and Stewart, 1974).

32 The buildings are described in n.a., "Hospital for Sick Children, Toronto" *Construction* 7 (October 1914): 378–81.

33 Stevens, *The American Hospital of the Twentieth Century*, 18.

34 On the architectural development of modern hospitals, see Adams, "Modernism and Medicine."

35 Alton Goldbloom, *Small Patients: The Autobiography of a Children's Doctor* (Toronto: Longmans, Green, 1959), 175–78. Goldbloom writes, "Children's Memorial was a most inactive hospital. Its outpatient department boasted two or three visits a day in fine weather, in winter often none for days. The few non-surgical patients were for the most part suffering from chronic disease and needed little more than nursing care. There were few facilities for special treatments. Any laboratory examinations beyond the very simplest were made through the courtesy of one of the larger hospitals. An ancient X-ray machine, operated usually by the intern, was used for the comparatively infrequent pictures that were taken" (176).

36 Montreal opened its *Gouttes de lait* system in 1901; by 1915 there were twenty-eight depots; see Duffin, *History of Medicine*, 319. See also Denyse Baillargeon, "Fréquenter les Gouttes de lait: L'expérience des mères montréalaises 1910–1965," *Revue d'histoire de l'Amérique française* 50 (Summer 1996): 29–68.

37 On the incubator, see Jeffrey P. Baker, *The Machine in the Nursery: Incubator Technology and the Origins of Newborn Intensive Care* (Baltimore: Johns Hopkins University Press, 1996).

38 Joel D. Howell, "Machines and Medicine: Technology Transforms the American Hospital," in *The American General Hospital: Communities and Social Contexts*, ed. Diana Elizabeth Long and Janet Golden (Ithaca: Cornell University Press, 1989), 132.

39 Goldbloom, *Small Patients*, 190.

40 On the significance of trained nurses to the twentieth-century hospital, see Kathryn McPherson *Bedside Matters: The Transformation of Canadian Nursing, 1900–1990* (Toronto: Oxford University Press, 1996).

41 See Jessie Boyd Scriver, *The Montreal Children's Hospital: Years of Growth* (Montreal: Montreal Children's Hospital and McGill-Queen's University Press, 1979), 84. *Modernization* here meant "specialization": the CMH no longer offered full training, but rather specialized in instruction, including lectures and demonstra-

tions, in medical, surgical, and orthopedic nursing, and infant feeding. For example, pediatric nursing was offered as a special three-month course for students at the RVH Training School; see Lynda deForest, *Proud Heritage: A History of the Royal Victoria Hospital Training School for Nurses, 1894–1972* (Montreal: The Alumnae Association of the Royal Victoria Hospital Training School for Nurses, 1994), 56–57.

42 On the importance of the architecture of nurses' residences, see Annmarie Adams, "Rooms of Their Own: The Nurses' Residences at Montreal's Royal Victoria Hospital," *Material History Review* 40 (Fall 1994): 29–41.

43 The Shriners' Hospital is an interesting example of a specialist children's hospital. On its design, see n.a., "The Shriners of Montreal Erecting Commodious Hospital for Crippled Children," *Contract Record and Engineering Review* (May 28, 1924), 540; and n.a., "Shriners' Hospital for Crippled Children, Montreal," *Journal Royal Architectural Institute of Canada* 4 (July 1927): 242–49.

44 Denise Lemieux, in *Une culture de la nostalgie: L'enfant dans le roman québecois de ses origines à nos jours* (Montreal: Boréal Express, 1984), writes of a "myth" of childhood that develops in Quebec literature between the wars, often centred on nostalgia and a romanticized folkloric past (12). In chapter 18 of Gabrielle Roy's *The Tin Flute* (1947), Rose-Anna visits her son Daniel Lacasse at the Children's Memorial Hospital (CMH); in the novel they lived in St. Henri, still today one of the city's poorest neighbourhoods.

45 A drawing in the Canadian Architecture Collection, McGill University (not yet catalogued), indicates that landscape architect Frederick Law Olmsted, designer of New York's Central Park and Montreal's Mount Royal Park, advised on the landscaping for the RVH, but it is unclear whether his design was executed.

46 This list of buildings has been pieced together from various sources, mostly "The Romance of a Great Idea," notes from a slide lecture given by nurse Dora Parry, probably in 1966, now in the Montreal Children's Hospital archive.

47 These "tents" were wooden structures with canvas, pull-down walls. Four are visible in a photo of Commencement Day published in the *Children's Memorial Hospital Annual Report* of 1912.

48 *MCH: The Children's Story*, a brochure published to celebrate the hospital's fiftieth anniversary, n.p.

49 Duffin, *History of Medicine*, 317. For a discussion of the ways early pediatricians justified their claim to a separate specialty, see Jonathan Gillis, "Bad Habits and Pernicious Results: Thumb Sucking and the Discipline of Late-Nineteenth-Century Paediatrics," *Medical History* 40 (January 1996): 55–73.

50 Edward H. Bensley, "Harold Beveridge Cushing (1873–1947)," *McGill Medical Luminaries* (Montreal: Osler Library, 1990), 95.

51 Lewis, *Royal Victoria Hospital*, 182. According to Martin Entin of the RVH, Ward N was on the third floor of Snell's East Wing, facing University Street.

52 On the early history of Ste-Justine, see Rita Desjardins, "Hôpital Sainte-Justine, Montréal, 1907–1921" (master's thesis, Université de Montréal, 1989); and Willie Major, "L'Hôpital Sainte-Justine," *L'Union Médicale* 69 (July 1940), 732–43.

53 For information on Sawyer's life and work, see *Architecture-Bâtiment-Construction*, 8 (janvier 1953), an issue devoted to Sawyer, "*un des architectes pionniers de la Province de Québec*" (13).

54 N.a., "St. Justine's Hospital, Montreal," *Construction* 21 (March 1928), 87.

55 N.a., "L'Hôpital Ste-Justine for Children, Montreal, Earns Splendid Reputation," *Canadian Hospital* 5 (October 1928), 20–21.

56 On the history of pediatrics in French-speaking Montreal, see Rita Desjardins, "L'institutionnalisation de la pédiatrie en milieu franco-montréalais 1880–1980: Les enjeux politiques, sociaux et biologiques" (PhD thesis, Université de Montréal, 1998).

57 The new pavilion was a merger of the former Montreal Maternity Hospital and the Royal Victoria. On its design, see n.a., "The Royal Victoria Maternity Hospital," *Canadian Hospital* 3 (October 1926): 11–15.

58 Goulet, Hudon, and Keel, *Histoire de l'Hôpital Notre-Dame de Montréal*, 108. On the impact of the relationship between pediatrics, obstetrics, and the trend towards in-hospital childbirth, see Veronica Strong-Boag, *The New Day Recalled: Lives of Girls and Women in English Canada, 1919–1939* (Mississauga: Copp Clark Pitman, 1988), 164.

59 The photo is in the Notman Photographic Archives, McCord Museum, VIEW-5025.

60 Patients at Ste-Justine were segregated according to their ages, and then by their sicknesses, separated by gender; at the CMH they seemed to be grouped in intimate, family-like clusters. In 1956 the hospital's director John De Belle looked forward to a new building in which the patients could be "segregated according to sex, age and disease groups." In particular he lamented that at the mountainside CMH it was "difficult to segregate older patients from young, boys from girls"; see "Children's Hospital Move Set for Dec. 1," *Montreal Daily Star*, October 26, 1956, 4.

61 Shelley Hornstein, "The Architecture of the Montreal Teaching Hospitals of the Nineteenth Century," *Journal of Canadian Art History* 14 (1991): 12–24.

62 One goal of recent writing on the history of medicine in Quebec has been to dispel this notion of the backwardness of francophone institutions; see Goulet et al., *Hôpital Notre-Dame*, 9–24. On recent historiography of Quebec medicine, see Marie-Josée Fleury and Guy Grenier, "La médicine et de la santé au Canada français: un bilan historiographique, 1987–2002," *Scientia Canadensis* 26 (2002): 29–58.

63 The Vivian Report, a survey of Montreal hospitals by a professor in McGill University's Department of Public Health, had recommended a change to a more accessible, larger downtown outdoor (emergency) department; see Scriver, *Montreal Children's Hospital*, 117–19. The CMH had absorbed the Montreal Children's (Vipond) Hospital, a small private children's hospital, and moved its outpatient department to the small hospital, a mansion renovated in 1932 by Huntly Ward Davis, the architect of the CMH, on St. Antoine near Guy Street. On the renovations, see n.a., "Remodelled and Re-Made Buildings," *Construction* 26 (May–June 1933): 71–74.

64 Scriver, *Montreal Children's Hospital*, 125–26.

65 McDougall also designed the Montreal General Hospital (1955), described in McDougall, Smith, and Fleming, Architects, "The Montreal General Hospital," *Journal Royal Architectural Institute of Canada* 32 (September 1955): 312–21, and the Montreal Chest Institute (1952 and 1955).

66 "Children's Hospital Move Set for Dec. 1," 4.

67 The Université de Montréal was originally intended to house a university hospital. On Cormier's design, see Isabelle Gournay, ed., *Ernest Cormier and the Université de Montréal* (Montreal: Canadian Centre for Architecture, 1990).

68 Quoted in Rosemary Stevens, *In Sickness and in Wealth*, 219–20.

69 In 1946 the U.S. government passed the *Hill-Burton Act*. Over the next twenty years, 4,678 projects in the United States received federal aid through its pro-

visions, with the ultimate goal of providing 4.5 hospital beds per 1,000 inhabitants throughout the country. See Stevens, *In Sickness and in Wealth*, 218.

70 The MCH sent children with infectious diseases to the Alexandra Hospital,
which had been established in 1904, three years before the Children's Memorial Hospital.

71 "Montreal Children's Hospital Becomes New Name of CMH," *Montreal Star*,
June 22, 1954, 6.

72 MCH pediatrician Alton Goldbloom's classic *The Care of the Child* (Toronto:
Longmans, Green), first appeared in 1928, was quickly translated into French,
and appeared in five editions by 1947. On the institutionalization of middle-class
nurturing, see Comacchio, *Nations Are Built of Babies*; Dianne Dodd, "Advice to
Parents: The Blue Books, Helen MacMurchy, M.D., and the Federal Depart-
ment of Health," *Canadian Bulletin of Medical History* 8 (1991): 203–30; Norah
Lewis, "Physical Perfection for Spiritual Welfare: Health Care for the Urban
Child, 1900–1939," in *Studies in Childhood History: A Canadian Perspective*, ed.
Patricia T. Rooke and R. L. Schnell (Calgary: Detselig Enterprises, 1982), 135–66;
and Neil Sutherland, *Children in English-Canadian Society: Framing the Twentieth-
Century Consensus* (Toronto: University of Toronto Press, 1976).

73 Joseph H.W. Bower, "Serving Sick Children," *Journal Royal Architectural Institute
of Canada* 28 (June 1951): 158.

74 See Jonathan Hughes, "The 'Matchbox on a Muffin': The Design of Hospitals
in the Early NHS," *Medical History*, 44 (January 2000), 21. Hughes points out that
a series of hospitals in the Southern United States followed hospital administrator Gordon Friesen's thorough attempt to use notions derived from industrial
production to lay out the planning and delivery of services in hospitals. The first
hospitals following his recommendations were completed in 1956, but by then
his ideas were already well known among hospital experts in North America and
Europe.

75 In fact another hospital McDougall designed in an aggressively modernist manner, the new Montreal General Hospital, opened in 1955 directly across Cedar
Avenue from the CMH. On its design, see note 64.

76 A view of the hospital showing the university tower accompanied an article on
the personnel building days before the hospital opened; see "Le pavilion du personnel à Sainte-Justine," *La Presse*, October 18, 1957, 18. See also the photo of
the ceremonies for the fiftieth anniversary of the Fondation de l'Hôpital Sainte-
Justine (May 21, 1957), in Nicolle Forget, Francine Harel Giasson, and Francine
Séguin, *Justine Lacoste-Beaubien et l'Hôpital Sainte-Justine* (Sainte Foy: Presses de
l'Université du Québec, 1995). The image features Justine Lacoste-Beaubien,
Cardinal Paul-Émile Léger, and pediatrician Edmond Dubé dining in a wing of
the hospital in front of a panoramic view of the Université.

77 See "Hospital Will Stand as Symbol of Hope," *Montreal Daily Star*, October 19,
1957, 4. The HSC in Toronto did not open a rooftop helioport until 1972.

78 Forget, Giasson, and Séguin, *Justine Lacoste-Beaubien*, 132.

79 "Hospital Will Stand as Symbol of Hope," 4. For a discussion of the significance
of the considerable architectural expertise of women in religious orders, see
Tania Martin, "Housing the Grey Nuns: Power, Religion and Women in Fin-de-
siècle Montréal" (master's thesis, McGill University, 1995).

80 See Bower, "Serving Sick Children," 158. These items were thus incorporated in
the design of a children's hospital absolutely contemporary with their introduction into Friesen's adult hospitals; see Hughes, "Matchbox on a Muffin," 40.

81 Gordon L. Wallace and Clare D. Carruthers, "Outline of Structure," *Journal
Royal Architectural Institute of Canada* 28 (June 1951), 172.

82 Butler and Erdman also advised that technical requirements, such as utility rooms, "do not vary much from any other service." See *Hospital Planning* (New York: F. W. Dodge, 1946), 60–61.

83 Bower, "Serving Sick Children," 157–58.

84 Bower, "Serving Sick Children," 156.

85 Hughes "Matchbox on a Muffin," 35.

86 On the pad and tower concept, see also Verderber and Fine, *Healthcare Architecture*, 48–50.

87 On the relationship between hospital design and civic design in postwar Britain, see Jonathan Hughes, "Hospital City," *Architectural History* 40 (1997): 266–88.

88 Scientific medicine meant an increasing level of standardization for hospital practices, equipment, and buildings, whether in general or specialist hospitals. From 1919 until 1951, hospitals in North America, including Canada, were accredited by the American College of Surgeons (ACS). In 1959 the Canadian Council on Hospital Accreditation took complete control and responsibility for accrediting hospitals in Canada. See George Harvey Agnew, *Canadian Hospitals, 1920–1970: A Dramatic Half Century* (Toronto: University of Toronto Press, 1974), 37–38.

89 Robert Venturi, Denise Scott Brown, and Steven Izenour, *Learning from Las Vegas* (Cambridge, MA: MIT Press, 1972).

90 See the discussion of the children's hospital as a fantasy environment in Jain Malkin, *Hospital Interior Architecture: Healing Environments for Special Patient Populations* (New York: Van Nostrand Rheinhold, 1992), 168–77.

91 Verderber and Fine, *Healthcare Architecture*, 157.

92 On interstitial space, see Verderber and Fine, *Healthcare Architecture*, 116–24, and Hughes, "Hospital City," 271–72.

93 Eberhard H. Zeidler, *Healing the Hospital: The McMaster Health Sciences Centre* (Toronto: Zeidler Partnership, 1974), 55–57.

94 For descriptions of the hospital, see Philip Arcidi, "P/A Inquiry: Hospitals Made Simple," *Progressive Architecture* 73 (March 1992), 92; and Mary Lou Lobsinger, "Animation for Sick Kids," *Canadian Architect* 38 (April 1993): 16–24.

95 Jim Murray described the elevation as "a lively facade with curiously Mackintosh implications," in the Canadian Architect Award of Excellence jury report; see Moira Farr, "1986 Awards of Excellence." *The Canadian Architect*, 31 (December 1986), 20.

96 Lobsinger, "Animation for Sick Kids," 21.

97 The McGill University Health Centre, "A Single Site, A Single Vision, A Singular Future," n.d., 14. Planning for the administrative merger began as early as 1993.

98 The Quebec government approved the project in June 2004. The proposal called for a hospital of just over 500 beds; however, the Montreal General Hospital would remain open with 300 beds. See "Superhospital funding clears final hurdle," *Montreal Gazette*, June 25, 2004, A1.

99 Susan Drouin, "The New Site Means New Configurations for Efficiency and Comfort Affair," *Montreal Gazette*, May 6, 2001. Drouin is associate director of MUHC Nursing—Obstetrics and Gynecology.

100 Jeff Heinrich, "Hospital Director Quits in Protest," *Montreal Gazette*, January 12, 2000, A1.

101 Funding for the $1.1 billion CHUM project was also approved in June 2004, but involved rebuilding on the current site of St. Luc Hospital. See "Superhospital funding clears final hurdle," A1.

102 His lecture was entitled "The Children's Hospital: Crown Jewel of a Medical Center."

103 Zeidler Roberts Partnership/Architects has recently been chosen as design architects for the $135 million Alberta Children's Hospital in Calgary, now under construction. See *Canadian Architect* 46 (May 2001): 11.

104 Charlotte Gray, "Focus Changing at Children's Hospitals," *Canadian Medical Association Journal* 158 (1998): 15.

105 See Robert Hamilton, "Planning of the Pre-Concept Architectural Design for the McGill University Health Centre, Montreal," in *Design and Health III: Health Promotion through Environmental Design*, ed. Alan Dilani (Stockholm: International Academy for Health and Design, 2004), 59–71.

106 Bruce King Komiske, "The Children's Hospital: Crown Jewel of a Medical Center," in *Healing by Design: Building for Health Care in the 21st Century* (Montreal: McGill University Health Centre, 2000), varied pagination. Komiske examines more images of the "best" children's hospitals in Bruce King Komiske, *Designing the World's Best Children's Hospitals* (Victoria, Australia: Images, 1999).

107 Komiske, "The Children's Hospital."

108 Verderber and Fine point out that health planners in the United States continue to have a "near obsession" (x) with the idea that every patient should be housed in a private room, whereas in the United Kingdom, by contrast, public, open wards are still considered both functional and ideal (196–200).

109 See Richard Lansdown, *Children in Hospital: A Guide for Family and Carers* (New York: Oxford University Press, 1996), 244–49.

110 Lansdown, *Children in Hospital*, 1996.

111 In fact, at the Healing by Design Colloquium, Wanda J. Jones, an expert in healthcare delivery systems, specifically warned against the campus plan of separate buildings; see Wanda J. Jones, "New Century Design for the McGill University Health Centre: From Negative to Positive Value in Health Facilities" (paper presented at Healing by Design, Montreal, September 20–21, 2000).

Frontier Health Services for Children

Alberta's Provincial Travelling Clinic, 1924–1942

⍥

Sharon L. Richardson

P roviding health services to sparsely populated, geographically isolated areas was a major challenge in many Canadian provinces
prior to the advent of universal hospital insurance in the late
1950s, and universal physician insurance in the late 1960s. The task
was especially daunting during the years of the Depression, which began
in Alberta and Saskatchewan in the late 1920s and continued until the
onset of the Second World War. Nonetheless, from 1924 to 1942, Alberta's
Department of Public Health sponsored a unique Travelling Clinic,
which conducted physical examinations, dental examinations and treatment, tonsillectomies and other minor surgery, and vaccination against
smallpox to children in frontier areas of the province. The purpose of
this article is to analyze Alberta's Provincial Travelling Clinic within the
context of public policy. Public policy is defined as a long series of more
or less related choices, including decisions not to act, which are made by
governments in response to public issues.[1] Health policy, one aspect of
public policy, focuses on government decisions related to goals for the
health of all the population of a jurisdiction and perceived priorities in
providing them health services.

Precursors of Alberta's Provincial
Travelling Clinic

Alberta's Travelling Clinic was one strategy used by the United Farmers
of Alberta (UFA) government to lessen public animosity after it dramatically curtailed provincially funded public health nursing services for
preschool and school-age children in 1923. The UFA government,
elected in 1921 on a platform of agrarian reform, replaced the Liberal
party, which had governed Alberta since its inception as a province in
1905. The UFA came to power at the beginning of a major farm crisis,
brought on by an economic recession combined with prolonged drought

in the southeast section of the province. To address Alberta's deteriorating economy, the newly elected UFA government curtailed spending for many government-sponsored programs and services, especially those deemed not essential to the provincial economy. Despite maintaining the existing level of overall funding of the Department of Public Health, as part of its program of fiscal restraint, the UFA government dramatically reduced the number of provincially employed public health nurses in 1922 from thirty to twenty. A year later, the UFA government further reduced these twenty positions to six. Since provincially employed public health nurses provided almost all of the health promotion and disease prevention programs for infants, preschool, and school-age children, as well as pre- and post-natal education for mothers, slashing their number severely curtailed availability of these services throughout the province.

The provincial Division of Public Health Nursing had been created in 1918 as a direct result of active and prolonged lobbying of the Liberal government for organized public health services for women and children by the United Farm Women of Alberta (UFWA).[2] The UFWA was the women's auxiliary of the United Farmers of Alberta (UFA), an Alberta populist political party that grew out of the agrarian reform movement shortly before the First World War. The UFA was led by Henry Wise Wood, an American and a member of the Disciples of Christ, a denomination that emphasized the need for Christian ethics in economic affairs. The UFA espoused democracy based on the Christian ethic.[3] Responding to political pressure from the UFWA, the Liberal government initiated and fully funded significant public health nursing services, with a particular focus on women and children living in rural Alberta.[4] These services included permanent Child Welfare Clinics in twelve rural districts, a summertime Travelling Child Welfare Clinic for more isolated and less densely populated rural areas of the province, and a District Nursing Service for settlers in frontier Alberta. Child Welfare Clinics for infants, preschool children, and expectant mothers in Edmonton, Medicine Hat, and Calgary were also staffed by provincially employed public health nurses who offered physical examination of infants and preschool children, and pre- and post-natal advice to mothers.[5] The Travelling Child Welfare Clinics, begun in 1920 to service remote rural areas, were staffed by two provincial public health nurses who delivered services similar to the permanent rural and urban Child Welfare Clinics. In addition to conducting Child Welfare Clinics, provincial public health nurses also made home visits, gave public lectures on health and home nursing, and provided physical examinations and immunization to school children upon request of rural school districts.[6] Physical examination and immunization of school children in Edmonton and Calgary was conducted by nurses employed by the respective school boards of these two cities.[7]

The District Nursing Service, created in 1919 under the Public Health Nurses Act, met needs for midwifery and emergency medical treatment in frontier communities with neither physicians nor hospitals. District nurses provided pre- and post-natal care, conducted home births, gave emergency medical treatment, held office hours for non-emergency care, prescribed and dispensed drugs, and also provided preventive public health services such as physical inspection and immunization of school children. The 1919 Public Health Nurses Act made legal the practice of midwifery by graduate nurses employed by the provincial Department of Public Health who had "taken a course in obstetrics" and who had permission of the minister of health.[8] Thus, within a few years, and in response to political pressure from the UFWA, Alberta's Liberal government established a province-wide preventive public health nursing service aimed at promoting the health of infants, preschool and school-age children, and prenatal and postnatal women throughout Alberta's urban and rural communities.[9]

As part of its fiscal policy of restraint, in 1922 the UFA government not only slashed the number of public health nurses it employed, but also implemented cost-sharing of public health nursing services on a fifty-fifty basis with municipalities. In a period of deepening economic recession, with reduced tax revenues, many municipalities could not afford to pay 50 per cent of the costs of public health nursing services, and had to forgo them entirely. As a consequence, province-wide programs of physical examination and immunization of infants, preschool and school-age children, provided by the provincial Division of Public Health Nursing, were dramatically curtailed in the rural regions where two-thirds of the population lived. Interestingly, District Nursing Services were gradually increased, suggesting the UFA government valued treatment more than prevention of illness and communicable disease control. Organized women's groups, such as the UFWA and the Women's Institutes (WI), as well as local school boards, were incensed by the government's reduction of health promotion and disease prevention services for women and children, and protested loudly.[10]

Despite their pre-election radical rhetoric, the newly elected UFA government failed to live up to its social reform promises. In part, this failure was associated with Alberta's faltering economy in the early 1920s. Farmers in southern Alberta pleaded for government relief to help them ride out the prolonged drought. Farmers in both southern and central Alberta demanded monetary reform, including a provincial bank that would operate on a service rather than a profit basis. Farmers in northern Alberta were preoccupied by the collapse of government-subsidized railways, which made it increasingly difficult to transport crops and live-stock to market. Throughout the province, farmers demanded reform in the grain marketing system. Addressing such major economic woes left the UFA government with few resources, monetary and human, to imple-ment its pre-election social reform promises. In part, however, failure to implement social reform also reflected the UFA's stress on the rights of the individual and its lingering reluctance to intrude into what it per-ceived as the private lives of citizens. Philosophically, the political lead-ers of the UFA exhibited concern with collective economic security and ambivalence about the role of government as a leader of social change.[11] For example, UFA leader Henry Wise Wood, influenced by his populist background in the United States, viewed government not as an initiator of social programs but as a force restraining social injustice.[12] Alberta was still something of a frontier province in the early 1920s, characterized by the rugged individualism of any frontier, coupled with a "live and let live" orientation to life. Acting cautiously and pragmatically, Premier Herbert Greenfield and his cabinet declined to engage in radical mon-etary reform, although they did permit drought-stricken southern farm-ers to renegotiate farm loans through a government-appointed com-missioner. The newly elected UFA government also reformed the grain marketing system by supporting creation of a cooperative wheat pool—the Alberta Wheat Pool—and began negotiating the sale of four incom-plete and unprofitable railways that had been heavily subsidized by the Liberal government.

When administratively inexperienced and ineffective Premier Green-field resigned in late 1925, he was replaced by Attorney-General John Brownlee, one of the major forces tempering the UFA's radicalism. Brownlee, an urban lawyer with social connection to Calgary's business and professional elite, had been legal advisor to the UFA prior to its elec-tion, and attorney general after 1921. As premier, Brownlee felt the major tasks facing the province were to balance the budget, continue attempts to dispose of the provincial railways, and secure from Ottawa provincial control of natural resources.[13] Expansion of social services, including health services, played no major part in Brownlee's plans for the province. His philosophy of economic development first, and social services later, was reinforced by George Hoadley, who held the dual portfolios of agriculture and public health throughout the UFA's four-teen years in power. Prior to joining the UFA, Hoadley had been the Alberta Conservative party leader. Hoadley's primary focus was improv-ing the agrarian economy of the province, rather than promoting the health of Albertans through publicly funded health services.

If Hoadley had not held the dual portfolios of public health and agri-culture, or if a more reform-minded member of the UFA party had held the dual portfolio, publicly funded preventive health services might have enjoyed more prominence during the UFA's years in government. Health care reform was a hotly debated topic during the provincial election campaign of 1921. In recognition that organized farm women had led health care reform, Irene Parlby, first president of the UFWA from 1915 to 1919, and later convenor of its public health committee, was rumoured to become minister of public health. Surprisingly, when the UFA was elected in 1921, she was passed over and made instead minister without portfolio. Parlby was designated special "women's minister," informally charged with acting on behalf of Alberta women and children. Without separate departmental responsibility or the budget that went with it, Parlby had no formal means of initiating programs or determining government policy on health care or social reform. Constrained by the rules of cabinet solidarity, she was compelled to support her cabinet colleagues in the UFA government. Subsequently, the UFA failed to live up to their pre-election promise to make public health care a priority "not only from the prevention but from the curative standpoint." Instead, the UFA government simply carried on health programs begun by the Liberal government under the spur of UFWA lobbying. In addition to a Division of Public Health Nursing established in 1918, and the Public Health Nurses Act passed in 1919, these programs included the Municipal Hospitalization Plan inaugurated in 1917 to assist municipalities to establish and operate hospitals through payment of hospital taxes by local ratepayers, and a tuberculosis sanatorium opened at Robertson in 1920 under the joint auspices of the federal Department of Soldiers Civil Re-establishment and the Alberta government.[14] The only new health programs begun by the UFA government were token efforts for rural and frontier areas—two experimental rural full-time health units in 1931, the Travelling Clinic in 1924, and a very limited District Physicians Plan in 1929, which saw three British doctors hired by the Department of Public Health sent to Notikewin, Kinuso and Slave Lake. Of these initiatives, only the rural full-time health units proved a permanent feature of Alberta's health care.[15] Both Brownlee and Hoadley were reluctant to expand the health care budget and eventually retreated fully from state medicine. A significant health policy problem that faced the UFA throughout its fourteen years in power, and which it failed to solve, was a marked discrepancy between health services available in the urban versus the rural and frontier areas of Alberta. UFA pre-election principles gave way to balanced budgets as the government's primary preoccupation.[16]

The UFA's fiscal policy of reducing the number of provincially employed public health nurses from thirty to six, and requiring municipalities to pay half the costs of public health nursing services, was a dramatic change from previous Liberal government preventive health policy. Not surprisingly, cities and municipalities resisted. Although the 1919 Public Health Act required a board of health in every district to be responsible for carrying out the provisions of the act, almost no rural municipalities, and only two of the urban municipalities—Edmonton and Medicine Hat—had functioning public health boards by 1922. By 1934, only three rural districts had organized public health boards that paid half the public health nursing service costs. These were the municipal districts served through Vegreville, Stanmore, and Milo. The municipal district of Marquis withdrew in 1934.[17] As Superintendent of the Provincial Department of Public Health Nursing Branch, Elizabeth Clark, commented in 1923, "While practically all [municipal councils] favour the scheme [of locally controlled public health nursing services], financial conditions proved the chief obstacle in not accepting it."[18] The financial conditions alluded to by Clark included reluctance to accept financial responsibility for a service previously provided without charge by the provincial government, as well as declining local revenues associated with poor prices for farmers' wheat and livestock.

Inception of Alberta's Travelling Clinic

In the unorganized regions of the province where population was too sparse, too dispersed, and/or too ethnically divergent to support any form of local government, it was impossible for settlers to organize preventive public health services. To the extent that pioneering Albertans perceived that their government "owed" them some kind of recompense for accepting the challenge to homestead in isolated areas that lacked even rudimentary services, the Travelling Clinic represented a politically motivated response. Almost from Alberta's inception as a province in 1905, its governments consistently made existing health problems worse by seeking to entice settlers into frontier areas it already knew itself incapable of servicing. As UFWA founding President Irene Parlby asserted at the 1919 UFA Annual Convention, "Since the [Liberal] government was responsible for inducing people to homestead in the wild areas of this province by often highly rose-coloured literature and propaganda, or the wiles of immigration agents,...it was the duty of the government to safeguard the lives of these people and their families" by "engage[ing] its own body of doctors and nurses; [and] provide[ing] them with adequate salaries and build[ing] homes for them in places where they are most needed."[19]

Following in the tradition of western "boosterism," which earlier lured settlers and investment into the arid southern prairies, Peace River promotional material of the 1920s promised free land, plentiful water, favourable climate, and good transportation. As Janice McGinnis notes in her "Introduction" to the letters of Mary Percy Jackson, "If such promises were not exactly a fabric of lies, they were certainly a fantasy of half-truths…and for women given the job of 'civilizing' the frontier, such misleading propaganda was particularly harmful."[20] Consequently, the UFA government was forced by the demands of organized women's groups to expand its District Nursing Service in these areas to meet needs for midwifery and emergency medical services, and to offer at least episodic physical examination and treatment of preschool and school-age children through the itinerant Travelling Clinic.

The notion of a provincially funded mobile clinic to provide medical and dental treatment to children in remote areas is variously attributed to a scheme operationalized in 1920 in Nova Scotia under the auspices of the Canadian Red Cross Society,[21] and to the 1923 initiative of Alberta District Nurse Olive Watherstone.[22] In his review of the public health policies of the UFA government, Collins described the 1920 Nova Scotia scheme, funded by the Canadian Red Cross, which sponsored two touring clinics whose staff comprised a "chest specialist, an eye, ear, nose and throat specialist, an orthopedist, a dentist, two public health nurses and a secretary," and who covered about forty-five points in forty-eight days throughout that province. He suggests that Nova Scotia's itinerant treatment team was well publicized and may have inspired the model subsequently adopted by the UFA government. In her history of district nursing in Alberta, Stewart presents the Alberta Travelling Clinic as a natural outgrowth of District Nurse Olive Watherstone's attempts to secure medical treatment services for children residing in her remote region. Watherstone was a British-trained nurse and midwife who served throughout the First World War as a nursing sister on British troop transport ships and in casualty clearing stations in France. She emigrated to Canada in 1921, and was appointed Alberta district nurse at Halcourt, fifty miles southwest of Grande Prairie, in the Peace River District, the same year. Her concern about the number of children in her area who required medical, surgical, and dental care, prompted Miss Watherstone to invite Dr. Carlisle of Lake Saskatoon to come into her district during the summer of 1923 to conduct a clinic for removal of tonsils and adenoids. Because of the distance from doctors and hospitals, and the expense involved, it was impossible for parents to obtain this treatment for their children outside the district. No statistics are available for this clinic, but it was reported as "very successful."[23]

Partly as a result of the success of Watherstone's local initiative, and partly in an attempt to ameliorate some of the deleterious effects of its severely reduced public health nursing service, in the summer of 1924, the Department of Public Health pilot-tested provincially funded public clinics at Halcourt and Wenham valley in the Peace District, Kinuso and Slave Lake, north of Edmonton, Rife, northeast of Edmonton, and Yeoford and Pendryl, southwest of Edmonton. It is not clear from archival records to what extent this "experiment," as it was later called, originated with Deputy Minister of Public Health W. C. Laidlaw, or with Elizabeth Clark, superintendent of the Public Health Nursing Branch; however, it must have had at least Laidlaw's tacit approval to recruit the necessary medical staff. Olive Watherstone organized the clinic at Halcourt at which nineteen children had their tonsils and adenoids removed. Elizabeth Clark, assisted by Slave Lake District Nurse Reid, organized the remaining clinics at which 264 children were physically examined and sixty-nine tonsillectomies and adenoidectomies and three circumcisions were conducted. Additionally, nine home visits were made, with four cases sent to hospital. R. G. Huckell, a surgeon from the University of Alberta Hospital, and A. E. Heacock, provincial dentist, comprised the medical staff.[24] Unlike Nova Scotia's 1920 touring clinic, no attempt was made in Alberta to screen for tuberculosis ("chest specialist") or to offer orthopedic services for crippled children ("orthopedist").

Deputy Minister of Public Health W. C. Laidlaw used his 1924 annual report to Minister Hoadley to praise the "experiment" of what he called the Travelling Clinic, noting, "We have received many letters from people in appreciation of the services rendered." Laidlaw further recommended that this service be increased in the summer of 1925, and that Drs. Huckell and Heacock, together with a nurse, "should start out in early May, or as soon as the roads are fit for driving," to visit all the established nursing districts. In advance of the Travelling Clinic, another nurse could be sent ahead to survey districts and organize "some local body to take charge of the details." Clearly, Laidlaw, who had been deputy minister since inception of the Alberta Department of Public Health in 1919, appreciated the potential for physical examinations of children done in conjunction with the Travelling Clinic to partially make up for preventive health services lost when the UFA government slashed the number of provincially employed public health nurses. Laidlaw was greatly respected by his medical colleagues in Alberta and likely provided the health promotion perspective that Minister of Agriculture and Public Health Hoadley lacked. Laidlaw's death in 1926 was recorded by his medical colleagues as "a great loss."[25] Throughout his 1924 annual report to Minister Hoadley, Laidlaw emphasized the benefits of preventive public health services and outlined strategies for achieving improved health throughout the province. For example, in reporting on the work of the Infectious Diseases Branch, Laidlaw specifically explained why general practitioners did not make competent public health officers, and recommended dividing the province into geographic public health districts, each with a provincially employed, specially trained full-time health officer in charge to coordinate disease prevention and health promotion.[26] Arguably, it was the political benefits, rather than the health benefits associated with the "experimental" Travelling Clinic, that garnered Minister Hoadley's endorsement of the innovation.

Capitalizing on the public relations value of the experimental Travelling Clinic, the UFA government continued to sponsor its summer visits to isolated communities from 1925 to 1931. Secretaries of school boards, women's organizations, and other interested bodies were notified of the conditions under which the clinic would visit their districts. One condition was that the Travelling Clinic had to be invited to visit. The other conditions were that at least twelve rural school districts had to combine for clinic purposes, and a local committee needed to form to arrange a suitable building, water supply, heat, beds, bedding, food, and coordinated transport of children to and from the clinic site. The Department of Public Health considered requests for clinic services during the winter and mapped a preliminary itinerary. Once the local committee completed its planning, a provincial public health or district nurse conducted preliminary physical examinations of all preschool and school children in the district and recommended who should be examined by Travelling Clinic physicians and dentists for further diagnosis and possible treatment. Communities requesting clinic visits were then notified regarding the clinic schedule and the date for their community's visit.[27]

Travelling Clinic staff usually consisted of one surgeon, one anesthetist, one or two dentists, two to four nurses, and one or two truck drivers. The surgeon was in charge of the Travelling Clinic. The surgeon was invariably a medical staff member of the University of Alberta Hospital in Edmonton, since the UAH was considered the "provincial hospital" and received an annual grant from the UFA government of $20 million over and above the usual per diem rate for patient occupancy. The anesthetist/examining physician was either a UAH medical staff member or, after 1929, one of the four doctors hired by George Hoadley to staff district stations at Battle River Prairie/Notikewin, in the northern Peace River country, Kinuso, on the southern shore of Lesser Slave Lake, and Lac La Biche, in northeastern Alberta. The dentists were either members of Dental Services at the University of Alberta, or employees of the provincial Department of Public Health. All of the nurses were provincially employed public health and district nurses. The truck drivers were either medical or dental students at the University of Alberta. None of the clinic staff received a special salary for their work, although their transportation, accommodation, and food was provided by the Department of Public Health.

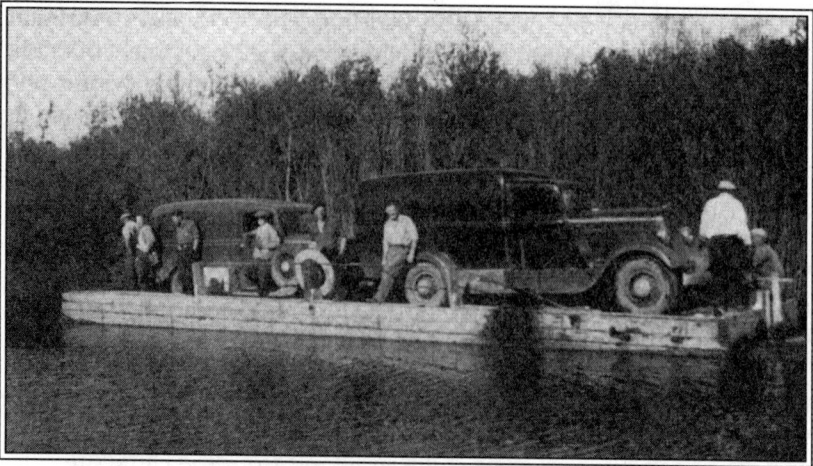

Ferry carrying two trucks on Wapiti River (1939) (Glenbow Archives, Calgary)

As photographs clearly show, the Travelling Clinic was very much a campers' expedition! Clinic staff travelled in two trucks into which they also packed sufficient tents, cooking utensils, food, clothing, and surgical equipment to be self-sustaining. When roads became impassable in the northern and Peace River district—as they often did when wet—equipment would be off-loaded into horse-drawn wagons or the Northern Alberta Railway, for transport to destination. The usual road-building method was to run two parallel ditches, piling the soil in the middle, which resulted in bottomless "gumbo" when it rained in these rich black clay areas. In southern and eastern Alberta the land was drier, but roads were rarely gravelled. Sometimes the trucks and staff travelled on river rafts, as shown en route to Slave Lake in 1936.

Whatever else they were, Travelling Clinic staff had to be able to manage life in the outdoors, and be enterprising and endlessly patient when plans didn't quite work out the first time. Some, like District Nurse Olive Watherstone—who served as nurse-in-charge from 1927 to 1931, and from 1934 to 1939—and provincial dentist Heacock—who served with the clinic each year from its inception in 1924—thoroughly enjoyed the itinerant summer employment. Others, like University Hospital Medical Superintendent Washburn—who wore a white shirt and bow tie on clinic expeditions—soon retired from the fray.[28]

On the local scene, community halls, churches, or schools were used for the clinic. Department instructions required that the building be house-cleaned, walls and windows washed, and the floor thoroughly scrubbed. One or two days before the Travelling Clinic arrived, local residents, armed with brooms, mops, pails, and scrub brushes cleaned the selected building. On the day of the clinic, a few local men and

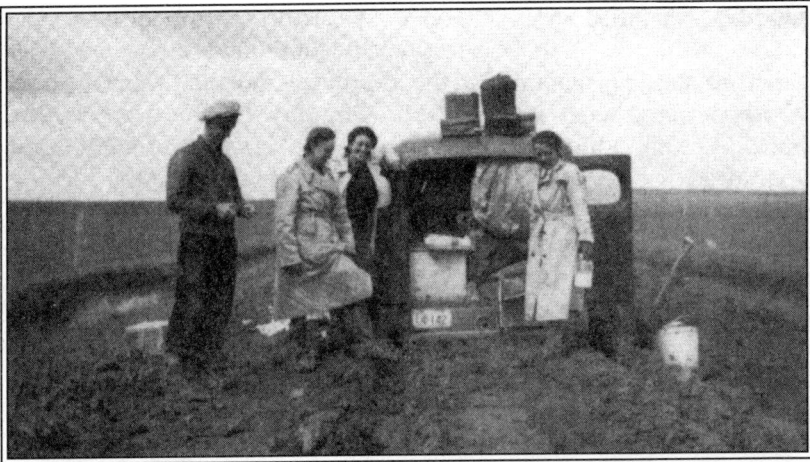

Clinic van mired in mud, Peace River area (1939) (Glenbow Archives, Calgary)

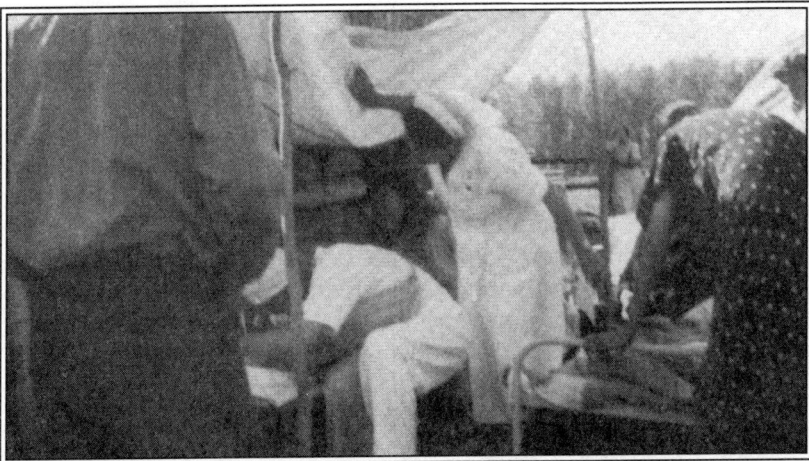

Travelling Clinic staff, Peace River (1935) (Glenbow Archives, Calgary)

women also assisted as janitors, registrars, and messengers. When the clinic staff arrived, they unloaded their equipment and prepared the room for the start of the clinic the following day. Then they set up their tents at a campsite nearby, if the weather was fine; if not, alternative accommodation would have been arranged in a hotel or private home. Arrangements would also have been made for meals for clinic staff, often provided by local women's organizations.[29]

The Travelling Clinic usually spent two full days at each site. On the first day of the clinic, both physicians and one dentist examined children and recommended to parents those requiring operations or dental treat-

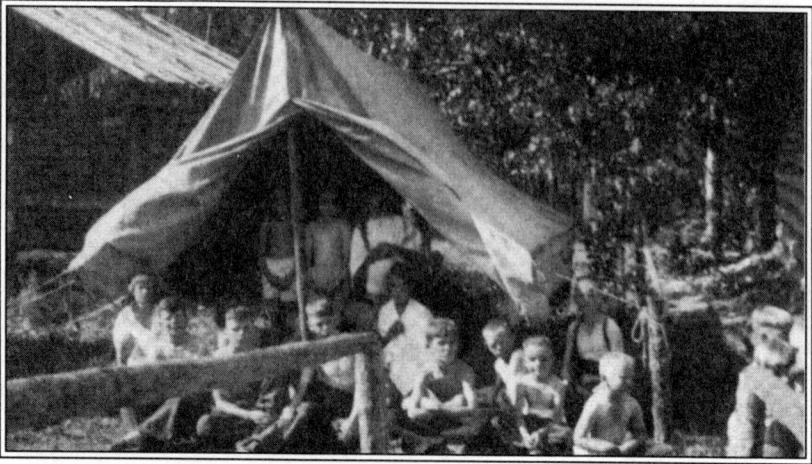

Children waiting examination, Pipeston Creek (1939) (Glenbow Archives, Calgary)

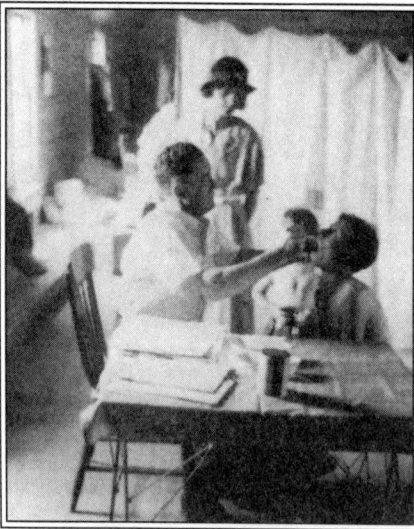

Dr. Gilchrist (dentist) examining two boys, Peace River area (1939) (Glenbow Archives, Calgary)

ment to return the following day. The second dentist carried on dental treatments, mostly fillings. The nurses were in charge of clerical work and overall clinic organization. On the second day, one dentist continued with dental treatments while the other dentist did extractions under general anesthesia. The surgeon, anesthetist, and scrub nurse conducted tonsillectomies and adenoidectomies and other minor surgical procedures. One nurse was in charge of sterilizing instruments and supplies, while the other one or two were responsible for patients before and

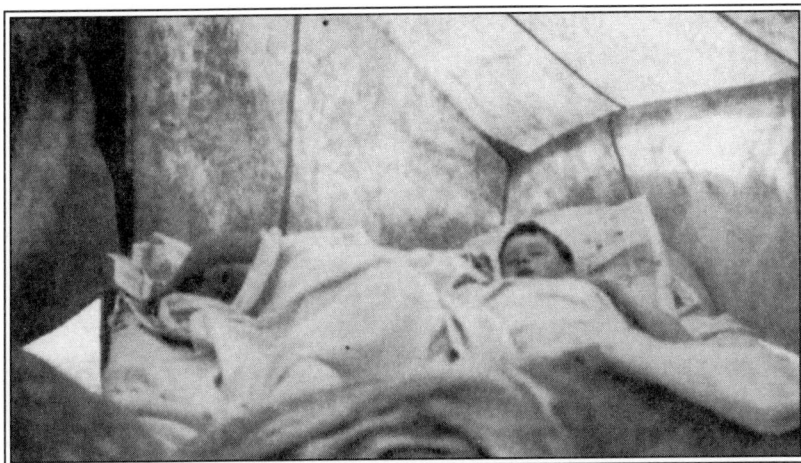

Children in recovery tent, Pipestone Creek (1939) (Glenbow Archives, Calgary)

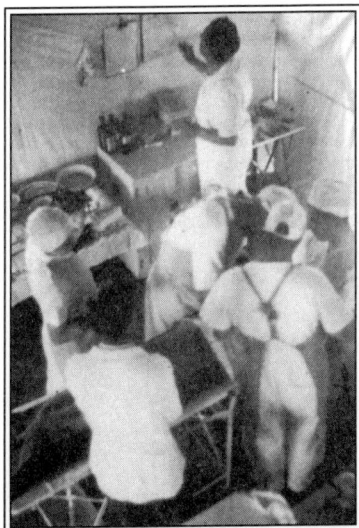

Operating team in theatre, Peace River area (1936) (Glenbow Archives, Calgary)

after operations. Patients remained in the improvised hospital ward—which was sometimes a tent—until the following day. On the third day the clinic moved on to the next site. Cots and blankets were brought in for the children by their parents, who camped on the site until the evening of the second day, when children were fit to be taken home. Some parents reportedly travelled thirty to forty miles in wagons drawn by horses, oxen, or mules to take advantage of the Travelling Clinics' services.[30]

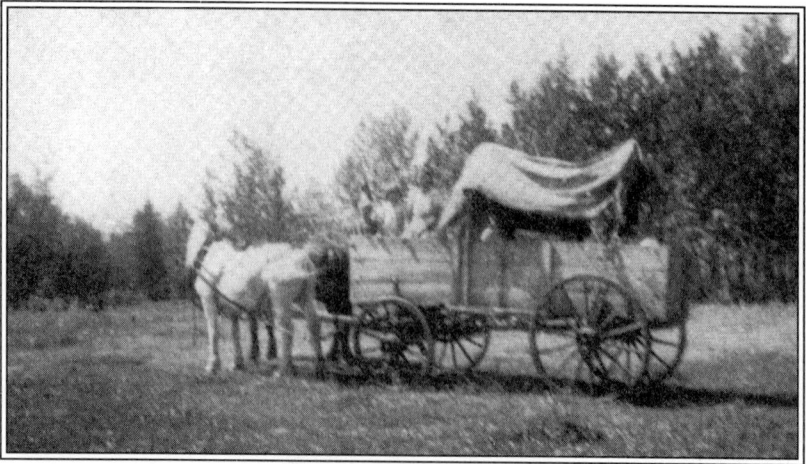

Parents taking children home after clinic in a horse-drawn grain wagon, Pipestone Creek (1939) (Glenbow Archives, Calgary)

The "experimental" Travelling Clinic proved so successful that in each of the succeeding four years the scope of its activities was increased. In 1925, the districts of Yeoford, Slave Lake, Halcourt, and Pendryl, which had been visited by the Travelling Clinic the preceding year, were revisited, and five additional clinics were held in the Peers district, west of Edmonton. A total of 335 children were medically examined and fifty-eight tonsillectomies and adenoidectomies performed; 819 children were examined dentally, with 656 cases treated. In her annual report, Elizabeth Clark, superintendent of the Public Health Nursing Branch, was at pains to point out that the Travelling Clinics "Do not in any way interfere with the local medical or dental services" because "they are only sent to districts in which no medical or dental services are available, and where the people are not able to provide for these services."[31] Clearly, the UFA government did not wish to compete with existing physician services or antagonize private physicians and dentists. Persuading physicians and dentists to establish practices in rural and frontier parts of Alberta was an ongoing challenge for Alberta governments; therefore, none wished to appear to be competing in any way with entrepreneurial medical and dental practitioners. The Department of Public Health in 1926 also implemented a partial fee structure for parents who, they believed, could afford to pay for Travelling Clinic services. Because many of the heads of families in the settlements of McLennan, Donnelly and Falher were employed, a "nominal cost" was levied for Travelling Clinic services, although a few cases were treated free on recommendations from reliable sources.[32] This practice appears to have continued throughout the UFA years of the Travelling Clinic, reflecting the UFA government's belief that whenever possible, recipients of government health services should contribute to their costs.

Despite the fact that the Travelling Clinic provided much-needed physical examination, immunization, and minor surgical treatment to children in isolated areas, when the UFA's financial situation worsened in the early 1930s, the Department of Public Health curtailed its activities. After the peak year of 1928, when eighty-eight centres were visited and 5,678 children were examined—more than twice the number of the preceding year—the duration and scope of the Travelling Clinic was reduced. During 1932 and 1933, as part of a "policy of economy," the Travelling Clinic did not operate. In fact, no reference is contained in the 1932 and 1933 annual reports of the Department of Public Health to the Travelling Clinic, at all.

Curtailment of Travelling Clinic activities reflected the UFA government's preoccupation with cutting costs and balancing the provincial budget as their primary strategy for dealing with a rapidly escalating financial crisis. Prices for wheat plummeted in 1930, drawing in the provincial government, which provided loan guarantees to the floundering wheat pools. The Brownlee government responded to the crisis with increased frugality, severely cutting back the civil service, shutting down agricultural colleges, shortening the school year, and reducing teachers' salaries.[33] Reeling under a reduced budget, the provincial Department of Public Health focused on preventive public health services in areas where population density was the greatest and services could be most efficiently delivered; that is, in the cities of Calgary, Edmonton, and Medicine Hat. In 1931, Alberta's total population was 730,000, with 84,000, 80,000, 10,000, and 10,000 residing in Calgary, Edmonton, Medicine Hat, and Lethbridge respectively. The southern city of Lethbridge did not participate in provincially sponsored public health services. Instead, beginning in 1909, Lethbridgeans supported a philanthropically funded visiting nursing service—the Lethbridge Nursing Mission—which continued as an independent nursing and welfare agency until 1954, when the Victorian Order of Nurses assumed responsibility for public health nursing.[34]

Throughout the Depression of the 1930s, the provincial Department of Public Health continued to provide public health nurses as supervisors of the permanent Child Welfare Clinics it had established in Edmonton in 1920, in Calgary and Medicine Hat in 1922, and in Vegreville in 1926. The Department of Public Health also continued to sponsor the summer Travelling Child Welfare Clinics begun in 1920 to serve more remote rural communities. In addition to maintaining these two health-promotion and disease-prevention programs aimed at infants, children, and mothers, in the field of public health, the UFA government established Alberta's first two full-time rural health units at Red Deer and Okotoks/High River (later renamed the Foothills H.U.) in 1931. These units comprised five rural municipalities and the eight or nine towns and villages within their boundaries. The Red Deer health unit served an area of approximately 1,700 square miles and a population of about 21,000. The Okotoks/High River health unit covered approximately 1,900 square miles and a population of about 15,000. Each health unit was administered by a volunteer board composed of representatives from each of the municipalities within the district. These rural full-time health units emphasized preventive health services, including physical examination of infants and children, pre- and post-natal advice to mothers, immunization for communicable diseases, general education on healthy living, and sanitary inspection for pure water, milk, and food. Each health unit was staffed by a specially trained medical officer of health, two public health nurses, a sanitary inspector, and a stenographer.[35] Funding from a special grant from the Rockefeller Foundation in the United States was critical to creation of these two permanent rural health units, which were intended to demonstrate the value of full-time preventive public health services in rural areas and small urban centres. The cost of approximately $10,000 per year was covered 50 per cent by the UFA government, 25 per cent by the participating municipalities, and 25 per cent by the Rockefeller Foundation.[36] At the expiration of the three-year trial period, when the Rockefeller Foundation withdrew its support, all the territory in both health units, with the exception of one town, agreed to continue operating the full-time rural health units.[37]

There was some justification for reduction in Travelling clinic services during the early 1930s, since despite an even more depressed provincial economy than what was experienced during the preceding two years, in 1932 the overall health of Albertans was maintained. For example, the combined death rate (deaths per 100,000 population) for diphtheria, scarlet fever, measles, and whooping cough was 8.3, as compared with the rate of 9.8 in 1931, and 20.5 as the average rate for the preceding five years. The infant mortality rate also declined to 58.62, as compared with the rate of 69.4 for 1931, and 72.22 as the average for the five years from 1927 to 1931. And although in 1932, sixty-four women died from conditions associated with childbirth, for a maternal death rate of 3.76 for every 1,000 children born, this was the lowest maternal death rate recorded in the history of the province.[38]

Persistent demands from settlers in isolated areas of the province for treatment services, coupled with the UFA government's dramatic decline in popularity after its re-election in June 1930,[39] stimulated expansion of the Department of Public Health's District Nursing Services and reinstatement of the Travelling Clinic in 1934. Premier Brownlee's retreat into fiscal conservatism as the full force of the Great Depression of the 1930s deepened, eroded support for the UFA government. In an attempt to limit settlers' increasingly vociferous complaints about inadequate health care, the Travelling Clinic was sent out late in 1934 to ten centres in northern Alberta. It examined 986 children, conducted 266 minor operations, and gave 262 dental treatments.[40] The same year the Travelling Clinic was reinstated, the UFA government was rocked by a sex scandal involving Premier Brownlee. Following his conviction for seducing a young government stenographer, Brownlee resigned as premier in July 1934.

When the Social Credit Party, led by fundamentalist lay preacher William Aberhart, ousted the UFA government in the 1935 provincial election, it inherited a massive public debt absorbing anywhere from one-third to more than half of the government's annual revenue.[41] Nonetheless, having been elected on a reform platform, Aberhart began almost immediately laying the framework for a social welfare state. Although his detractors considered Aberhart a vain, authoritarian, short-tempered man whose oratorical abilities far exceeded his intellectual capabilities, he was deeply distressed by the poverty and hopelessness that surrounded him and genuinely committed to seeking solutions to Depression conditions.[42] Under Aberhart, state-supported medicine and hospitalization was an integral part of the Social credit platform from 1935 until his death in office in 1943. For example, beginning in 1936, diagnosis and sanatorium treatment of pulmonary tuberculosis was made free of charge for all Alberta residents when the Tuberculosis Act came into force. Previously, municipalities were held responsible for maintaining their residents in the sanatorium, at a daily cost of $1.50, with any balance owing assumed by the Department of Public Health. Beginning in 1936, with the opening of a branch tuberculosis clinic in the Edmonton General Hospital, provincial TB bed capacity increased 78 per cent from 210 to 374. The same year, diagnostic services were expanded, and in 1937, there was an increase of 240 per cent over 1936 in TB diagnostic examinations.[43] Similarly, in 1938, the Poliomyelitis Sufferers Act gave free hospital, medical, and surgical care to Albertans suffering from the after-effects of polio, as well as supplying orthopedic appliances and academic or vocational training for employment. In 1940, the Cancer Treatment and Prevention Act created two provincial clinics—one in Calgary and one in Edmonton—where patients could be examined and could obtain authorization for further diagnostic and treatment services at no direct cost to themselves. Diagnostic services included tissue and X-ray examination and minor or major surgery, while treatment services included X-ray and radium therapy and surgical intervention, including operating room and anesthetic fees.[44]

The Social Credit government under Aberhart also expanded preventive public health services soon after coming to power. Public health services for mothers, infants, and children were reinstated by increasing the number of provincially employed public health nurses from seven to fifteen in 1935, and twenty-one in 1936. In 1938, a new rural health unit encompassing four municipalities and six villages in northeastern Alberta was established with headquarters at Lamont. This full-time rural health unit covered about 1,170 square miles with a population of 20,000 and a school population of approximately 5,000.[45] Another reflection of Aberhart's commitment to state medicine was increasing treatment services to Albertans in isolated areas. Consequently, both the District Nursing Service, which provided emergency medical and midwifery services, and the Travelling Clinic, which provided itinerant preventive and treatment services to children, were dramatically expanded after 1935.[46]

During 1935, the Travelling Clinic was in the field for four months from May 20 to September 28, visiting thirty-four centres throughout the drought-stricken and economically devastated southeast and east-central regions of the province, and the sparsely populated northeast. A total of 5,105 children were physically examined, with 888 minor operations, 2,149 dental treatments, and 2,238 dental extractions following.[47] Except for 1936, when the Travelling Clinic focused on fifteen centres in the Peace River District of northwestern Alberta, the clinic operated annually from mid-May to mid-August, physically examining and treating between 3,000 and 4,000 preschool and school-age children.[48] The Peace River District of northwestern Alberta, and the southeast, southcentral, and northeastern regions of the province continued to be visited at least every second year from 1935 through 1942. In 1943, the Travelling Clinic did not operate, ostensibly "owing to the impossibility of obtaining the medical, dental and nursing staff required" as physicians and graduate nurses left Alberta to serve in the military during the Second World War. Further, in his 1943 annual report to the provincial minister of public health, Deputy Minister Malcolm Bow remarked, "There appears to be little prospect of resuming this service until the medical, dental and nursing personnel required is available after the war."[49] Citing difficulty obtaining health care personnel to staff the Travelling Clinic for 1943 may have been at least partly a ruse used by the Social Credit government to disguise a significant change in policy direction that followed Premier Aberhart's death in office in May 1943. Aberhart's successor, Ernest Manning, began his twenty-five-year career as premier by steering Alberta public policy further right and assuming an anti-socialist stance. Manning's avowed anti-socialist, anti-unionist support of individualism promoted entrepreneurial enterprise in Alberta, while at the same time the Social Credit party grappled with demands to expand education and health services and aid farmers. Social Credit's swing to the right under Premier Manning was significantly aided by the resurgence of the provincial economy brought about by the Second World War. The Second World War can be credited with pulling Alberta out of the economic depression of the 1930s, and creating an affluence that supported ongoing health and social services reform. Agriculture, the mainstay of the Alberta economy, flourished during the war as farmers diversified to supply British markets. Extensive military involvement in the British Commonwealth Air Training Plan and participation in U.S. defence plans to protect Alaska, prompted Alberta's construction and air transportation industries and promoted rapid economic growth. The war also created a new national interest in Alberta's energy supplies—coal, conventional oil, and the oil sands. By the end of the Second World War, the province's per capita income equalled the national average.[50]

Not surprisingly, during and immediately after the Second World War, the Social Credit government could afford to extend public health services for mothers, as well as infants and children. Under the Maternity Hospitalization Act of 1944, free maternity hospital services became available to Albertans who had resided in the province for twelve consecutive months, or who were wives of servicemen resident in the province at the date of their enlistment. The only stipulations were that the woman had passed twenty-eight weeks of gestation and that the period of hospitalization did not exceed twelve days. This legislation was intended to further reduce the provincial maternal death rate, which was three times higher in home deliveries than in those conducted in hospital.[51] Five additional full-time rural health units opened in 1944, in the districts surrounding Stettler, Didsbury, rural Edmonton, Holden, and Two Hills. These health units offered a full range of disease-prevention and health-promotion services for all residents, including communicable disease control through immunization and case finding; sanitary inspection of water, milk, and food; pre- and post-natal advice to mothers; infant and child welfare clinics; school health services; and promotion of mental hygiene and nutrition. Half of the budget of each full-time rural health unit, up to a maximum of $7,000, was provided by the provincial Department of Public Health, while the district served provided the balance. The estimated cost per capita for public health service in the districts receiving it was approximately seventy-two cents. In addition, basic public health programs were begun in Rocky Mountain House, Macleod/Pincher Creek, Brooks, Strathmore, Westlock, Athabasca, Wainwright, McLennan, and Spirit River school divisions by the "one-nurse health units." These units were begun pending increased availability of full-time medical and nursing staff after the war.[52]

In expanding public health, medical treatment, and hospitalization services, the Social Credit government benefited significantly from discoveries of large reserves of oil and gas during the immediate post–Second World War period of reconstruction. These discoveries, which heralded an unprecedented era of prosperity in Alberta, began in 1947 at Leduc, south of Edmonton, and continued throughout the 1950s and into the 1960s. Many new hospitals were built and existing hospitals expanded. Health care became hospital based and available in all but the most isolated areas of northern Alberta. Fed in part on the wealth generated by the petroleum industry, northern Alberta developed rapidly. With improvements in roads, communication, and transportation, access to doctors and hospitals became easier, even in the most isolated districts of the Peace River. The rapid expansion of rural health units in the 1960s also meant that preventive health services previously provided by the Travelling Clinic, such as physical examination and immunization of preschool and school-age children, increasingly came under the sponsorship of local health units. By 1962, there were twenty-four local health units, each with a staff of medical officer of health, four public health nurses, a sanitary inspector, a secretary-technician, and a part-time secretary-treasurer, to serve an average population of 27,000.[53] In point of fact, 1942 was the last year of operation of the Travelling Clinic. A colourful era in travelling treatment services for children in isolated parts of Alberta had ended.

Overall Impact of Provincial Travelling Clinic

What, then, can be said about the overall impact of the provincial Travelling Clinic on the health of Alberta children from 1924 to 1943? Certainly the clinic provided physical examination of preschool and school-age children in some isolated parts of the province where this service was not otherwise available. It also ensured at least a minimum level of immunization against smallpox in these areas during the years after decimation of the provincial public health nursing service in 1923 and prior to the availability of communicable disease control services offered by expanding rural health units during the post–Second World War period of reconstruction. Probably, too, the dental treatment and minor surgical procedures done by the Travelling Clinic helped forestall more serious dental and medical problems. In the years before the advent of antibiotics, removal of offending teeth, tonsils, and adenoids was considered standard treatment to control repeated ear, nose, and throat infections. The extent to which the large number of tonsillectomies and adenoidectomies were beneficial probably remains a point of some conjecture, given the almost routine use of this treatment modality;

however, the disease prevention work of the Travelling Clinic is less disputable.

What the Travelling Clinic could not do was provide dependable, routine, and regularly scheduled preventive health and treatment services for children in remote areas of the province. By its very nature, the clinic was an ad hoc endeavour, largely dependent on political whim and travelling conditions. It reflected government public policy in a unique way. Neither the UFA nor the Social Credit governments under Aberhart developed long-range, coherent public policy on health and social services. By and large, public policy affecting health and social services in Alberta during the 1920s and 1930s was reactive, rather than proactive; that is, health policy evolved in response to intermittent and often iterative demands for treatment services, such as those provided by physicians and hospitals. Government health policy reflected limited long-range planning for improvement in overall health services, including preventive public health measures. The notion of long-range planning for health services for all citizens, regardless of their geographic locale, ethnicity, or ability to pay, was slow to root in Alberta, for at least three reasons.

First, neither the UFA nor the Social Credit parties had well-developed health platforms prior to coming to power in 1921 and 1935, respectively. Both parties were elected in reaction to pervasive dissatisfaction with their predecessors, rather than because of the soundness of their policy platforms. Neither the UFA nor the Social Credit party expected to be elected when it was, and certainly not in such sweeping numbers. In the July 1921 election, the UFA won thirty-eight seats, nearly two-thirds of the sixty-one seats, taking virtually all the rural constituencies in southern and central Alberta. In August 1935, Social Credit swept into power with fifty-six of sixty-three seats and 54 per cent of the popular vote. Further, both the UFA and Social Credit government under Aberhart, were composed predominantly of political neophytes with no prior experience of governing, and a limited grasp of public policy issues that did not directly affect them as individuals. Consequently, policy issues affecting economic growth preoccupied both governments, especially as they related to farming and transportation. Health and social welfare policy was far down the list of priorities for the UFA government, and for the early Social Credit government, formulation of health policy tended to be piecemeal and episodic.

Second, both the UFA and Social Credit governments under Aberhart were forced to address economic crises centred on farm and labour problems that devoured both time and fiscal resources, leaving very little left over for non-economic policy issues, such as health and social services. Despite its early rhetoric, under Premier Brownlee, the UFA government adhered to conservative public policy and rejected any radical innovations, such as expansion of government-sponsored preventive public health measures. Palmer attributes the conservatism of the provincial UFA to inexperience of new members, the underlying conservatism of founding leader Henry Wise Wood and subsequent leader Premier Brownlee, concern about fiscal solvency, and the declining radicalism of Alberta farmers in the late 1920s. Fiscal solvency preoccupied the UFA government from 1930 to 1935, when the interest from Alberta's massive public debt absorbed anywhere from one-third to more than half of the UFA government's annual revenue.[54] Similarly, Aberhart's Social Credit party came to power at a time of economic crisis, in the depths of the Great Depression, when low grain prices, coupled with drought and soil drifting in southern and east-central Alberta, brought many farmers to the brink of disaster. During the depression of the 1930s, average per capita income of Albertans fell well below the national average. Having promised sweeping economic and social reform, but lacking practical experience in governing, Aberhart stumbled through the late 1930s and early 1940s, attempting to balance the provincial budget while laying the framework for a social welfare state and initiating major educational reforms that reflected his own background and the strong contingent of teachers in the government. Under Aberhart, Alberta politics were highly volatile, due in large part to eccentricities such as government-issued script to augment legal currency, putting the banks under provincial control (with legislation that was subsequently disallowed by the federal government) and attempting to legislatively limit freedom of the press (also disallowed by the federal government). Had it not been for the Second World War lifting Alberta out of its economic doldrums, the Social Credit government might very well have been turned out of office by the early 1940s.

Third, the North American public health reform movement of the early twentieth century was adopted with varying speed and commitment by Canadian municipal and provincial governments. Not all citizens welcomed public health initiatives intended to "spread the social gospel of healthful living." This "social gospel" was intended to link proposed reform through the political system with the religious heritage of the nation for the "salvation of society."[55] For example, some parents perceived physical examination of school children by doctors and nurses as interference with parental rights and invasion of family privacy. Others opposed preventive measures such as immunization for communicable diseases as infringement of religious rights and unwarranted strategies to prevent illness.[56] The perceived role of children and their families, and elected governments' responsibility to ensure a minimum standard of living, was equivocal under both the UFA and early Social Credit governments. Although both the UFA and Social Credit parties had a Christian base that supported the notion of helping others less fortunate than oneself, they also stressed the rights of the individual. Consequently, the home was perceived as sacrosanct and family matters only to be interfered with in cases of extreme poverty or demonstrated immorality. The strong rural base of both parties reinforced their conservative values on children and family life, thereby limiting public policy that might be perceived as intrusive to the sanctity of the home. Consequently, health and social service policy under both the UFA and early Social Credit governments focused on those children perceived as in great need, and not children whose families could reasonably be expected to care for them adequately. Further, since Alberta public health nurses were primarily white, middle-class, and Anglo-Saxon, and their health teaching was coloured both by moral reform and enthusiasm for technological solutions administered by experts, they were often viewed with suspicion by other ethnic groups, including French Canadians from Quebec, German-speaking and communal Mennonites and Hutterites, and the large population of Ukrainians who homesteaded north-central Alberta.

The UFA government's wariness about government interference in the life of the individual not only reduced preventive public health services, but also limited adoption of a fully funded system of state medicine.[57] Under the UFA, in 1928 the concept of "state medicine" was initially declared impractical by Minister George Hoadley. Following repeated lobbying by the provincial Labour party and support by UFA party members M. McKeen and Irene Parlby, in March 1932, the UFA government finally agreed to re-examine ways in which adequate medical and health services could be made equally available to all Albertans. In its final report in 1934, a legislative committee defined state medicine as "a system of medical administration by which the state provides medical services for the entire population, and under which *all* practitioners are employed, directed and paid by the state on a salary basis." In comparison, state health insurance was defined as "a system of state insurance for health purposes. Under such a system a non-profit, state-supervised organization administers a fund provided for the mutual provision of medical services for the beneficiaries included under the system." Having clarified this important distinction, the legislative committee rejected the concept of state medicine on the grounds "that the general [medical] practitioner should be retained as the family physician in order that a close personal contact may be maintained between physician and patient." This rejection was in spite of the fact that more than half of all Alberta physicians practised exclusively in the major cities of Calgary and Edmonton and that many rural communities had limited or no access to local physician services.[58] Nonetheless, the UFA government in 1934 pro-

posed one urban and one rural trial project to test the feasibility of a
health insurance scheme. Later, in the spring of 1935, the UFA government, now headed by R. G. Reid, introduced a bill to create a provincial
health insurance plan as a way of minimizing individual costs of medical
care and promoting access. The bill proposed geographic health insurance districts in which all citizens contributed at least 50 per cent of
insurance costs, the state contributed 20 per cent, and employers contributed at least 20 per cent. If insured individuals, such as most farmers, were not employees, they would be required to pay the employer's
portion. Physicians' fees were to be reimbursed by a provincial body of
three, one of whom was a doctor.[59] The act was passed; however, the
UFA government did not put it into operation prior to its defeat in the
1935 election.[60] Possibly because of the significant proportion of the
costs proposed to be born by individuals, the Social Credit government
ignored the act. The Social Credit government only initiated a province-
wide hospital insurance plan for all Albertans in 1958, in conjunction with
the federal government's Hospitals and Diagnostic Services Act.[61]

Under both the UFA and Social Credit governments, the Provincial
Travelling Clinic was essentially a stopgap and expedient measure to
assuage complaints from isolated settlers about lack of access to health
services. It was especially useful in addressing demands of settlers in
the Peace River district, which endured limited health and social services throughout the 1920s, 1930s and 1940s. Northern Alberta, in general, and the Peace River district in particular, comprised Alberta's pioneer fringe until well into the 1950s, when oil and gas exploration
boosted the economy. Alberta's Provincial Travelling Clinic provided a
health service at nominal cost to both the UFA and Social Credit governments. All staff were already either provincial government employees,
or, in the case of physicians "borrowed" from the University of Alberta
Hospital, did not require additional salary. The provincial government
had only to supply the two vehicles, gasoline, and supplies for the itinerant clinic. Local residents ensured clean buildings for physical examinations and operative and dental procedures, as well as many of the
meals and accommodation for clinic staff at each site. With minimal
financial outlay, the Provincial Travelling Clinic comprised a financially
and a politically expedient temporary solution to essentially flawed public policy affecting the health of Alberta children.

Acknowledgement

Research funding for this article was provided by an operating grant
from the Alberta Association of Registered Nurses.

Notes

1 William Dunn, *Public Policy Analysis: An Introduction* (Englewood Cliffs, NJ: Prentice-Hall, 1981), 46–47.

2 Sharon Richardson, "Political Women, Professional Nurses, and the Creation of Alberta's District Nursing Service, 1919–1925," *Nursing History Review* 6 (1998): 25–50.

3 See Howard Palmer and Tamara Palmer, *Alberta: A New History* (Edmonton: Hurtig Publishers, 1990), 182–97, for a succinct discussion of the agrarian reform movement in Alberta and the creation of the UFA party.

4 Elizabeth Clark, "Public Health Nursing Branch," *Annual Report of the Department of Public Health, Including Vital Statistics Branch, 1923*, 21, Provincial Archives of Alberta (hereafter cited as PAA).

5 Elizabeth Clark, "Annual Report of the Public Health Nursing Branch," *Report of the Department of Public Health 1922*, 27–34, PAA.

6 W. C. Laidlaw, *Report of the Department of Public Health, 1924*, 12, PAA.

7 Adelaide Schartner, *Health Units of Alberta* (Edmonton: Co-op Press, 1982), 36, 46–47.

8 *The Public Health Nurses Act*, file 8, box 1, RG 52, chapter 7, Faculty of Nursing Collection, University of Alberta Archives (hereafter cited as UAA).

9 Clark, "Public Health Nursing Branch," 21.

10 Catherine A. Cavanaugh, "In Search of a Useful Life: Irene Marryat Parlby, 1868–1965" (PhD dissertation, University of Alberta, 1994), 89–99, 112–14.

11 Palmer and Palmer, *Alberta: A New History*, 278–80.

12 W. L. Morton, "The Social Philosophy of H. W. Wood, the Canadian Agrarian Leader," *Agricultural History* (April 1948): 116.

13 Palmer and Palmer, *Alberta: A New History*, 195–96, 210–12, 214–18.

14 M. G. McCallum, "The Alberta Department of Public Health," in *The Federal and Provincial Health Services in Canada*, ed. R. D. Defries, 2nd ed. (Ottawa: Canadian Public Health Association, 1962), 111–13.

15 Department of Public Health, *On the Alberta Health Horizon* (Edmonton: Government of Alberta, 1945).

16 Cavanaugh, "Irene Marryat Parlby," 112–14.

17 Kate S. Brighty, "Public Health Nursing Division, *Sixteenth Annual Report of the Department of Public Health, 1934*, 35, PAA.

18 Clark, "Public Health Nursing Branch," 21.

19 Irene Parlby, "Report of the U.F.W.A. President to the U.F.A.," *Annual Report and Year Book 1919*, 11–12 (Edmonton: United Farmers of Alberta, 1919).

20 Janice Dickin McGinnis, "Introduction," *Suitable for the Wilds: Letters from Northern Alberta, 1929–1931* (Toronto: University of Toronto Press, 1995), 16.

21 Paul Victor Collins, "The Public Health Policies of the United Farmers of Alberta Government, 1921–1935" (master's thesis, University of Western Ontario, 1969), 65.

22 Irene Stewart, *These Were Our Yesterdays: A History of District Nursing in Alberta* (Altona, MB: D. W. Friesen & Sons, 1979), 45–52, 63–74.

23 Stewart, *These Were Our Yesterdays*, 64, 75–78.

24 Elizabeth Clark, "Report of the Public Health Nursing Branch," *Annual Report of the Department of Public Health 1924*, 38–39, PAA.

25 Heber Jamieson, *Early Medicine in Alberta: The First Seventy-Five Years* (Edmonton: Douglas Printing, 1947), 75; and Malcolm R. Bow and F. T. Cook, "Public Health

in Alberta," in *The Development of Public Health in Canada*, ed. R. D. Defries (Ottawa: Canadian Public Health Association, 1940), 118.

26 W. C. Laidlaw, "Deputy Minister," *Annual Report of the Department of Public Health 1924*, 12–13, PAA.

27 Bow and Cook, "Public Health in Alberta," 123–24; Stewart, *These Were Our Yesterdays*, 64–65.

28 Malcolm R. Bow, "Public Health Services in Alberta," *Canadian Public Health Journal* 21 (1930): 590–600; and Bow and Cook, "Public Health in Alberta," 115–129; "Social Legislation in the Province of Alberta, Canada," n.d., J. M. MacEachern Papers, 1910–1968, UAA; [no title] item number 868B, accession number 69.289, Premiers Papers, PAA; Stewart, *These Were Our Yesterdays*, 63–74.

29 Stewart, *These Were Our Yesterdays*, 65.

30 Stewart, *These Were Our Yesterdays*, 65.

31 Clark, "Public Health Nursing Branch," *Annual Report 1925*, 29.

32 Elizabeth Clark, "Report of the Public Health Nursing Branch," *Annual Report of the Department of Public Health, 1926*, 23, PAA.

33 Palmer and Palmer, *Alberta: A New History*, 254.

34 "Forty-Seventh Annual Report of the Welfare Mission, Lethbridge, Alberta, 1956," *Annual Reports and History of the Lethbridge Nursing Mission Collection*, City of Lethbridge Archives.

35 Malcolm R. Bow, *Thirteenth Annual Report of the Provincial Department of Public Health 1931*, 13–14, PAA.

36 Department of Public Health, Province of Alberta, *History, Administration, Organization and Work of Provincial Department of Public Health and Boards of Health.* (Edmonton: King's Printer, 1937), 10.

37 Bow and Cook, "Public Health in Alberta," 128–29.

38 Malcolm R. Bow, *Fourteenth Annual Report of the Provincial Department of Public Health, Including the Vital Statistics Report 193*, 10–13, PAA.

39 Palmer and Palmer, *Alberta: A New History*, 254–56.

40 Malcolm R. Bow, *Sixteenth Annual Report of the Provincial Department of Public Health, Including the Vital Statistics Branch, 1934*, 14, PAA.

41 Palmer and Palmer, *Alberta: A New History*, 269.

42 Palmer and Palmer, *Alberta: A New History*, 662.

43 Bow and Cook, "Public Health in Alberta," 124–25.

44 Department of Public Health, *On the Alberta Health Horizon*, 5, 7, 21, 37–38.

45 Bow and Cook, "Public Health in Alberta," 128–29.

46 Malcolm Bow, *Sixteenth Annual Report of the Department of Public Health, 1934*, 13–14; Kate Brighty, "Public Health Nursing Division," *Sixteenth Annual Report of the Department of Public Health, 1934*, 36, PAA; Malcolm Bow, *Eighteenth Annual Report of the Provincial Department of Public Health, 1936*, 16; and Kate Brighty, "Public Health Nursing Division," *Eighteenth Annual Report of the Provincial Department of Public Health, 1936*, 36–38, PAA.

47 Kate S. Brighty, "Public Health Nursing Division," *Seventeenth Annual Report of the Provincial Department of Public Health, Including the Vital Statistics Branch, 1935*, 37–39, PAA.

48 *Annual Reports of the Department of Public Health, 1936, 1937, 1938, 1939, 1940, 1941, 1942*, PAA.

49 Malcolm R. Bow, *Twenty-Fifth Annual Report of the Provincial Department of Public Health, Including the Vital Statistics Branch, 1943*, 21, PAA.

50 Palmer and Palmer, *Alberta: A New History*, 281–88.

51 Department of Public Health, *On the Alberta Health Horizon*, 35.
52 Department of Public Health, *On the Alberta Health Horizon*, 14–15, 17.
53 Annual Reports of the Director of Public Health Nursing, *Annual Reports of the Department of Public Health*, 1951 to 1968, PAA.
54 Palmer and Palmer, *Alberta: A New History*, 269.
55 R. Allen, "The Social Gospel and the Reform Tradition in Canada, 1890–1928," *Canadian Historical Review* 49 (December 1968): 381–84.
56 Kari Dehli, "'Health Scouts' for the State? School and Public Health Nurses in Early Twentieth-Century Toronto," *Historical Studies in Education* 2 (1990): 247–64; Mona Gleason, "Race, Class, and Health: School Medical Inspection and 'Healthy' Children in British Columbia, 1890 to 1930," *Canadian Bulletin of Medical History* 19, 1 (2002): 105–106; and Susan Riddell, "Curing Society's Ills: Public Health Nurses and Public Health Nursing in Rural British Columbia, 1919–1946" (master's thesis, Simon Fraser University, 1991): 63–76.
57 Collins, "Public Health Policies," 136.
58 Government of Alberta, *Final Report of the Legislative Commission on Medical Health Service* (Edmonton: Government of Alberta, 1934).
59 Malcolm Bow, *Seventeenth Annual Report of the Department of Public Health, 1935*, PAA.
60 Collins, "Public Health Policies," 130.
61 McCallum, "Alberta Department of Public Health," 120–21.

Selected Bibliography in the History
of Children's Health

☙

Articles

Adams, Annmarie. "Modernism and Medicine: The Hospitals of Stevens and Lee, 1916–1932." *Journal of the Society of Architectural Historians* 58 (March 1999): 42–61.

Alaimo, K. "Shaping Adolescence in the Popular Milieu: Social Policy, Reformers, and French Youth, 1870–1920." *Journal of Family History* 17, 4 (1992): 420.

Allen, R. "The Social Gospel and the Reform Tradition in Canada, 1890–1928." *Canadian Historical* Review 49 (December1968): 381–84.

Andrews, Margaret W. "Sanitary Conveniences and the Retreat of the Frontier: Vancouver, 1886–1926." *BC Studies* 87 (Autumn, 1990): 3–22.

Apple, Rima. "To Be Used Only under the Direction of a Physician: Commercial Infant Feeding and Medical Practice, 1870–1940." *Bulletin of the History of Medicine* 54 (1980): 402–406.

Armitage, Andrew. "Lost Vision: Children and the Ministry for Children and Families." *BC Studies* 118 (Summer 1998): 93–108.

Aronson, N. "Nutrition as a Social Problem: A Case Study of Entrepreneurial Strategy in Science." *Social Problems* 29, 5 (1982): 474–87.

Atkins, P. J. "White Poison? The Social Consequences of Milk Consumption, 1850–1930." *Social History of Medicine* 5 (1992): 216–17.

Baillargeon, Denyse. «'Fréquenter les Gouttes de lait'. L'expérience des mères montréalaises, 1910-1965». *Revue d'histoire de l'Amérique française* 50, 1 (été 1996) : 29–68.

Baillargeon, Denyse. «Gouttes de lait et soif de pouvoir. Les dessous de la lutte contre la mortalité infantile à Montréal, 1910–1953». *Bulletin canadien d'histoire de la médecine/Canadian Bulletin of Medical History* 15, 1 (1998) : 27–57.

Baillargeon, Denyse. «Les rapports médecins-infirmières et l'implication de la Métropolitaine dans la lutte contre la mortalité infantile, 1909-1953». *Canadian Historical Review* 77, 1, (mars 1996) : 33–61.

Baker, Maureen, and David Tippin. "Fighting 'Child Poverty': The Discourse of Restructuring in Canada and Australia." *Australia-Canadian Studies* 17, 2 (1998): 121–31.

Banister, P. "Too Many Children or Too Many Pediatricians?" *Canadian Medical Association Journal* 103, 7 (July 1970): 157–59.

Barbaut, Jacques. *Histoires de la naissance.* Paris: Editions Plume, 1990. «Un accouchement traditionnel : une affaire de femmes». Dans *Le corps des femmes,* sous la direction de Edward Shorter, 57–73. Paris : Le Seuil, 1984.

Barrett, Mark, and Kim Connolly-Stone. "The Treaty of Waitangi and Social Policy." *Social Policy Journal of New Zealand* 11 (December 1998): 31.

Birn, A. E. "Six Seconds per Eyelid: The Medical Inspection of Immigrants at Ellis Island, 1892–1914." *Dynamis. Acta. Hosp. Med. Sci. Hist. Illus.* 17 (1997): 281–316.

Birn, Anne-Emanuelle. "Skirting the Issue: Women and International Health in Historical Perspective." *American Journal of Public Health* 89 (1999): 399–407.

Braithwaite, Catherine, Peter Keating et Sandi Viger. «The Problem of Diptheria in the Province of Quebec : 1894-1909». *Histoire sociale/Social History* 29, 57 (mai 1996) : 71–95.

Brosco, Jeffrey P. "Weight Charts and Well Child Care: How the Pediatrician Became the Expert in Child Health." *Archives of Pediatrics and Adolescent Medicine* 155 (2001): 1385–89.

Brumberg, J. "Chlorotic Girls, 1870–1920: A Historical Perspective on Female Adolescence." *Child Development* 53 (1982): 1468–77.

Buck, Peter. "'Why Not the Best? Some Reasons and Examples from Child Health and Rural Hospitals.'" *Journal of Social History* 18 (1985): 413–31.

Coburn, D., G. M. Torrance, and J. M. Kaufert. "Medical Dominance in Canada, in Historical Perspective: The Rise and Fall of Medicine?" *International Journal of Health Services Research* 13, 3 (1981): 407–28.

Cohen, Yolande, et Louise Bienvenue. «Émergence de l'identité professionnelle chez les infirmières professionnelles, 1890–1927», *Bulletin canadien d'histoire de la médecine/Canadian Bulletin of Medical History* 11,1 (1994) : 119–51.

Cohen, Yolande, et Michèle Gélinas. «Les infirmières hygiénistes de la Ville de Montréal : du service privé au service civique». *Histoire sociale/Social History* 22, 44 (novembre 1989) : 219–46.

Cohen, Yolande. «La contribution des sœurs de la Charité à la modernisation de l'Hôpital Notre-Dame 1880-1940. *The Canadian Historical Review* 77, 2 (June 1996) : 185–220.

Cohen, Yolande. «La modernisation des soins infirmiers dans la province de Québec (1880–1930). Un enjeu de négociation entre professionnels». *Sciences sociales et santé* 13, 3 (1995) : 11–32.

Comacchio, C. R. "Dancing to Perdition: Adolescence and Leisure in Interwar English Canada." *Journal of Canadian Studies* 32, 3 (Fall 1997): 5–27.

Connor, J. T. H. "Hospital History in Canada and the United States." *Canadian Bulletin of Medical History/Bulletin canadien d'histoire de la médecine* 7 (1990): 93–104.

Costa, Dora, and Richard Steckel. "Long Term Trends in Health, Welfare, and Economic Growth in the United States." *Working Papers Series on Historical Factors in Long Run Growth,* Historical Paper 76: 12–15 Cambridge, MA: National Bureau of Economic Research, 1995.

Davin, Anna. "Imperialism and Motherhood." *History Workshop Journal* 5 (1978): 9–65.

Dehli, Kari. "'Health Scouts' for the State? School and Public Health Nurses in Early Twentieth-Century Toronto." *Historical Studies in Education* 2 (1990): 247–64.

De Jonge, James J. "Metamorphosis of a Public Institution: The Early Buildings of the Kingston General Hospital." *Society for the Study of Architecture in Canada Bulletin* (September 22, 1997): 74–82.

Desrosiers, Georges. «Joseph-Albert Baudoin (1875-1962) : Professeur d'hygiène». *Canadian Bulletin of Medical History/Bulletin canadien d'histoire de la médecine* 10 (1993) : 251-68.

Desrosiers, Georges, Benoit Gaumer, François Hudon et Othmar Keel. «Les renforcements des interventions gouvernementales dans le domaine de la santé entre 1922 et 1936 : Le Service provincial d'Hygiène de la province de Québec». *Bulletin canadien d'histoire de la médecine/Canadian Bulletin of Medical History* 17, 1 (2001) : 205–40.

Dodd, Dianne. "The Blue Books, Helen MacMurchy, M.D., and the Federal Department of Health." *Canadian Bulletin of Medical History/Bulletin canadien d'histoire de la médecine* 8 (1991): 203–30.

Dubé, J.-E. «Les débuts de la lutte contre la mortalité infantile à Montréal. Fondation de la première Goutte de lait». *L'Union médicale du Canada* 65 (1936) : 879–91.

Duffy, John. "School Vaccination: The Precursor to School Medical Inspection." *Journal of the History of Medicine and Allied Sciences* 33 (1978): 344–55.

Duffy, John. "School Buildings and the Health of American School Children in the Nineteenth Century. " In *Healing and History: Essays for George Rosen*, edited by C. E. Rosenberg, 161–78. New York: Science History Publications, 1979.

Dupuis, Jean-Claude. «La pensée économique de l'Action française, 1917-1928». *Revue d'historie de l'Amerique Francaise* 47, 2 (automne 1993) : 193-291.

Dwork, Deborah. "Health Conditions of Immigrant Jews on the Lower East Side of New York: 1880–1914. " *Medical History* 24 (1981): 1–40.

Ebbs, J. H. "The Canadian Paediatric Society: Its Early Years." *Canadian Medical Association Journal* 126, 12 (1980): 235.

Elder, G. "Adolescence in the Life Cycle." In *Adolescence in the Life Cycle*, edited by G. Elder and S. E. Dragastin, 1–3. New York: Cambridge University Press, 1974.

Elliot, Susan J., and Leslie T. Foster. "Mind-Body-Place: A Geography of Aboriginal Health in British Columbia." In *A Persistent Spirit: Towards Understanding Aboriginal Health in British Columbia*, edited by Peter H. Stephenson, Susan J. Elliott, Leslie T. Foster, and Jill Harris, 95–127. Victoria: University of Victoria Western Geographical Press, 1995.

Evans, Hughes. "The Discovery of Child Sexual Abuse in America." In *Formative Years: Children's Health in the United States, 1880–2000*, edited by Alexandra Minna Stern and Howard Markel, 233–59. Ann Arbor: University of Michigan Press, 2002.

Farley, Michael, Peter Keating et Othmar Keel. «Les origines de l'action publique dans le domaine de la santé au Québec : Une critique du modèle explicatif par l'intervention de l'Etat à partir de la Révolution Tranquille». *Communication au Congrès de l'Association canadienne d'histoire de la science, de la médecine et de la technologie*, Kingston, 1984.

Farley, Michael, Peter Keating et Othmar Keel. «La vaccination à Montréal dans la seconde moitié du XIXᵉ siècle : pratiques, obstacles et résistances». Dans *Sciences et médecine au Québec. Perspectives socio-historiques*, sous la direction de

Marcel Fournier, Yves Gingras et Othmar Keel. Québec : Institut québécois de recherche sur la culture, 1987.

Farley, Michael, Othmar Keel et Camille Limoges. «Les commencements de l'administration montréalaise de la santé publique (1865–1885)». Dans *Science, Technology, and Medicine in Canada's Past : Selections from Scientia Canadensis*, sous la direction de Richard A. Jarrel et James P. Hull, 269–308. Thornhill : Scientia Press, 1991.

Featherstone, Lisa. "Whose Breast Is Best? The Wet Nurse in Late Nineteenth Century Australia." *Birth Issues Journal* 11 (2002): 41–46.

Fleury, Marie-Josée, and Guy Grenier. "La Médicine et de la santé au Canada français: un bilan historiographique, 1987–2002." *Scientia Canadensis* 26 (2002) : 29–58.

Fildes, V. "Infant Feeding Practices and Infant Mortality in England, 1900–1919." *Continuity and Change* 13, 2 (1998): 251–80.

Fingard, Judy. "'The Winter's Tale': The Seasonal Contours of Pre-Industrial Poverty in British North America, 1815–1860." Canadian Historical Association, *Historical Papers* (1974): 65–94.

Fiske, Jo-Anne. "Carrier Women and the Politics of Mothering." In *Rethinking Canada: The Promise of Women's History*, edited by Veronica Strong-Boag, Mona Gleason, and Adele Perry, 235–48. Toronto: Oxford University Press, 2002.

Folbre, Nancy. "The Unproductive Housewife: Her Evolution in Nineteenth Century Economic Thought." *Signs* 16 (1991): 463–84.

Fournier, Marcel, Annick Germain, Yves Lamarche et Louis Maheu. «Le champ scientifique québécois : Structure, fonctionnement et fonctions», *Sociologie et sociétés* 7, 1 (mai 1975) : 119–32.

Fox, Daniel M., and James Terry. "Photography and the Self-Image of American Physicians, 1880–1920." *Canadian Bulletin of Medical History/Bulletin canadien d'histoire de la médecine* 52 (1978): 435–57.

Gagan, David. "For 'Patients of Moderate Means': The Transformation of Ontario's Public General Hospitals, 1880–1950." *Canadian Historical Review* 70 (1989): 151–79.

Garn, Stanley, and Diane Clark. "Nutrition, Growth, Development, and Maturation: Findings from the Ten-State Nutrition Survey of 1968–70." *Pediatrics* 56 (1975): 306–18.

Garrett, Elidh, and Andrew Wear. "Suffer the Little Children; Mortality, Mothers and the State." *Continuity and Change* 9, 2 (1994): 179–84.

Garrison, Fielding H. "History of Pediatrics." In *Abt-Garrison History of Pediatrics*, edited by Isaac A. Abt, 2. Philadelphia: W. B. Saunders, 1965.

Gaumer, Benoît et al., «Le service de santé de Montréal, de l'établissement au démantèlement (1865-1975)». *Cahiers du centre de recherches historiques* 12 (avril 1994) : 132.

Gillis, Jonathan. "Bad Habits and Pernicious Results: Thumb Sucking and the Discipline of Late-Nineteenth-Century Pediatrics." *Medical History* 40 (January 1996): 55–73.

Gleason, Mona. "'Disciplining the Student Body: Schooling and the Construction of Canadian Children's Bodies, 1930–1960.'" *History of Education Quarterly* 41, 2 (Summer, 2001): 189–215.

Gleason, Mona. "Race, Class, and Health: School Medical Inspection and 'Healthy' Children in British Columbia, 1890 to 1930." *Canadian Bulletin of Medical History/Bulletin canadien d'histoire de la médecine* 19 (2002): 95–112.

Goldbloom, Alton. "A Twenty-Five-Year Retrospective on Infant Feeding." *Journal of the Maine Medical Association* 45 (1954): 267.

Goulet, Denis, et Othmar Keel. «Généalogie des représentations et des attitudes face aux épidémies au Québec depuis le XIXe siècle». *Anthropologie et Société* 15 (1991) : 205–28

Goulet, Denis, et Othmar Keel. «Les hommes-relais de la bactériologie en territoire québécois et l'introduction de nouvelles pratiques diagnostiques et thérapeutiques (1890–1920)». *Revue d'histoire de l'Amérique française* 46, 3 (1993) : 417–42.

Goulet, Denis, et Othmar Keel. «Santé publique, histoire des travailleurs et histoire hospitalière : Sources et méthodologie». *Bulletin du Regroupement des chercheurs–chercheuses en histoire des travailleurs et travailleuses du Québec* 16, 2-3 (1990) : 47–48 et 67–80.

Goulet, Denis, Gilles Lemire et Denis Gauvreau. «Des bureaux d'hygiène municipaux aux unités sanitaires. Le Conseil d'hygiène de la province de Québec et la structuration d'un système de santé publique 1886–1926». *Revue d'histoire d'Amérique française* 49, 4 (printemps 1996) : 491–520.

Granshaw, Lindsay. "Fame and Fortune by Means of Bricks and Mortar." In *The Hospital in History*, edited by Lindsay Grandshaw and Roy Porter, 202. London: Routledge, 1989.

Guérard, François. «Ville et santé au Québec. Un bilan de la recherche historique», *Revue d'Histoire de l'Amérique française* 53, 1 (1999) : 19–46.

Guérard, François. «L'histoire de la santé au Québec : filiations et spécificités». *Bulletin canadien d'histoire de la médecine/Canadian Bulletin of Medical History* 17, 1–2 (2000) : 55–72.

Guy, Donna J. "The Pan American Child Congresses, 1916 to 1942: Pan Americanism, Child Reform, and the Welfare State in Latin America." *Journal of Family History* 23 (1998): 274.

Hadwiger, Don. "Nutrition, Food Safety, and Farm Policy." *Proceedings of the Academy of Political Science* 34 (1982): 8–12.

Haimes, Erica V. "When Transgressions Become Transparent: Limiting Family Forms in Assisted Conception." *Journal of Law and Medicine* 9 (2002): 438–48.

Haine, W. S. "The Development of Leisure and the Transformation of Working-class Adolescence in France." *Journal of Family History* 17, 4 (1992): 451.

Hanawalt, B. "Historical Descriptions and Prescriptions for Adolescence." *Journal of Family History* 17, 4 (1992): 341–44.

Hastrup, Kirsten. "A Question of Reason: Breast-feeding Patterns in Seventeenth and Eighteenth Century Iceland." In *The Anthropology of Breast-Feeding: Natural Law or Social Construct*, edited by Vanessa Maher, 91–108. Providence: Berg, 1992.

Henripin, Jacques, et Yves Peron. «La transition démographique de la province de Québec». Dans *La population du Québec : études et perspective*, sous la direction de Hubert Charbonneau. Montréal : Boréal Express, 1973.

Hornstein, Shelley. "The Architecture of the Montreal Teaching Hospitals of the Nineteenth Century." *Journal of Canadian Art History* 14 (1991): 12–24.

Howell, Joel D. "Machines and Medicine: Technology Transforms the American Hospital." In *The American General Hospital: Communities and Social Contexts*, edited by Diana Elizabeth Long and Janet Golden, 132. Ithaca: Cornell University Press, 1989.

Hughes, Jonathan. "Hospital City." *Architectural History* 40 (1997): 266–88.

Hulbert, Ann. "Dr. Spock's Baby: Fifty Years in the Life of a Book and the American Family." *New Yorker* 20 (1996): 82–92.

Hunt, Mary. "Scientific Temperance, and the Dilemma of Democratic Education in America, 1879–1906." *History of Education Quarterly* 32 (Spring 1992): 1–30.

Hymel, Kent, and Carol Jenny. "Child Sexual Abuse." *Pediatrics in Review* 17 (1996): 236–50.

James, C. L. "Practical Diversions and Educational Amusements: Evangelia Home and the Advent of Canada's Settlement Movement, 1902–09." *Historical Studies in Education* 10, 1–2 (Spring/Fall 1998): 49–51.

Jasen, Patricia. "Race, Culture, and the Colonization of Childbirth in Northern Canada." *Social History of Medicine* 10, 3 (1997): 383–400.

Jones, J. A., G. W. Pipe, and V. L. Matthews. "A Student-Directed Program in Smoking Education." *Canadian Public Health Journal* 61, 3 (May/June 1970): 253–56.

Jones, Kathleen W. "Sentiment and Science: The Late Nineteenth Century Pediatrician as Mother's Advisor." *Journal of Social History* (Fall 1983): 81.

Jones, Wanda J. "New Century Design for the McGill University Health Center: From Negative to Positive Value in Health Facilities." *Healing by Design: Building for Health Care in the 21st Century*. Montreal: McGill University Health Centre, 2000.

Juhasz, A. N. "Sex Knowledge of Prospective Teachers and Graduate Nurses." *Canadian Nurse* 63 (1967): 48–50.

Kiple, Kenneth, and Virginia Kiple. "Deficiency Diseases in the Caribbean." *Journal of Interdisciplinary History* 11 (1980): 197–215.

Kiple, Kenneth. "A Survey of Recent Literature on the Biological Past of the Black." *Social Science History* 10 (1986): 343–68.

Komlos, John, and Joo Han Kim. "On Estimating Trends in Historical Heights." *Historical Methods* 23 (1990): 116–20.

Kunkel, H. O., and P. B. Thompson. "Interests and Values in National Nutrition Policy in the United States." *Journal of Agricultural Ethics* 1 (1988): 241–65.

Lavigne, Marie. «Réflexions féministes autour de la fertilité des Québécoises». Dans *Maîtresses de maison, maîtresses d'école; Femmes, famille et éducation dans l'histoire du Québec* sous la direction de Micheline Dumont et Nadia Fahmy-Eid. Montréal : Boréal Express, 1983.

Lefaucheur, Nadine. "La puériculture d'Adolphe Pinard." In *Darwinisme et Societé*, edited by Patrick Tort, 413-36. Paris: Presses Universitaires de France, 1992.

Lesser, Arthur. "The Origin and Development of Maternal and Child Health Programs in the United States." *American Journal of Public Health* 75 (1985): 590–98.

Lewis, Jane. "The Social History of Social Policy: Infant Welfare in Edwardian England." *Journal of Social Policy* 9, 4 (1980): 463–86.

Lewis, Norah. "Physical Perfection for Spiritual Welfare: Health Care for the Urban Child, 1900–1939." In *Studies in Childhood History: A Canadian Perspective*, edited by Patricia T. Rooke and R. L. Schnell, 135–66. Calgary: Detselig, 1982.

Link, William A. "Privies, Progressivism, and Public Schools: Health Reform and Education in the Rural South, 1909–1920." *The Journal of Southern History* 54, 4 (November 1988): 623–42.

Lloyd, Josephine. "The 'Languid Child' and the Eighteenth-Century Man-Mid-wife." *Bulletin of the History of Medicine* 75 (2001): 641–79.

Maher, Vanessa. "Breast-feeding in Cross Cultural Perspective." In *The Anthropology of Breast-Feeding: Natural Law or Social Construct*, 1–36. Providence: Berg, 1992.

Maher, Vanessa. "Breast-feeding and Maternal Depletion: Natural Law or Cultural Arrangements." In *The Anthropology of Breast-Feeding: Natural Law or Social Construct*. 151–79. Providence: Berg, 1992.

Markel, Howard, and Henry Koplik, M.D. "The Good Samaritan Dispensary of New York City and the Description of Koplik's Spots." *Archives of Pediatrics and Adolescent Medicine* 150 (1996): 535–39.

Marland, Hilary. "A Pioneer in Infant Welfare: The Huddersfield Scheme 1903–1920." *Social History of Medicine* 6, 1 (1993): 25–50.

McCuaig, K. "From Social Reform to Social Service: The Changing Role of Volunteers; The Anti-Tuberculosis Campaign, 1900–30." *Canadian Historical Review* 61, 4 (1980): 485.

McKeown, T., and R. G. Record. "The Reason for the Decline of Mortality in England and Wales during the Nineteenth Century." *Population Studies* 16 (1962): 94–122.

Moffat, Tim, and Ann Herring. "The Historical Roots of High Rates of Infant Death in Aboriginal Communities in Canada in the Early Twentieth Century: The Case of Fisher River, Manitoba." *Social Science & Medicine* 48 (1999): 1821–32.

Monnais-Rousselot, Laurence. «Colonisation et problèmes sociaux : une intervention médicale. L'expérience de l'Indochine française, 1860–1954». Dans *Nouvelles configurations des problèmes sociaux et l'intervention*, sous la direction de Henri Dorvil et Robert Mayeur. Sainte Foy : Presses de l'Université du Québec à Montréal, 2001.

Monnais-Rousselot, Laurence. «La professionnalisation du «médecin indochinois» au XXe siècle : Des paradoxes d'une médicalisation coloniale». *Actes de la Recherche en Sciences Sociales* 143 (2002) : 36–43.

Morton, W. L. "The Social Philosophy of H. W. Wood, the Canadian Agrarian Leader." *Agricultural History* (April 1948): 116.

Myers, A. W. "Breast-feeding: A Canadian Perspective on a Global Priority." *Canadian Medical Association Journal* 125 (1981): 1078–1142.

Petersen, Alan. "The New Genetics and the Politics of Public Health." *Critical Public Health* 8, 1 (March 1998): 59–71.

Pilcher, Jeffry. "Food Fads." In *The Cambridge World History of Food*, edited by Kenneth Kiple and Kriemhild Ornelas, 1486–95. Cambridge, UK, and New York: Cambridge University Press, 2000.

Prior, Lindsay. "The Architecture of the Hospital: A Study of Spatial Organization and Medical Knowledge." *British Journal of Sociology* 39 (1988): 86–113.

Richardson, Sharon. "Political Women, Professional Nurses, and the Creation of Alberta's District Nursing Service, 1919–1925." *Nursing History Review* 6 (1998): 25–50.

Richardson, Theresa. "Ambiguities in the Lives of Children: Postmodern Views on the History and Historiography of Childhood in English Canada." *Pedagogica Historica* 32 (1996): 363–93.

Rogers, Naomi. "Germs with Legs: Flies, Disease, and the New Public Health." *Canadian Bulletin of Medical History/Bulletin canadien d'histoire de la médecine* 63 (1989): 599–617.

Rooke, Patricia T., and Rudy L. Schnell. "'Uncramping Child Life': International Children's Organisations, 1914–1939." In *International Health Organisations and Movements, 1918–1939*, edited by Paul Weindling, 180. Cambridge: Cambridge University Press, 1995.

Rosen, George. "Early Medical Photography." *Ciba Symposium* 4 (1942): 1344–55.

Rosen, George. "The First Neighborhood Health Center Movement: Its Rise and Fall." In *Sickness and Health in America*, edited by J. W. Leavitt and R. L. Numbers, 185–99. Madison: University of Wisconsin Press, 1997.

Rosenberg, C. E. "Social Class and Medical Care in 19th Century America: The Rise and Fall of the Dispensary." In *Sickness and Health in America*, edited by J. W. Leavitt and R. L. Numbers, 157–71. Madison: University of Wisconsin Press, 1997.

Rosen, George. "The First Neighborhood Health Center Movement: Its Rise and Fall." In *Sickness and Health in America*, edited by J. W. Leavitt and R. L. Numbers, 185–99. Madison: University of Wisconsin Press, 1997.

Rosselot, V., Jorge. "UNICEF y la Protección de la Infancia 1946–1990." *Revista de Pediatría* (Santiago) 33 (1990): 165–77.

Sacco, Lynn. "Sanitized for Your Protection: Medical Discourse and the Denial of Incest in the United States, 1890–1940." *Journal of Women's History* 14 (2002): 80–104.

Saillant, Francine. *Accoucher autrement. Repères historiques, sociaux et culturels de la grossesse et de l'accouchement au Québec*. Montréal: Editions St Martin, 1987.

Saint-Germain, Yves. «La société québécoise et la vie économique : quelques échos de la décennie de la «grande ambivalence 1920-1929». Dans *Économie québécoise,* sous la direction de Robert Comeau, 439–64. Montréal : Presses de l'Université du Québec, 1969.

Sangster, Joan. "Masking and Unmasking the Sexual Abuse of Children: Perceptions of Violence against Children in 'The Badlands' of Ontario, 1916–1930." *Journal of Family History* 25, 4 (October 2000): 504–26.

Scheper-Hugers, N., and C. Sargent. "Introduction: The Cultural Politics of Childhood." In *Small Wars: The Cutural Politics of Childhood*, edited by N. Scheper-Hughes and C. Sargent, 1–33. Berkeley: University of California Press, 1998.

Schneider, William H. "Puericulture and the Style of French Eugenics." *History and Philosophy of the Life Sciences* 8 (1986): 265–77.

Schnell, R. L. "A Children's Bureau for Canada: The Origins of the Canadian Council on Child Welfare, 1913–1921." In *The Benevolent State: The Growth of Welfare in Canada*, edited by A. Moscovitch and J. Alberts. Toronto: Garamond, 1987.

Scott, Susan. "Malnutrition, Pregnancy and Infant Mortality: A Biometric Model." *Journal of Interdisciplinary History,* 30 (1999): 54–56.

Sears, Alan. "Before the Welfare State: Public Health and Social Policy." *CRSA/RCSA* 32, 2 (1995): 169–88.

Seidler, Edward. "The Historical Survey of Children's Hospitals." In *The Hospital in History*, edited by Lindsay Granshaw and Roy Porter, 181–97. London: Routledge, 1989.

Sethna, C. "Men, Sex and Education: The Ontario Women's Temperance Union and Children's Sex Education, 1900–20." *Ontario History* 88, 3 (September 1996): 186–206.

Sethna, C. "Wait till Your Father Gets Home: Absent Fathers, Working Mothers and Delinquent Daughters in Ontario during World War II." In *Family Matters: Papers in Post-Confederation Canadian Family History*, edited by E. A. Montigny and L. Chambers, 19–38. Toronto: Canadian Scholars Press, 1998.

Sgroi, Suzanne M. "'Kids with Clap': Gonorrhea as an Indicator of Child Sexual Assault." *Victimology: An International Journal* 2 (1977): 251–67.

Shakespeare, Tom. "Manifesto for Genetic Justice." *Social Alternatives* 18, 1 (January 1999): 29–32.

Shortt, S. E. D. "The Canadian Hospital in the Nineteenth Century: An Historiographic Lament." *Journal of Canadian Studies* 18 (Winter 1982–84): 3–14.

Smith, Michael J. "Dampness, Darkness, Dirt, Disease: Physicians and the Promotion of Sanitary Science in Public Schools." In *Profiles of Science and Society in the Maritimes Prior to 1914*, edited by Paul A. Bogaard, 200–203. Halifax: Acadiensis, 1990.

Solis-Cohen, Rosebud T. "The Exclusion of Aliens from the United States for Physical Defects." *Canadian Bulletin of Medical History/Bulletin canadien d'histoire de la médecine* 21 (1947): 33–50.

Sproule-Jones, Megan. "Crusading for the Forgotten: Dr. Peter Bryce, Public Health, and Prairie Native Residential Schools." *Canadian Bulletin of Medical History/Bulletin canadien de l'histoire de la médecine* 13, 2 (1996): 199–224.

Steckel, Richard. "Heights, Living Standards, and History: A Review Essay." *Historical Methods* 24 (1991): 183–87.

Stehin, Isadora. "Infant Formula: Second Best, But Good Enough." *FDA Consumer, The Magazine of the U.S. Food and Drug Administration* 30 (1996): 17.

Stern, Alexandra. "Responsible Mothers and Normal Children: Eugenics, Nationalism, and Welfare in Post-Revolutionary Mexico, 1920–1940." *Journal of Historical Sociology* 12 (1999): 369–97.

Sutherland, Neil. "When You Listen to the Winds of Childhood, How Much Can You Believe?" *Curriculum Inquiry* 22, 3 (1992): 235–56.

Szreter, Simon. "The Importance of Social Intervention in Britain's Mortality Decline, 1850–1914: A Reinterpretation of the Role of Public Health." *Social History of Medicine* 1 (1988): 1–37.

Taylor, Karen J. "Venereal Disease in Nineteenth Century Children." *Journal of Psychohistory* 12 (1985): 431–63.

Thapa, S., R. V. Short, and M. Potts. "Breastfeeding, Birth Spacing and Their Effects on Child Survival." *Nature* 335, 6192 (20 October 1988): 679–82.

Thompson, Angela. "To Save the Children: Smallpox Inoculation, Vaccination, and Public Health in Guanajuato, Mexico, 1797–1840." *The Americas* 49 (1993): 431–55.

Thornton, Patricia, Sherry Olson et Quoc Thuy Thach. «Dimensions sociales de la mortalité infantile à Montréal au milieu du XIXe siècle». *Annales de démographie historique* (1988) : 299–325.

Thornton, Patricia A. and Sherry Olson. «Family Contexts of Fertility and Infant Survival in Nineteenth Century Montreal». *Journal of Family History* 16, 4 (1991) : 401–17.

Tomes, Nancy. "Merchants of Health: Medicine and Consumer Culture in the United States, 1900–1940." *Journal of American History* 1 (2001): 519–47.

Valverde, Mariana, and Lorna Weir. "Regulating New Reproductive and Genetic Technologies: A Feminist View of Recent Canadian Government Initiatives." *Feminist Studies* 23, 2 (Summer 1997): 419–23.

Vogel, Morris J. "The Transformation of the American Hospital, 1850–1920." In *Health Care in America*, edited by Susan Reverby and David Rosner, 105–16. Philadelphia: Temple University, 1979.

Ward, W. P., and P. C. Ward. "Infant Birth Weight and Nutrition in Industrializing Montreal." *American Historical Review* 89, 2 (1984): 324–45.

Wasserman, M. J. "Henry Coit and the Certified Milk Movement in the Development of Modern Pediatrics." *Canadian Bulletin of Medical History/Bulletin canadien d'histoire de la médecine* 46 (1972): 359–90.

Weigley, Emma. "It Might Have Been Euthenics: The Lake Placid Conferences and the Home Economics Movement." *American Quarterly* 26 (1974): 79–96.

White, P. L. "Nutrition: A Medical, Political, and Public Issue." *Journal of the American Medical Association* 241 (1979): 1407–08.

Whitehead, Margaret. "Women Were Made for Such Things: Women Missionaries in British Columbia 1850s to 1940s." *Atlantis* 14 (Fall 1988): 141–50.

Whitehead, Margaret. "'A Useful Christian Woman': First Nations Women and Protestant Missionary Work in British Columbia." *Atlantis* 18 (Fall–Summer 1992–93): 142–66.

Woods, Pamela J. "Hazardous to Children's Health? New Zealand Primary Schools, 1890 to 1914." *Historical News* 66, 4 (May, 1993): 4–8.

Woods, R. I., P. A. Watterson, and J. H. Woodward. "The Causes of Rapid Infant Mortality Decline in England and Wales 1861–1921, Part: I." *Population Studies*, 42 (1988): 349.

Worboys, Michael. "Tuberculosis and Race in Britain and Its Empire, 1900–1950." In *Race, Science and Medicine, 1700–1960*, edited by Ernest Waltraud and Bernard Harris, 144–66. London, New York: Routledge, 1999.

Yew, Elizabeth. "Medical Inspection of Immigrants at Ellis Island, 1891–1924." *Bulletin of the New York Academy of Medicine* 56 (1980): 488–510.

Yourk, Darren. "Poverty, abuse the main concerns of children." *Globe and Mail*, August 14, 2001.

Zelmanovits, Judith Bender. "'Midwife Preferred': Maternity Care in Outpost Nursing Stations in Northern Canada 1945–1988." In *Women, Health and Nation: Canada and the United States since 1945*, edited by Georgina Feldberg, 161–189. Montreal and Kingston: McGill-Queen's University Press, 2003.

Books

Abbott, Maude. *History of the Medicine in the Province of Quebec.* Montréal: McGill-Queen's University Press, 1931.

Abel, Kerry. *Drum Songs: Glimpses of Dene History.* Montreal and Kingston: McGill-Queen's University Press, 1993.

Adams, Annmarie. *Architecture in the Family Way: Doctors, Houses, and Women, 1870–1900.* Montreal: McGill-Queen's University Press, 1996.

Adams, M. L. *The Trouble with Normal: Postwar Youth and the Making of Heterosexuality.* Toronto: University of Toronto Press, 1997.

Addams, Jane. *Twenty Years at Hull House, with Autobiographical Notes.* 1910; reprint, Chicago: University of Illinois Press, 1990.

Ageron, Charles-Robert, Catherine Coquery-Vidrovitch, Gilbert Meynier, Jacques Thobie, *Histoire de la France coloniale.* Paris: Armand Colin, 1991.

Agnew, Harvey. *Canadian Hospitals, 1920–1970: A Dramatic Half Century.* Toronto: University of Toronto Press, 1974.

Allahar, A. L. *Generation on Hold: Coming of Age in the Late 20th Century.* Toronto: Stoddart, 1994.

Allen, Peter Lewis. *The Wages of Sin: Sex and Disease, Past and Present.* Chicago and London: University of Chicago Press, 2000.

Allen, R. *The Social Passion: Religion and Social Reform in Canada 1914–28.* Toronto: University of Toronto Press, 1997.

Anctil, Hervé, et Marc-André Bluteau, *La santé et l'assistance publique au Québec, 1886–1986* Québec: Santé Société, édition spéciale, 1986.

Anderson, Kay. *Vancouver's Chinatown: Racial Discourse in Canada, 1875–1980.* Montreal: McGill-Queen's University Press, 1991.

Apple, Rima D. *Mothers and Medicine: A Social History of Infant Feeding.* Madison: University of Wisconsin Press, 1987.

Apple, Rima D., and Janet Golden. *Mothers and Motherhood: Readings in American History.* Columbus: Ohio State University Press, 1997.

Ariès, Philippe. *Histoire des populations françaises.* Paris: Le Seuil, 1971.

Arnup, Katherine *Education for Motherhood. Advice for Mothers in Twentieth-Century Canada* Toronto: University of Toronto Press, 1994.

Ashby, LeRoy. *Endangered Children: Dependency, Neglect and Abuse in American History.* New York: Twayne, 1997.

Bailey, B. *From Front Porch to Back Seat.* Baltimore: Johns Hopkins University Press, 1988.

Baillargeon, D. *Making Do: Home and Family in Montreal during the Great Depression.* Waterloo: Wilfrid Laurier University Press, 1998.

Baker, Jeffrey P. *The Machine in the Nursery: Incubator Technology and the Origins of Newborn Intensive Care.* Baltimore: John Hopkins University Press, 1996.

Balinska, Marta. *Une vie pour l'humanitaire: Ludwik Rajchman 1881–1965.* Paris: Éditions la découverte, 1995.

Bates, Barbara. *Bargaining for Life: A Social History of Tuberculosis, 1876–1938.* Philadelphia: University of Pennsylvania Press, 1992.

Baumslag, N., and D. L. Michels. *Milk, Money, and Madness: The Culture and Politics of Breastfeeding.* Westport, CT: Bergin and Garvey, 1993.

Bensley, Edward H. *McGill Medical Luminaries.* Montreal: Olsen Lebiany, 1990.

Bernier, Jacques. *La médecine au Québec. Naissance et évolution d'une profession* Québec : Les Presses de l'Université Laval, 1989.

Bideau, Alain, Bertrand Desjardins, and Hector Perez-Brignoli, eds. *Infant and Child Mortality in the Past*. Oxford: Clarendon Press, 1997.

Black, Maggie. *Children First: The Story of UNICEF, Past and Present*. New York: Oxford University Press, 1996.

Blee, Kathleen M. *Women of the Klan: Racism and Gender in the 1920s*. Berkeley: University of California Press, 1991.

Blumin, Stuart. *The Emergence of the Middle Class: Social Experience in the American City*. Cambridge, MA: Cambridge University Press, 1989.

Bock, Gisela, and Pat Thane, eds., *Maternity and Gender Policies. Women and the Rise of the European Welfare States 1880s–1950s*. London and New York: Routhledge, 1994.

Bodnar, J. *The Transplanted: A History of Immigrants in Urban America*. Bloomington: University of Indiana Press, 1985.

Bolt, Clarence. *Thomas Crosby and the Tsimshian: Small Shoes for Feet Too Large*. Vancouver: UBC Press, 1992.

Boomgaard, Peter. *Children of the Colonial State. Population Growth and Economic Development in Java, 1795–1880*. Amsterdam: Center for Asian Studies, 1990.

Bradbury, Dorothy. *Four Decades of Action for Children: A Short History of the Children's Bureau, 1903–46*, no. 358. Washington, DC: U.S. Govt. Print, 1956.

Brandt, Allan M. *No Magic Bullet: A Social History of Venereal Disease in the United States since 1880*. New York: Oxford University Press, 1987.

Brocheux, Pierre, and Daniel Hémery, *Indochine. La colonisation ambiguë, 1858–1954*. Paris: La Découverte, 2002, 2ᵉ éd.

Brumberg, Joan Jacobs. *Fasting Girls: The Emergence of Anorexia Nervosa as a Modern Disease*. Cambridge: Harvard University Press, 1988.

Brumberg, Joan Jacobs. *The Body Project: An Intimate History of American Girls*. New York: Random House, 1997.

Bryder, Linda. *Below the Magic Mountain: A Social History of Tuberculosis in Twentieth-Century Britain*. Oxford: Oxford University Press, 1988.

Burnham, John. C. *How Superstition Won and Science Lost: Popularizing Science and Health in the United States*. New Brunswick: Rutgers University Press, 1987.

Burns, Stanley. *Early Medical Photography in America*. New York: Burns Archive, 1983.

Christophers, Brett. *Positioning the Missionary: John Booth Good and the Confluence of Cultures in Nineteenth-Century British Columbia*. Vancouver: UBC Press, 1998.

Coates, Ken S. *Best Left as Indians: Native–White Relations in the Yukon Territory, 1840–1973*. Montreal and Kingston: McGill-Queen's University Press, 1991.

Cohen, R., and J. Heimlich *Milk: The Deadly Poison*. New York: Argus, 1998.

Cohen, Yolande. *Profession infirmière. Une histoire des soins dans les hôpitaux du Québec*. Montréal: Les Presses de l'Université de Montréal, 2000.

Cohen, Yolande, Jacinthe Pépin, Esther Lamontagne et André Duquette, *Les sciences infirmières. Genèse d'une discipline*. Montréal: Les Presses de l'Université de Montréal, 2002.

Collin, Johanne, et Denis Béliveau, *Histoire de la pharmacie au Québec*. Montréal: Musée de la pharmacie du Québec, 1994.

Comacchio, Cynthia R. *Nations Are Built of Babies: Saving Ontario's Mothers and Children, 1900–1940*. Montreal: McGill-Queen's University Press, 1994.

Cone, Thomas E., Jr., *History of American Pediatrics*. Boston: Little Brown, 1979.

Connor, J. T. H. *Doing Good: The Life of Toronto's General Hospital.* Toronto: University of Toronto Press, 2000.

Cooper, Donald B. *Epidemic Disease in Mexico City, 1716–1813: An Administrative, Social, and Medical Study.* Austin: Institute of Latin American Studies, University of Texas Press, 1965.

Cooter, Roger, ed. *In the Name of the Child: Health and Welfare 1880–1940.* London: Routledge, 1992.

Copp, Terry. *Classe ouvrière et pauvreté, les conditions de vie des travailleurs montréalais 1897–1929* Montréal : Boréal Express, 1978.

Costin, Lela B. *Two Sisters of Social Justice: A Biography of Grace and Edith Abbott.* Urbana: University of Illinois Press, 1983.

Crossman, Kelly. *Architecture in Transition: From Art to Practice, 1885–1906.* Montreal: McGill-Queen's University Press, 1987.

Cunningham, Hugh, and Pier Paolo Viazzo, eds. *Child Labour in Historical Perspective, 1800–1985: Case Studies from Europe, Japan and Colombia.* Florence: UNICEF and the Instituto degli Innocenti, 1996.

Currie, Dawn. *Girl Talk: Adolescent Magazines and Their Readers.* Toronto: University of Toronto Press, 1999.

Dalley, Bronwyn. *Family Matters: Child Welfare in Twentieth-Century New Zealand.* Auckland: Auckland University Press, 1998.

Danbom, David. *Born in the Country: A History of Rural America.* Baltimore: Johns Hopkins University Press, 1995.

Davis, Susan G. *Parades and Power: Street Theater in Nineteenth-Century Philadelphia.* Philadelphia: Temple University Press, 1986.

Davidson, Roger, and Lesley A. Hall. *Sex, Sin and Suffering: Venereal Disease and European Society since 1870.* London and New York: Routledge, 2001.

Dawley, Alan. *Struggles for Justice: Social Responsibility and the Liberal State.* Cambridge: Belknap Press of Harvard University Press, 1991.

Deforest, Lynda. *Proud Heritage: A History of the Royal Victoria Hospital Training School for Nurses, 1894–1972.* Montreal: The Alumnae Association of the Royal Victoria Hospital Training School for Nurses, 1994.

Democratic Republic of Vietnam, *La protection de la mère et de l'enfant au Vietnam.* Hanoi: Editions en Langues Etrangères, 1979.

Demos, John. *Past, Present, and Personal: The Family and the Life Course in American History.* New York: Oxford University Press, 1986.

Desrosiers, Georges, Benoît Gaumer et Othmar Keel. *La santé publique au Québec. Histoire des unités sanitaires de comtés, 1926–1975,* Montréal, Presses de l'Université de Montréal, 1998.

Desjardins, Édouard, Ellen C. Flanagan et Suzanne Giroux, *Heritage: History of the Nursing Profession in Quebec from the Augustinians and Jeanne Mance to Medicare.* Montréal: The Association of Nurses of the Province of Quebec, 1971.

Dormandy, T. *The White Death: A History of Tuberculosis.* New York: New York University Press, 2000.

Dorrey, Annette K. Vane. *Better Baby Contests: The Scientific Quest for Perfect Childhood Health in the Early Twentieth Century.* Jefferson, NC: McFarland, 1999.

Dow, Derek. *Safeguarding the Public Health: A History of the New Zealand Department of Health.* Wellington: Victoria University Press, 1995.

Duffin, Jacalyn. *History of Medicine: A Scandalously Short Introduction.* Toronto: University of Toronto Press, 1999.

Duffy, John. *The Sanitarians: A History of American Public Health*. Urbana: University of Illinois Press, 1990.

Dupuis, E. M. *Nature's Perfect Food: How Milk Became America's Drink*. New York: New York University Press, 2002.

Durie, Mason. *Whaiora: Maori Health Development*. Auckland: Oxford University Press, 1994.

Dwork, Deborah. *Companion Encyclopedia of the History of Medicine*. Vol. 2. London: Routledge, 1993.

Dwork, Deborah. *War Is Good for Babies and Other Children: A History of the Infant and Child Welfare Movement in England, 1898–1918*. London: Tavistock, 1987.

Ehrenreich, Barbara, and Deidre English. *For Her Own Good: 150 Years of the Experts' Advice to Women*. London: Pluto Press, 1979.

Ettling, John. *The Germ of Laziness: Rockefeller Philanthropy and Public Health in the New South*. Cambridge: Harvard University Press, 1981.

Ewen, Elizabeth. *Immigrant Women in the Land of Dollars.: Life and Culture on the Lower East Side, 1890–1925*. New York: Monthly Review Press, 1985.

Faber, H. K., and R. McIntosh. *History of the American Pediatric Society, 1887–1965*. New York: McGraw-Hill, 1965.

Feldberg, Georgina D. *Disease and Class: Tuberculosis and the Shaping of Modern American Society*. New Brunswick: Rutgers University Press, 1995.

Felt, Jeremy P. *Hostages of Fortune: Child Labor Reform in New York State*. Syracuse, NY: Syracuse University Press, 1965.

Fildes, Valerie. *Breasts, Bottles and Babies: A History of Infant Feeding*. Edinburgh: Edinburgh University Press, 1986.

Fildes, Valerie. *Wet Nursing: A History from Antiquity to the Present*. Oxford: Basil Blackwell, 1988.

Fitzgerald, Frances. *America Revised: History Schoolbooks in the Twentieth Century*. Boston: Little, Brown, 1979.

Fleras, Augie, and Paul Spoonley. *Recalling Aotearoa: Indigenous Politics and Ethnic Relations in New Zealand*. Auckland: Oxford University Press, 1999.

Forget, Nicolle, Francine Harel Giasson, and Francine Seguin. *Justine Lacoste-Beaubien et l'Hôpital Sainte-Justine*. Sainte Foy: Presses de l'Université du Québec, 1995.

Foucault, Michel. *Naissance de la clinique*. Paris: Les Presses universitaires de France, 1963.

Fournier, S., and E. Crey, Jr. *Stolen from Our Embrace: The Abduction of First Nations Children and the Restoration of Aboriginal Communities*. Vancouver: Douglas & McIntyre, 1997.

Fowke, V. C. *Canadian Agricultural Policy: The Historical Pattern*. Toronto: University of Toronto Press, 1947.

Fox, Daniel M., and Christopher Lawrence. *Photographing Medicine: Images and Power in Britain and America since 1940*. New York: Greenwood Press, 1988.

Fox, Richard Wightman, and T. J. Jackson Lears, eds. *The Culture of Consumption: Critical essays Essays in American History 1880–1980*. New York: Pantheon Books, 1983.

Friedman, Reena S. *These Are Our Children: Jewish Orphanages in the United States, 1880–1925*. Hanover, NH: Brandeis University Press/University Press of New England, 1994.

Fuchs, Rachel G. *Poor and Pregnant in Paris: Strategies for Survival in the Nineteenth Century*. New Brunswick: Rutgers University Press, 1992.

Gagan, David, and Rosemary Gagan. *For Patients of Moderate Means: A Social History of the Voluntary Public General Hospital in Canada, 1890–1950*. Montreal: McGill-Queen's University Press, 2002.

Gaskell, Jane. *Gender Matters from School to Work*. Philadelphia: Open University Press, 1982.

Gaumer, Benoit, Georges Desrosiers et Othmar Keel, *Histoire du Service de santé de la Ville de Montréal*. Québec : Les éditions de l'IQRC, 2002.

Gélis, Jacques. *L'arbre et le fruit. La naissance dans l'Occident moderne, XVIe-XIXe siècles*. Paris: Fayard, 1984.

Georges Desrosiers, Benoit Gaumer et Othmar Keel, *La santé publique au Québec. Histoire des unités sanitaires de comté : 1926–1975* Montréal: Les Presses de l'Université de Montréal, 1998.

Glassberg, David. *American Historical Pageantry: The Uses of Tradition in the Early Twentieth Century*. Chapel Hill: University of North Carolina Press, 1990.

Gleason, Mona. *Normalizing the Ideal: Psychology, the School, and the Family in Post-World War II Canada, 1945–1960*. Toronto: University of Toronto Press, 1999.

Goldbloom, Alton. *Small Patients: The Autobiography of a Children's Doctor*. Toronto: Longmans, Green, 1959.

Golden, Janet. *A Social History of Wet-nursing in America: From Breast to Bottle*. Cambridge: Cambridge University Press, 1996.

Golden, Janet, and Charles E. Rosenberg. *Pictures of Health: A Photographic History of Philadelphia Health Care, 1862–1945*. Philadelphia: University of Pennsylvania Press, 1991.

Golden, Janet. *Infant Asylums and Children's Hospitals: Medical Dilemmas and Developments 1850–1920; An Anthology of Sources*. New York: Garland, 1989.

Gordon, Linda. *Heroes of Their Own Lives: The Politics and History of Family Violence, Boston, 1880–1960*. New York: Viking, 1988.

Gordon, Linda. *Pitied but Not Entitled: Single Mothers and the History of Welfare, 1890–1935*. Cambridge: Harvard University Press, 1994.

Goulet, Denis, et André Paradis, *Trois siècles d'histoire médicale au Québec. Chronologie des pratiques et des institutions* Montréal: VLB éditeur, 1992.

Goulet, Denis, François Hudon et Othmar Keel, *Histoire de l'Hôpital Notre-Dame de Montréal, 1880–1980*. Montréal: VLB éditeur, 1993.

Goulet, Denis. *Histoire de la Faculté de Médecine de l'Université de Montréal, 1843–1993*. Montréal : VLB éditeur, 1993.

Gove, Thomas. *Gove Inquiry into Child Protection: Final Report*. Vol. 1, *Matthew's Story*. Vol. 2, *Matthew's Legacy*. Victoria: Queen's Printer, 1995.

Gow, James I. *Histoire de l'administration publique québécoise de 1867–1970* Toronto, Montréal: L'Institut d'administration publique du Canada/ Les Presses de l'Université de Montréal, 1986.

Grant, Julia. *Raising Baby by the Book: The Education of American Mothers*. New Haven: Yale University Press, 1998.

Green, Harvey. *Fit for America: Health, Fitness, Sport and American Society*. New York: Pantheon, 1986.

Green, Harvey. *The Light of the Home: An Intimate View of the Lives of Women in Victorian America*. New York: Pantheon, 1983.

Grossberg, Michael. *Governing the Hearth: Law and Family in Nineteenth-Century America*. Chapel Hill: University of North Carolina Press, 1985.

Guérard, François. *Histoire de la santé au Québec* Montréal: Boréal, 1996: François Guérard, «La formation des grands appareils sanitaires, 1800–1945». Dans *L'institution médicale, Atlas historique du Québec*, sous la direction de Normand Séguin. Sainte-Foy: Les Presses de l'Université Laval, 1998: 75–106.

Guest, Dennis. *The Emergence of Social Security in Canada*. Vancouver: University of British Columbia Press, 1980.

Guimond, James. *American Photography and the American Dream*. Chapel Hill: University of North Carolina Press, 1991.

Gutman, Herbert. *The Black Family in Slavery and Freedom*. New York: Pantheon, 1976.

Gutman, Judith M. *Lewis Hine and the American Social Conscience*. New York: Walker, 1967.

Gutman, Judith M. *Lewis Hine: Two Perspectives*. New York: Grossman, 1974.

Haig-Brown, Celia. *Resistance and Renewal: Surviving the Indian Residential School*. Vancouver: Tillacum, 1988.

Hale, Thomas W. *Medications and Mothers' Milk*. Texas: Pharmasoft Medical Publishing, 2002.

Hales, Peter Bacon. *Silver Cities: The Photography of American Urbanization*. Philadelphia: Temple University Press, 1984.

Halpern, Sydney A. *American Pediatrics: The Social Dynamics of Professionalism, 1880–1980*. Berkeley: University of California Press, 1988.

Hammonds, Evelynn Maxine. *Childhood's Deadly Scourge: The Campaign to Control Diphtheria in New York City, 1880–1930*. Baltimore: Johns Hopkins University Press, 1999.

Handlin, Oscar. *The Uprooted: The Epic Story of the Great Migrations That Made the American People*. Boston: Atlantic Monthly Books, 1973.

Hardy, Anne. *The Epidemic Streets: Infectious Disease and the Rise of Preventive Medicine*. Oxford: Clarendon Press, 1993.

Hartmann, Mary S., and Lois Banner, eds. *Clio's Consciousness Raised: New Perspectives on the History of Women*. New York: Harper and Row, 1974.

Haskell, Thomas L. *The Authority of Experts: Studies in History and Theory*. Bloomington: University of Indiana Press, 1984.

Havemann, Paul. *Indigenous Peoples' Rights in Australia, Canada and New Zealand*. Auckland: Oxford University Press, 1999.

Heinze, Andrew R. *Adapting to Abundance: Jewish Immigrants, Mass Consumption, and the Search for American Identity*. New York: Columbia University Press, 1990.

Hendrick, H. *Images of Youth*. London: Oxford University Press, 1990.

Henripin, Jacques *Naître ou ne pas être*, Québec, IQRC, coll. Diagnostic, 1989.

Hicks, Neville. *"This Sin and Scandal": Australia's Population Debate 1891–1911*. Canberra: ANU Press, 1978.

Higham, John. *Strangers in the Land: Patterns of American Nativism, 1860–1925*. New York: Atheneum, 1963.

Hofstadter, Richard H. *The Age of Reform: From Bryan to F. D. R.* New York: Alfred A. Knopf, 1956.

Holcombe, Lee. *Victorian Ladies at Work: Middle Class Working Women in England and Wales 1850–1914*. London: Newton Abbot, 1973.

Howe, K. R. *Race Relations: Australia and New Zealand*. Wellington/Sydney: Methuen, 1977.

Hoy, Suellen. *Chasing Dirt: The American Pursuit of Cleanliness*. New York: Oxford University Press, 1995.

Hulbert, Ann. *Raising America: Experts, Parents, and a Century of Advice about Children*. New York: Alfred A. Knopf, 2003.

Hunt, Lynn, ed. *The New Cultural History*. Berkeley: University of California Press, 1989.

Jakle, John, and Keith Sculle. *Fast Food: Roadside Restaurants in the Automobile Age*. Baltimore: Johns Hopkins University Press, 1999.

Jamieson, Heber. *Early Medicine in Alberta: The First Seventy-Five Years*. Edmonton: Douglas Printing, 1947.

Jenkins, Philip. *Moral Panic: Changing Concepts of the Child Molester in Modern America*. New Haven and London: Yale University Press, 1998.

Jenkins, Reese. *Images and Enterprise: Technology and the American Photographic Industry*. Baltimore: Johns Hopkins University Press, 1975.

Jones, Kathleen W. *Taming the Troublesome Child: American Families, Child Guidance, and the Limits of Psychiatric Authority*. Cambridge: Harvard University Press, 1999.

Jones, Norman Howard. *The Pan American Health Organization: Origins and Evolution*. Geneva: World Health Organization, 1981.

Kanigel, Robert. *The One Best Way: Frederick Winslow Taylor and the Enigma of Efficiency*. New York: Viking, 1997.

Katz, Michael B. *In the Shadow of the Poorhouse: A Social History of Welfare in America*. New York: Basic Books, 1986.

Katz, Michael. *Poverty and Policy in American History*. New York: Academic Press, 1983.

Katz, Michael, ed. *The "Underclass" Debate: View from History*. Princeton: Princeton University Press, 1993.

Keating, Peter, et Othmar Keel, dir., *Santé et société au Québec, XIXᵉ–XXᵉ siècle*. Montréal: Boréal, 1995.

Kelm, Mary-Ellen. *Colonizing Bodies: Aboriginal Health and Healing in British Columbia*. Vancouver: UBC Press, 1998.

Kemp, John R. *Lewis Hine: Photographs of Child Labor in the New South*. Jackson: University Press of Mississippi, 1986.

Kennedy, John F. *A Nation of Immigrants*. New York: Harper Perennial Library, 1986.

Kett, J. *Rites of Passage: Adolescence in America*. New York: Basic Books, 1977.

Kincaid, James R. *Child-Loving: The Erotic Child and Victorian Culture*. New York and London: Routledge, 1992.

Kincaid, James R. *Erotic Innocence: The Culture of Child Molesting*. Durham: Duke University Press, 1998.

King, Alan J. C., and Beverly Coles. *The Health of Canada's Youth: Views and Behaviours of 11-, 13- and 15-Year-Olds from 11 Countries*. Ottawa: National Health and Welfare, 1992.

King, Charles R. *Children's Health in America: A History*. New York: Twayne, 1993.

Kirk, Sylvia Van. *Many Tender Ties: Women in Fur Trade Society in Western Canada, 1670–1830*. Winnipeg: Watson & Dwyer, 1980.

Klaus, Alsia. *Every Child a Lion: The Origins of Maternal and Infant Health Policy in the United States and France*. Ithaca: Cornell University Press, 1993.

Kline, Wendy. *Building a Better Race: Gender, Sexuality, and Eugenics from the Turn of the Century to the Baby Boom.* Berkeley: University of California Press, 2001.

Komiske, Bruce King. *Designing the World's Best Children's Hospitals.* Victoria, Australia: Images, 1999.

Komlos, John, ed. *Stature, Living Standards, and Economic Development: Essays in Anthropometric History.* Chicago: University of Chicago Press, 1994.

Kostash, Myrna. *No Kidding: Inside the World of Teenage Girls.* Toronto: McClelland & Stewart, 1987.

Koven, Seth, and Sonya Michel, eds., *Mothers of a New World. Maternalist Politics and the Origins of Welfare States.* New York et Londres: Routledge, 1993.

Kraut, A. M. *Silent Travelers: Germs, Genes and the Immigrant Menace.* New York: Basic Books, 1994.

Ladd-Taylor, Molly. *Mother-Work: Women, Child Welfare, and the State, 1890–1930.* Urbana: University of Illinois Press, 1994.

Ladd-Taylor, Molly. *Raising a Baby the Government Way: Mothers' Letters to the Children's Bureau, 1915–1932.* New Brunswick: Rutgers University Press, 1986.

Law Commission of Canada. *Restoring Dignity: Responding to Child Abuse in Canadian Institutions.* Ottawa: Law Commission of Canada, 2000.

Leach, William. *Land of Desire: Merchants, Power and the Rise of a New American Culture.* New York: Pantheon Books, 1993.

Leavitt, Judith Walzer. *Typhoid Mary: Captive to the Public's Health.* Boston: Beacon Press, 1996.

Lederer, Susan, and Naomi Rogers. *Medicine in the Twentieth Century* (London: Harwood Academic, 2000.

Lemieux, Denise. *Une culture de la nostalgie: L'enfant dans le roman québecois de ses origines à nos jours.* Montreal: Boreal Express, 1984.

Levenstein, Harvey. *Revolution at the Table: The Transformation of the American Diet.* New York: University of California Press, 1988.

Levenstein, Harvey. *Paradox of Plenty: A Social History of Eating in Modern America.* New York: University of California Press, 1993.

Lewis, Sclater D. *Royal Victoria Hospital 1887–1947.* Montreal: McGill University Press, 1969.

Lindenmeyer, Kristie. *A "Right to Childhood": The U.S. Children's Bureau and Child Welfare, 1912–1946.* Urbana: University of Illinois Press, 1997.

Linton, D. *Who Has the Youth Has the Future.* Cambridge, MA: Harvard University Press, 1990.

Little, Margaret. *No Car, No Radio, No Liquor Permit: The Moral Regulation of Single Mothers in Ontario, 1920–1997.* Toronto: University of Toronto Press, 1998.

Lomax, Elizabeth M. R. *Small and Special: The Development of Hospitals for Children in Victorian Britain.* London: Wellcome Institute for the History of Medicine, 1996.

Lubove, Roy. *The Professional Altruist: The Emergence of Social Work as a Career 1880–1930.* New York: Atheneum, 1980.

Lux, Maureen. *Medicine That Walks: Disease, Medicine and Canadian Plains Native People, 1880–1940.* Toronto: University of Toronto Press, 2001.

MacDonald, Robert A. J. *Making Vancouver, 1863–1913* (Vancouver: University of British Columbia Press, 1996.

MacDougall, H. *Activists and Advocates: Toronto's Health Department, 1883–1983.* Toronto: Dundurn Press, 1990.

Malkin, Jain. *Hospital Interior Architecture: Healing Environments for Special Patient Populations*. New York: Van Nostrand Rheinhold, 1992.

Marchand, Roland. *Advertising the American Dream: Making Way for Modernity, 1920–1940*. Berkeley: University of California Press, 1985.

Markel, Howard. *Quarantine! East European Jewish Immigrants and the New York City Epidemics of 1892*. Baltimore: Johns Hopkins University Press, 1997.

Markel, Howard, and Frank A. Oski. *The H. L. Mencken Baby Book: Comprising the Contents of H. L. Mencken's What You Ought to Know about Your Baby, with Commentaries*. Philadelphia: Hanley and Belfus, 1990.

Marshall, Dominique. *Aux origins sociales de l'Etat-providence*. Montreal: Les Presses de l'Université de Montréal, 1998.

Mason, Mary Ann. *From Father's Property to Children's Rights: The History of Child Custody in the United States*. New York: Columbia University Press, 1994.

Matthews, Jill Julius. *Good and Mad Women: The Historical Construction of Femininity in Twentieth Century Australia*. Sydney: George Allen and Unwin, 1984.

McClintock, Anne. *Imperial Leather: Race, Gender, and Sexuality in Colonial Conquest*. New York: Routledge, 1995.

McCuaig, Katherine. *The Weariness, the Fever, and the Fret: The Campaign against Tuberculosis in Canada, 1900–1950*. Montreal: McGill-Queen's University Press, 1999.

McGinnis, Janice Dickin. *Suitable for the Wilds: Letters from Northern Alberta, 1929–1931*. Toronto: University of Toronto Press, 1995.

McKeown, T. *The Modern Rise of Population*. New York: Academic Press, 1976.

McLaren, A. *Our Own Master Race: Eugenics in Canada, 1885–1945*. Toronto: McClelland and Stewart, 1990.

McPherson, Kathryn. *Bedside Matters: The Transformation of Canadian Nursing, 1900–1990*. Toronto: Oxford University Press, 1996.

Meckel, Richard. *Save the Babies: American Public Health Reform and the Prevention of Infant Mortality, 1850–1929*. Baltimore: Johns Hopkins University Press, 1990.

Melosi, Martin. *Garbage in the Cities: Refuse, Reform, and the Environment, 1800–1980*. College Station, Texas A&M Press, 1981.

Melosi, Martin V. *The Sanitary City: Urban Infrastructure in America from Colonial Times to the Present*. Baltimore: Johns Hopkins University Press, 2000.

Metzker, Isaac, ed. *A Bintel Brief: Sixty Years of Letters from the Lower East Side to the Daily Forward*. Garden City, NY: Doubleday, 1971.

Migozzi, Jacques. *Les facteurs du développement démographique au Cambodge*, Paris: CNRS, 1971.

Miller, Francesca. *Latin American Women and the Search for Social Justice*. Hanover: University Press of New England, 1991.

Miller, J. R. *Shingwauk's Vision: A History of Native Residential Schools*. Toronto: University of Toronto Press, 1996.

Milroy, John. *"A National Crime": The Canadian Government and the Residential School System 1879–1986*. Winnipeg: University of Manitoba Press, 1999.

Mitchinson, Wendy. *Giving Birth in Canada 1900–1950*. Toronto: University of Toronto Press, 2002.

Modell, J. *Into One's Own: From Youth to Adulthood in the United States*. Berkeley: University of California Press, 1988.

Monnais-Rousselot, Laurence. *Médecine et colonisation. L'aventure indochinoise, 1860–1939*. Paris: CNRS Editions, 1999.

Morantz-Sanchez, Regina Markell. *Sympathy and Science: Women Physicians in American Medicine*. New York: Oxford University Press, 1985.

Moscovitch, A., and G. Drover. *The Benevolent State: The Growth of Welfare in Canada*. Toronto: Garamond Press, 1987.

Muncy, Robyn. *Creating a Female Dominion in American Reform, 1890–1935*. New York: Oxford University Press, 1991.

Nasaw, David. *Children of the City: At Work and at Play*. New York: Oxford University Press, 1985.

Nestle, M. *Food Politics: How the Food Industry Influences Nutrition and Health*. Los Angeles: University of California Press, 2002.

Neubauer, J. *The Fin-de-Siècle Culture of Adolescence*. New Haven: Yale University Press, 1992.

Odem, Mary E. *Delinquent Daughters: Protecting and Policing Adolescent Female Sexuality in the United States, 1885–1920*. Chapel Hill and London: University of North Carolina Press, 1995.

Ogle, Maureen. *All the Modern Conveniences: American Household Plumbing, 1840–1890*. Baltimore: Johns Hopkins University Press, 1997.

Owen, Norman G. *Death and Disease in South East Asia: Explorations in Social, Medical and Demographic History*. Singapore: Oxford University Press, 1987.

Parr, J. *Domestic Goods*. Toronto: University of Toronto Press, 1999.

Parr, J., ed. *A Diversity of Women*. Toronto: University of Toronto, 1995.

Parr, Joy, ed. *Childhood and Family in Canadian History*. Toronto: McClelland and Stewart, 1982.

Patterson, James T. *America's Struggle against Poverty, 1900–1980*. Cambridge: Harvard University Press, 1981.

Pearson, Howard, with the assistance of A. K. Brown. *The Centennial History of the American Pediatric Society, 1888–1988*. New Haven: Yale University Printing Service, 1988.

Pernick, Martin S. *The Black Stork: Eugenics and the Death of ' "Defective' " Babies in American Medicine and Motion Pictures Since since 1915*. New York: Oxford University Press, 1996.

Petitat, André, *Les infirmières de la vocation à la profession*. Montréal: Boréal, 1989.

Phillips, Jock. *A Man's Country? The Image of the Pakeha Male: A History*. Auckland: Penguin Books, 1997.

Pillsbury, Richard. *No Foreign Food: The American Diet in Time and Place*. Boulder, CO: Westview Press, 1998.

Pleck, Elizabeth. *Domestic Tyranny: The Making of Social Policy against Family Violence from Colonial Times to the Present*. New York: Oxford University Press, 1987.

Poovey, Mary. *Uneven Developments: The Ideological Work of Gender in Mid-Victorian England*. London: Virgo, 1989.

Popkin, Barry M., Tamar Lasky, Deborah Spicer, and Monica E. Yamamoto. *The Infant-Feeding Triad: Infant, Mother and Household*. New York: Gordon and Breach, 1986.

Prescott, H., Munro. *A Doctor of Their Own: The History of Adolescent Medicine*. Cambridge, MA: Harvard University Press, 1998.

Preston, Samuel H., and Michael R. Haines. *Fatal Years: Child Mortality in Late-Nineteenth-Century America*. Princeton: Princeton University Press, 1991.

Prout, James A. *Constructing and Reconstructing Childhood: Contemporary Issues in the Sociological Study of Childhood.* London: Falmer, 1990.

Razzell, Peter. *Essays in English Population History.* London: Caliban Books, 1994.

Reiger, Kerreen M. *The Disenchantment of the Home: Modernising the Australian Family 1880–1940.* Melbourne: Oxford University Press, 1985.

Richardson, Harriet. *English Hospitals 1660–1948.* Swindon: Royal Commission on the Historical Monuments of England, 1998.

Riis, Jacob A. *How the Other Half Lives: Studies among the Tenements of New York.* New York: Charles Scribner's Sons, 1890.

Risse, Guenter B. *Mending Bodies, Saving Souls: A History of Hospitals.* New York: Oxford University Press, 1999.

Roe, Jill, ed., *Twentieth Century Sydney. : Studies in Urban and Social History.* Sydney: Hale and Ironmonger, 1980.

Rollet-Échalier, Catherine *La politique à l'égard de la petite enfance sous la IIIᵉ République.* Paris: INED, 1990.

Rooke, Patricia, and R. L. Schnell. *Discarding the Asylum: From Child Rescue to the Welfare State in English Canada (1800–1950).* Lanham, MD: University Press of America, 1983.

Rooke, Patricia T., and R. L. Schnell, eds. *Studies in Canadian Childhood: A Canadian Perspective.* Calgary: Detselig Enterprises, 1982.

Rosen, George. *A History of Public Health.* New York: MD Publications, 1958.

Rosenberg, Charles. *The Care of Strangers: The Rise of America's Hospital System.* New York: Basic Books, 1987.

Rothman, Sheila. *Woman's Proper Place: A History of Changing Ideas, 1870 to the Present.* New York: Basic Books, 1978.

Roy, Fernande. *Histoire des Idéologies au Québec aux XIXᵉ et XXᵉ siècle.* Montréal: Boréal, 1993.

Rutherdale, Myra. *Women and the White Man's God: Gender and Race in Canada's Mission Field.* Vancouver: University of British Columbia, 2002.

Ryan, Ben. *Women in Public: Between Banners and Ballots, 1825–1880.* Baltimore: Johns Hopkins University Press, 1990.

Scriver, Jessie Boyd. *The Montreal Children's Hospital: Years of Growth.* Montreal: McGill-Queen's University Press, 1979.

Schartner, Adelaide. *Health Units of Alberta.* Edmonton: Co-op Press, 1982.

Showalter, Elaine. *The Female Malady: Women, Madness, and English Culture, 1830–1980.* New York: Pantheon Books, 1985.

Shui Meng, Nguyen. *The Population of Indochina.* Singapore: Institute for the South East Asian Studies, 1974.

Sims, Laura. *The Politics of Fat: Food and Nutrition Policy in America.* New York: M.E. Sharpe, 1998.

Skogstad, G. *The Politics of Agricultural Policy-making in Canada.* Toronto: University of Toronto Press, 1987.

Smith, Susan L. *Sick and Tired of Being Sick and Tired: Black Women's Health Activism in America, 1890–1950.* Philadelphia: University of Pennsylvania Press, 1995.

Smolen, Rick, and Phillip Moffitt. *Medicine's Greatest Journey: One Hundred Years of Healing.* Boston: Bullfinch Press, 1992.

Sontag, Susan. *On Photography.* New York: Farrar, Straus & Giroux, 1973.

Speck, Dara Culhane. *An Error in Judgement: The Politics of Medical Care in an Indian/White Community.* Vancouver: Talon Books, 1987.

Springhall, J. *Coming of Age: Adolescence in Britain, 1860–1960.* London: Oxford University Press, 1986.

Stange, Maren. *Symbols of Ideal Life: Social Documentary Photography in America, 1890–1950.* New York: Cambridge University Press, 1989.

Stearns, Peter N. *Anxious Parents: A History of Modern Childrearing in America.* New York and London: New York University Press, 2003.

Stepan, Nancy Leys. *The Hour of Eugenics: Race, Gender, and Nation in Latin America.* Ithaca: Cornell University Press, 1991.

Stern, Alexandra Minna, and Howard Markel. *Formative Years: Children's Health in the United States, 1880–2000.* Ann Arbor: University of Michigan Press, 2002.

Stevens, Edward Flecher. *The American Hospital of the Twentieth Century.* 3rd ed. New York: Dodge, 1928.

Stevens, Rosemary. *In Sickness and in Wealth: American Hospitals in the Twentieth Century.* New York: Basic Books, 1989.

Stewart, Irene. *These Were Our Yesterdays: A History of District Nursing in Alberta.* Altona, MB: D. W. Friesen & Sons, 1979.

Stilz, Gerhardt. *Colonies, Missions, Cultures in the English-Speaking World: General and Comparative Studies.* Tübingen: Stauffenburg Verlag, 1999.

Strong-Boag, Veronica. "Intruders in the Nursery: Childcare Professionals Reshape the Years from One to Five, 1920–1940." In *Childhood and Family in Canadian History,* edited by Joy Parr. Toronto: McClelland & Stewart, 1982.

Strong-Boag, Veronica. *The New Day Recalled: Lives of Girls and Women in English Canada, 1919–1939.* Mississauga: Copp Clark Pitman, 1988.

Stuart-Macadam, P., and K. A. Dettwyler. *Breastfeeding: Biocultural Perspectives.* New York: Aldine de Gruyter, 1995.

Sussman, George D. *Selling Mother's Milk: The Wet-nursing Business in France, 1715–1914.* Urbana: University of Illinois Press, 1982.

Sutherland, Neil. *Children in English-Canadian Society: Framing the Twentieth Century Consensus.* Waterloo: Wilfrid Laurier University Press, 2000.

Sutherland, Neil. *Growing Up: Childhood in English Canada from the Great War to the Age of Television.* Toronto: University of Toronto Press, 1997.

Taylor, Jeremy. *The Architect and the Pavilion Hospital: Dialogue and Design Creativity in England 1850–1914.* Leicester: Leicester University Press, 1997.

Teller, Michael E. *The Tuberculosis Movement: A Public Health Campaign in the Progressive Era.* Westport, CT: Greenwood, 1988.

Tiffin, Susan. *In Whose Best Interest: Child Welfare Reform in the Progressive Era.* Westport, CT: Greenwood, 1982.

Tomes, Nancy. *The Gospel of Germs: Men, Women and the Microbe in American Life.* Cambridge, MA: Harvard University Press, 1998.

Trachtenberg, Alan. *Reading American Photographs: Images as History, Mathew Brady to Walker Evans.* New York: Hill and Wang, 1989.

Trattner, Walter I. *From Poor Law to Welfare State: A History of Social Welfare in America.* New York: Free Press, 1974.

Trofimenkoff, Susan Mann. *The Dream of Nation: A Social and Intellectual History of Quebec.* Toronto: MacMillan, 1982.

Valverde, Mariana. *The Age of Light, Soap, and Water. Moral Reform in English Canada, 1885-1925.* Toronto: McClelland and Stewart, 1991.

Vien, Nguyên Khac. *Vietnam, une longue histoire.* Hanoi: The Gioi, 1993.

Vinikas, Vincent. *Soft Soap, Hard Sell: American Hygiene in an Age of Advertisement.* Ames: Iowa State University Press, 1992.

Verderber, Stephen, and David J. Fine. *Healthcare Architecture in an Era of Radical Transformation.* New Haven: Yale University Press, 2000.

Waldram, J. B., D. A. Herring, and T. K. Young. *Aboriginal Health in Canada: Historical, Cultural and Epidemiological Perspectives.* Toronto: University of Toronto Press, 1995.

Ward, Colin, and Dennis Hardy. *Goodnight Campers! The History of the British Holiday Camp.* London: Mansell, 1986.

Wegs, R. *Growing Up Working Class: Youth in Vienna, 1870–1920.* Philadelphia: University of Pennsylvania Press, 1989.

Weindling, Paul, ed. *International Health Organisations and Movements, 1918–1939.* Cambridge: Cambridge University Press, 1995.

Weiner, Deborah. *Architecture and Social Reform in Late-Victorian London.* Manchester: Manchester University Press, 1994.

Wiebe, Robert H. *The Search for Order, 1877–1920.* New York: Hill and Wang, 1967.

Wilkerson, Karen Buhler. *False Dawn: The Rise and Decline of Public Health Nursing, 1900–1930.* New York: Garland, 1989.

Wilson, J. Donald, ed., *Children, Teachers, and Schools in the History of British Columbia.* Calgary: Detselig, 1995, 209–234.

Wrigley, E. A. *Population and History.* New York: McGraw-Hill, 1969.

Yee, Paul. *Saltwater City: An Illustrated History of the Chinese in Vancouver.* Vancouver and Toronto: Douglas and McIntyre, 1988.

Yule, Peter. *The Royal Children's Hospital: A History of Faith, Science and Love.* Sydney: Halstead, 1999.

Yuval-Davis, Nira, and Floya Anthias. *Woman-Nation-State.* London: Macmillan, 1989.

Zelizer, Viviana. *Pricing the Priceless Child: The Changing Social Value of Children.* New York: Basic Books, 1985.

Zmora, Nurith. *Orphanages Reconsidered: Child Care Institutions in Progressive Era Baltimore.* Philadelphia: Temple University Press, 1994.

Theses & Dissertations

Bienvenue, Louise «Le rôle du Victorian Order of Nurses dans la croisade hygiéniste montréalaise (1877–1925)», mémoire de MA, Université du Québec à Montréal, 1995.

Bliss, Katherine Elaine. "Prostitution, Revolution and Social Reform in Mexico City, 1918–1940." PhD dissertation, University of Chicago, 1996.

Blum, Ann S. "Children without Parents: Law, Charity, and Social Practice, Mexico City, 1870–1940." PhD dissertation, University of California, Berkeley, 1997.

Brosco, Jeffrey P. "Sin or Folly? Child and Community Health in Philadelphia, 1900–1930." PhD dissertation, University of Pennsylvania, 1994.

Cavanaugh, Catherine A. "In Search of a Useful Life: Irene Marryat Parlby, 1868–1965." PhD dissertation, University of Alberta, 1994.

Collins, Paul Victor. "The Public Health Policies of the United Farmers of Alberta Government, 1921–1935." Master's thesis, University of Western Ontario, 1969.

Deslauriers, Lucie «Histoire de l'Hôpital Notre-Dame, 1880–1924», mémoire de MA, Université de Montréal, 1985.

Desjardins, Rita. «Hopital Sainte-Justine, Montreal, 1907-1921», mémoire de MA, Université de Montréal, 1989.

Desjardins, Rita «L'Institutionnalisation de la pédiatrie en milieu franco-montréalais, 1880–1980. Les enjeux politiques, sociaux et biologiques», thèse de doctorat, Université de Montréal, 1999

Déziel, Céline. «L'enseignement clinique à l'Hôpital Notre-Dame de 1880 à 1924», mémoire de MA, Université de Montréal, 1992.

Dupuis, Jean-Claude «Nationalisme et catholicisme. L'Action française de Montréal, 1917-1938», mémoire de MA, Université de Montréal, 1992.

Fleming, Phillip. "Eugenics in New Zealand 1900–1940." Master's thesis, Massey University, 1981.

Fleury, Marie-Josée «L'Hôpital Saint-Paul (1905–1934) et sa contribution à la prévention et à la lutte contre les maladies contagieuses», mémoire de MA, Université de Montréal, 1993.

Gagnon, Ginette «L'aqueduc de Montréal au tournant du siècle (1890–1914): L'établissement de la purification de l'eau potable», mémoire de MA, Université de Montréal, 1998.

Guérard, François «La santé publique dans deux villes du Québec de 1887 à 1939. Trois-Rivières et Shawinigan», thèse de doctorat, UQAM, 1993.

Hudon, François «L'Hôpital comme microcosme de la société: Enjeux institutionnels et besoins sociaux à l'Hôpital Notre-Dame de Montréal, 1880–1960», thèse de doctorat, Université de Montréal, 1997.

Lewis, Milton James. "'Populate or Perish': Aspects of Infant and Maternal Health in Sydney, 1870–1939." PhD dissertation, Australian National University, 1976.

Malissard, Pierrick «Quand les universitaires se font entrepreneurs. Les laboratoires Connaught et l'Institut de microbiologie et d'hygiène de l'Université de Montréal», thèse de doctorat, Université du Québec à Montréal, 1999.

Monnais-Rousselot, Laurence. «Médecine coloniale, pratiques de santé et sociétés en Indochine française (1860–1939)», thèse de doctorat, Université Paris VII-Denis Diderot, 1997.

Pottisham, Nancy. "'Save the Children: A History of the Children's Bureau, 1903–1918.'" PhD dissertation, University of California at Los Angeles, 1974.

Riddell, Susan. "Curing Society's Ills: Public Health Nurses and Public Health Nursing in Rural British Columbia, 1919–1946." Master's thesis, Simon Fraser University, 1991.

Schiff, Noah. "The Sweetest of All Charities: The Toronto Hospital for Sick Children's Medical and Public Appeal, 1875–1905." Master's thesis, University of Toronto, 1999.

Sloane, David Charles. "Caring for the Children: The Emergence of the Modern Children's Hospital, 1890–1930." Unpublished, 2000.

Tétreault, Martin «L'état de santé des Montréalais de 1880 à 1914», mémoire de MA, Université de Montréal, 1979.

Toon, Elizabeth. "'Managing the Conduct of the Individual Life: Public Health Education and American Public Health, 1910–1940.'" PhD dissertation, University of Pennsylvania, 1998.

Wilson, S. K. "The Aims and Ideology of Cora Wilding and the Sunlight League 1930–36." Master's extended essay, Canterbury University, 1980.

Yee, Paul. "Chinese Business in Vancouver, 1886–1914." Master's thesis, University of British Columbia, 1978.

List of Contributors

෴

CHERYL KRASNICK WARSH teaches history at Malaspina University-College in Nanaimo, British Columbia, and is editor-in-chief of the *Canadian Bulletin of Medical History/Bulletin canadien d'histoire de la médecine*. She is the author of *Moments of Unreason: The Practice of Canadian Psychiatry and the Homewood Retreat, 1883–1923* and the forthcoming *Women's Health in North America, 1800–2000*.

VERONICA STRONG-BOAG is a Fellow of the Royal Society of Canada, a former president of the Canadian Historical Association and teaches in Women's Studies and Educational Studies at the University of British Columbia. She is the author of *Finding Families, Finding Ourselves: English Canada Confronts Adoption from the 19th Century to the 1990s* (forthcoming) and, with Carole Gerson, *Paddling Her Own Canoe: The Times and Texts of E. Pauline Johnson (Tekahionwake)*.

ANNMARIE ADAMS is an associate professor in the School of Architecture at McGill University. She is the author of *Architecture in the Family Way: Women, Houses, and Doctors, 1870-1900* and co-author of *Designing Women: Gender and the Architectural Profession*.

DENYSE BAILLARGEON est professeure au département d'histoire de l'Université de Montréal. Elle est l'auteure de *Un Québec en mal d'enfants. La médicalisation de la maternité, 1910-1970*.

ANNE-EMANUELLE BIRN is Canada Research Chair in International Health at the University of Toronto. Her forthcoming book is *Marriage of Convenience: Rockefeller International Health and Revolutionary Mexico*.

CYNTHIA COMACCHIO teaches history at Wilfrid Laurier University; her forthcoming book is *The Dominion of Youth: Adolescence in English Canada, 1920–1950*.

HUGHES EVANS, MD, PhD, is a practising general pediatrician and a medical historian. Her historical interest in child sexual abuse is complemented by clinical practice in that area.

LISA FEATHERSTONE is a member of the Department of Modern History at Macquarie University, Sydney, where she teaches gender history and Australian history. Her research interests include reproduction, pediatrics, and sexuality.

MARIE-JOSÉE FLEURY est professeur adjoint au Département de psychiatrie de l'Université McGill et chercheur au Centre de recherche de l'Hôpital Douglas à Montréal. Elle etait publié au *Ruptures, Revue transdisciplinaire en santé, Health Services management Research,* et *The International Journal of Health Planning and Management.*

MONA GLEASON is a faculty member in Educational Studies, University of British Columbia, the author of *Normalizing the Ideal: Psychology, Schooling, and the Family in Postwar Canada*, and co-editor of *Children, Teachers, and School in the History of British Columbia, 2nd Edition* and *Rethinking Canada: The Promise of Women's History, 4th Edition*.

JANET GOLDEN teaches history at Rutgers University, Camden, and is the author of *Message in a Bottle: The Making of Fetal Alcohol Syndrome*. She is currently working on a history of children's experiences of illness in the United States from 1865 to 1945.

GUY GRENIER détient un doctorat en histoire de la médecine à l'Université de Montréal. Il est présentement agent de recherche au l'Hôpital Douglas à Montréal. Il etait publié *Les monstres, les fous et les autres*, et *Cent ans de médecine francophone, Histoire de l'Association des médecins de langue française du Canada*.

HOWARD MARKEL, MD, PhD is the George E. Wantz Professor of the History of Medicine and professor of Pediatrics and Communicable Diseases at the University of Michigan, where he directs the Center for the History of Medicine. He is the author of *When Germs Travel* and *Quarantine! East European Jewish Immigrants and the New York City Epidemics of 1892*, and co-editor of *Formative Years: Children's Health in the United States, 1880–2000*.

LAURENCE MONNAIS is an assistant professor, Department of History and Centre for East Asian Studies, University of Montreal. Her first book was entitled, *Médecine et colonisation. L'aventure indochinoise, 1869-1939*.

ALECK OSTRY is an associate professor in the Department of Healthcare and Epidemiology, Faculty of Medicine, University of British Columbia, and is the recipient of a Canadian Institute for Health Research New Investigator award.

SHARON L. RICHARDSON, past president of the Alberta Association of Registered Nurses, is an associate professor of Nursing, University of Alberta.

NAOMI ROGERS is an associate professor in the History of Medicine and Women's, Gender and Sexuality Studies at Yale University. She is the author of *Dirt and Disease: Polio before FDR* and *An Alternative Path: The Making and Remaking of Hahnemann Medical School and Hospital in Philadelphia*.

MYRA RUTHERDALE is the author of *Women and the White Man's God: Gender and Race in the Canadian Mission Field* and an assistant professor of history at York University in Toronto.

JUDITH SEALANDER is a professor of history at Bowling Green State University, Bowling Green, Ohio. She is the author of five books, most recently *The Failed Century of the Child: Governing America's Young in the Twentieth Century*.

MARGARET TENNANT is a professor of history at Massey University, New Zealand. She has primarily published in the areas of women's and welfare history, and recently co-edited *Past Judgement: Social Policy in New Zealand History*.

DAVID THEODORE is a research associate on the project Medicine by Design at the School of Architecture, McGill University. He is a regular contributor to *Azure*, *Architecture*, and *Canadian Architect*.

Index

CR

Page numbers in italics refer to photographs.

Abbreviations: ACHA (American Child Health Association), b.c. (British Columbia), CHO (Child Health Organization), PASB (Pan American Sanitary Bureau), UFA (United Farmers of Alberta), USDA (U.S. Department of Agriculture)

Aberhart, William, 495–96, 499, 500. *See also* Social Credit Party

Aboriginal children: as adversely affected by European contact, 4–5; bathing of, 314–15; daily schedules, as imposed on, 317–18; delivery of, 306–11; health of, 4–5, 7; personal hygiene of, 313–18, 319–20; placement of, with non-Aboriginal families, 7; poverty among, 2; resistance of, to Western intervention, 319–20; in residential schools, 6, 322n9; treatment of, by Aboriginal community, 4, 318; Western dress, as imposed on, 311–13, *312*. *See also* First Nations children; Inuit children; Maori

Aboriginal peoples: as adversely affected by European contact, 4–5; birthing practices of, 306–11; child poverty among, 2; clothing of babies by, 312–13; evacuation of, for medical treatment, 310–11; treatment of children by, 4, 318. *See also* First Nations peoples; Inuit; Maori

Action française, L' (Quebec nationalist magazine), 102, 106

Addams, Jane, 76, 216, 358

adolescence: adult fascination with, 376; and child labour, 366–68; medicalization of, 355–56, 357–58; theories about, 357; as time of physical and

psychological upheaval, 358–59, 376–77; of women, 360, 362, 367–68, 370. *See also* health education; high schools

adolescents: and child labour, 366–68; drug use by, 375–76; earlier physical maturity of, in postwar years, 372–73; health education for, 363–66, 368–69, 373, 377; rebelliousness of, 366–67; school health inspections of, 365, 366, 368; sex education for, 362–63, 373–74; sexuality of, 360–63, 373; smoking among, 374; specialized medical care for, as proposed by pediatricians, 371, 377–79; venereal disease among, 370

African Americans: perceived promiscuity of, 340–41, 347n10; portrayal of, as unclean, 51, 52; racism towards, as unchallenged by interwar child health movement, 49–52; support of, for health promotion activities, 51

Agriculture, Department of (Canada): milk consumption campaigns by, 199, 202–203; nutrition science professionals, as employed by, 202; support and regulation of dairy industry by, 196–97

Agriculture, U.S. Department of (USDA), 163, 170–71, 392

Alberta: during Depression and Second World War, 493–97; economic recession of, after First World War, 479–80,